Analytical Techniques for Biomedical Nanotechnology

Online at: https://doi.org/10.1088/978-0-7503-3379-5

Analytical Techniques for Biomedical Nanotechnology

Edited by
Ajeet Kaushik
NanoBioTech Laboratory, Department of Environmental Engineering, Florida Polytechnic University, Lakeland, FL 33805, USA

Sesha S Srinivasan
Department of Engineering Physics, Florida Polytechnic University, Lakeland, FL 33805, USA

Yogendra Kumar Mishra
Mads Clausen Institute, NanoSYD, University of Southern Denmark, Alison 2, 6400 Sønderborg, Denmark

IOP Publishing, Bristol, UK

ISBN 978-0-7503-3379-5 (ebook)
ISBN 978-0-7503-3377-1 (print)
ISBN 978-0-7503-3380-1 (myPrint)
ISBN 978-0-7503-3378-8 (mobi)

DOI 10.1088/978-0-7503-3379-5

Version: 20230701

IOP ebooks

British Library Cataloguing-in-Publication Data: A catalogue record for this book is available from the British Library.

Published by IOP Publishing, wholly owned by The Institute of Physics, London

IOP Publishing, No.2 The Distillery, Glassfields, Avon Street, Bristol, BS2 0GR, UK

US Office: IOP Publishing, Inc., 190 North Independence Mall West, Suite 601, Philadelphia, PA 19106, USA

The authors dedicate this book to every analytical technology making the science of spatial impact by providing information and knowledge to understand the existing state-of-the-art technology and explore future technology for a sustainable society.

Contents

Preface

This book is an effort to explore 'analytical techniques', at both, the fundamental as well as the applied level, for biomedical applications. It aims to provide a broad perspective about the development of analytical methods involved in materials science and electronics, especially in the field of nano-enabled biomedical sciences. It will highlight the fundamentals and systematic developments in analytical techniques to achieve better characterization, providing more scientific information, rapid diagnostics, cost-effective, user-friendly approaches, and most importantly the *state-of-art* developing methodologies for personalized health management. Moreover, it will give an adequate understanding of the imposed limitations and propose the future perspectives and challenges associated with analytical methods to achieve the desired performance in targeted biomedical applications.

Recently, nanotechnology has emerged as a necessary vehicle for the development of advanced technologies for healthcare and wellness. Such developments require advanced surface functionalized hybrid materials for targeted biomedical applications. Nano-biotechnology assisted methodologies are gaining attention due to desired performance, which can be useful to detect, monitor, and manage targeted diseases. Moreover, the significant advancements in developing 'holy grail' materials for biomedical applications often demand the availability of advanced analytical techniques, which are the key factors to understanding the followings aspects.

1. To identify the fundamental knowledge of the various analytical techniques and procedures with reference to targeted biomedical applications.
2. To explore alteration in properties of materials, bio-systems, and involved interfaces in the nano–bio-systems.
3. To demonstrate whether the as-developed nano-system and devices are useful for health and wellness or otherwise need more developments.
4. To develop the miniaturized, reliable, and efficient systems of high sensitivity and selectivity needed for complex disease managements.
5. To discover the knowledge of the nano–bio interface to assess the potential of techniques and the corresponding developed prototypes.

As objectives, it has been noted that on-going nano-biotechnology related research involves multidisciplinary science and simultaneous expertize from various fields on a single platform. The role of analytical science has improved the performance of devices, which have been developed for biomedical applications. Despite significant advances, there is a gap between chemists, biologists, physicists, mathematicians, engineers, and information technologists (internet of things) and bridging that gap is essential for adequate realizations of advanced biomedical technological breakthroughs. To develop the next generation technologies, this book is crucial to bridge the gap and connect experts. The major objectives of this book will be:

(a) to investigate the analytical techniques for targeted biomedical applications,
(b) to introduce the fundamental insights and mechanisms for conceptual understanding,
(c) to identify the prospects and perspectives of analytical tools and techniques,
(d) to demonstrate the challenges and involve experts of different disciplines to develop innovative and precise measurement systems, and
(e) to explore the multidisciplinary research for developing advanced systems for improved performance with respect to targeted nanomaterials-based biomedical applications.

This book will educate the scholars (students, researchers, post-docs, scientists, academicians, industrialists, government) and experts who belong to different disciplines and conducting multidisciplinary research. The knowledge of this book will be useful to translate fundamental research to applied nano-enabled biomedical research. In addition to fundamental knowledge at deep levels, this book will be an ideal platform to explore appropriate single or combinational techniques to improve the system's performance as per requirements, i.e., point-of-care health wellness.

Ajeet Kaushik
Sesha S Srinivasan
Yogendra K Mishra

Acknowledgements

This compilation would have been impossible without the support of contributors. The editors sincerely acknowledge the hard, sincere, and dedicated work of each contributor to make this book of high significance like one of its types. We are also very thankful to the Institute of Physics (IOP), UK for providing us an opportunity to edit a book of wide interest, especially useful for every scholar. Additionally, the affiliated institutions, namely Florida Polytechnic University, USA, and the University of Southern Denmark (SDU) Denmark, including the families and friends of authors are also acknowledged for providing facilities, motivation, and invaluable support.

Editor biographies

Ajeet Kaushik

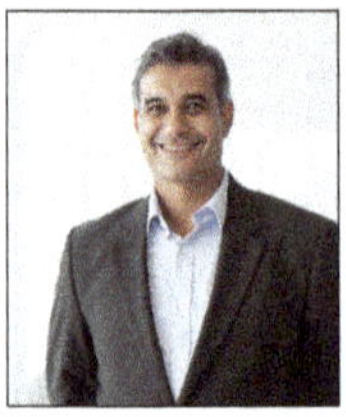

Ajeet Kaushik is an assistant professor of Chemistry at the Department of Environmental Engineering of Florida Polytechnic University. He has over 15 years of experience in exploring analytical techniques for the characterisation of nanostructures, bio/chemical sensors fabrication confirmation, and nanomedicine optimization. Prior to joining Florida Polytechnic University in 2019, he worked as a faculty member at the Medical College of Florida International University.

Sesha S Srinivasan

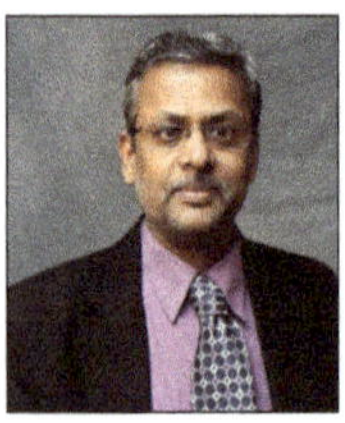

Sesha Srinivasan is an assistant professor of Engineering Physics at Florida Polytechnic University. He has more than two decades of research and project management experience with expertise in the analytical characterization and synthesis of novel materials for emerging applications in hydrogen storage, catalysis, thermochemical and thermal energy, thermochromic coatings, advanced oxidation and biofuel generation. Srinivasan was a Postdoc (2002–2004) at the University of Hawaii, Research Assistant Professor (2004–2009) at the University of South Florida, and on the Faculty of Physics (2009–2014) at Tuskegee University.

Yogendra K Mishra

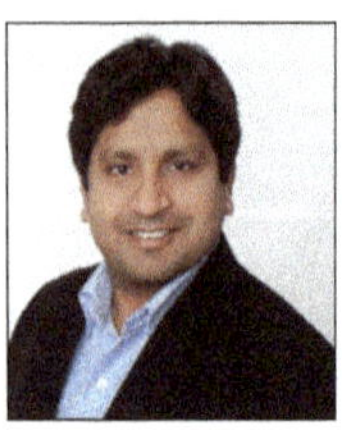

Yogendra Mishra is a professor and leader of Smart Materials at University of Southern Denmark. He was an Alexander von Humboldt Fellow and later a Group Leader at Kiel University, Germany, from 2009 to 2019. He joined University of Southern Denmark as a professor in 2019. He is known world-wide for tetrapod-based 3D materials engineering and translational materials-based research activities.

List of contributors

Tansir Ahamad
Department of Chemistry, College of Science, King Saud University, PO Box 2455, Riyadh 11451, Saudi Arabia

Md. Mottahir Alam
Department of Electrical and Computer Engineering, Faculty of Engineering, King Abdulaziz University, PO Box 80204, Jeddah 21589, Saudi Arabia

Radheka Bhaduri
St. Xaviers College, Kolkata (Autonomous), West Bengal, India

Shilpa Bhatkande
Arts and Science Department, University of Houston-Victoria Katy Campus, 22400 Grand Cir Blvd Suite 206, Katy, TX 77449, USA

Rahul Bhattacharjee
KIIT School of Biotechnology, Kalinga Institute of Industrial Technology (KIIT-DU), Bhubaneswar, Odisha, India

Hima Sree Buddhiraju
Department of Biomedical Engineering, Indian Institute of Technology Hyderabad, Kandi 502 284, India

Srija Chakrabarty
St. Xaviers College, Kolkata (Autonomous), West Bengal, India

Soumalya Chakraborty
Department of Pharmaceutics, National Institute of Pharmaceutical Education and Research (NIPER), Sector 67, S.A.S. Nagar, Mohali 160062, Punjab, India

Sanjoy Kumar Das
Institute of Pharmacy, Jalpaiguri, West Bengal 735101, India

Abhijit Dey
Department of Life Sciences Presidency University 86/1 College Street, Kolkata 700073, West Bengal, India

Swapnil Dharaskar
Nano-Research Group, Department of Chemical Engineering, School of Technology, Pandit Deendayal Energy University, Raisan, Gandhinagar, Gujarat 382426, India

Jaspreet Dhau
Research and Development, Molekule Inc, 3802 Spectrum BLVD, Tampa, FL 33612, USA

Neeraj Dilbaghi
Department of Bio and Nano Technology, Guru Jambheshwar University of Science and Technology, Hisar-Haryana 125001, India

Shraddha Dorlikar
Department of Microbiology, Rashtrasant Tukadoji Maharaj Nagpur University, India

Hardik Gohel
Arts and Science Department, University of Houston-Victoria Katy Campus, 22400 Grand Cir Blvd Suite 206, Katy, TX 77449, USA

Akhilesh Kumar Gupta
Department of Physics, University of Nebraska Omaha, NE 68182, USA

Gaurav Hitkaric
School of Applied Sciences, Shri Venkateshwara University, Rajabpur Gajraula Amroha 244236, India

Mohd Imran
Department of Chemical Engineering, Faculty of Engineering, Jazan University, PO Box 706, Jazan 45142, Saudi Arabia

Sulagna Kar
KIIT School of Biotechnology, Kalinga Institute of Industrial Technology (KIIT-DU), Bhubaneswar, Odisha, India

Sandeep Kaushik
Department of Environmental Science, Indira Gandhi National Tribal University, Amarkantak, MP 484887, India

Afzal Khan
State Key Laboratory of Silicon Materials, School of Materials Science and Engineering, Zhejiang University, Hangzhou 310027, China

Kamil Reza Khondakar
School of Health Sciences and Technology, University of Petroleum and Energy Studies, Dehradun 248007, Uttarakhand, India

N Y Kim
RFIC Center, Kwangwoon University, Seoul 139-701, Republic of Korea

Rajeev Kumar
Department of Environment Studies, Panjab University, Chandigarh 160014, India

Sandeep Kumar
Department of Bio and Nano Technology, Guru Jambheshwar University of Science and Technology, Hisar-Haryana 125001, India

Saurabh Kumar
Centre for Nano Science and Engineering (CeNSE), Indian Institute of Science, Bengaluru, India
Department of Medical Devices, National Institute of Pharmaceutical Education and Research, Guwahati, India

Vijay Kumar
Department of Physics, National Institute of Technology Srinagar, Jammu and Kashmir 190006, India

Chinmaya Mahapatra
Department of Biotechnology, National Institute of Technology Raipur, Raipur, Chhattisgarh 492010, India

Vidhu Malik
Department of Chemistry, DCRUST Murthal, Sonipat, Haryana, India

Priyanka Mankotia
Institute of Forensic Science & Criminology, Panjab University, Chandigarh 160014, India

Hirak Mazumdar
Woxsen University, Hyderabad 502345, India

Bhaskar Mazumder
Department of Pharmaceutical Sciences, Dibrugarh University, Dibrugarh 786004, Assam, India

Jyotsana Mehta
Department of Bio and Nano Technology, Guru Jambheshwar University of Science and Technology, Hisar-Haryana 125001, India

Priya Mitra
KIIT School of Biotechnology, Kalinga Institute of Industrial Technology (KIIT-DU), Bhubaneswar, Odisha, India

Sayan Mukherjee
School of Medical Sciences and Technology, Indian Institute of Technology, Kharagpur, India

Vivek Kumar Nautiyal
Department of Physics, Gaya College Gaya, a constituent unit of Magadh University, BodhGaya, Bihar 823001, India

Vanya Nayak
Department of Chemistry, Banaras Hindu University, Varanasi, Uttar Pradesh 221005, India

Karishma Niveria
Nanobiotech Lab, Department of Zoology, Kirori Mal College, University of Delhi, Delhi 110007, India

Ritesh Palkar
Department of Chemical Engineering, Faculty of Technology, Marwadi University, Rajkot, Gujarat 360003, India

Shashank S Pawitwar
Department of Cellular Biology and Pharmacology, Herbert-Wertheim College of Medicine, Florida International University, Miami, FL, USA

G Qiao
School of Materials Science and Engineering, Jiangsu University, Zhenjiang 212013, China

Rajan Rajabalaya
PAPRSB Institute of Health Sciences, University Brunei Darussalam, Brunei Darussalam

Pooja Rawat
Department of Applied Physics and Institute of Natural Sciences, Kyung Hee University, Yong-in 17104, Republic of Korea

Syed S Razia
Department of Chemistry, Gaya College Gaya, a constituent unit of Magadh University, BodhGaya, Bihar 823001, India

Aravind Kumar Rengan
Department of Biomedical Engineering, Indian Institute of Technology Hyderabad, Kandi 502 284, India

Jong Soo Rhyee
Department of Applied Physics and Institute of Natural Sciences, Kyung Hee University, Yong-in 17104, Republic of Korea

Nitish Sagar
Centre for Nano Science and Engineering (CeNSE), Indian Institute of Science, Bengaluru, India

Ishwar Prasad Sahu
Department of Physics, Indira Gandhi National Tribal University, Amarkantak, MP 484887, India

K Saremi
Institute of Biological Science, Faculty of Science, University of Malaya, 50603 Kuala Lumpur, Malaysia

S V Satya Prasad
Department of Production and Industrial Engineering, National Institute of Technology Jamshedpur, Jharkhand 831014, India

Rakesh Sehgal
Department of Mechanical Engineering, National Institute of Technology Srinagar, Jammu and Kashmir 190006, India

Prosenjit Sen
Centre for Nano Science and Engineering (CeNSE), Indian Institute of Science, Bengaluru, India

Z Shahnavaz
School of Materials Science and Engineering, Jiangsu University, Zhenjiang 212013, China

Kashma Sharma
Institute of Forensic Science & Criminology, Panjab University, Chandigarh 160014, India

Parshant Kumar Sharma
RFIC Bio Centre, Kwangwoon University, 20 Kwangwoon-ro, Nowon-gu, Seoul 01897, South Korea
Department of Electronics Engineering, Kwangwoon University, 20 Kwangwoon-ro, Nowon-gu, Seoul 01897, South Korea

Vishal Sharma
Institute of Forensic Science & Criminology, Panjab University, Chandigarh 160014, India

Poonam Shashidhar
TERI-Deakin Nanobiotechnology Centre, The Energy and Resource Institute, Gurugram, Haryana 122001, India
Deakin University, Geelong, Waurn Ponds, VIC, Australia

M J A Shiddiky
School of Environment and Science (ESC) and Queensland Micro- and Nanotechnology Centre (QMNC), Griffith University, Nathan, QLD 4111, Australia

Ravikumar B Shinde
Department of Zoology, Shri Pundlik Maharaj Mahavidyalaya, Nandura, MS, India

Vikas Shukla
Nanobiotech Lab, Department of Zoology, Kirori Mal College, University of Delhi, Delhi 110007, India

S Shweta
Department of Botany, Guru Ghasidas University, Bilasur, Chattisgarh 495009, India

Amritpal Singh
Department of Chemistry, Mata Gujri College, Fatehgarh Sahib 140406, India

Avtar Singh
Research and Development, Molekule Inc, 3802 Spectrum BLVD, Tampa, FL 33612, USA
Department of Chemistry, Sri Guru Teg Bahadur Khalsa College, Anandpur Sahib, Punjab 140118, India

Kirandeep Singh
Physical and Material Chemistry Divison, CSIR-National Chemical Laboratory, Pune 411008, India

Kshitij RB Singh
Department of Chemistry, Banaras Hindu University, Varanasi, Uttar Pradesh 221005, India

Poonam Singh
Department of Applied Chemistry, Delhi Technological University, Delhi, India

Ravindra Pratap Singh
Department of Biotechnology, Indira Gandhi National Tribal University, Amarkantak, MP 484887, India

Subhash Singh
Department of Production and Industrial Engineering, National Institute of Technology Jamshedpur, Jharkhand 831014, India

Anindita Tarafdar
Department of Biomedical Engineering, Indian Institute of Technology Hyderabad, Kandi, 502 284 India

Yash Thakare
Department of Chemical Engineering, Sinhgad College of Engineering, Pune, Maharashtra, India

Anita Kamra Verma
Nanobiotech Lab, Department of Zoology, Kirori Mal College, University of Delhi, Delhi 110007, India

Kartikey Verma
Department of Chemical Engineering, Indian Institute of Technology Kanpur, Kanpur 208016, Uttar Pradesh, India

IOP Publishing

Ajeet Kaushik, Sesha S Srinivasan and Yogendra Kumar Mishra

Chapter 1

Emergence of analytical techniques

Kamil Reza Khondakar

The impact of nanotechnology and the development of micro/nano sensors has significantly enhanced the discovery of new therapeutic and diagnostic approaches. The emergence of precision medicine towards developing personalized healthcare systems have been achieved by high throughput analytical systems. Current analytical systems are the integration of multiple fields like material science, biology, electronics, MEMS, physics, computer, chemical science, etc towards developing a better diagnostic system. There are many versatile techniques available that have transformed the healthcare sector in many ways. Some of the well-known techniques are electrochemical, Raman, mass spectroscopy, SEM/TEM, fluorescence, NMR, MEMS, artificial intelligence (AI), etc. These systems are highly sensitive and accurate; however, an ideal analytical system would consist of multiple characterization tools providing more scientific information for rapid diagnostics and quicker analysis. These innovative biosensing platforms need to be cost-effective, user friendly and allow real time monitoring, particularly for point-of-care applications. The emergence of nanotechnology and nanobiotechnology along with the significant advancements in material science (nanomaterials, nanomedicine) has provided reliable, ultra-high sensitivity, high selectivity and efficient portable sensors to screen, monitor and treatment of diseases in real time. Current researchers are looking ahead to build a multidisciplinary system for developing advanced diagnostics systems for all in one chip technology for personalized healthcare management.

1.1 Introduction

The rapid developments and innovations in nanotechnology/nanomaterials have opened up several opportunities in all technological fields such as electronics, energy, agriculture, and the healthcare sector [1]. Further, the unique properties of the nanomaterials like larger active surface atoms, tunable optical and chemical properties, variable size and shape have provided significant advances in biomedical applications [2–4]. Recent years have witnessed significant progress in precision

doi:10.1088/978-0-7503-3379-5ch1

medicine for developing more efficient and multi-analysis immunoassay/biomedical systems by combining nanotechnology with nanomaterials [2, 5, 6]. These newly decorated and advanced systems have revolutionized the healthcare systems from developing ultrasensitive medical devices to point-of-care tools for clinical practice in hospitals/houses [7, 8].

Immunoassay/biomedical tools are one of the most advanced tools for the quantitative detection of biochemical targets (e.g., pathogens, bacteria, cells, nucleic acids, proteins, etc) [8, 9]. Most of these analytes are extracted from body fluids like saliva, urine, blood/plasma, etc for clinical investigation. There are various assays/tools that have progressed from the traditional ones performed on tubes/glass plates/microplates to sophisticated miniaturized platforms using various kinds of readout signals. The current technique for detection and analysis of analytes which include electrochemistry, Raman, electronics, magnetic, UV, FTIR, optical microscopy, surface plasmon resonance, fluorescence and mass spectroscopy, etc are the frontiers of the traditional disciplines in science and engineering [10, 11]. These amazing analytical techniques allow better characterization to be achieved, providing more accurate clinical information, rapid diagnostics, cost-effective, user friendly approaches, and state-of-the-art facilities for personalized health management [12–14].

This chapter discusses different emerging and existing techniques to prepare nanostructures and the benefits/limitations of each type along with their application. Next, various approaches to prepare different types of systems, their characteristics in generating nanomaterials with desired properties are presented. The chapter also focuses on existing and new tools combined with nanostructures for development of ultrasensitive instruments for health management. Further, current immunoassay/tools like ELISA (the enzyme-linked immunosorbent assay), PCR (polymerase chain reaction), FACS (fluorescence-activated cell sorting), clustered regularly interspaced short palindromic repeats (CRISPR) as sophisticated analyte-detecting tools composed of biological, chemical, electrical, optical, computational or combination techniques have provided a rapid diagnostic system in hospitals and medical research facilities [8, 15–17]. However, the human effort in improving the diagnostic system is a continuous process and many factors contribute to achieving these milestones. Now, we will summarize some of the factors that have contributed immensely for developing advanced healthcare systems.

1.2 Nanomaterials

We will discuss some of the well-known characteristics of nanostructures that led to the development of better healthcare systems [18]. Some of the characteristics of nanostructures are unique in nature that can be controlled or tuned as per the requirement. (i) The shape and size of nanomaterial: the better control over the size and shape of nanomaterials leads to various novel properties [19]. The size tuneability has control over the color of the quantum dots such as CdSe emits multiple color over a nanometer range of particle size. Also, different shapes of gold nanomaterials (rod, dumbbell, triangle, flower, etc) provide their unique surface resonance plasmonic effect. (ii) Non-toxic and biocompatibility: these unique characteristics of nanoparticles are an important factor in the biomedical sector for *in vitro* usage as well as drug development. (iii) Stability: stable nanoparticles are a necessity to avoid aggregation and provide the same characteristics every time for sophisticated tool development. (iv) Versatility: this factor is important as nanomaterials can be used for multipurpose utilities like coating, drug delivery, magnetic separation, imaging, etc. Iron oxide is one such nanomaterial which can serve all the above purposes for developing biomedical devices. Hence this versatile nanomaterial was approved by the FDA for human usage.

1.2.1 Analyte/biomarker

An analyte/biomarker is a substance which may or may not be present in human fluids (blood, saliva, urine, etc) and can be measured/quantified for the detection of disease [20, 21]. Consequently, the outcome of these investigations leads to proper prognostic or diagnostic steps for the precise management of the disease. For example, cancer biomarkers which are present in blood or other body fluids can be traced through the detection of cells, proteins, nucleic acids, enzymes, exosomes, lipids, etc [22]. The purpose of tracing the cancer biomarker is to develop a reliable, highly sensitive and selective sensor for early cancer detection, monitoring and treatment strategy. Various promising detection methods based on the specific recognition of biomarkers or analytes have been developed to manage various diseases. Figure 1.1 depicts some of the recently developed techniques like artificial intelligence, lab on chip, nanomedicine, smart nanomaterials, bioimaging tools, etc have revolutionized the personal healthcare system for investigation of diseases by integrating multiple analytical systems (optical, electrochemical, microscopy, MEMS, etc).

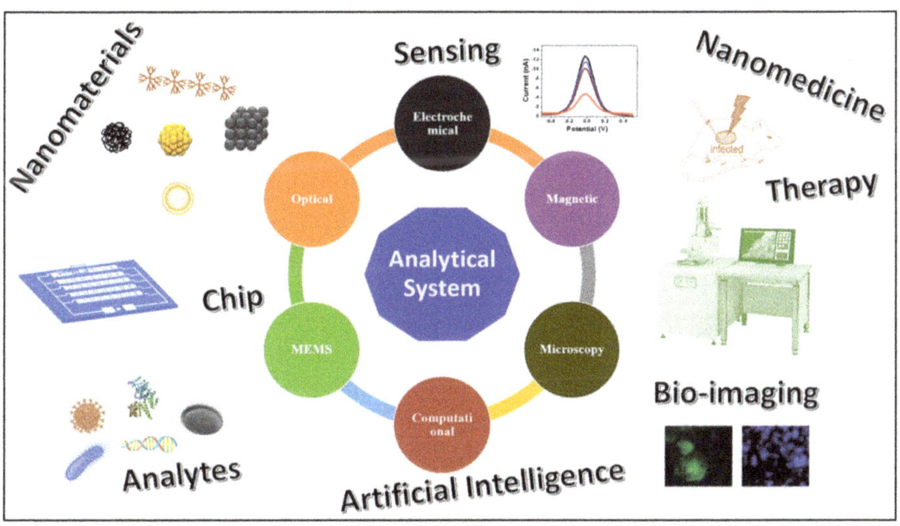

Figure 1.1. Schematic illustration of analytical system integrating multiple platforms for biomedical application.

1.3 Electrochemical system

One of the earliest analyte detection systems (or immunoassays) developed by researchers and scientists was electrochemical techniques which can quantify the analytes by measuring the changes in electrical signals such as potential, current, resistance, and capacitance and has gained a wide variety of applications in biosensor arena [23]. Electrochemical assay has been prevalent in the market for its simplicity and high sensitivity for providing quick diagnostics to millions of people. The sensitivity of amperometric immunoassays is significantly affected by the conductivity and specific area of the sensing interface as well as the electrochemical activity of redox species [23]. The large specific area, good electron conductivity, biocompatibility, and catalytic performance of the redox species led to excellent electrochemical activity. Some of the well-known devices available in the market are glucose sensors, cholesterol sensors, tumor markers etc [24]. It offers quick, simple and sensitive detection but has some clinical limitation of interference, long-term stability and non-specific adsorption.

1.3.1 Optical systems (fluorescence, SPR, Raman, mass spectroscopy)

The optical properties of nanomaterials such as fluorescence spectra, colorimetry, and Raman scattering properties are being developed to construct medical devices. Depending on the type of optical material used, color-based fluorescent (dye, quantum dots) and non-fluorescent nanomaterials (gold, silver, graphene, etc) are being continuously explored in order to design ultrasensitive higher resolution imaging systems [25].

In the last few decades, the invention of the laser and extensive research on optical nanomaterials have led to many optical sensors. Hence, the optical detection technique has become one of the most popular methods for immunoassay development. Popular simple colorimetric assay like pregnancy test strips have been employed in various hospitals and maternity centers for initial screening. Similarly, UV–visible spectroscopy, FTIR techniques and chemiluminescence immunosensors are being utilized in clinical diagnosis for its simplicity and ease of handling [26].

Recently, fluorescence immunoassays have revolutionized the health industry for improved sensitivity and fast readout process. Molecular fluorescence imaging has achieved a new height of success as they can image a single molecule with high precision [27, 28]. Fluorescence microscopy utilizes an imaging agent known as fluorescent dye tagged with target antibodies (proteins) that binds with target analyte to capture the highlighted image. For example, they can image protein agglomeration present on human cell surface through a fluorescence dye tagged antibody [4]. One of the pioneering works performed by Koller *et al* demonstrated the first clinical trials of investigating fluorescence-guided surgery in humans [29]. They reported the clinical translation and evaluation of tumor-targeted fluorescent tracers for molecular fluorescence imaging of tumors in breast cancer.

Surface plasmon resonance (SPR) immunoassays provides a label-free optical sensing platform [30]. The working principle for measuring the analyte is to measure the absorption index and the specific interactions between antibodies and antigens can be determined by the changes in reflective index. This system provides *in situ* monitoring of analyte through the adsorption of analyte onto a gold or silver metal surface for various biosensor applications.

Raman spectroscopy has significantly changed the vibrational spectroscopic techniques for its versatile application like materials characterization, material detection, diagnostics system, etc [31, 32]. Among the various Raman spectroscopy variants, surface enhanced Raman spectroscopy (SERS) has been a promising tool development as a result of significant progress of nanomaterial as it provide single molecule sensitivity in molecular diagnostics [4, 33]. Some of the technical benefits of SERS as a clinical assay are minimal sample preparation and the ability to detect target molecules in aqueous samples, as water exhibits very weak Raman scattering due to its small Raman cross-section. These qualities have enabled Raman spectroscopy to construct multiplex detection platforms for point-of-care application [34].

Mass spectroscopy (MS) is another powerful analytical technique to quantify biomolecules and to identify unknown samples [35]. Under the influence of external electric and magnet field, MS disintegrates compounds or molecules into charged species and categorized them according to their mass and charge ratio. They are extensively used in lipid and protein analysis for understanding the basic human metabolic system. It provides precise determination of the molecular mass of target molecule for various proteins/peptides identification.

1.3.2 Electron microscope (SEM, TEM, AFM, EDX, XPS)

The most advanced imaging system such as scanning electron microscopy (SEM), transmission electron microscopy (TEM), atomic force microscopy (AFM), energy-dispersive x-ray spectroscopy (EDX), and are more frequently used for imaging as well as disease evaluation [36, 37]. They offer qualitative, quantitative and/or structural information regarding changes that occur in nanomaterials/biomaterials/thin film sensors/interfacial areas of devices. SEM/TEM/AFM provide micro- and nanoscale characterization of nanomaterials/biological structures, internal shape and size, surface topology for in-depth analysis. The compositional and elemental analysis of nanostructures are facilitated by EDX. These highly sensitive imaging techniques have found application in biomolecule (cells, proteins, bacteria, etc) structure evaluation, nano biomaterial-interface determination, nano-enabled drug delivery systems, targeted therapy, nanomedicine, etc [38]. Another useful photoelectron based system known as x-ray photoelectron spectroscopy (XPS) has been widely used for measuring surface chemistry of a few nanometers width of solid surface to extract information about the chemical state of the nanostructures.

1.3.3 Magnetic systems (NMR, VSM)

Nuclear magnetic resonance (NMR) and vibrating sample magnetometer (VSM) techniques are based on magnetic properties of nanomaterials. NMR is a physical phenomenon where the nuclei of nanomaterial oscillates with external weak magnetic field to determine the structure of organic molecules whereas VSM measures magnetic moment as a function of an applied magnetic field in solid and liquid samples. They are utilized to explore magnetic properties of nanomaterials/micro-nano systems to understand molecular dynamics, determining purity of sample, understanding biomolecule structures, probing magnetic activity at drug target sites. Recently, the microfabrication technique has enabled miniaturization of the NMR system using immuno-magnetic labeling as well as label-free biomolecule detection [39]. Magnetic systems have wide applications in medical diagnostics as magnetic sensors, magnetic material as probes, brain mapping in nanomedicine, etc. Another lesser known technique electron paramagnetic resonance (EPR) spectroscopy is used to study the free radicals and paramagnetic species in nano-biomaterials when the spin states of an electron oscillate under an applied magnetic field. One of the interesting areas that has changed the biomedical sector is nanomedicine due to significant progression of magnetic nanoparticles and their diagnostic applications in human organ imaging (liver, lymph node, inflammation and vascular imaging, etc) [40, 41]. Iron oxide nanoparticles are one of the most sought nanomaterials as image-guided drug delivery, magnetic particle imaging, image-guided and microbubble-mediated opening of the blood–brain barrier, and theranostic tissue engineering [42].

1.3.4 Microfluidic system

Microfluidic chip-based point-of-care assays are gaining popularity for the concept of developing a lab-on-a-chip device [43]. These platforms can perform multitasks in one assay procedure for rapid diagnosis and quicker decision making. It consumes a minute quantity of reagents and analytes to perform quantitative, rapid, automated and high-yield measurement [44]. These novel prototypes have revolutionized the clinical settings in hospitals, diagnostics centers as well as personalized medicine development. Further, microfluidics can be easily integrated within standard detection systems and opened new possibilities for multiplexed detection of diseases with minimal requirement of essential reagents for constructing a cost-effective and portable device. For example, Trau *et al* fabricated a gold electrode-based lab-on-a-chip devices combining hydrodynamic microfluidic flow with multiple detection systems for various disease screening, monitoring, detection and quantification (pathogens, bacteria, cancer biomarkers, etc) [8, 45–47]. This versatile nanoshearing chip has evolved as a lab-on-a- chip multifunctional platform. They have integrated this chip successfully with electrochemical systems, colorimetric assay, fluorescence technique and SERS instrument for biomolecule identification, immunoassays development, drug monitoring tool, and individual analyte imaging.

1.4 Conclusion and future direction

The future of the biomedical sector is very promising. This chapter has summarized the existing technologies and has reported the potential of nano-enabled multidisciplinary smart platforms for personalized healthcare management. The immediate future in clinical pathology is to build multiple detection of analytes in a single run of assay. This will have myriad advantages over single assay systems. A multiplexed system provides simultaneous measurement of multiple analytes and provides valuable information to reduce false positive results and is able to design a more accurate system for better disease diagnosis. This single platform for multiple assay performance would reduce medical expenses and analysis time. This would be a valuable step forward for constructing a point-of-care system.

The imaging applications of nanostructures in the health sector is immense. The imaging systems have great advantages due to their nanoscale dimensions suitable for biomolecule labelling and monitoring. The imaging applications depend on several factors such as shape, biocompatibility, biodegradability, and stability of nanostructures. One of the key areas in developments would be high-resolution imaging of biomolecules for targeted drug delivery. This would allow specific drug delivery treatments to be safer and more accessible to all patients [48].

Dr Francis Collins, a renowned American scientist who led the 'Human Genome Project' shared his vision about the precision medicine initiative and remarked that the next generation of scientists would create new approaches for detecting, measuring, and analyzing a wide range of biomedical information—including molecular, genomic, cellular, clinical, behavioral, physiological, and environmental parameters [49]. Based on that concept many opportunities have evolved and AI is one of the prodigies in this area to achieve this feat. AI is the future of smart healthcare system. Medical technology will revolutionize as AI can assimilate billions of data related to health including patient data such as medical imaging, drug data, treatment procedure, electronic records, etc. In this way, AI with the help of human intelligence can create a predictable algorithm to manage and combat deadly diseases for better health management.

Acknowledgement

The author acknowledges respective departments and institutions for providing support and facilities.

References

[1] Bhushan B 2017 Introduction to nanotechnology *Springer Handbook of Nanotechnology* (Berlin: Springer) pp 1–19

[2] Bhardwaj V and Kaushik A 2017 *Biomedical Applications of Nanotechnology and Nanomaterials* (Basel: Multidisciplinary Digital Publishing Institute)

[3] Reza K K, Ali M A, Srivastava S, Agrawal V V and Biradar A 2015 Tyrosinase conjugated reduced graphene oxide based biointerface for bisphenol A sensor *Biosens. Bioelectron.* **74** 644–51

[4] Reza K K, Dey S, Wuethrich A, Sina A A I, Korbie D, Wang Y and Trau M 2018 Parallel profiling of cancer cells and proteins using a graphene oxide functionalized ac-EHD SERS immunoassay *Nanoscale* **10** 18482–91

[5] Adlakha-Hutcheon G, Khaydarov R, Korenstein R, Varma R, Vaseashta A, Stamm H and Abdel-Mottaleb M 2009 Nanomaterials, nanotechnology *Nanomaterials: Risks and Benefits* (Berlin: Springer) pp 195–207

[6] Reza K K, Sina A A I, Wuethrich A, Grewal Y S, Howard C B, Korbie D and Trau M 2019 A SERS microfluidic platform for targeting multiple soluble immune checkpoints *Biosens. Bioelectron.* **126** 178–86
[7] Kaminski T S and Garstecki P 2017 Controlled droplet microfluidic systems for multistep chemical and biological assays *Chem. Soc. Rev.* **46** 6210–26
[8] Khondakar K R, Dey S, Wuethrich A, Sina A A I and Trau M 2019 Toward personalized cancer treatment: from diagnostics to therapy monitoring in miniaturized electrohydrodynamic systems *Acc. Chem. Res.* **52** 2113–23
[9] Kamil Reza K, Wang J, Vaidyanathan R, Dey S, Wang Y and Trau M 2017 Electrohydrodynamic-induced SERS immunoassay for extensive multiplexed biomarker sensing *Small* **13** 1602902
[10] Yakoh A, Pinyorospathum C, Siangproh W and Chailapakul O 2015 Biomedical probes based on inorganic nanoparticles for electrochemical and optical spectroscopy applications *Sensors* **15** 21427–77
[11] Anik Ü, Timur S and Dursun Z 2019 Metal organic frameworks in electrochemical and optical sensing platforms: a review *Microchim. Acta* **186** 196
[12] Zhang L and Webster T J 2009 Nanotechnology and nanomaterials: promises for improved tissue regeneration *Nano Today* **4** 66–80
[13] Wuethrich A, Rajkumar A R, Shanmugasundaram K B, Reza K K, Dey S, Howard C B, Sina A A I and Trau M 2019 Single droplet detection of immune checkpoints on a multiplexed electrohydrodynamic biosensor *Analyst* **144** 6914–21
[14] Dey S *et al* 2019 A microfluidic-SERSplatform for isolation and immuno-phenotyping of antigen specific T-cells *Sensors Actuators* A **284** 281–88
[15] Rodríguez-Rodríguez D R, Ramírez-Solís R, Garza-Elizondo M A, Garza-Rodríguez M D L and Barrera-Saldaña H A 2019 Genome editing: a perspective on the application of CRISPR/Cas9 to study human diseases (review) *Int. J. Mol. Med.* **43** 1559–74
[16] Li H, Bai R, Zhao Z, Tao L, Ma M, Ji Z, Jian M, Ding Z, Dai X and Bao F 2018 Application of droplet digital PCR to detect the pathogens of infectious diseases *Biosci. Rep.* **38** BSR20181170
[17] Shinkins B, Nicholson B D, Primrose J, Perera R, James T, Pugh S and Mant D 2017 The diagnostic accuracy of a single CEA blood test in detecting colorectal cancer recurrence: results from the FACS trial *PLoS One* **12** e0171810
[18] Yin Y and Talapin D 2013 The chemistry of functional nanomaterials *Chem. Soc. Rev.* **42** 2484–87
[19] Roduner E 2006 Size matters: why nanomaterials are different *Chem. Soc. Rev.* **35** 583–92
[20] Wu L and Qu X 2015 Cancer biomarker detection: recent achievements and challenges *Chem. Soc. Rev.* **44** 2963–97
[21] Hanash S M, Baik C S and Kallioniemi O 2011 Emerging molecular biomarkers—blood-based strategies to detect and monitor cancer *Nat. Rev. Clin. Oncol.* **8** 142–50
[22] Ludwig J A and Weinstein J N 2005 Biomarkers in cancer staging, prognosis and treatment selection *Nat. Rev. Cancer* **5** 845–56
[23] Tang Z and Ma Z 2017 Multiple functional strategies for amplifying sensitivity of amperometric immunoassay for tumor markers: a review *Biosens. Bioelectron.* **98** 100–12
[24] Ali M A, Kamil Reza K, Srivastava S, Agrawal V V, John R and Malhotra B D 2014 Lipid–lipid interactions in aminated reduced graphene oxide interface for biosensing application *Langmuir* **30** 4192–201

[25] Shikha S, Salafi T, Cheng J and Zhang Y 2017 Versatile design and synthesis of nano-barcodes *Chem. Soc. Rev.* **46** 7054–93
[26] Orrit M, Ha T and Sandoghdar V 2014 Single-molecule optical spectroscopy *Chem. Soc. Rev.* **43** 973–76
[27] Platnich C M, Rizzuto F J, Cosa G and Sleiman H F 2020 Single-molecule methods in structural DNA nanotechnology *Chem. Soc. Rev.* **49** 4220–33
[28] Jung S-R, Fujimoto B S and Chiu D T 2017 Quantitative microscopy based on single-molecule fluorescence *Curr. Opin. Chem. Biol.* **39** 64–73
[29] Koller M *et al* 2018 Implementation and benchmarking of a novel analytical framework to clinically evaluate tumor-specific fluorescent tracers *Nat. Commun.* **9** 3739
[30] Moran K L M, Lemass D and O'Kennedy R 2018 Surface plasmon resonance-based immunoassays: approaches, performance, and applications *Handbook of Immunoassay Technologies* ed S K Vashist and J H T Luong (New York: Academic) ch 6 pp 129–56
[31] Krafft C and Popp J 2015 The many facets of Raman spectroscopy for biomedical analysis *Anal. Bioanal. Chem.* **407** 699–717
[32] Zhang X, Tan Q-H, Wu J-B, Shi W and Tan P-H 2016 Review on the Raman spectroscopy of different types of layered materials *Nanoscale* **8** 6435–50
[33] Laing S, Gracie K and Faulds K 2016 Multiplex *in vitro* detection using SERS *Chem. Soc. Rev.* **45** 1901–18
[34] Cialla-May D, Zheng X-S, Weber K and Popp J 2017 Recent progress in surface-enhanced Raman spectroscopy for biological and biomedical applications: from cells to clinics *Chem. Soc. Rev.* **46** 3945–61
[35] Rajawat J and Jhingan G 2019 Mass spectroscopy *Data Processing Handbook for Complex Biological Data Sources* (Amsterdam: Elsevier) pp 1–20
[36] Xu M, Liu J, Sun J, Xu X, Hu Y and Liu B 2020 Optical microscopy and electron microscopy for the morphological evaluation of tendons: a mini review *Orthop. Surg.* **12** 366–71
[37] Spence J C 2013 *High-Resolution Electron Microscopy* (Oxford: Oxford University Press)
[38] Oxley M P, Lupini A R and Pennycook S J 2016 Ultra-high resolution electron microscopy *Rep. Prog. Phys.* **80** 026101
[39] Dupré A, Lei K-M, Mak P-I, Martins R P and Peng W K 2019 Micro- and nanofabrication NMR technologies for point-of-care medical applications—a review *Microelectron. Eng.* **209** 66–74
[40] Wu K, Su D, Liu J, Saha R and Wang J-P 2018 *Magnetic nanoparticles in nanomedicine* arXiv preprint (arXiv:1811.01418)
[41] Tomitaka A, Kaushik A, Kevadiya B D, Mukadam I, Gendelman H E, Khalili K, Liu G and Nair M 2019 Surface-engineered multimodal magnetic nanoparticles to manage CNS diseases *Drug Discovery Today* **24** 873–82
[42] Dadfar S M, Roemhild K, Drude N I, von Stillfried S, Knüchel R, Kiessling F and Lammers T 2019 Iron oxide nanoparticles: diagnostic, therapeutic and theranostic applications *Adv. Drug Delivery Rev.* **138** 302–25
[43] Sun J, Xianyu Y and Jiang X 2014 Point-of-care biochemical assays using gold nanoparticle-implemented microfluidics *Chem. Soc. Rev.* **43** 6239–53
[44] Nge P N, Rogers C I and Woolley A T 2013 Advances in microfluidic materials, functions, integration, and applications *Chem. Rev.* **113** 2550–83

[45] Wang Y, Vaidyanathan R, Shiddiky M J A and Trau M 2015 Enabling rapid and specific surface-enhanced Raman scattering immunoassay using nanoscaled surface shear forces *ACS Nano* **9** 6354–62

[46] Dey S, Vaidyanathan R, Carrascosa L G, Shiddiky M J A and Trau M 2016 Electric field induced isolation, release, and recapture of tumor cells *ACS Sens.* **1** 399–405

[47] Grewal Y S, Shiddiky M J, Mahler S M, Cangelosi G A and Trau M 2016 Nanoyeast and other cell envelope compositions for protein studies and biosensor applications *ACS Appl. Mater. Interfaces* **8** 30649–64

[48] Medlock J, Das A A K, Madden L A, Allsup D J and Paunov V N 2017 Cancer bioimprinting and cell shape recognition for diagnosis and targeted treatment *Chem. Soc. Rev.* **46** 5110–27

[49] Collins F S and Varmus H 2015 A new initiative on precision medicine *New Engl. J. Med.* **372** 793–95

IOP Publishing

Analytical Techniques for Biomedical Nanotechnology

Ajeet Kaushik, Sesha S Srinivasan and Yogendra Kumar Mishra

Chapter 2

Electrochemical techniques for biomedical nanotechnology

Jyotsana Mehta, Neeraj Dilbaghi and Sandeep Kumar

The growing diversity in analytical techniques has greatly impacted our healthcare and overall quality of life. The key issues that are to be considered while developing analytical platforms are low development cost, high sensitivity, appreciable selectivity, easy interpretation of results, and applicability for real-time analysis, particularly in point-of-care devices which require simple integration. In the light of these factors, electrochemical analytical techniques are of great utility and act as the most promising candidates attributed to their simplicity, high specificity and sensitivity fast analysis, reduced consumption of solvent and sample, low operational cost along with being easily readable and having easily understandable results. The main focus of this chapter is towards highlighting the application of advanced nanomaterials based electrochemical analytical approaches for the diagnosis of analytes of biomedical importance. The analytical capacities of electrochemical sensors have been improved drastically due to the attractive properties of nanomaterials, thereby, opening up the possibilities of developing new technologies facilitating early detection of different disease biomarkers.

2.1 Introduction

The prompt expansion of knowledge and technology in human society offers development of highly specific, sensitive, cost-effective, rapid, and robust analytical methods which can facilitate efficient monitoring of biomedical analytes. Electrochemical sensors are the most attractive research areas holding a leading position amongst all chemical sensors. Electrochemistry is a powerful analytical technique that encompasses the advantages of moderate cost, instrumental simplicity, and portability. The electrochemical techniques are selective, sensitive, facile, and rapid enough for efficient applicability in biomedical fields, and indeed in almost all the analytical chemistry areas. In an electrochemical sensor, an electrode

doi:10.1088/978-0-7503-3379-5ch2

transduces a chemical or biological signal into an electrical one via a large variety of electrochemical strategies such as potentiometry, voltammetry, amperometry, and impedimetry as shown in figure 2.1. Potentiometry has found widespread applicability as an electrochemical sensing technique since the early 1930s. Potentiometric sensors provide the qualitative and quantitative information about the composition of the sample to be analyzed via measuring the potential between the two electrodes. Voltammetry has shown its potential for measurement of levels of metabolites, disease markers, and even minute doses of drugs, to mention a few in blood and urine. The two types of voltammetry techniques namely, linear sweep voltammetry (LSV) and cyclic voltammetry (CV) have attracted great attention for the exposition of redox mechanisms and electrode processes. On the other hand, square wave voltammetry (SWV) and differential pulse voltammetry (DPV) have attracted interest to be used in the quantification of electroactive analytes in biological fluids. A highly sensitive electrochemical approach, stripping voltammetry is particularly useful in ultrasensitive detection as it has the ability to preconcentrate analytes. Amperometry is another widely employed electrochemical technique for the development of electrochemical sensors of biomedical importance. Amperometric sensors measure current response at the electrode at a fixed potential in order to measure the

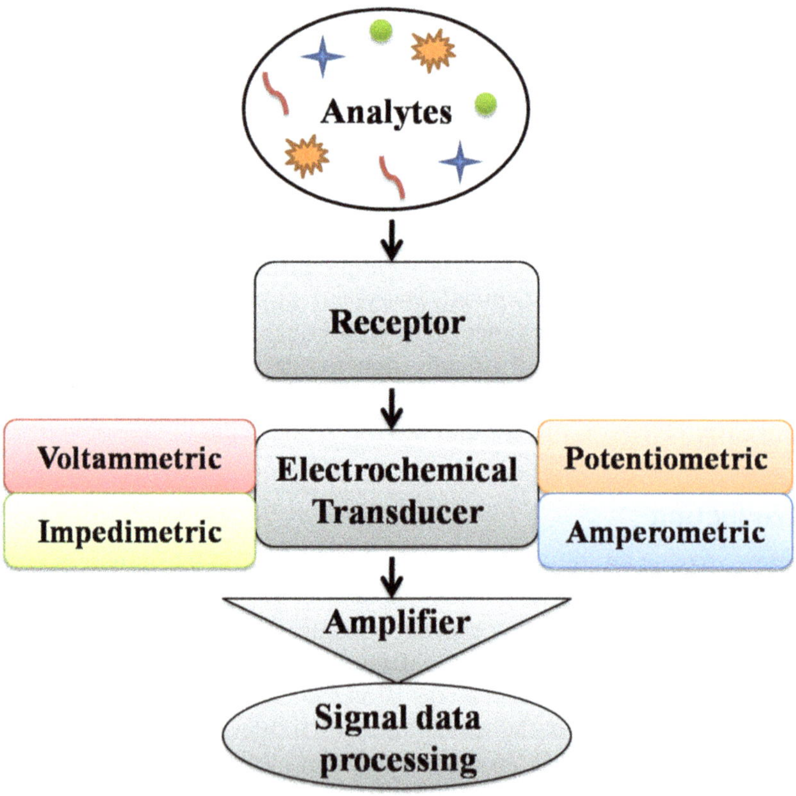

Figure 2.1. Basic principle of electrochemical sensors.

concentration of an analyte. Impedance is also an excellent electrochemical technique explored for the determination of bulk and electrode interface properties which further measure the analyte concentration in terms of electrochemical quantitative parameters.

The last two decades have witnessed the integration of nanomaterials into sensing platforms. The advances in synthesis methods of nanomaterials have provided better control over size, shape, charge, and other physicochemical properties. The composite formation of nanomaterials with polymers and bioactive molecules has enhanced their biocompatibility and analyte targeting. Functionalization has also resulted in better transmission of recognition events into electronic signal transduction for the development of electronic sensing devices with novel functions. The important characteristics of nanomaterials which collectively influence the electron transport mechanisms for improved electrochemical characteristics are chemical composition, quality of crystal structure, surface chemistry, and axis orientation, etc. The major advantages of incorporating nanomaterials into electrochemical analysis systems are their easy implementation as non-invasive diagnostic tools and their potential to combine multiple modalities into a single detection probe. This has enabled the fabrication of an electrochemical diagnostic tool exhibiting higher sensitivity and selectivity along with miniaturization and point-of-care applicability.

The intent of this chapter is to provide impending information regarding electrochemical sensors integrated with nanomaterials, and to exemplify their prospective application and benefits in biomedical diagnostic tools. The most promising analytical applications of such sensors encompass detection of disease and cancer biomarkers, monitoring of general health parameters (ions, lactate, glucose, and neurotransmitters, to mention a few) as well as pathogenic microorganisms. The chapter starts with the introduction of different electrochemical techniques followed by their application in collaboration with nanomaterials for the determination of healthcare related analytes. Further, new sophisticated electrochemical sensing devices such as planar, wearable, microfluidic, and molecularly imprinted platforms are summarized. The challenges, opportunities, and future prospects regarding development of advanced electrochemical nanosensors for biomedical diagnostics are also discussed.

2.2 Principles of electrochemical analytical methods

2.2.1 Potentiometry-based analysis

Potentiometry has been the most conventional electrochemical analytical technique since the 1930s which uses ion selective electrode (ISE) as the indicator electrode and measures the activity of ionic analyte species. ISEs are membranous and the binding of analyte ions to the membrane is based on its composition resulting in highly specific and sensitive binding to respective ions leaving behind the co-ions. The wide usage of potentiometry-based ISEs in almost all the laboratories is attributed to cost-effectiveness, simplicity, wide linear dynamic detection range, rapid response, and non-destructive nature. The techniques also offer straightforward measurement and easy interpretation of ionic content in real or synthetic samples by non-expert users via quantification of acquired signal in the form of electromotive force (EMF) versus time near to zero-current conditions. Technically, a potentiometric sensor consists of a reference electrode and potential measuring device along with an ISE. Three distinct charge transfer processes take place in the electrochemical cell. For example, the electrons move between electrodes and wires, ions move in solutions, and the electrons are transferred to ions or vice versa on the surface of electrodes. The charge transfer event is translated into a voltage signal through which analytical information is obtained. The potentiometric readout of the electrochemical cell in the form of EMF is detected as difference between the reference electrode and the measured membrane potential. The Nernst equation (equation (2.1)) describes the ideal response of a potentiometric electrochemical cell as a variation of potentiometric signal with activity of the analyte ion. Ion activity is described as the free concentration of the analyte ion which is the recognized driving force in any electrochemical (chemical or biological) reaction. The magnitude of ion activity may be of smaller magnitude than that of total analyte ion concentration in the presence of complexing agent in the sample. Further, the calibration graph between EMF and logarithmic activity is used to calculate the analyte ion concentration in the sample.

$$\mathrm{EMF} = K + RT/zF \ln a_{\mathrm{I}} \tag{2.1}$$

where the EMF isoelectromotive force, i.e., observed potential at zero current; K is potential of reference electrode at liquid junction; a_{I} is the activity of the primary ion; z is the charge of ion; F, R, and T are Faraday constant, gas constant, and absolute temperature, respectively.

2.2.2 Voltammetry-based analysis

Voltammetry is a type of electrochemical analytical technique in which current–voltage measurement is performed at a given electrode. Polarography is the first developed voltammetry-based technique developed by Czech chemist Jaroslav Heyrovsky in 1922 for which he received the Nobel Prize in chemistry in 1959. In polarography, current–voltage is measured using a mercury dropping electrode having fixed flow of mercury drop. Current–voltage measurements in voltammetry take place in an electrochemical cell consisting of three-electrode configuration, namely, auxillary/counter, reference, and working electrode. On applying the potential (E or V) to the working electrode, the current flows through the cell which is recorded. The applied potential is a controllable parameter and acts as the driving force which either oxidizes or reduces the chemical species present in the solution. The current–voltage measurements are displayed in the form of voltammogram, a plot of current versus potential.

Cyclic voltammetry (CV) is the most commonly used electrochemical analytical technique for studying the various aspects of redox reactions. In CV, the potential is applied in both the forward and reverse directions at the working electrode, i.e., the direction of voltage scan is reversed and the resulting current is recorded. However, the scan rate is kept the same in both directions. The effect of scan rate on peak current i_{p} is determined using the Randles–Sevcik equation. For example, in ferrocene/ferrocenium couple involving redox events, i_p depends on the scan rate along with the diffusional properties and concentration of electroactive species as per the equation:

$$i_p = 0.4463nFAC\left(\frac{nFvD}{RT}\right)^{1/2}$$

Or if the solution is at 25 °C

$$i_p = 2.69 \times 10^5 n^{3/2} A D^{1/2} C v^{1/2}$$

where A—electrode area (cm^2), C—concentration (mol cm^{-3}), D—diffusion coefficient (cm^2 s^{-1}), F—Faraday constant (C mol^{-1}), i_p—current maximum (amps), n—number of electrons transferred in the redox event, v—scan rate (V s^{-1}), R—gas constant (J K^{-1} mol^{-1}), T—temperature (K). In electrochemistry, the interpretations of this equation appear counter-intuitive, i.e., i_p increases at faster voltage scan rates. In cyclic voltammetry, the current passing through the electrode is dependent on the diffusion of species across the electrode surface. This diffusion flux is further influenced by the concentration gradient near the electrode which is affected by the concentration of species at the electrode, and diffusion of the species through solution. The change in cell voltage changes the concentration of the species at the surface of the electrode as per the Nernst equation. Overall, a faster voltage sweep causes a larger concentration gradient near the electrode, resulting in a higher current.

A special case of voltammetry is stripping voltammetry analysis which can measure even sub-nanogram concentration of analyte with sufficient accuracy. Such a high level of sensitivity is achieved due to analyte preconcentration onto the surface of the working electrode prior to the measurement of current in the potential scan. The preconcentration step also reduces the background noise, thereby, improving the signal-to-noise ratio. Other modern variants of voltammetric analysis are linear sweep, square wave, and pulse voltammetry. In linear sweep voltammetrty (LSV), the current at the working electrode is measured while the potential is swept linearly between working and reference electrode. The potentials at which the species are electrolyzed (oxidized or reduced) are depicted as a peak or trough in the current signal in a voltammogram. Square wave voltammetry (SWV) is a modified form of LSV in which the potential between working and reference electrode is applied in the square wave's form. The current so produced is measured twice—initially at the finish of forward potential pulse followed by a second measurement at the termination of the reverse potential pulse. The differential current is obtained as the difference between the reverse current waveform and the forward current waveform. The peaks and their magnitude in the different current versus applied voltage graphs are indicative of redox processes and concentration of redox species, respectively. Another form of LSV is DPV which comprises of series of applied uniform voltage pulses. The current is recorded prior to every potential change which reduces the effect of the charging current. The difference in current value is then plotted against the applied potential. The reversible reactions in DPV have symmetric peaks and the peak current is directly proportional to the analyte ion concentration.

2.2.3 Amperometry-based analysis

Amperometry is another electrochemical analytical technique based on the measurement of a steady state current resulting from the use of an oxidizing or reducing potential applied to the working electrode. The basic principle of these measurements relies on quantification of current generated upon oxidation or reduction of electroactive species. The term amperometry has been coined using the words *ampere* (current measurement unit) and *meter* (measurement device). It differs from the voltammetry technique wherein the current measurements are recorded over a controlled range of applied potential whereas in the ase of amperometry the current is measured at a constant voltage.

An amperometry measurement cell comprises a working and a reference electrode along with the instrumentation to control the applied potential and measure the analyte signal (output current) as a function of time. For measurement, a constant potential with respect to the reference electrode is applied to the working electrode (upon which the analyte is deposited) and the corresponding change in the steady state current is recorded. Note that the output current is a measure of rate of oxidation or reduction of the electroactive species (deposited over the working electrode) which varies in direct correspondence to the mass analyte concentration making the method suitable for diverse analytical applications.

The output current varies with the concentration of the analyte according to the Cottrell equation:

$$i = \frac{nFAc_0\sqrt{D}}{\sqrt{\pi t}}$$

where A—area of electrode (cm^2), c_0—initial conc. of analye (mol ml^{-1}), D—diffusion coefficient (cm^2 s^{-1}), F—Faraday constant (96 487 C mol^{-1}), i—current (A), n—number of electrons transferred, and t—time. Through intelligent selection of the electrode material as well as the potential applied the amperometry technique can be used to distinguish various electroactive species in a solution. In the case of amperometric titrations, the voltage applied across the working and reference electrodes is kept constant followed by measurement of the diffusion current passing through the cell and plotting against the volume of the reagent added. The analytical method finds great relevance in biomedicine and environmental and industrial applications in the form of amperometric sensors.

2.2.4 Impedimetry-based analysis

Impedimetry analysis is a potent analytical technique and has been broadly employed for detecting interfacial binding events. Impedance is a measure of electric circuit opposition to the current on the application of voltage. The interfacial impedance is measured by tracking the current response on the application of sinusoidal voltage perturbations during electrochemical impedance spectroscopy

(EIS) measurements. A typical EIS system is composed of a three-electrode configuration—working, reference, and auxiliary/counter electrode. The auxiliary electrode exhibits polarity exactly equal and opposite to that of the working and reference electrode and is set at the fixed potential. The potentiostat/galvanostat in addition to a frequency response analyzer (FRA) are also components of the instrument. The FRA provides an AC current sine wave of particular amplitude to the potentiostat. During impedance measurements, AC current applied to the working electrode changes its polarity from positive to negative in a periodic manner and subsequent current response is measured.

The term spectroscopy signifies the analysis of a particular event over a frequency range (generally between 10 mHz and 100 kHz). On drifting AC current across the network consisting of capacitor, inductor, and resistors, the resulting total complex resistance, i.e., impedance is noted whose phase and magnitude depends on the frequency sweep range and electronic components. In yhe majority of cases, only the capacitive and real resistive but not inductive behaviors of the electrochemical cell are considered. Further, the complex impedance (Z') is calculated as the ratio of excitation voltage w.r.t. time function V(t) to current–time function I(t) as response signal.

- Excitation voltage signal, $V(t) = V_{\mathrm{m}}.\sin(\omega t)$,
- Response current signal, $I(t) = I_{\mathrm{m}}.\sin(\omega t + \phi)$ and
- Calculated impedance, $Z = V(t)/I(t) = V_{\mathrm{m}}.\sin(\omega t)/I_{\mathrm{m}}.\sin(\omega t + \phi)$

where I_{m} and V_{m} are the maximum current and voltage signals, t is the time, ω is the angular frequency ($\omega = 2\pi$f), and ϕ is the shift phase.

The results of EIS measurements can be represented in two ways: (i) Bode plot and (ii) Nyquist plot. A Bode plot depicts the frequency information with log scale of frequency on x-axis and magnitude along with phase of impedance (complex quantity) on the y-axis. However, in a Nyquist plot, the real component of impedance is plotted on the x-axis and the imaginary component is plotted on the y-axis. Each individual point on the Nyquist plot gives impedance at that particular frequency.

EIS has been employed in a variety of applications such as pathogen detection, health analysis, food and environmental monitoring, to mention a few. It facilitates the label-free bioaffinity detection between biological probes and their specific analytes. EIS is a comparatively less destructive technique applied for studying biological interactions and interface characteristics of the modified electrodes.

2.3 Status of electrochemical analytical techniques in biomedical nanotechnology

Electrochemical analytical techniques offer the advantages that they are rapid, simplified, cost-effective, and easy to use and making them selective and sensitive for the analyte of interest is an attractive research area. The rapidity achieved in the electrochemical sensors is appealing for their use in medical diagnostic applications where test results are required in a very short time span to understand the diseases molecular dynamic changes and ensure a timely cure. The electrodes used in electrochemical sensors are small enough to be applicable for use with different types of samples such as electrodes for blood and cell culture samples, tattoo based electrodes for monitoring via skin surface, and implantable electrodes for determining brain activity parameters. The applications of electrochemical sensors in biomedical diagnostics range from detecting drugs, identifying disease biomarkers, monitoring levels of neurotransmitters to detection of pathogenic microorganisms and other general health parameters (such as glucose, lactate, metabolic products, and enzymes, to mention a few).

The quantification of glucose levels in diabetic patients is the leading area of development of highly efficient, cost-effective, and portable sensors. The integration of nanomaterials in electrochemical sensors employed for monitoring glucose has surged in the last decade. For example, single-walled carbon nanotubes (SWCNTs) and nafion modified electrodes have been employed for the highly sensitive amperometric detection of glucose at low potential. Disease biomarker detection is a major medical application of electrochemistry. Prostate-specific antigen (PSA) is one such biomarker detected for the diagnosis of prostate cancer [1]. Nanomaterial based amplification strategy has been employed for increasing the sensitivity of electrochemical detection of PSA. Singh and co-workers have investigated the use of $ZnSnO_3$ perovskite nanomaterials for highly sensitive and selective detection of cardiac biomarkers [2]. Molybdenum disulfide nanosheets have also been reported for the electrochemical based quantification of the genetic biomarker of breast cancer demonstrating the potential of electrochemical detection at the level of nucleic acids [3].

Rapid detection of drugs in blood or urine samples is another major biomedical application of electrochemical analytical techniques. For instance, screen-printed electrodes coated with iron oxide nanocubes have been investigated for quantification of an antihistamine, meclizine [4]. A polyethylenimine-based electrochemical sensor has been developed to measure the quantity of the anti-coagulant drug, heparin in plasma which is indicative of hemostasis [5]. Neurochemistry is also an upcoming research area for the application of electrochemical analytical methods and one such example is the use of carbon electrodes as reviewed by Venton *et al* [6]. Another interesting review summarizing the use of electrodes for *in vivo* detection of different neurotransmitters (e.g., dopamine and epinephrine) has been published in the literature [7]. Zestos and group have developed polymer coated electrochemical sensor electrodes for the detection of dopamine metabolite, 3,4-dihydroxyphenylacetic acid (DOPAC) [8]. Pathogenic microorganism detection is also a prospective biomedical application of the electrochemical analytical technique. Different research groups have developed electrochemistry based surface-enhanced Raman spectroscopy (SERS), aptamer, antibody, and nucleic acid based highly sensitive bacterial sensors with the aid of nanomaterials as either immobilization substrates and transducer materials or both [9, 10].

Many research articles are based on the development of complete sensing platforms for different analytes of biomedical importance using recent technological advancements. Mo and co-workers have developed an electrochemical detection platform for studying the parameters involved in skin physiology via an electrode attached to the skin in the form of an epidermal tattoo [10]. The detection of nitrite ions in macrophages has been facilitated by combining electrochemical detection with microchip electrophoresis system [11]. A large number of noteworthy reviews have also been published highlighting the detection of autoantibodies present in autoimmune disorders and a variety of cancers, alkaline phosphatase enzyme useful both as disease markers and labels in electrochemical sensing, and also on antifouling coating of electrodes required for usage in monitoring of biological samples.

The following section recapitulates the electrochemical analytical platforms employing nanomaterials reported so far taking into consideration neurotransmitters, glucose, and cancer biomarkers as analytes.

2.3.1 Electrochemical analysis of neurotransmitters

Neurotransmitters are the key components of the neural network that control physiological conditions and behavior through communication regulation. These molecules are either directly or indirectly involved in all the neurophysiological processes ranging from sleep, appetite, learning, and memory [12]. Hindrance in production, transport, secretion, uptake, or destruction of neurotransmitters results in a variety of adverse health effects such as depression, neurogenerative disorders, and addiction [13]. Therefore, measurement of neurotransmitter levels is essential for studying neural functions, the effect of neurotransmitters on various organs, and early diagnosis of neurological diseases. Electrochemical analytical devices are an important means for *in vivo* and *in vitro* monitoring of neurotransmitters attributed to simple design, low cost, real-time detection, and high sensitivity.

Dopamine was the first neurotransmitter to be detected electrochemically *in vivo* in 1972, following which various electrochemical and electrode modifications have been investigated [14]. Most commonly explored electrochemical techniques for *in vivo* monitoring of dopamine levels are differential pulse voltammetry, fixed potential amperometry, paired pulse voltammetry, and rapid scan cyclic voltammetry [15–18]. Amongst all available electrode materials, carbon-based microelectrodes and metal (Au and Pt) electrodes are extensively used transducer materials [19, 20]. The electrochemical detection of dopamine under physiological conditions is facilitated by the 2e/2H$^+$ redox reaction of this neurotransmitter. Since the pioneering work of Wightman, dopamine sensors based on rapid scan cyclic voltammetry via direct electrochemical oxidation of analyte at carbon-based microelectrode are the methods of choice for determining brain dopamine levels *in vivo* [19, 21].

Enzymes (e.g., laccase, polyphenol oxidase, or tyrosinase) are also employed for the direct electrochemical sensing of dopamine. These enzymes convert dopamine molecules into dopaquinone which is electrochemically reduced, detected electrochemically at low potential of 0.1 V, and co-related to the actual concentration of dopamine present. The use of enzymes reduced the noise signals produced from the interfering molecules, eliminates the problem of consecutive reactions that arise in the case of dopamine oxidation, and also protects electrodes from passivation [22, 23]. Enzyme immobilization is an important aspect taken into consideration while developing enzyme based electrochemical sensing platforms. A variety of materials such as conducting polymers, carbon-based materials, mesoporous materials, and metal or oxide nanoparticles have been investigated to provide sufficient surface area for high density enzyme immobilization, stability to enzyme, and enhanced conductivity to the electrode surface in electrochemical sensors [24–27]. Njagi and group have explored ceria-based metal oxide and chitosan co-immobilized tyrosinase enzyme for developing carbon fiber microeletrode (CFME) for highly sensitive *in vivo* detection of dopamine down to 1 nM concentration [25]. The sensor exhibited high specificity in the presence of common interfering molecules including nomifensine, a dopamine uptake inhibitor. The same is demonstrated in figure 2.2. The treatment with nomifensine increased the stimulation of median forebrain bundle on high frequency signal recording. The control condition demonstrates the dopamine response temporal specificity in response to stimulation. The dopamine biosensor was placed in each animal's striatum and sites of stimulation were confirmed as being close to median forebrain bundle (figure 2.2(b)).

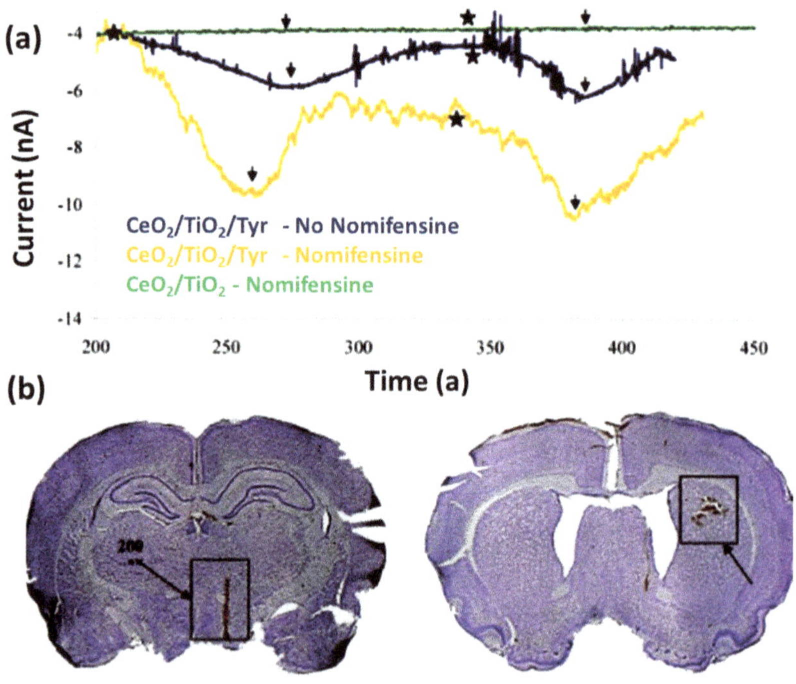

Figure 2.2. (a) Amperometric sensor for dopamine made up of cerium oxide/titanium dioxide/tyrosinase (CeO_2/TiO_2/Tyr) modified carbon fiber microelectrode (CFME). *In vivo* measurements obtained at a potential of −150 mV against Ag/AgCl electrode. Enzyme free sensor (green line) exhibited no signal. (b) Images of histological section of rat brain with stimulation site at the left and biosensor placement or measurement site at right. Reprinted with permission from [25], copyright (2010) American Chemical Society.

Graphene based electrochemical sensors have shown promising results towards highly sensitive and specific detection of dopamine in human serum and urine samples, mouse hippocampaus, and rat striatum [28–30]. The carbon electrodes modified with ioinic liquids and molecular sieves have achieved very low detection limits for dopamine in human serum samples [31–33]. The integration of metal nanoparticles and semiconducting metal oxides exhibiting catalytic or conducting properties has also enhanced the dopamine detection sensitivity and the most promising results are obtained using poly(3,4-ethylenedioxythiophene) or PEDOT which is a conducting polymer [34, 35]. A Cu nanoparticles and polypyrrole modified electrode has been reported for the simultaneous detection of dopamine and uric acid with sufficiently high sensitivity in the presence of interfering molecules [36].

Serotonin is another important neurotransmitter detected most commonly using amperometry and voltammetry (cyclic voltammetry and differential pulse voltammetry) based electrochemical detection methods along with CFME as the working electrodes. Nafion coated CFME has been reported to monitor changes in serotonin levels in dissected central nervous system (CNS) of fruit fly post pharmaceutical and genetic alterations [37]. For this, rapid scan cyclic voltammetry was performed at 0.5 V oxidation potential against an Ag/AgCl electrode and 400 V s^{-1} scan rate [38]. A similar type of electrode modified with carbon nanotubes and Nafion has also been demonstrated to monitor changes in serotonin concentrations in digestive system of zebrafish embryos 5 days after fertilization [39]. The linear response was achieved between 5 and 200 nM using the fabricated microelectrode with detection limit of 1 nM. Further, 1% chitosan modification (prevents non-specific protein adsorption) of a similar electrode was investigated for the detection of serotonin at low oxidation potential of 0.36 V in zebrafish embryos [40]. The sensing electrode displayed detection limit of 1.6 nM within linear range of 2–100 nM for serotonin in genetically engineered zebrafish embryos. Boron-doped diamond microelectrodes have also facilitated *in vitro* detection of serotonin [41].

Electrochemical analytical methods have enabled detection of epinephrine neurotransmitters at nanomolar level. A carbon nanotube and 2-(4-oxo-3-phenyl-3,4-dihydroquinazolinyl)-*N*′-phenyl-hydrazinecarbothioamidemodified carbon electrode have been investigated for quantification of epinephrine [42]. Another nanocomposite film made up of SWCNTs, gold nanoparticles (AuNPs), and polypyrrole has been used to develop electrochemical sensing electrodes for the measurement of epinephrine [43]. The sensor exhibited high sensitivity and specificity in the presence of other interfering molecules including ascorbic acid and uric acid. Similarly, a glassy carbon electrode (GCE) functionalized with over-oxidized composite of polypyrolle-multiwalled carbon nanotubes (MWCNTs) has also been investigated for the detection of epinephrine [44]. Epinephrine specific molecularly imprinted has been employed as electrode material for electrochemical detection of epinephrine through differential pulse voltammetry and impedimetry. A GCE modified with electro-deposited nanocomposite hybrid film of platinum–gold has been reported for the quantification of both epinephrine and norepinephrine individually with great specificity [45]. Another nanocomposite of MWCNT modified pyrolytic graphite electrode has been investigated for simultaneous square wave voltammetry-based electrochemical detection of epinephrine and norepinephrine [46]. Nanomaterials have also been explored for their dual functionality as immobilization substrates for neurotransmitter specific biolomolecules and transducer materials. For instance, a norepinephrine specific DNA molecule-AuNPs modified electrode has been used as an electrochemical sensing platform for quantification of norepinephrine [47].

Enzymatic electrochemical biosensors have also been investigated for the detection of glutamate using glutamate dehydrogenate or oxidase enzyme immobilized on an electrodes surface along with coenzyme, and electron mediator. Carbon paste wax based electrodes have efficiently achieved linear response between 0.3 and 5 mM for glutamate via amperometry in flow injection analysis [48]. A mediator free voltammetry-based glutamate biosensor has been developed using glutamate dehydrogenase enzyme immobilized carbon nanotubes attached to silicon substrate [49]. The biosensor exhibited a low detection limit of 57 nM within the linear range of 0.1–20 μM. Another sensor composed of glutamate oxidase immobilized on platinum electrodes has been reported for ultrasensitive detection of electroactive H_2O_2 produced as a result of enzymatic reaction. The cerium oxide nanoparticles exhibiting oxygen storage capability have also been employed for developing an enzymatic microbiosensor for the monitoring of glutamate levels in rat brains during brain hypoxia (figure 2.3) [50]. The nanoparticles act as a source of oxygen for the oxidase enzyme which allows the biosensor to work efficiently under non-oxygenic conditions like ischemic hypoxia associated with neurological disorders such as Alzheimer's, cerebral ischemia, and Parkinson's disease.

Various enzyme-based electrochemical biosensors have been designed for acetylcholine neurotransmitter which gets converted into electrochemically active product

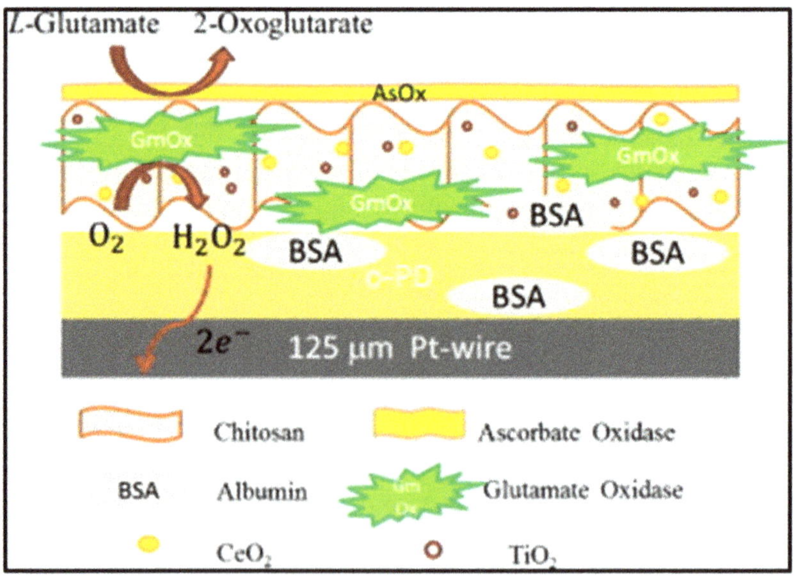

Figure 2.3. Schematic of cerium oxide nanoparticles-based biosensor design and the GluA detection principle. Reprinted with permission from [50], copyright (2014), with permission from Elsevier.

choline and hydrogen peroxide through catalytic activity of acetylcholinesterase (AChE) and choline oxidase (ChOx) [51]. A compact device has been fabricated by co-immobilizing two enzymes on a platinum electrode for the detection of acetylcholine in biological fluids and tissues via amperometry [52]. Nano-biosensors have been reported for electrochemical detection of acetylcholine with the use of an electrode composed of cadmium sulfide nanocrystals, carbon fibers, glassy carbon, metal nanoparticles, mesoporous silica, and MWCNTs transducer materials [53–57]. Nafion modified Pt/Ir microelectrodes have been investigated for real-time amperometric detection of nitric oxide (NO), an electrochemically active gaseous neurotransmitter in cerebral fluids [58]. The linear response for nitric oxide was achieved using the sensing electrode between 0.01 and 600 M in response time of less than 8 s at potential of 0.9 V required for NO reduction. A NO microsensor composed of carbon fibers modified with chitosan, hemin, and MWCNTs has been reported for square wave voltammetry-based detection at −0.762 V potential against Ag/AgCl [59]. The sensor achieved a detection limit of 25 nM within a linear range of 0.25–1 M with high selectivity. Another amperometric NO sensor has been fabricated using metallo 4,4,4,4-tetra-amine phthalocyanine (MTAPc) electropolymerized on Pt-modified nano-alumina oxide template [60]. The sensor exhibited high sensitivity for NO with linear detection range between 10 and 100 nM.

2.3.2 Electrochemical analysis of glucose

Glucose is the main metabolite present in the human body, whose proper absorption is of great significance, failure of which can lead to diabetes. Diabetes is a collective term for metabolic diseases causing the largest number of deaths and leading to disabilities such as nerve degeneration, blindness, and kidney failure, to mention a few. Therefore, precise monitoring of glucose levels in diabetic patients is essential for efficient treatment, avoiding long-term complications, and diabetic emergencies. The past two decades have witnessed a surge in use of nanomaterials for enzymatic and non-enzymatic platforms in the development of glucose sensors.

Nanomaterial based electrochemical sensors have achieved very high sensitivity for glucose measurement with or without the aid of enzymes. The non-enzymatic sensing of glucose is a fast and cost-effective approach. Noble metal nanoparticles such as platinum and gold along with their composites have been employed for conventional non-enzymatic sensing of glucose [61–63]. However, this method suffers from limitation low sensitivity due to slow kinetics of electrocatalytic oxidation of glucose on conventional electrodes and impairment of noble metal electrodes due to adsorbed oxidation intermediates [64]. Nanomaterials such as boron-doped diamond nanorods, Cu nanoclusters/multiwalled carbon nanotubes (MWCNTs) composite, nanofibers electrospun using palladium (IV)-doped copper oxide composite, nanoporous Au, palladium nanoparticles modified functional carbon nanotubes, polycrystalline Pt electrodes, Ti/TiO_2 nanotube array/Ni composites, 3D ordered microporous platinum templates, and dispersible Ni nanoparticles embedded carbon film electrodes similar to graphite electrodes have been explored as electrocatalysts for non-enzymatic detection of glucose [65–70]. It has been observed that enhanced electro-oxidation is observed at Cu and Ni electrodes as compared to Au and Pt electrodes due to electrocatalysis mediated by Cu^{2+}/Cu^{3+} and Ni^{2+}/Ni^{3+} redox couples bound on the surface [71, 72]. Highly ordered array electrodes made up of Pt-nanotubes have been reported as highly selective, sensitive, and stable electrode materials for non-enzymatic sensing of glucose [73]. Other nanomaterials such as mesoporous Pt and Pt–Pb networks have been investigated for achieving a more stable and efficient sensing response towards glucose [73, 74]. Pt_2Pb alloy based electrodes have shown electro-oxidation of glucose at more negative potentials as compared to pure Pt surface for better performance of sensing platform due to the exceptionally favorable nanostructure and high roughness factor of the surface [75]. Graphene and Pt–Ni alloy composite, platinum/copper sulfide/tin oxide nanoparticles-CNTs structured composite, pallidium-SWCNTs hybrid nanostructures, and Cu micropuzzles made up of high quality Cu-microplates have also been used in the non-enzymatic electrochemical detection of glucose in which puzzle-like patterns are assembled into Cu-microplates with the help of glucose [61, 63, 76, 77]. However, reactive active metals can dissolve easily into electrochemical solution even at very low potentials, thus, limiting their applicability at high potential.

Au-based nanomaterials exhibit high stability and excellent catalytic effects similar to glucose oxidase enzyme which promotes their usage in glucose sensors. For instance, small Au-nanoclusters of 3.6 nm size and glucose oxidase imitating Au nanoparticles have been reported in the literature that facilitate catalytic oxidation of glucose and have been efficiently employed in the development of non-enzymatic amperometric glucose sensors. A carbon cloth integrated electrode modified with Au nanoparticles/polyaniline (AuNPs/PANI/CC) has been employed for construction of a flexible glucose sensor (figure 2.4) [78]. The vertical arrays of PANI with 200 nm height and 100 nm diameter have been grown over the surface of flexible CC electrode followed by deposition of electrocatalytically active AuNPs of 20 nm diameter. The developed glucose sensor showed a detection limit of 3.08 μM within a linear range of 10.26–10.0 mM via cyclic voltammetry measurements. An electrochemical sensor based on graphene oxide-molecular imprinted polymer (GO-MIP) has been developed for non-enzymatic detection of glucose [79]. The fabricated electrode exhibited excellent selectivity and electrocatalytic activity similar to a glucose oxidase enzyme towards glucose oxidation. The sensor achieved 0.1 nM detection limit within a 2 min response time. Another amperometric sensor based on nanocomposite of Ag nanoparticles entrapped in polyaniline with reduced graphene oxide (Ag-PANI/rGO) has been reported for glucose monitoring [80]. The electrochemical response yielded a detection limit of 0.79 μM in the linear range between 50 and 0.1 μM in a few seconds response time. The detection is based on the interaction of Ag species with nitrogen atoms of PANI for improved electron transfer during glucose electrochemical reduction which is detected at the electrode.

A hierarchical nanocomposite of CuO/NiO-carbon derived from Cu–Ni–metal organic framework and deposited over cellotapes has been exploited as highly sensitive and specific electrochemical probe for non-enzymatic detection of

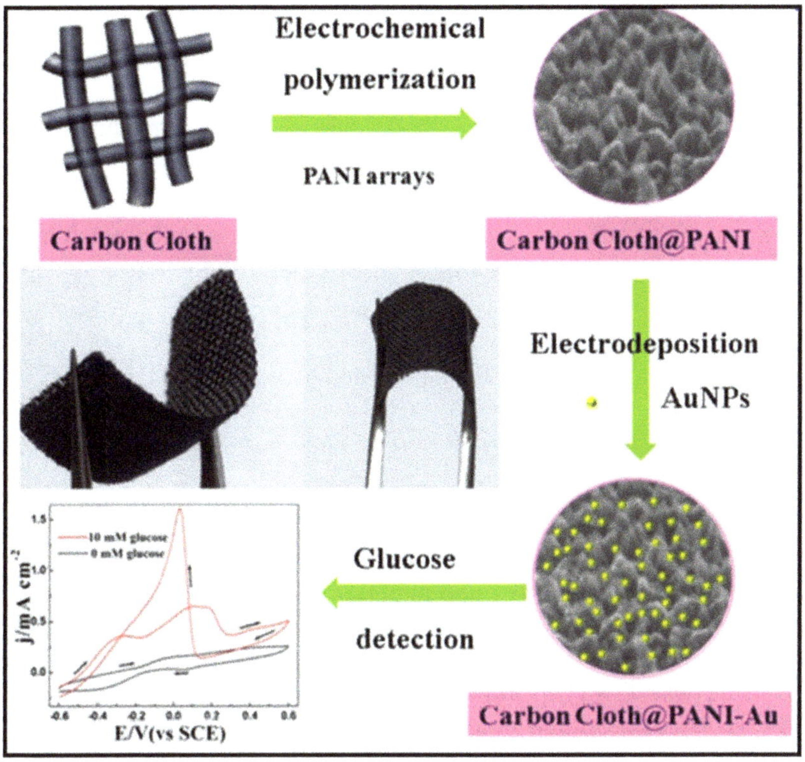

Figure 2.4. Representation of a flexible AuNPs/PANI/Carbon cloth based electrochemical sensor for glucose. Reprinted from [78], copyright (2017), with permission from Elsevier.

glucose [81]. The sensing platform overcomes the impediments of high cost, repeated electrode cleaning and modification, use of inactive swellable binders, and time depletion. The amperometric measurement of glucose at 0.65 V versus Ag/AgCl electrode provided linear range of 100 nM to 4.5 nM with detection limit of 37 nM in 5 s. A sandwich like nanocomposite of CuO nanowires grown over Cu_2O nanofilm (CuO/Cu_2O) exhibiting enhanced electrocatalytic activity towards glucose oxidation has also been investigated for glucose sensing [82]. The developed platform is able to sense glucose down to 1 μM concentration within a linear range of 0.1–6 mM in a response time of 1.5 s. The improved electrocatalytic activity and subsequent sensitivity of nanocomposite is attributed to high surface area of CuO nanowires and synergistic effect from Cu_2O nanofilm. A nickel–cobalt carbonate hydroxysulfide multistage nanowire array deposited onto the carbon cloth-based electrode has also been explored for glucose sensing [83]. The leaves-on-brachlet structure of nanocomposite provided a higher number of active sites along with improved specific capacitance and the introduction of sulfur further enhanced the electron transfer for better performance of sensing film. The sensor exhibited a wide linear detection range between 0.25 and 3308 μM with a 0.25 μM detection limit with high selectivity, stability, and reproducibility.

The electrochemical detection of glucose using enzymes is based on the principle given in the original work of Clark and Lyons with the use of glucose oxidase (GO_x) enzyme [84] as per the equation:

$$\text{D-glucose} + O_2 + H_2O + \text{Glucose oxidase} \rightarrow \text{D-gluconic acid} + H_2O_2$$

$$H_2O_2 \rightarrow 2H^+ + O_2 + 2e^-$$

To perform an electrochemical reaction with the use of glucose dehydrogenase (GDH), the electron transfer mediator is required and the reaction is depicted as:

$$GDH_{(ox)} + \text{D-glucose} \rightarrow GDH_{(red)} + \delta\text{-glucolactone}$$

$$\text{Mediator}_{(ox)} + GDH_{(red)} \rightarrow \text{Mediator}_{(red)} + GDH_{(ox)}$$

$$\text{Mediator}_{(red)} \rightarrow \text{Mediator}_{(ox)} + e^-$$

A GCE modified with nanodendrite of poly[meso-tetrakis(2-thienyl)porphyrinato] cobalt(II)-single-walled carbon nanotubes (SWCNTs)-nafion-GO_x has been employed for cyclic voltammetry-based glucose detection [85]. The synergistic effect of enzyme and nanostructures resulted in better performance of sensor as compared to other control electrode systems with a detection limit of 5.33 μM within a linear concentration range of 0–1 mM. Another sensing device composed of chitosan–Prussian blue–MWCNTs–hollow platinum cobalt nanochains (CS–PB–MWCNTs–H-PtCo) modified gold electrode with immobilized GO_x enzyme has been demonstrated for glucose monitoring [86]. The electrode exhibited detection over a wide linear range of 1.5 μM with 0.47 μM limit of detection (LOD) at very low potential 0.6–0.8 V. A GCE has also been cast with hollow nanostructures of MWCNTs decorated with platinum (HPt-MWCNTs) for sensing of glucose [87]. The covalent immobilization of GO_x enzyme was facilitated using negatively charged L-cysteine and positively charged poly(diallydimethylammonium) chloride (PDDA) encapsulated AuNPs (PDDA-Au). The complete schematic of the so developed three-electrode system along with conceptualized structure of HPt-MWCNTs based enzyme immobilized working electrode and three probable type of electrochemical reactions facilitating detection of glucose are shown in figure 2.5. The detection limit of 0.4 μM was achieved within 1.2 μM–8.4 mM linear concentration range for glucose.

An example of cyclic voltammetry and impedance based measurement of glucose levels has been reported using GCE with electro-deposited Pt nanoparticles chitosan nanocomposite followed by specific enzyme immobilization [88]. Another highly conductive platform has been designed using Au thin film deposited on GCE for physisorption of GO_x enzyme for facilitating improved electron transfer and better sensitivity [89]. Nano-complexes of hydroxyl fullerenes, poly (diallyldimethylammonium chloride) (PDDA)-capped gold nanoparticles (AuNPs) functionalized graphene (G)/MWCNTs, nafion coated reduced graphene oxide with GO_x, have also been investigated for sensitive and specific glucose sensing [90, 91]. A lab-on-chip has been devised for detecting very low levels of glucose in saliva using

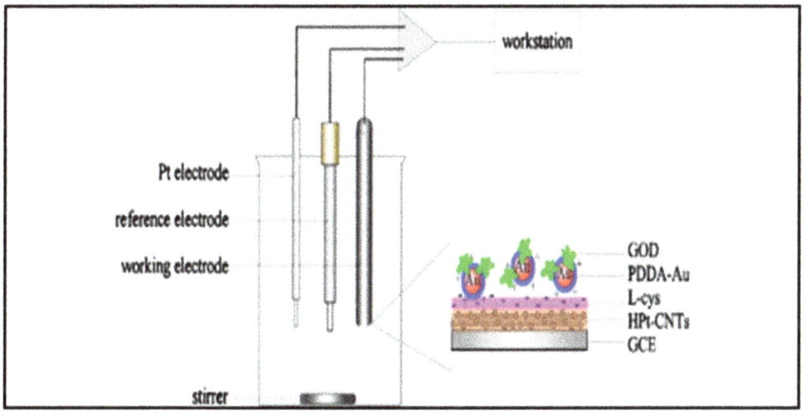

Figure 2.5. Schematic of three-electrode system of HPt-MWCNTs based glucose sensor with conceptualized image of enzyme immobilized working electrode. Reprinted from [87], copyright (2011), with permission from Elsevier.

polysilicon nanogap modified with GO_x via (3-aminopropyl)truethoxysilane (APTES) [92]. A working electrode in tri-electrode configuration has been fabricated using AgNPs and nanowires derived biologically from genetically modified filamentous phage (fd-tet-p8MMM) along with a specific enzyme for sensing glucose [93]. In another example, template assisted CuO nanoleaves have been synthesized from polyethylene glycol on a gold coated glass substrate and co-immobilized with glucose oxidase enzyme for the monitoring of glucose levels [94]. The sensor exhibited linear response within a concentration range of 10 μM–20 mM with a detection limit of 5 μM. A glucose enzyme based electrochemical sensor has been fabricated using three-dimensional nanoneedles of $NiCo_2O_4$ deposited on nickel foam [95]. The potentiometric measurements using the developed sensing platform demonstrated high sensitivity, specificity, stability, reproducibility, and good practical applicability. Another glucose biosensor has been investigated using ZnO nanorods grown over the borosilicate glass capillary tip for electrostatic immobilization of a glucose specific enzyme [96]. The sensor has been exploited for the determination of glucose levels in frog oocytes and human adipocytes.

Another interesting approach for glucose detection has been demonstrated using glucose oxidase and hybrid nanostructures of palladium helical carbon nanofiber (Pd-HCNF) immobilized with nafion on GCE [97]. The nanomaterial exhibited electrocatalytic activity towards glucose oxidation resulting into production of H_2O_2 which is detected and subsequently co-related to glucose concentration in the sample to be analyzed. Pt nanoparticles have also been exploited in combination with PANI to form hydrogel nanostructures for detection of glucose [97]. The combination offered advantage of conductivity of hydrogel, catalytic property of nanoparticles, and increased surface area for high density immobilization of enzyme. This leads to the enhanced catalytic oxidation of glucose and subsequent improved sensor performance with detection limit of 0.7 μM over a linear concentration range of 0.01–8 mM.

2.3.3 Electrochemical analysis of cancer biomarkers

Cancerous cell tissues produce and secrete cancer biomarkers such as α-fetoprotein (AFP), breast cancer antigen 1 (BRCA1), carbohydrate antigen-125 (CA 125), carbohydrate antigen-153 (CA 153), carcinoembryonic antigen (CEA), epidermal growth factor receptor (EGFR), epithelial cancer biomarker (EpCAM) and prostate-specific antigen (PSA), to mention a few at higher levels as compared to normal cells [98]. Electrochemical analytical methods have attracted research attention for the detection of cancer biomarkers even in low concentration with high sensitivity, specificity, and reproducibility. For the development of highly sensitive electrochemical sensors for cancer biomarker detection, nanomaterials are employed either as surface modifiers to improve conductivity and/or surface area of electrodes or as signaling labels. Such sensors can be operated using different electrochemical modes in the form of amperometry, potentiometry, and impedimetry [99]. For amperometric and voltammetric measurements, enzymes and redox probes are immobilized on the conducting electrode surface. However, impedimetric sensors require the redox ions to be present in the sample solution for recording the output signal.

An AuNPs modified GCE has been functionalized with horseradish peroxidase (HRP) conjugated anti-AFP antibodies and protein A to develop a sandwich immunoassay for AFP, a cancer biomarker [100]. The sensor achieved a linear detection range of 5–80 ng ml^{-1} with a detection limit of 3.7 ng ml^{-1} via the voltammetry principle. A nanocomposite of porous zinc oxide (ZnO) modified with AuNPs, anti-AFP antibodies, and HRP enzyme has been reported as a signaling label for electrochemical sensing of AFP [101]. The paper-based sensor has been developed by growing branched zinc oxide nanorods (BZR) arrays exhibiting high charge carrying capacity on the working electrode composed of reduced graphene oxide (rGO). Further, labeling of antigen and horseradish peroxidase (HRP) enzyme has been facilitated with a composite of porous zinc oxide and gold nanoparticles (PZS@AuNPs). The competitive binding takes place between AFP and the labeled signaling molecule for attachment to an anti-AFP modified electrode surface. After a competitive reaction, the enzyme participates in biocatalytic process on introduction of signal labels into the immunosensor. The schematic representation of the competitive binding of the immunosensor is depicted in figure 2.6. The density of signal is influenced by the concentration of AFP in the sample which is recorded by incubating the electrode in a solution containing H_2O_2 and 4-chloro-1-napththol (4CN). The reaction of the redox couple is blocked on the HRP catalyzed production of benzo-4-chlorohexadienone (B4CH) which is correlated to initial concentration of AFP. The developed sensor observed detection limit of 0.08 pg ml^{-1} within a linear concentration range of 0.2 pg ml^{-1}–500 ng ml^{-1}.

Carbon nanohorns (CNHs) exhibiting structural similarity to SWCNTs have also been reported for detection of AFP employing anti-AFP antibodies, HRP, and GO_x [102]. The cyclic voltammetry and impedimetry-based electrochemical response to AFP was obtained in glucose solution with 0.33 pg ml^{-1} detection limit and 0.001–60 ng ml^{-1} linear response range. A similar CNHs-based platform has been investigated for immunosensing of AFP with much higher sensitivity and a low

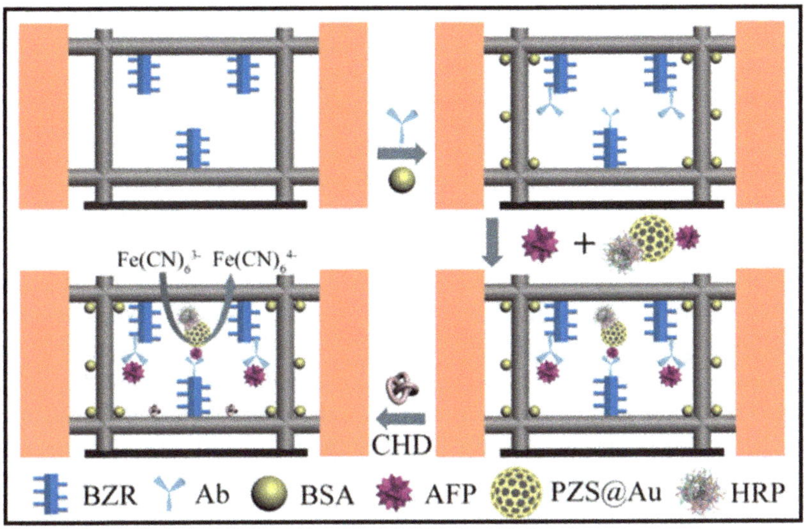

Figure 2.6. Schematic representation of competitive immunoassay based sensor for AFP, a cancer biomarker using branched zinc oxide nanorods (BZR) modified rGO electrode and AFP-porous zinc oxide (PZS)@Au-HRP as signal labels. Reprinted from [101], copyright (2015), with permission from Elsevier.

detection limit of 0.07 pg ml^{-1} [103]. In this sensor, a SPCE modified with anti-AFP antibodies was firstly incubated in an AFP containing sample having a known concentration of CNH molecules that bind to the label and analyte AFP competitively resulting in change in the electrochemical response. A graphene oxide (GO)-based electrochemical detection platform has been explored for detection of AFP. For instance, carboxy-functionalized GO attached to Prussian blue (PB) has been employed to modified GCE for DPV based detection of AFP down to 0.05 ng ml^{-1} concentration over a linear range of 0.5–60 ng ml^{-1} [104]. A nanocomposite of GO/PB/AuNPs/ionic liquid has also been investigated for ultrasensitive detection of AFP down to 4.6 pg ml^{-1} concentration [105]. Copper sulfide as a redox catalyst has been deposited on GO nanosheets to serve as signal labels for AFP detection [106]. The performance of the sensor improved due to the increased presence of H_2O_2 related to the AFP concentration facilitated by CuS/Cu_2S redox couple originated catalytic current. The sensor achieved a detection limit of 0.5 pg ml^{-1} and a linear detection range of 0.001–10 ng ml^{-1}.

An immunosensor for a prostate cancer biomarker, PSA has been prepared using specific antibodies immobilized AuNPs along with a ferrocene-tagged label [107]. The voltammetric measurements resulted in the detection of PSA down to 0.5 pg ml^{-1} detection limit over a linear range of 2.0 pg ml^{-1}–10 ng ml^{-1}. AgNPs conjugated with ZnO nanospheres have been investigated as signaling labels for the development of a PSA immunosensing platform [108]. As Ag is easily electrochemically oxidized to Ag_2O resulting in the formation of a reduction current of H_2O_2 which is detected as an output signal for PSA and detected through cyclic voltammetry. The redox active organometallic compounds such as iron oxide have also been employed as signaling labels in conjugation with anti-PSA antibody and ferrocene to fabricate electrochemical sandwich immunoassay for PSA [109]. The sensor achieved a detection limit of 2 pg ml^{-1} within a linear range of 0.01–40 ng ml^{-1} via voltammetry for PSA. Another sandwich immunoassays for PSA has been reported using carboxy-functionalized MWCNTs modified Au electrodes [110]. The PSA analyte present in the sample to be analyzed attaches to anti-PSA antibodies conjugated with HRP molecules that are immobilized onto MWCNTs. The sensor observed voltammetric linear response towards PSA between 1 pg ml^{-1} and 10 ng ml^{-1} concentration with 0.4 pg ml^{-1} detection limit. The higher sensitivity of the sensor is attributed to the enhanced binding of HRP molecules to MWCNTs modified labels. In another report, graphene oxide/cobalt hexacyanoferrate nanocomposite thin film modified GCE has been employed for highly sensitive voltammetric detection of PSA [111]. The use of graphene oxide improved the redox signal, thereby, achieving a detection limit of 0.01 ng ml^{-1} over a linear range of 0.02–2 ng ml^{-1}.

An amperometric immunosensor for carcinoembryonic antigen (CEA) has been reported using carboxyl-functionalized CNT modified conductive paper covalently immobilized with anti-CEA antibodies [112]. The paper-based sensor showed an impedimetric response towards CEA with a detection limit of 1 ng ml^{-1} within the physiological range of 2–15 ng ml^{-1}. The use of CdSe QD nanocomposites with CuO nanoparticles and secondary antibodies has also been reported for the detection of CEA antigenic biomarker [113]. A voltammetric sensor employing macroporous three-dimensional graphene oxide foam has been applied for highly sensitive detection of CEA down to 90 pg ml^{-1} concentration over a linear range of 0.1–750 ng ml^{-1}. The use of carboxy-functionalized graphene oxide sheets as signaling probes has been reported for further sensitive immunosensing of CEA via toluidine blue (TB) modification with detection limit of 0.1 ng ml^{-1} [114]. The sensitivity of the graphene based sensor of CEA has been improved with the usage of the redox active compound thionine with an achieved detection limit of 0.65 pg ml^{-1} and a linear concentration range of 0.01–300 ng ml^{-1} [115].

A DNA-based biosensor has also been reported for the quantification of the breast cancer biomarker, BRCA1. For this, a single stranded 19-mer oligonucleotide specific to BRCA1 has been immobilized onto AuNPs functionalized GCE [116]. The change in the impedance values observed during hybridization of the oligonucleotide probe with BRCA1 analyte present in the sample resulted in a detection limit of 1.72 fM for BRCA1 between the linear concentration range of 5 fM to 1 nM. Another AuNPs modified gold electrode has been employed for impedimetric detection of epidermal growth factor receptor, EGFR down to concentration of 0.34 pg ml^{-1} within a wide linear range of 1 pg ml^{-1}–1 μg ml^{-1} [117]. Epidermal growth factor receptor (EGFR) is an overexpressed biomarker in a variety of tumors such as breast, colorectal, gastric, ovarian, pancreatic, and renal. The immunosensor employed immobilized protein G and anti-EGFR antibodies for enhanced specificity towards the analyte. Nanocomposites in the form of AuNP–graphene silica sol–gel and AgNP–polydopamine–thionine have been used as electrode surface modifiers for the construction of electrochemical biosensors [118]. AgNP–chitosan nanocomposite modified electrode has been employed as a voltammetric immunosensor for the detection of EpCAM, an epithelial cancer biomarker with an achievable detection limit of 2.7 pg ml^{-1} [119].

Highly stable hybrid nanostructures composed of carboxy-functionalized CdSe quantum dots and silica coated amine functionalized AuNPs have been employed for impedimetric immunosensing of carbohydrate antigen-125 (CA 125), an ovarian cancer biomarker [120]. The biosensor exhibited detection limit of 1.6 mU ml^{-1} within a linear concentration range of 1–0.1 U ml^{-1}. The sensitivity of CNTs based biosensors has been improved with the aid of ZnO nanowires embedded with MWCNTs [121]. The so-developed sensing platform has been exploited for the detection of CA125 biomarker down to 1.13 mU ml^{-1} concentration over a wide linear range of 1 mU ml^{-1}–1000 U ml^{-1}. A reduced graphene oxide modified SPCE has been reported for highly sensitive voltammeric detection of CA125 with a detection limit of 1 pg ml^{-1} and wide linear concentration range of 0.001–100 ng ml^{-1} [122]. The voltammetric determination of golgi protein 73 (GP73) which is a significant biomarker for biliary tract cancer has also been facilitated using CdSe quantum dots [123]. In this sensor, CdSe QD-tagged lectin has been used as a signaling label with a detection limit of 12 pM over a linear concentration range of 20–5000 pM in human serum samples. The differential pulse voltammetric detection of α2,3-sialylated glycans, a carcinoma diagnostic marker in serum has been facilitated using CNT modified glassy carbon electrodes [124]. The sensor exhibited detection limit of 3 fg ml^{-1} for α2,3-sialylated over a linear concentration range of 10 fg ml^{-1}–50 ng ml^{-1}.

In another report, ferritin modified MWCNTs have been used as signaling labels along with a secondary antibody to develop a highly sensitive immunosensor for CA153, breast cancer biomarker [125]. The voltammetric sensor achieved a detection limit of 9 mU ml^{-1} over a linear range of 50 mU ml^{-1}–100 U ml^{-1}. Reduced graphene oxide and *N*-doped reduced graphene oxide (rGO) have also been explored for voltammetric detection of the carbohydrate antigen-153 (CA153) biomarker down to 1 and 5 pg ml^{-1} detection limit, respectively 102. A highly sensitive sensor for 8-hydroxy-2′-deoxyguanosine (8-OHdG), a biomarker significantly expressed oxidative stress and cancer has been reported using sulfur-doped rGO synthesized using lenthionine, a biomass precursor [98]. With the regulation of the amount of sulfur doping (2.2.8%), the detection limit of 1 nM was achieved over wide detection window of 20–0.002 μM with good specificity, stability, and reproducibility. The improved electrochemical activity is attributed to the high electron-donating capability of the doped sulfur atoms to facilitate transfer of electrons to the specific biomolecules. A prostate cancer biomarker, PCA3 has been detected efficiently using a single stranded DNA probe based bionsensor employing layer-by-layer deposited chitosan and MWCNT film [126]. The presence of specific BRCA1 gene sequence results in hybridization to the immobilized complementary probe and subsequent change at the electrode interface monitored electrochemically (figure 2.7). The electrochemical impedance measurements resulted in detection of the PCA3 biomarker down to 0.128 nM concentration with high selectivity. Very recently, an electrochemical biosensor has been reported for ultrasensitive detection

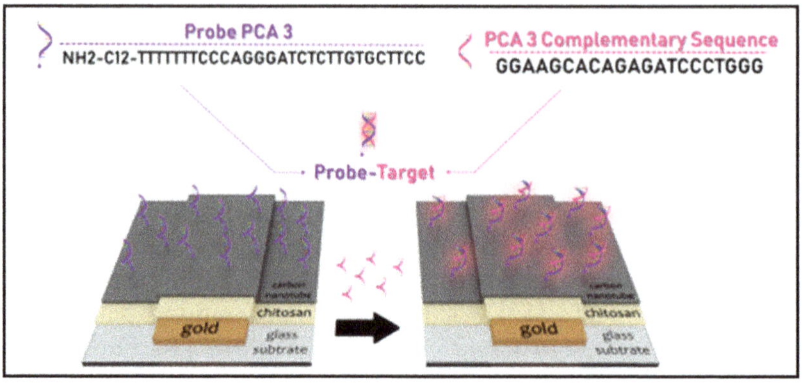

Figure 2.7. Schematic of chitosan/MWCNTs modified gold electrode-based DNA biosensor for PAC3, cancer biomarker along with hybridization based detection. Reprinted with permission from [126], copyright (2019) American Chemical Society.

of the PIK3CA gene associated with lung cancer using MoS_2 nanosheets functionalized with riboflavin 5′-monophosphate sodium salt (FMNs) [127]. The nanocomposite of FMNs/MoS_2 nanocomposite exhibited very fine electrochemical activity along with rich phosphonate groups for covalent attachment of amine functionalized DNA probe complementary to PIK3CA gene. The sensor achieved detection limit of 0.0012 fM with high stability, reproducibility and excellent selectivity for early detection of lung cancer.

2.4 Recent nanotechnological advancement of electrochemical sensors in biomedicine

2.4.1 Wearable electrochemical sensors

Wearable sensors have attracted considerable research attention owing to their wide potential for applicability in the determination of a variety of physiological and clinical parameters. Wearable sensors can be defined as devices worn by someone that use chemical or physical methods to monitor health and fitness without the aid of a sample pretreatment step, heavy instrumentation, and trained personnel. To date, most of the wearable sensors are predominantly used for fitness and well-being monitoring. However, the research, development, and commercialization of devices dedicated to the measurement of clinical parameters have seen a notable growth in the last 5 years. The wearable sensor global market is expected to exceed USD 2.86 billion by 2025 at an increasing rate of 38.8% with investment from big brands such as Apple® and Google® [128].

The major advantages of wearable sensors are in terms of monitoring of vital body functions and clinical diagnostics in real time without the need of heavy and sophisticated instruments which is what people desire. The sample collection is also either non-invasive or minimally invasive in the case of wearable sensors. Wearable electrochemical sensors (WES) reported in last few years dedicated to the biomedical diagnostics are majorly based on amperometry, potentiometry, and voltammetry principles [128]. The wearable sensors working with potentiometry have been applied for measurement of electrolytes and pH in biological fluids such as sweat, interstitial fluids, and saliva [129–131]. The diagnosis of cystic fibrosis, a genetic disorder related to mucus thickening due to changes in the pancreas is dependent on the quantification of Na^+ and Cl^- ions. Three types of wearable devices have been reported for analysis of these ions in sweat: epidermal patches, sweatbands, and wristbands [128, 132–134]. The materials such as carbon fiber and textiles in the form of eyeglasses have also been investigated [135–137]. Most studies concentrating on wearable potentiometric devices have been performed only *in vivo* with only few reports serving the accuracy of results to determine the reliability of the proposed devices. Diamond and group designed the first prototype of wearable potentiometric sensor in 2010 consisting of inner-filling solution type sodium ion selective electrode (ISE) embedded in a belt with adsorbent patches for cthe ollection of sweat [138]. Today, all-solid-state ISEs have replaced the solution based ISEs. The general strategy is to incorporate conductive film on the flexible substrate along with ion-to-electron transducer and sensing element. ISEs comprising of polyaniline (PANI) or iridium oxide based solid electrodes have been exploited for pH determination in sweat [139].

The wearable potentiometric sensors are dedicated to the determination of small ions, on the other hand, amperometric devices focus on the detection of organic molecules of clinical relevance such as glucose, lactate, and uric acid [128, 129, 135, 139–141]. Considering the alarming increase in the number of diabetic patients, wearable sensors have been developed for real-time glucose monitoring in biological fluids such as blood, interstitial fluid, saliva, sweat, and tears. An amperometric wearable glucose sensor made of gold electrodes printed on a poly(dimethylsiloxane) (PDMS) substrate has been reported for quantification of glucose in sweat (figure 2.8) [142]. The fabricated sensor offers various advantages such as good skin compatibility, easy usage, and sufficient accuracy. The wearable devices for simultaneous analysis of multiple analytes have also been designed by arrangement of electrodes with different specificities printed on PDMS substrate [143]. The device is based on amperometric detection of glucose along with potentiometric measurement of cations (Na^+, K^+, and H^+). A wireless flexible electronic circuit and battery free communication incorporated into the sensors enables data feeding and collection using a smartphone only.

Pulsed electrochemical techniques such as differential pulse and square wave voltammtery have been explored in wearable devices for analysis of cortisol, heavy metals, and different organic molecules [144–147]. The level of metals (e.g., Zn and Cu) in the body is significant for strengthening of the immune system and functioning of enzymes. A wearable tattoo based electrochemical device has been fabricated for simultaneous analysis of different ions such as Cd^{2+}, Cu^{2+}, Hg^{2+}, Pb^{2+}, and Zn^{2+} in sweat and urine. It should be noted that potentiometric sensors are able to detect high concentration of ions in biological fluids, however, amperometric or voltammetric techniques along with preconcentration steps need to be considered in cases where detection of trace amounts is expected [128]. Dual electrochemical and colorimetric wearble sensors have also gained considerable

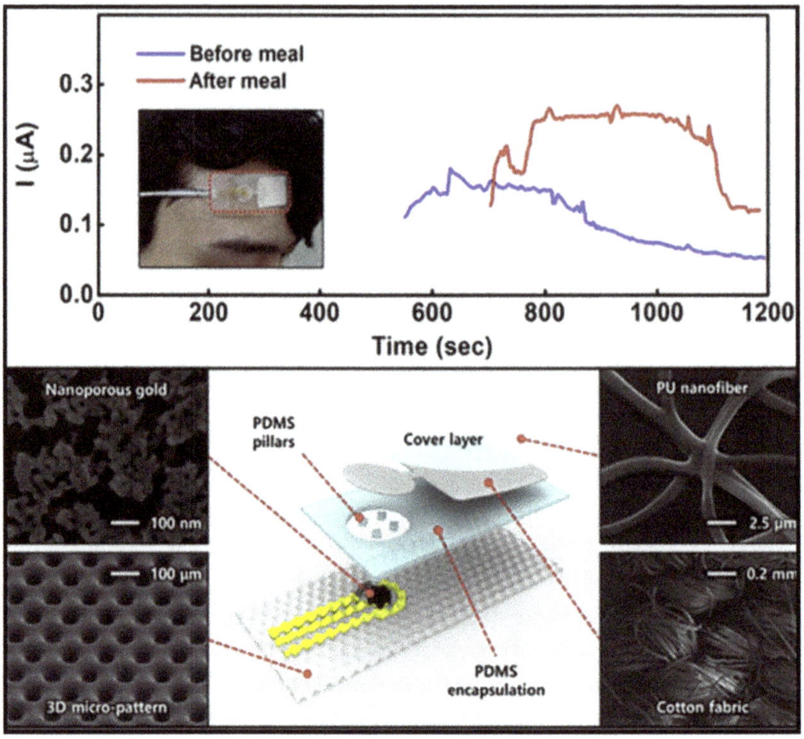

Figure 2.8. Wearable device attached to the patient's skin to record glucose levels in the sweat before and after having a meal along with micrographic details of the parts of the sensor. Reprinted with permission from [142], copyright (2019) American Chemical Society.

interest in recent years. For instance, a wearble device based on both electrochemical and colorimetric detection has been reported for monitoring of chloride, glucose, lactate, and pH in sweat [147]. The developed sensor requires only a smartphone to analyze the data collected and recorded by the sensing device.

Overall, point-of care personal monitoring of clinical parameters is essential and can be achieved using wearable electrochemical sensing devices for early disease diagnosis and subsequent treatment. These devices can further reduce healthcare costs and mortality rates. The main challenges with wearable sensors are human body integration and miniaturization of such devices, transmission and proper validation of extracted results, and correlation of real-time results with conventional and well-established techniques.

2.4.2 Planar electrochemical sensors

Planar electrochemical devices are one-dimensional sensors which meet the new-age requirements of miniaturization, portability, and robustness. There are three major categories of planar sensors, namely, thick film, thin film, and field effect transistors-based sensors.

Thick film technology is a very popular means of developing hybrid circuits which was introduced about three decades ago. Thick film devices are comprised of thick films, semiconducting material, and monolithic integrated circuits along with other discrete devices [148]. Screen printing is the oldest method of deposition of thick films which offers advantages in terms of flexible materials and design choice, low manufacturing cost, and fabrication automation [149]. A thick film sensor is composed of layers of special pastes or inks that are sequentially deposited into an insulating substrate as shown in figure 2.9 [148]. The desired patterns on the thick film are obtained using the mask. Thick film electrochemical sensors are divided into two categories: impedance based sensors (capacitance and resistance variations used to measure analyte) and one with current or potential variations.

The most researched application of screen-printed thick film based sensors in biomedical diagnostics is the determination of blood glucose levels in diabetic people

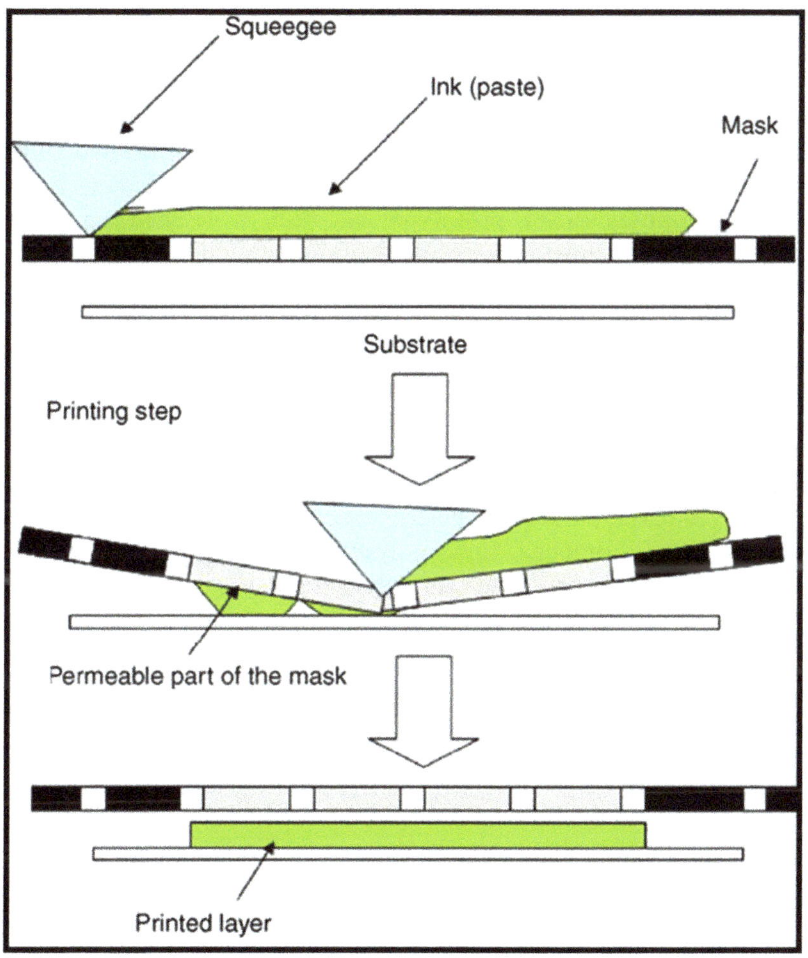

Figure 2.9. Schematic of different steps of screen-printed for producing thick films. Reprinted with permission from [149], copyright (2006), with permission from Elsevier.

[150]. The well-known electrochemical sensor for glucose is the simplified combination of the glucose oxidase (GOD) enzyme with a screen-printed electrode which meets the monitoring requirements of people with diabetics efficiently. The first commercialized amperometric glucose sensor pen-sized, Exatech™ was launched by Genetics International, Boston in 1987 [151]. The device is a small, disposable glucose sensitive electrode made up of mixture of GOD and a mediator screen-printed onto a carbon substrate and a pen-sized meter with an electronic circuit and LCD display. With a simple finger prick, the blood oozes out and can be used to measure blood glucose level in duration of 20–30 s. Thick film technology has also been employed to develop a portable, disposable amperometric sensor for measuring oxygen levels transcutaneously [152]. The fabricated sensor works on the principle of a Clark cell using a three-electrode configuration (screen-printed gold counter and working electrode along with Ag/AgCl reference electrode). The sensor achieved result accuracy and fast response, thus, facilitating continuous monitoring of oxygen levels.

Screen printing has also been investigated for the development of biosensors exploiting bioaffinity between biomolecules and analytes for detection. Immunosensors are the extensively reported screen-printed biosensors in which the antigen/analyte specific antibodies attached to the screen-printed substrate are used as recognition molecules to qualitatively and quantitatively detect analyte. An electrochemical immunosensor prototype has been developed for progesterone hormone using passively adsorbed specific antibodies onto the screen-printed carbon electrode (SPCE) via a competitive immunoassay platform [153]. The competitive binding takes place between the unlabeled progesterone present in the sample to be analyzed and alkaline phosphatase (ALP) enzyme labeled progesterone which generates the signal. The electrochemical signal is produced by the enzymatic cleavage of the phosphorylated enzyme substrate and the signal is reduced with the increasing concentration of progesterone present in the sample. Another electrochemical immunoassay for human chorionic gonadotrophin (hCG) hormone has been reported based on two-site heterogeneous enzyme platform [154]. For this, nafion coated SPCE attached to a polystyrene microwell has been used for streptavidin–biotin chemistry based immobilization of ALP label. The analytical signal produced by the formation of hydrolysis product of enzymatic substrate, phosphorylated [(4-hydroxyphenyl) aminocarbonyl]-cobaltocenium. The so obtained cyclic voltammograms observed peak current at potential of 0.5 V against Ag/AgCl electrode with 100 mIU ml^{-1} detection limit over linear range of 200–10 000 mIU ml^{-1} (1 mg = 9825 IU).

A potentiometric immunosensor has also been described allowing the detection of insulin down to 20 nM concentration of insulin [155]. Such platforms of immunosensors have also been employed for the detection of immunoglobulin molecules. A homogeneous separation-free method has been reported for the detection of rabbit IgG based on competitive immunoassay between free and glucose oxidase enzyme labeled antigen for binding the immobilized antibody [156]. The introduction of substrate glucose into the system catalytically produces H_2O_2 which can be detected by measuring the current generated at a reduction potential of 20.35 V. The sensor achieved detection limit of 0.33 mg ml^{-1} within a linear range of 0.5–2 mg ml^{-1}. A heterogeneous electrochemical immunosensing platform for IgG has been designed using gold colloidal particles for labeling the antibody probes (figure 2.10) [157]. The gold labels are detected via anodic stripping voltammetry (ASV) post oxidative dissolution of gold metal in acidic solution. The detection limit for IgG reached down to 3 pM concentration which is remarkable. A direct non-competitive immunoassay for mouse IgG has been investigated using a mixture of ferrocene labeled antibody and IgG antigenic analyte along with gold plated SPCE [158]. The mixture is separated electrophoretically to obtain the labeled antigen/antibody complex and labeled free antibody followed by anodic quantification of the ferrocene tracer with detection limit of 2.5 pg ml^{-1}.

A novel approach to detect anti-DNA antibodies has also been described with the use of DNA and enzyme (cholinesterase or peroxidase) modified graphite SPCEs [159]. The platform has been employed for the detection of anti-DNA antibodies in the serum for diagnosis of bronchial asthma and systemic lupus erythematosus (SLE). The addition of the enzyme substrate acetylcholine or hydroquinone followed by redox conversion of products results in the decrease in the amperometric signal on incubation of sensing platform with samples containing anti-DNA antibodies. This decrease is observed as the access of substrate to active site of enzyme is restricted. Screen-printed DNA biosensors are another type of bioaffinity-based electrochemical sensors that have enormous application in early diagnosis of genetic disorders. DNA biosensors make use of nucleic acid as recognition probes and work on the principle of hybridization to the complementary nucleic acid to be detected. A disposable electrochemical sensor for bacteria has been constructed after the PCR amplification step [160]. For this, a screen-printed graphite electrode immobilized (at a fixed potential) with specific oligonucleotide sequence against *Chlamydia trachomatis* bacteria has been evaluated using chrono-potentiometric stripping analysis (PSA). Within 2 min of incubation, the guanine residues of the probe immobilized on the surface are oxidized and observed via PSA. The signal is correlated inversely to the concentration of specific DNA analyte present in the sample due to complementary binding and subsequent non-availability of guanine residues.

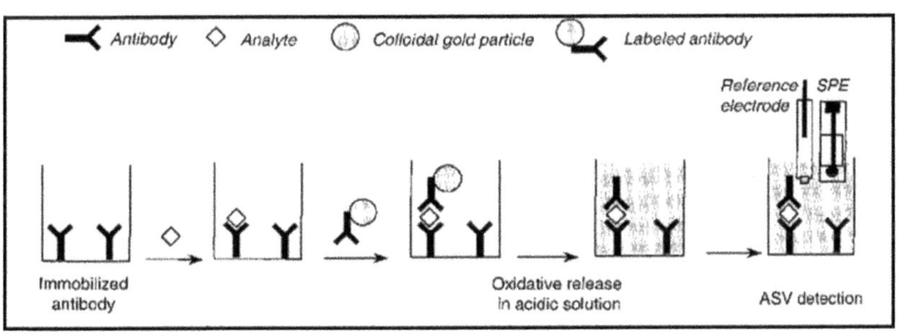

Figure 2.10. Schematic representation of the screen-printed electrode-based electrochemical immunoassay using colloidal gold label. Reprinted with permission from [157], copyright (2000) American Chemical Society.

Thin film technology is another way to develop planar electrochemical sensors that produce microelectrode systems having a reproducible and well defined interface between sensor recognition and transduction sites [161]. A variety of thin film based microelectrodes have been fabricated for development of conductometric, potentiometric, and voltammetric sensors of biomedical diagnostic applications [162]. The most frequently used method for developing patterns on thin film sensors is photolithography in which geometric shapes present on the masks are transferred onto the silicon wafer surface (figure 2.11).

An amperometric sensor for real-time lactate detection has been developed using lactate oxidase enzyme mixed with polyurethane matrix for deposition onto the working electrode [163]. The two-electrode configured structure comprised of SiO_2 covered glass slide of 0.7 mm thickness, titan layer for stable adhesion of platinum. Potentiometric thin film based sensors for detecting pH have also been reported for biological, clinical, and dermatological applications [164]. The sensors are composed of electropolymerized films of polyethylenimine and polypropylenimine, synthetic enzyme mixed with biocompatible polymers immobilized on platinum working electrodes. Many commercial electrode arrays have been exploited as thin film sensors for clinical analysis. A multilayer gold nanocomposite microarray has been devised for simultaneous detection of glucose, pyruvate, and lactate.

Interdigitated electrodes or interdigitated electrode arrays (IDAs) are a type of thin film microelectrode made up of interconnected parallel microbands of alternating anodic and cathodic configuration. The IDAs are advantageous over conventional microelectrodes as their specific geometric differences provide specific electrochemical behavior and quasi-steady-state currents due to non-planar diffusion to each microelectrode. Interdigitated structures are cast in metal as well in mono- or polycrystalline silicon [149]. The most common use of IDAs is in the development of enzymatic biosensors. A conductometric urea biosensor has been investigated by functionalizing the IDAs with clay gel entrapped urease enzyme

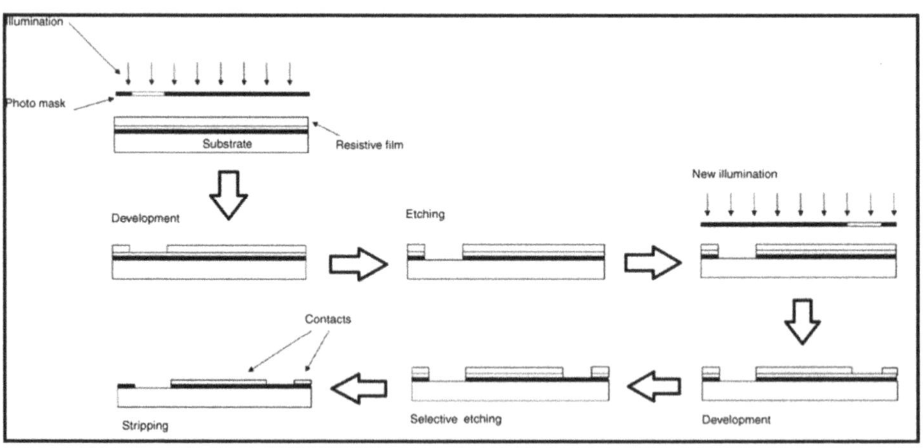

Figure 2.11. Schematic for development of thin film using photolithography and selective etching. Reprinted with the permission from [149], copyright (2006), with permission from Elsevier.

crosslinked using glutaraldehyde and adsorbed into poly(pyrroledyridiunium) film [165]. Nanodimensional IDAs have also been used to construct bioaffinity based impedimetric sensors exhibiting improved sensitivity when compared to other impedimetric sensor arrangements. The binding of analyte to the biological recognition probe brings about the change in a very small region just above the surface as shown in figure 2.12. This change can be efficiently scanned by nanoscaled electrodes resulting in high sensitivity. Another advantage of IDAs is the structuring of large active areas at once, therefore, multiple sensors can be put in a single array. Gold interdigitated nanoeleectrodes modified with DNA have been fabricated to study the hybridization event using a mediator via square wave voltammetry technique [166]. The hybridization event was observed with 10%–40% increase in electrochemical signal when compared to other macro- and microelectrode structures.

Recently, silicon technology has gained popularity for commercial production of electrochemical devices due to performance improvement along with cost and size reduction. The technology has resulted in the development of relatively new field effect transistors (FET) sensors. The integration of potentiometric ion selective electrodes with FET has been realized in the form of ion selective field effect transistors (ISFET) having potential difference as the output signal [167]. The magnitude of surface potential changes with change in the activity or concentration of analyte ion. The enzymatic ISFET based biosensors have been designed by immobilizing specific enzymes onto an ISFET gate. An enzymatic biosensor based on enzyme modified pH sensitive silicon nitride ISFET has been reported for the detection of urea with high sensitivity and reproducibility with a linear detection range covering the pathophysiological as well as physiological ranges [168]. The fabricated device has been used for bedside monitoring of critical patients via integration into commercial devices. A variety of immunosensors have also been developed using ISFET technology. For instance, a pH-FET based immunosensor

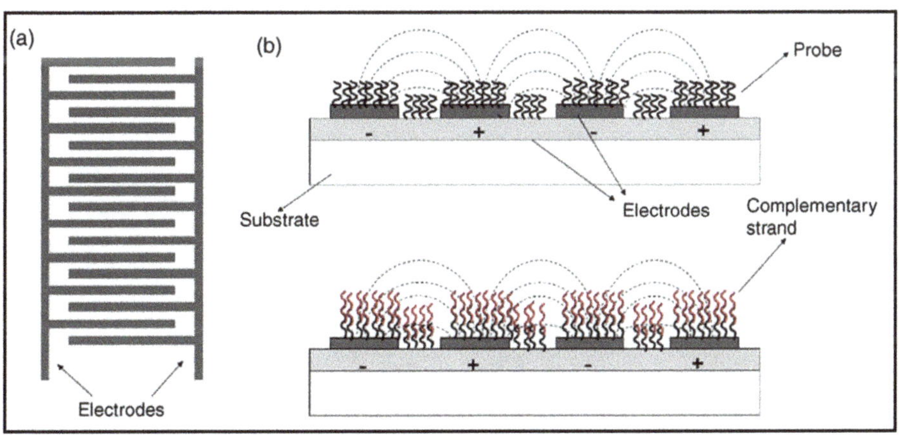

Figure 2.12. (a) Representation of an interdigitated electrode. (b) Change in the electric field of an affinity biosensor upon binding of probe complementary DNA analyte. Reprinted with permission from [149], copyright (2006), with permission from Elsevier.

has been investigated for the detection of interferon in broth [169]. The sensor is composed of interferon immobilized onto the pH-FET gate which when brought into contact with lactamase enzyme linked anti-interferon antibody brings about local change in pH. The change is proportional to the analyte concentration present in the sample and is detected potentiometrically within dynamic range of 10–100 μg ml^{-1}. Another ISFET based immunosensor has been reported for detection of a potent neurotoxin, bungarotoxin down to concentration of 16 ng ml^{-1}.

2.4.3 Microfluidic electrochemical sensors

Microfluidics is a technology used to process a minimal amount of fluid using micrometer-scale channels. Integration of microfluidics with point-of-care (POC) diagnostics offers advantages of portability, requirement of very small amount of sample, cost-effectiveness along with high sensitivity and specificity. It can also facilitate high-throughput analysis of multiple reactions simultaneously and integrate multiple steps of sample pretreatment, reaction, separation, and detection onto a single microfluidic chip. Therefore, microfluidic chips have been employed extensively for the detection of proteins, nucleic acids, cells and other small molecules for diagnosis of cancers and other diseases. A typical microfluidic chip is composed of inlet, mixing channel, and outlet integrated with signal detector (figure 2.13). The materials suitable for microfluidic platforms are inorganic (glass and silica), organic (polydimethylsiloxane—PDMS, polymethyl methacrylate—PMMA, polystyrene—PS and paper), and composite materials.

Roche developed a microfluidic POC, COBAS B101 for simultaneous detection of C-reactive protein (CRP), hemoglobin A1c (HbA1c), and lipid profile. The results are obtained within minutes using only 2 μl of sample [170]. An aptamer based microfluidic device has been developed for the quantification of cortisol levels in which complex procedures of immobilizing capture probe, target labeling, and washing before obtaining electrochemical signal have been eliminated. The results

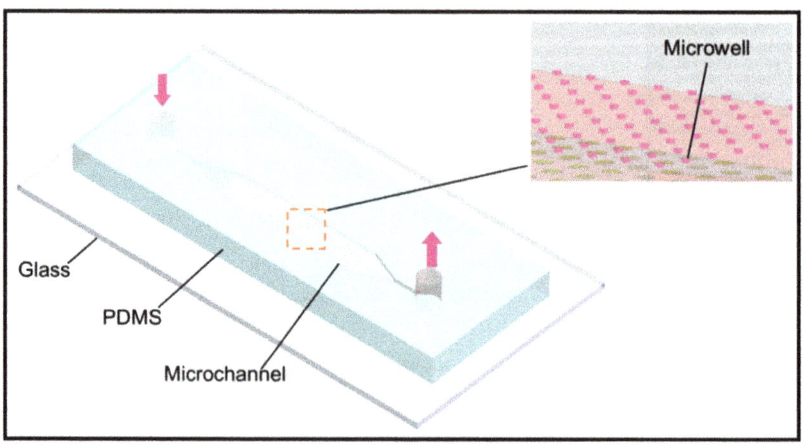

Figure 2.13. Representation of a microfluidic chip.

were comparable to those derived using enzyme linked immunosorbent assay (ELISA) but in a short assay time of 2.5 min with only 1 μl of sample. Microfluidic devices have also been used for cancer biomarker detection. An integrated microfluidic 'sample-to-targeted gene analysis' biochip has been reported for the detection of prostate cancer on genetic level from body fluids (serum liquid biopsies and urine) of patients [171]. The sensing platform is designed to detect multiple prostate cancer specific genes, namely, *KLK2*, *PCA3*, *SChLAP1*, and *TMPRSS2–ERG* gene fusion (figure 2.14). The biochip has different functional domains for (a) lysing cells to extract the genetic material, (b) amplification of targeted gene via nanofluidic manipulation, (c) peroxidase imitating nanozyme labeling, and (d) electrochemical detection of target gene. The developed microfluidic device completes the detection in only 30 min and is able to detect even 50 copies of target genes.

A microfluidic chip has been employed for the transdermal detection of glucose [172]. The device is made up of flexible three-electrode configuration with a graphene and gold nanoparticle modified working electrode. The sensor detects glucose levels with high sensitivity down to concentration of 0.3 mg dl^{-1} with a linear range between 0 and 40 mg dl^{-1}. The same group of researchers has improved the linear detection range for glucose using the similar microfluidic platform composed of graphene and gold nanoparticles but with the addition of glucose oxidase enzyme [173]. Another microfluidic enzymatic electrochemical biosensor has been developed using glucose oxidase enzyme and three-dimensional porous graphene aerosol. High electrical conductivity, biocompatibility, and increased surface area of graphene aerosol improved the performance of the sensor. Further, incorporation of microfluidics reduced the amount of sample consumed. The amperometric measurements

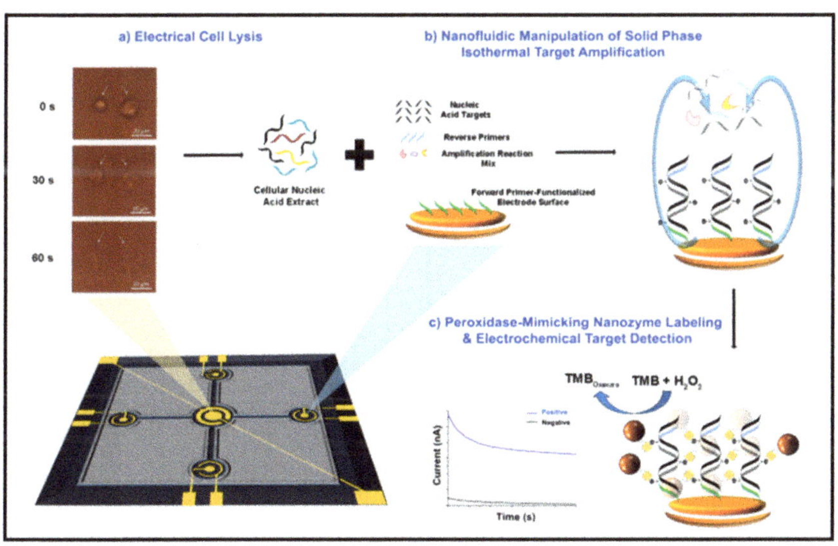

Figure 2.14. Integrated microfluidic chip having a single central lytic chamber along with four fluidic channels linked amplification/detection chambers for analysis of targeted prostate cancer genes in liquid biopsies. Reprinted with permission from [171], copyright (2018) American Chemical Society.

achieved the detection limit of 0.87 mM within a linear range of 1–18 mM with remarkable specificity and response stability [174]. A 3D paper-based screen-printed microfluidic electrochemical sensor has been designed for glucose monitoring in human sweat and blood as shown in figure 2.15. The highly conducting paper modified with Prussian blue/reduced graphene oxide–tetraethylene pentamine (PB/rGO–TEPA) has been employed based on electrochemical detection of H_2O_2 released as the catalytic product of immobilized glucose oxidase. The linear detection range between 0.1 mM and 25 mM with a limit of detection of 25 μM for glucose has been observed using the developed sensor [175].

Cancer diagnosis has also been efficiently facilitated using microfluidic electrochemical sensing platforms. For instance, an electrochemical gold electrode array-based microfluidic chip has been devised for multiplexed, high-throughput, simple and fast cancer biomarker detection. The array features an 8-port manifold multiplexed 32 individual microelectrodes for providing 2256 individual sensors. The system is capable of detecting multiple cancer biomarker proteins, namely, interleukin-6 (IL-6), platelet factor-4 (PF-4), prostate-specific antigen (PSA), and prostate-specific membrane antigen (PSMA) in serum within a clinically relevant detection limit of 0.05–2 pg ml^{-1} within a dynamic range from sub pg ml^{-1} to ng ml^{-1} [176]. A multi-sensor microarray microfluidic chip for detection of three DNA biomarkers of bladder cancer (DAPK, *E. Cad* and *RARβ*) has been reported [177]. The hairpin structured DNA probe is immobilized onto the gold working electrode via four stable sulfur–gold bonds. The change in current signal is obtained when the molecular beacon attached to DNA probe hybridizes with target DNA strand and subsequent change in structure. The sensor is able to detect markers down to a concentration of 250 fM in urine samples within a linear range of 100 nM to 200 fM within 20 min by cyclic voltammetry and impedance principles of electrochemistry. A disposable microfluidic electrochemical array device (μFED) has been developed and tested successfully for the detection of a breast cancer biomarker, estrogen receptor alpha (ERα) [178]. The device is composed of eight

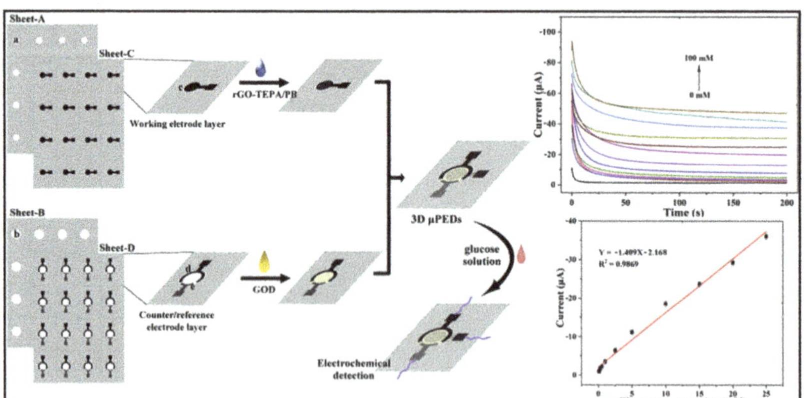

Figure 2.15. 3D paper-based microfluidic electrochemical biosensor for detection of glucose. Reprinted with permission from [175], copyright (2020) with permission from Elsevier.

carbon working electrodes along with reference and counter electrode. The working electrodes are modified with ERα specific DNA sequences for providing specificity. Anti-ERα antibodies and horseradish peroxidase enzyme (HRP) are immobilized onto paramagnetic particles for capturing and pre-concentrating the analyte from the solution. Antibody and enzyme bio-conjugated paramagnetic particles are injected into fabricated μFED and ERα is detected amperometrically at applied voltage of −0.2 V against Ag/AgCl. An ultralow detection limit of 10 fg ml^{-1} has been achieved using the developed device. A low cost fabricated microfluidic electrochemical sensor chip has been reported for the detection of breast cancer biomarkers, CA 15–3 in less than 2 min using 5 μl of sample [179]. The electrodes are composed of bare stainless steel capillaries which are cost-effective and already being mass produced. On the other hand, microfluidic chips consist of electrical double-layer capillary capacitors due to which neither redox probes nor amplification strategies are required, thereby reducing cost.

2.5 Conclusion

Development of highly sensitive sensors that are able to detect extremely low levels of disease markers at an early stage is considered to be the most recognized research area in biomedicine for improving the health status and decreasing the mortality rate. Electrochemical sensors are efficient candidates possessing desirable characteristics such as portability, rapid response, real-time monitoring, label-free detection along with high sensitivity and specificity. Nanotechnological advancements in the form of incorporated nanomaterials and nanodevices have further been investigated to improve the performance of electrochemical sensors in the field of biomedical diagnostics. Nanomaterials such as metal nanoparticles, metal oxides, carbon nanotubes, graphene, and quantum dots have been explored as recognition probes, signaling molecules, transducer materials, and immobilization substrates for bioprobes in electrochemical sensors for analytes of biomedical significance. Integration of nanotechnology and electrochemical sensing in medical diagnostics endows rapid, highly accurate, real-time, and personalized monitoring of health parameters. Significant efforts have been made to translate such advancements into compact devices in the form of wearable, planar, and microfluidic sensors which can be easily commercialized and made available to the patients for point-of-care applications.

Acknowledgements

JM is grateful to CSIR for SRA fellowship (No. B-12587 dated 01-08-2019). SK would like to thank the HSCST, Government of Haryana, India (research grant vide letter No. HSCST/R&D/2018/2103 dated 01-08-2018).

References

[1] Liu L, Zhao G, Dong X, Li X, Wei Q and Cao W 2018 An electrochemical immunosensor based on a multiple signal amplification strategy for highly sensitive detection of prostate specific antigen *Anal. Methods* **10** 4917–25

[2] Supraja P, Sudarshan V, Tripathy S, Agrawal A and Singh S G 2019 Label free electrochemical detection of cardiac biomarker troponin T using $ZnSnO_3$ perovskite nanomaterials *Anal. Methods* **11** 744–51

[3] Yang J, Yin X and Zhang W 2019 Electrochemical determination of PIK3CA gene associated with breast cancer based on molybdenum disulfide nanosheet-supported poly (indole-6-carboxylic acid) *Anal. Methods* **11** 157–62

[4] Khorshed A A, Khairy M, Elsafty S A and Banks C E 2019 Disposable screen-printed electrodes modified with uniform iron oxide nanocubes for the simple electrochemical determination of meclizine, an antihistamine drug *Anal. Methods* **11** 282–7

[5] Tian L, Zhao H, Zhao Z, Zhai J and Zhang Z 2019 A facile voltammetric method for detection of heparin in plasma based on the polyethylenimine modified electrode *Anal. Methods* **11** 1324–30

[6] Cao Q, Puthongkham P and Venton B J 2019 new insights into optimizing chemical and 3D surface structures of carbon electrodes for neurotransmitter detection *Anal. Methods* **11** 247–61

[7] Ou Y, Buchanan A M, Witt C E and Hashemi P 2019 Frontiers in electrochemical sensors for neurotransmitter detection: towards measuring neurotransmitters as chemical diagnostics for brain disorders *Anal. Methods* **11** 2738–55

[8] Raju D, Mendoza A, Wonnenberg P, Mohanaraj S, Sarbanes M, Truong C and Zestos A G 2019 Polymer modified carbon fiber-microelectrodes and waveform modifications enhance neurotransmitter metabolite detection *Anal. Methods* **11** 1620–30

[9] McLeod K E, Lynk T P, Sit C S and Brosseau C L 2019 On the origin of electrochemical surface-enhanced Raman spectroscopy (EC-SERS) signals for bacterial samples: the importance of filtered control studies in the development of new bacterial screening platforms *Anal. Methods* **11** 924–9

[10] Mo X, Wu Z, Huang J, Zhao G and Dou W 2019 A sensitive and regenerative electrochemical immunosensor for quantitative detection of *Escherichia coli* O157: H7 based on stable polyaniline coated screen-printed carbon electrode and rGO-NR-Au@ Pt *Anal. Methods* **11** 1475–82

[11] Siegel J M, Schilly K M, Wijesinghe M B, Caruso G, Fresta C G and Lunte S M 2019 Optimization of a microchip electrophoresis method with electrochemical detection for the determination of nitrite in macrophage cells as an indicator of nitric oxide production *Anal. Methods* **11** 148–56

[12] Heng J I T, Moonen G and Nguyen L 2007 Neurotransmitters regulate cell migration in the telencephalon *Eur. J. Neurosci.* **26** 537–46

[13] Sheikh S, Haque E and Mir S S 2013 Neurodegenerative diseases: multifactorial conformational diseases and their therapeutic interventions *J. Neurodegener. Dis.* **2013** 536481

[14] Blank C, Murrill E and Adams R 1972 Central nervous system effects of 6-aminodopamine and 6-hydroxydopamine *Brain Res.* **45** 635–7

[15] Shon Y-M, Lee K H, Goerss S J, Kim I Y, Kimble C, Van Gompel J J, Bennet K, Blaha C D and Chang S-Y 2010 High frequency stimulation of the subthalamic nucleus evokes striatal dopamine release in a large animal model of human DBS neurosurgery *Neurosci. Lett.* **475** 136–40

[16] Suzuki A, Ivandini T A, Yoshimi K, Fujishima A, Oyama G, Nakazato T, Hattori N, Kitazawa S and Einaga Y 2007 Fabrication, characterization, and application of boron-doped diamond microelectrodes for *in vivo* dopamine detection *Anal. Chem.* **79** 8608–15

[17] Yoshimi K, Naya Y, Mitani N, Kato T, Inoue M, Natori S, Takahashi T, Weitemier A, Nishikawa N and McHugh T 2011 Phasic reward responses in the monkey striatum as detected by voltammetry with diamond microelectrodes *Neurosci. Res.* **71** 49–62
[18] Jang D P, Kim I, Chang S-Y, Min H-K, Arora K, Marsh M P, Hwang S-C, Kimble C J, Bennet K E and Lee K H 2012 Paired pulse voltammetry for differentiating complex analytes *Analyst* **137** 1428–35
[19] Robinson D L, Hermans A, Seipel A T and Wightman R M 2008 Monitoring rapid chemical communication in the brain *Chem. Rev.* **108** 2554–84
[20] Zachek M K, Hermans A, Wightman R M and McCarty G S 2008 Electrochemical dopamine detection: Comparing gold and carbon fiber microelectrodes using background subtracted fast scan cyclic voltammetry *J. Electroanal. Chem.* **614** 113–20
[21] Cheer J F, Wassum K M, Sombers L A, Heien M L, Ariansen J L, Aragona B J, Phillips P E and Wightman R M 2007 Phasic dopamine release evoked by abused substances requires cannabinoid receptor activation *J. Neurosci.* **27** 791–5
[22] Majewska U E, Chmurski K, Biesiada K, Olszyna A R and Bilewicz R 2006 Dopamine oxidation at per (6-deoxy-6-thio)-α-cyclodextrin monolayer modified gold electrodes *Electroanalysis* **18** 1463–70
[23] Freeman R, Elbaz J, Gill R, Zayats M and Willner I 2007 Analysis of dopamine and tyrosinase activity on ion-sensitive field-effect transistor (ISFET) devices *Chem. Eur. J.* **13** 7288–93
[24] Maciejewska J, Pisarek K, Bartosiewicz I, Krysiński P, Jackowska K and Biegunski A 2011 Selective detection of dopamine on poly (indole-5-carboxylic acid)/tyrosinase electrode *Electrochim. Acta* **56** 3700–6
[25] Njagi J, Chernov M M, Leiter J and Andreescu S 2010 Amperometric detection of dopamine *in vivo* with an enzyme based carbon fiber microbiosensor *Anal. Chem.* **82** 989–96
[26] Tang H, Lin P, Chan H L and Yan F 2011 Highly sensitive dopamine biosensors based on organic electrochemical transistors *Biosens. Bioelectron.* **26** 4559–63
[27] Wang Y, Zhang X, Chen Y, Xu H, Tan Y and Wang S 2010 Detection of dopamine based on tyrosinase-Fe3O4 nanoparticles-chitosan nanocomposite biosensor *Am. J. Biomed. Sci.* **2** 209–16
[28] Wang Z, Xia J, Zhu L, Chen X, Zhang F, Yao S, Li Y and Xia Y 2011 A selective voltammetric method for detecting dopamine at quercetin modified electrode incorporating graphene *Electroanalysis* **23** 2463–71
[29] Kim Y-R, Bong S, Kang Y-J, Yang Y, Mahajan R K, Kim J S and Kim H 2010 Electrochemical detection of dopamine in the presence of ascorbic acid using graphene modified electrodes *Biosens. Bioelectron.* **25** 2366–9
[30] Hou S, Kasner M L, Su S, Patel K and Cuellari R 2010 Highly sensitive and selective dopamine biosensor fabricated with silanized graphene *J. Phys. Chem.* C **114** 14915–21
[31] Chang J-L, Wei G-T and Zen J-M 2011 Screen-printed ionic liquid/preanodized carbon electrode: effective detection of dopamine in the presence of high concentration of ascorbic acid *Electrochem. Commun.* **13** 174–7
[32] Li Y, Liu X and Wei W 2011 Square wave voltammetry for selective detection of dopamine using polyglycine modified carbon ionic liquid electrode *Electroanalysis* **23** 2832–8
[33] Zhu Z, Qu L, Guo Y, Zeng Y, Sun W and Huang X 2010 Electrochemical detection of dopamine on a Ni/Al layered double hydroxide modified carbon ionic liquid electrode *Sensors Actuators* B **151** 146–52

[34] Celebanska A, Tomaszewska D, Lesniewski A and Opallo M 2011 Film electrode prepared from oppositely charged silicate submicroparticles and carbon nanoparticles for selective dopamine sensing *Biosens. Bioelectron.* **26** 4417–22
[35] García M, Armendáriz G, Godínez L A, Torres J, Sepúlveda-Guzmán S and Bustos E 2011 Detection of dopamine in non-treated urine samples using glassy carbon electrodes modified with PAMAM dendrimer–Pt composites *Electrochim. Acta* **56** 7712–7
[36] Ulubay Ş and Dursun Z 2010 Cu nanoparticles incorporated polypyrrole modified GCE for sensitive simultaneous determination of dopamine and uric acid *Talanta* **80** 1461–6
[37] Wood K M and Hashemi P 2013 Fast-scan cyclic voltammetry analysis of dynamic serotonin reponses to acute escitalopram *ACS Chem. Neurosci.* **4** 715–20
[38] Fang H, Vickrey T L and Venton B J 2011 Analysis of biogenic amines in a single *Drosophila* larva brain by capillary electrophoresis with fast-scan cyclic voltammetry detection *Anal. Chem.* **83** 2258–64
[39] Njagi J, Ball M, Best M, Wallace K N and Andreescu S 2010 Electrochemical quantification of serotonin in the live embryonic zebrafish intestine *Anal. Chem.* **82** 1822–30
[40] Özel R E, Wallace K N and Andreescu S 2014 Alterations of intestinal serotonin following nanoparticle exposure in embryonic zebrafish *Environ. Sci. Nano* **1** 27–36
[41] Singh Y S, Sawarynski L E, Michael H M, Ferrell R E, Murphey-Corb M A, Swain G M, Patel B A and Andrews A M 2010 Boron-doped diamond microelectrodes reveal reduced serotonin uptake rates in lymphocytes from adult rhesus monkeys carrying the short allele of the 5-HTTLPR *ACS Chem. Neurosci.* **1** 49–64
[42] Beitollahi H, Karimi-Maleh H and Khabazzadeh H 2008 Nanomolar and selective determination of epinephrine in the presence of norepinephrine using carbon paste electrode modified with carbon nanotubes and novel 2-(4-oxo-3-phenyl-3,4-dihydro-quinazolinyl)-*N*′-phenyl-hydrazinecarbothioamide *Anal. Chem.* **80** 9848–51
[43] Lu X, Li Y, Du J, Zhou X, Xue Z, Liu X and Wang Z 2011 A novel nanocomposites sensor for epinephrine detection in the presence of uric acids and ascorbic acids *Electrochim. Acta* **56** 7261–6
[44] Shahrokhian S and Saberi R-S 2011 Electrochemical preparation of over-oxidized polypyrrole/multi-walled carbon nanotube composite on glassy carbon electrode and its application in epinephrine determination *Electrochim. Acta* **57** 132–8
[45] Thiagarajan S and Chen S-M 2009 Applications of nanostructured Pt–Au hybrid film for the simultaneous determination of catecholamines in the presence of ascorbic acid *J. Solid State Electrochem.* **13** 445–53
[46] Goyal R N and Bishnoi S 2011 Simultaneous determination of epinephrine and norepinephrine in human blood plasma and urine samples using nanotubes modified edge plane pyrolytic graphite electrode *Talanta* **84** 78–83
[47] Lu L-P, Wang S-Q and Lin X-Q 2004 Fabrication of layer-by-layer deposited multilayer films containing DNA and gold nanoparticle for norepinephrine biosensor *Anal. Chim. Acta* **519** 161–6
[48] Pasco N, Jeffries C, Davies Q, Downard A, Roddick-Lanzilotta A and Gorton L 1999 Characterisation of a thermophilic L-glutamate dehydrogenase biosensor for amperometric determination of L-glutamate by flow injection analysis *Biosens. Bioelectron.* **14** 171–8
[49] Gholizadeh A, Shahrokhian S, Mohajerzadeh S, Vosoughi M, Darbari S and Sanaee Z 2012 Mediator-less highly sensitive voltammetric detection of glutamate using glutamate dehydrogenase/vertically aligned CNTs grown on silicon substrate *Biosens. Bioelectron.* **31** 110–5

[50] Özel R E, Ispas C, Ganesana M, Leiter J and Andreescu S 2014 Glutamate oxidase biosensor based on mixed ceria and titania nanoparticles for the detection of glutamate in hypoxic environments *Biosens. Bioelectron.* **52** 397–402
[51] Larsson N, Ruzgas T, Gorton L, Kokaia M, Kissinger P and Csöregi E 1998 Design and development of an amperometric biosensor for acetylcholine determination in brain microdialysates *Electrochim. Acta* **43** 3541–54
[52] Gunaratna P C and Wilson G S 1990 Optimization of multienzyme flow reactors for determination of acetylcholine *Anal. Chem.* **62** 402–7
[53] Guerrieri A, Lattanzio V, Palmisano F and Zambonin P 2006 Electrosynthesized poly (pyrrole)/poly (2-naphthol) bilayer membrane as an effective anti-interference layer for simultaneous determination of acethylcholine and choline by a dual electrode amperometric biosensor *Biosens. Bioelectron.* **21** 1710–8
[54] Lee S-R, Rahman M M, Ishida M and Sawada K 2009 Development of a highly-sensitive acetylcholine sensor using a charge-transfer technique on a smart biochip *TrAC Trends Anal. Chem.* **28** 196–203
[55] Shimomura T, Itoh T, Sumiya T, Mizukami F and Ono M 2009 Amperometric biosensor based on enzymes immobilized in hybrid mesoporous membranes for the determination of acetylcholine *Enzyme Microb. Technol.* **45** 443–8
[56] Xue W and Cui T 2008 A high-resolution amperometric acetylcholine sensor based on nano-assembled carbon nanotube and acetylcholinesterase thin films *J. Nano Res.* **1** 1–9
[57] Wang C-I, Chen W-T and Chang H-T 2012 Enzyme mimics of Au/Ag nanoparticles for fluorescent detection of acetylcholine *Anal. Chem.* **84** 9706–12
[58] Wynne A M, Reid C H and Finnerty N J 2014 In vitro characterisation of ortho phenylenediamine and Nafion®-modified Pt electrodes for measuring brain nitric oxide *J. Electroanal. Chem.* **732** 110–6
[59] Santos R M, Rodrigues M S, Laranjinha J and Barbosa R M 2013 Biomimetic sensor based on hemin/carbon nanotubes/chitosan modified microelectrode for nitric oxide measurement in the brain *Biosens. Bioelectron.* **44** 152–9
[60] Yap C, Xu G and Ang S 2013 Amperometric nitric oxide sensor based on nanoporous platinum phthalocyanine modified electrodes *Anal. Chem.* **85** 107–13
[61] Myung Y, Jang D M, Cho Y J, Kim H S, Park J, Kim J-U, Choi Y and Lee C J 2009 Nonenzymatic amperometric glucose sensing of platinum, copper sulfide, and tin oxide nanoparticle-carbon nanotube hybrid nanostructures *J. Phys. Chem.* C **113** 1251–9
[62] Xia Y, Huang W, Zheng J, Niu Z and Li Z 2011 Nonenzymatic amperometric response of glucose on a nanoporous gold film electrode fabricated by a rapid and simple electrochemical method *Biosens. Bioelectron.* **26** 3555–61
[63] Gao H, Xiao F, Ching C B and Duan H 2011 One-step electrochemical synthesis of PtNi nanoparticle-graphene nanocomposites for nonenzymatic amperometric glucose detection *ACS Appl. Mater. Interfaces* **3** 3049–57
[64] Chen C, Xie Q, Yang D, Xiao H, Fu Y, Tan Y and Yao S 2013 Recent advances in electrochemical glucose biosensors: a review *RSC Adv.* **3** 4473–91
[65] Luo D, Wu L and Zhi J 2009 Fabrication of boron-doped diamond nanorod forest electrodes and their application in nonenzymatic amperometric glucose biosensing *ACS Nano* **3** 2121–8
[66] Song Y Y, Zhang D, Gao W and Xia X H 2005 Nonenzymatic glucose detection by using a three-dimensionally ordered, macroporous platinum template *Chem. Eur. J.* **11** 2177–82

[67] Wang C, Yin L, Zhang L and Gao R 2010 Ti/TiO_2 nanotube array/Ni composite electrodes for nonenzymatic amperometric glucose sensing *J. Phys. Chem.* C **114** 4408–13
[68] Yin H, Zhou C, Xu C, Liu P, Xu X and Ding Y 2008 Aerobic oxidation of D-glucose on support-free nanoporous gold *J. Phys. Chem.* C **112** 9673–8
[69] Kang X, Mai Z, Zou X, Cai P and Mo J 2007 A sensitive nonenzymatic glucose sensor in alkaline media with a copper nanocluster/multiwall carbon nanotube-modified glassy carbon electrode *Anal. Biochem.* **363** 143–50
[70] You T, Niwa O, Chen Z, Hayashi K, Tomita M and Hirono S 2003 An amperometric detector formed of highly dispersed Ni nanoparticles embedded in a graphite-like carbon film electrode for sugar determination *Anal. Chem.* **75** 5191–96
[71] Luo P F and Kuwana T 1994 Nickel–titanium alloy electrode as a sensitive and stable LCEC detector for carbohydrates *Anal. Chem.* **66** 2775–82
[72] Zhao J, Wang F, Yu J and Hu S 2006 Electro-oxidation of glucose at self-assembled monolayers incorporated by copper particles *Talanta* **70** 449–54
[73] Yuan J, Wang K and Xia X 2005 Highly ordered platinum-nanotubule arrays for amperometric glucose sensing *Adv. Funct. Mater.* **15** 803–9
[74] Park S, Chung T D and Kim H C 2003 Nonenzymatic glucose detection using mesoporous platinum *Anal. Chem.* **75** 3046–9
[75] Sun Y, Buck H and Mallouk T E 2001 Combinatorial discovery of alloy electrocatalysts for amperometric glucose sensors *Anal. Chem.* **73** 1599–604
[76] Meng L, Jin J, Yang G, Lu T, Zhang H and Cai C 2009 Nonenzymatic electrochemical detection of glucose based on palladium–single-walled carbon nanotube hybrid nanostructures *Anal. Chem.* **81** 7271–80
[77] Pang H, Lu Q, Wang J, Li Y and Gao F 2010 Glucose-assisted synthesis of copper micropuzzles and their application as nonenzymatic glucose sensors *Chem. Commun.* **46** 2010–12
[78] Xu M, Song Y, Ye Y, Gong C, Shen Y, Wang L and Wang L 2017 A novel flexible electrochemical glucose sensor based on gold nanoparticles/polyaniline arrays/carbon cloth electrode *Sensors Actuators* B **252** 1187–93
[79] Alexander S, Baraneedharan P, Balasubrahmanyan S and Ramaprabhu S 2017 Highly sensitive and selective non enzymatic electrochemical glucose sensors based on graphene oxide-molecular imprinted polymer *Mater. Sci. Eng.* C **78** 124–9
[80] Deshmukh M A, Kang B-C and Ha T-J 2020 Non-enzymatic electrochemical glucose sensors based on polyaniline/reduced-graphene-oxide nanocomposites functionalized with silver nanoparticles *J. Mater. Chem.* C **8** 5112–23
[81] Archana V, Xia Y, Fang R and Gnana Kumar G 2019 Hierarchical CuO/NiO–carbon nanocomposite derived from metal organic framework on cello tape for the flexible and high performance nonenzymatic electrochemical glucose sensors *ACS Sustain. Chem. Eng.* **7** 6707–19
[82] Li R, Liu X, Wang H, Wu Y, Chan K and Lu Z 2019 Sandwich nanoporous framework decorated with vertical CuO nanowire arrays for electrochemical glucose sensing *Electrochim. Acta* **299** 470–8
[83] Zhang Y, Ma Y, Li Y, Zhu W, Wei Z, Sun J, Li T and Wang J 2020 Ambient self-derivation of nickel–cobalt hydroxysulfide multistage nanoarray for high-performance electrochemical glucose sensing *Appl. Surf. Sci.* **505** 144636

[84] Clark L C Jr and Lyons C 1962 Electrode systems for continuous monitoring in cardiovascular surgery *Ann. N. Y. Acad. Sci.* **102** 29–45

[85] Chen W, Ding Y, Akhigbe J, Brückner C, Li C M and Lei Y 2010 Enhanced electrochemical oxygen reduction-based glucose sensing using glucose oxidase on nanodendritic poly [meso-tetrakis (2-thienyl) porphyrinato] cobalt (II)-SWNTs composite electrodes *Biosens. Bioelectron.* **26** 504–10

[86] Che X, Yuan R, Chai Y, Li J, Song Z, Li W and Zhong X 2011 A glucose biosensor based on chitosan–Prussian blue–multiwall carbon nanotubes–hollow PtCo nanochains formed by one-step electrodeposition *Colloids Surf.* B **84** 454–61

[87] Wang Y, Yuan R, Chaia Y, Li W, Zhuo Y, Yuan Y and Li J 2011 Direct electron transfer: electrochemical glucose biosensor based on hollow Pt nanosphere functionalized multiwall carbon nanotubes *J. Mol. Catal.* B **71** 146–51

[88] Li J, Yuan R, Chai Y, Che X and Li W 2012 Construction of an amperometric glucose biosensor based on the immobilization of glucose oxidase onto electrodeposited Pt nanoparticles-chitosan composite film *Bioprocess. Biosyst. Eng.* **35** 1089–95

[89] Qiu C, Wang X, Liu X, Hou S and Ma H 2012 Direct electrochemistry of glucose oxidase immobilized on nanostructured gold thin films and its application to bioelectrochemical glucose sensor *Electrochim. Acta* **67** 140–6

[90] Yu Y, Chen Z, He S, Zhang B, Li X and Yao M 2014 Direct electron transfer of glucose oxidase and biosensing for glucose based on PDDA-capped gold nanoparticle modified graphene/multi-walled carbon nanotubes electrode *Biosens. Bioelectron.* **52** 147–52

[91] Gao Y-F, Yang T, Yang X-L, Zhang Y-S, Xiao B-L, Hong J, Sheibani N, Ghourchian H, Hong T and Moosavi-Movahedi A A 2014 Direct electrochemistry of glucose oxidase and glucose biosensing on a hydroxyl fullerenes modified glassy carbon electrode *Biosens. Bioelectron.* **60** 30–4

[92] Balakrishnan S R, Hashim U, Letchumanan G, Kashif M, Ruslinda A, Liu W, Veeradasan P, Prasad R H, Foo K and Poopalan P 2014 Development of highly sensitive polysilicon nanogap with APTES/GOx based lab-on-chip biosensor to determine low levels of salivary glucose *Sensors Actuators* A **220** 101–11

[93] Kang Y R, Hwang K H, Kim J H, Nam C H and Kim S W 2010 Disposable amperometric biosensor based on nanostructured bacteriophages for glucose detection *Meas. Sci. Technol.* **21** 105804

[94] Ibupoto Z, Khun K, Lu J and Willander M 2013 The synthesis of CuO nanoleaves, structural characterization, and their glucose sensing application *Appl. Phys. Lett.* **102** 103701

[95] Hussain M, Ibupoto Z H, Abbasi M A, Liu X, Nur O and Willander M 2014 Synthesis of three dimensional nickel cobalt oxide nanoneedles on nickel foam, their characterization and glucose sensing application *Sensors* **14** 5415–25

[96] Asif M H, Elinder F and Willander M 2011 Electrochemical biosensors based on ZnO nanostructures to measure intracellular metal ions and glucose *J. Anal. Bioanal. Tech* S7–003

[97] Jia X, Hu G, Nitze F, Barzegar H R, Sharifi T, Tai C-W and Wågberg T 2013 Synthesis of palladium/helical carbon nanofiber hybrid nanostructures and their application for hydrogen peroxide and glucose detection *ACS Appl. Mater. Interfaces* **5** 12017–22

[98] Shahzad F, Zaidi S A and Koo C M 2017 Highly sensitive electrochemical sensor based on environmentally friendly biomass-derived sulfur-doped graphene for cancer biomarker detection *Sensors Actuators* B **241** 716–24

[99] Wang B, Akiba U and Anzai J-I 2017 Recent progress in nanomaterial-based electrochemical biosensors for cancer biomarkers: a review *Molecules* **22** 1048

[100] Giannetto M, Elviri L, Careri M, Mangia A and Mori G 2011 A voltammetric immunosensor based on nanobiocomposite materials for the determination of alpha-fetoprotein in serum *Biosens. Bioelectron.* **26** 2232–6

[101] Sun G, Yang H, Zhang Y, Yu J, Ge S, Yan M and Song X 2015 Branched zinc oxide nanorods arrays modified paper electrode for electrochemical immunosensing by combining biocatalytic precipitation reaction and competitive immunoassay mode *Biosens. Bioelectron.* **74** 823–9

[102] Yang F, Han J, Zhuo Y, Yang Z, Chai Y and Yuan R 2014 Highly sensitive impedimetric immunosensor based on single-walled carbon nanohorns as labels and bienzyme biocatalyzed precipitation as enhancer for cancer biomarker detection *Biosens. Bioelectron.* **55** 360–5

[103] Zhao C, Lin D, Wu J, Ding L, Ju H and Yan F 2013 Nanogold-enriched carbon nanohorn label for sensitive electrochemical detection of biomarker on a disposable immunosensor *Electroanalysis* **25** 1044–9

[104] Jia X, Liu Z, Liu N and Ma Z 2014 A label-free immunosensor based on graphene nanocomposites for simultaneous multiplexed electrochemical determination of tumor markers *Biosens. Bioelectron.* **53** 160–6

[105] Gao Q, Liu N and Ma Z 2014 Prussian blue–gold nanoparticles-ionic liquid functionalized reduced graphene oxide nanocomposite as label for ultrasensitive electrochemical immunoassay of alpha-fetoprotein *Anal. Chim. Acta* **829** 15–21

[106] Li L, Zhang L, Yu J, Ge S and Song X 2015 All-graphene composite materials for signal amplification toward ultrasensitive electrochemical immunosensing of tumor marker *Biosens. Bioelectron.* **71** 108–14

[107] Yang K, Qi L, Gao Z, Zu X and Chen M 2014 A novel electrochemical immunosensor for prostate-specific antigen based on noncovalent nanocomposite of ferrocene monocarboxylic acid with graphene oxide *Anal. Lett.* **47** 2266–80

[108] Sun G, Liu H, Zhang Y, Yu J, Yan M, Song X and He W 2015 Gold nanorods-paper electrode based enzyme-free electrochemical immunoassay for prostate specific antigen using porous zinc oxide spheres–silver nanoparticles nanocomposites as labels *New J. Chem.* **39** 6062–7

[109] Li H, Wei Q, He J, Li T, Zhao Y, Cai Y, Du B, Qian Z and Yang M 2011 Electrochemical immunosensors for cancer biomarker with signal amplification based on ferrocene functionalized iron oxide nanoparticles *Biosens. Bioelectron.* **26** 3590–5

[110] Akter R, Rahman M A and Rhee C K 2012 Amplified electrochemical detection of a cancer biomarker by enhanced precipitation using horseradish peroxidase attached on carbon nanotubes *Anal. Chem.* **84** 6407–15

[111] Li T, Yang M and Li H 2011 Label-free electrochemical detection of cancer marker based on graphene–cobalt hexacyanoferrate nanocomposite *J. Electroanal. Chem.* **655** 50–5

[112] Kumar S, Willander M, Sharma J G and Malhotra B D 2015 A solution processed carbon nanotube modified conducting paper sensor for cancer detection *J. Mater. Chem.* B **3** 9305–14

[113] Wen G, Yang X and Xi X 2015 Cathode photoelectrochemical immunoassay based on analyte-induced formation of exciton trapping for carcinoembryonic antigen detection *J. Electroanal. Chem.* **757** 192–7

[114] Chen X, Jia X, Han J, Ma J and Ma Z 2013 Electrochemical immunosensor for simultaneous detection of multiplex cancer biomarkers based on graphene nanocomposites *Biosens. Bioelectron.* **50** 356–61

[115] Song Z, Yuan R, Chai Y, Zhuo Y, Jiang W, Su H, Che X and Li J 2010 Horseradish peroxidase-functionalized Pt hollow nanospheres and multiple redox probes as trace labels for a sensitive simultaneous multianalyte electrochemical immunoassay *Chem. Commun.* **46** 6750–2

[116] Wang W, Fan X, Xu S, Davis J J and Luo X 2015 Low fouling label-free DNA sensor based on polyethylene glycols decorated with gold nanoparticles for the detection of breast cancer biomarkers *Biosens. Bioelectron.* **71** 51–6

[117] Elshafey R, Tavares A C, Siaj M and Zourob M 2013 Electrochemical impedance immunosensor based on gold nanoparticles–protein G for the detection of cancer marker epidermal growth factor receptor in human plasma and brain tissue *Biosens. Bioelectron.* **50** 143–9

[118] Peng H-P, Hu Y, Liu A-L, Chen W, Lin X-H and Yu X-B 2014 Label-free electrochemical immunosensor based on multi-functional gold nanoparticles–polydopamine–thionine–graphene oxide nanocomposites film for determination of alpha-fetoprotein *J. Electroanal. Chem.* **712** 89–95

[119] Ortega F G, Fernández-Baldo M A, Serrano M J, Messina G A, Lorente J A and Raba J 2015 Epithelial cancer biomarker EpCAM determination in peripheral blood samples using a microfluidic immunosensor based in silver nanoparticles as platform *Sensors Actuators* B **221** 248–56

[120] Johari-Ahar M, Rashidi M, Barar J, Aghaie M, Mohammadnejad D, Ramazani A, Karami P, Coukos G and Omidi Y 2015 An ultra-sensitive impedimetric immunosensor for detection of the serum oncomarker CA-125 in ovarian cancer patients *Nanoscale* **7** 3768–79

[121] Paul K B, Singh V, Vanjari S R K and Singh S G 2017 One step biofunctionalized electrospun multiwalled carbon nanotubes embedded zinc oxide nanowire interface for highly sensitive detection of carcinoma antigen-125 *Biosens. Bioelectron.* **88** 144–52

[122] Wu Y, Xue P, Kang Y and Hui K M 2013 Paper-based microfluidic electrochemical immunodevice integrated with nanobioprobes onto graphene film for ultrasensitive multiplexed detection of cancer biomarkers *Anal. Chem.* **85** 8661–8

[123] Yu Y, Gao T, Li H, Ye Z, Chen Z and Li G 2014 A novel electrochemical immunosensor for Golgi Protein 73 assay *Electrochem. Commun.* **42** 6–8

[124] Niu Y, He J, Li Y, Zhao Y, Xia C, Yuan G, Zhang L, Zhang Y and Yu C 2016 Determination of α2,3-sialylated glycans in human serum using a glassy carbon electrode modified with carboxylated multiwalled carbon nanotubes, a polyamidoamine dendrimer, and a glycan-recognizing lectin from *Maackia amurensis Microchim. Acta* **183** 2337–44

[125] Akter R, Jeong B, Choi J-S and Rahman M A 2016 Ultrasensitive nanoimmunosensor by coupling non-covalent functionalized graphene oxide platform and numerous ferritin labels on carbon nanotubes *Biosens. Bioelectron.* **80** 123–30

[126] Soares J C, Soares A C, Rodrigues V C, Melendez M E, Santos A C, Faria E F, Reis R M, Carvalho A L and Oliveira O N Jr 2019 Detection of the prostate cancer biomarker PCA3 with electrochemical and impedance-based biosensors *ACS Appl. Mater. Interfaces* **11** 46645–50

[127] Zhang W, Yang J and Wu D 2020 Surface-functionalized MoS_2 nanosheets sensor for direct electrochemical detection of PIK3CA gene related to lung cancer *J. Electrochem. Soc.* **167** 027501

[128] Ferreira P C, Ataide V N, Chagas C L S, Angnes L, Coltro W K T, Paixão T R L C and de Araujo W R 2019 Wearable electrochemical sensors for forensic and clinical applications *TrAC Trends Anal. Chem.* **119** 115622

[129] Nyein H Y Y, Gao W, Shahpar Z, Emaminejad S, Challa S, Chen K, Fahad H M, Tai L-C, Ota H and Davis R W 2016 A wearable electrochemical platform for noninvasive simultaneous monitoring of Ca^{2+} and pH *ACS Nano* **10** 7216–24

[130] Gao W, Emaminejad S, Nyein H Y Y, Challa S, Chen K, Peck A, Fahad H M, Ota H, Shiraki H and Kiriya D 2016 Fully integrated wearable sensor arrays for multiplexed *in situ* perspiration analysis *Nature* **529** 509–14

[131] Lee Y, Howe C, Mishra S, Lee D S, Mahmood M, Piper M, Kim Y, Tieu K, Byun H-S and Coffey J P 2018 Wireless, intraoral hybrid electronics for real-time quantification of sodium intake toward hypertension management *Proc. Natl Acad. Sci.* **115** 5377–82

[132] Glennon T, O'Quigley C, McCaul M, Matzeu G, Beirne S, Wallace G G, Stroiescu F, O'Mahoney N, White P and Diamond D 2016 'SWEATCH': a wearable platform for harvesting and analysing sweat sodium content *Electroanalysis* **28** 1283–9

[133] Bariya M, Shahpar Z, Park H, Sun J, Jung Y, Gao W, Nyein H Y Y, Liaw T S, Tai L-C and Ngo Q P 2018 Roll-to-roll gravure printed electrochemical sensors for wearable and medical devices *ACS Nano* **12** 6978–87

[134] Sempionatto J R, Martin A, García-Carmona L, Barfidokht A, Kurniawan J F, Moreto J R, Tang G, Shin A, Liu X and Escarpa A 2019 Skin-worn soft microfluidic potentiometric detection system *Electroanalysis* **31** 239–45

[135] Sempionatto J R, Nakagawa T, Pavinatto A, Mensah S T, Imani S, Mercier P and Wang J 2017 Eyeglasses based wireless electrolyte and metabolite sensor platform *Lab Chip* **17** 1834–42

[136] Parrilla M, Ferré J, Guinovart T and Andrade F J 2016 Wearable potentiometric sensors based on commercial carbon fibres for monitoring sodium in sweat *Electroanalysis* **28** 1267–75

[137] Zamora M L, Domínguez J M, Trujillo R M, Goy C B, Sanchez M A and Madrid R E 2018 Potentiometric textile-based pH sensor *Sensors Actuators* B **260** 601–8

[138] Schazmann B, Morris D, Slater C, Beirne S, Fay C, Reuveny R, Moyna N and Diamond D 2010 A wearable electrochemical sensor for the real-time measurement of sweat sodium concentration *Anal. Methods* **2** 342–8

[139] Cuartero M, Parrilla M and Crespo G A 2019 Wearable potentiometric sensors for medical applications *Sensors* **19** 363

[140] Choi D-H, Kim J S, Cutting G R and Searson P C 2016 Wearable potentiometric chloride sweat sensor: the critical role of the salt bridge *Anal. Chem.* **88** 12241–7

[141] Yao H, Liao Y, Lingley A, Afanasiev A, Lähdesmäki I, Otis B and Parviz B 2012 A contact lens with integrated telecommunication circuit and sensors for wireless and continuous tear glucose monitoring *J. Micromech. Microeng.* **22** 075007

[142] Bae C W, Toi P T, Kim B Y, Lee W I, Lee H B, Hanif A, Lee E H and Lee N-E 2019 Fully stretchable capillary microfluidics-integrated nanoporous gold electrochemical sensor for wearable continuous glucose monitoring *ACS Appl. Mater. Interfaces* **11** 14567–75

[143] Xu G, Cheng C, Liu Z, Yuan W, Wu X, Lu Y, Low S S, Liu J, Zhu L and Ji D 2019 Battery-free and wireless epidermal electrochemical system with all-printed stretchable electrode array for multiplexed *in situ* sweat analysis *Adv. Mater. Technol.* **4** 1800658
[144] Gao W, Nyein H Y, Shahpar Z, Fahad H M, Chen K, Emaminejad S, Gao Y, Tai L-C, Ota H and Wu E 2016 Wearable microsensor array for multiplexed heavy metal monitoring of body fluids *ACS Sens.* **1** 866–74
[145] Tai L C, Gao W, Chao M, Bariya M, Ngo Q P, Shahpar Z, Nyein H Y, Park H, Sun J and Jung Y 2018 Methylxanthine drug monitoring with wearable sweat sensors *Adv. Mater.* **30** 1707442
[146] Parlak O, Keene S T, Marais A, Curto V F and Salleo A 2018 Molecularly selective nanoporous membrane-based wearable organic electrochemical device for noninvasive cortisol sensing *Sci. Adv.* **4** eaar2904
[147] Bandodkar A J, Gutruf P, Choi J, Lee K, Sekine Y, Reeder J T, Jeang W J, Aranyosi A J, Lee S P and Model J B 2019 Battery-free, skin-interfaced microfluidic/electronic systems for simultaneous electrochemical, colorimetric, and volumetric analysis of sweat *Sci. Adv.* **5** eaav3294
[148] White N and Turner J 1997 Thick-film sensors: past, present and future *Meas. Sci. Technol.* **8** 1
[149] Laschi S and Mascini M 2006 Planar electrochemical sensors for biomedical applications *Med. Eng. Phys.* **28** 934–43
[150] Wang J and Chen Q 1994 Enzyme microelectrode array strips for glucose and lactate *Anal. Chem.* **66** 1007–11
[151] Higgins I J, Hill H A and Plotkin E V 1985 Sensor for components of a liquid mixture *US Patent* US4545382A
[152] Lam Y-Z L and Atkinson J 2002 Disposable screen-printed biosensor for transcutaneous oxygen measurement *Meas. Sci. Technol.* **13** 2074
[153] Hart J, Pemberton R, Luxton R and Wedge R 1997 Studies towards a disposable screen-printed amperometric biosensor for progesterone *Biosens. Bioelectron.* **12** 1113–21
[154] Bagel O, Degrand C, Limoges B, Joannes M, Azek F and Brossier P 2000 Enzyme affinity assays involving a single-use electrochemical sensor. Applications to the enzyme immunoassay of human chorionic gonadotropin hormone and nucleic acid hybridization of human cytomegalovirus DNA *Electroanalysis* **12** 1447–52
[155] Wang J, Mo J W and Erdem A 2002 Single-use thick-film electrochemical sensor for insulin *Electroanalysis* **14** 1365–8
[156] Darain F, Park S-U and Shim Y-B 2003 Disposable amperometric immunosensor system for rabbit IgG using a conducting polymer modified screen-printed electrode *Biosens. Bioelectron.* **18** 773–80
[157] Dequaire M, Degrand C and Limoges B 2000 An electrochemical metalloimmunoassay based on a colloidal gold label *Anal. Chem.* **72** 5521–8
[158] Wang J, Ibáñez A and Chatrathi M P 2002 Microchip-based amperometric immunoassays using redox tracers *Electrophoresis* **23** 3744–9
[159] Evtugyn G, Mingaleva A, Budnikov H, Stoikova E, Vinter V and Eremin S 2003 Affinity biosensors based on disposable screen-printed electrodes modified with DNA *Anal. Chim. Acta* **479** 125–34

[160] Wang J, Rivas G, Cai X, Palecek E, Nielsen P, Shiraishi H, Dontha N, Luo D, Parrado C and Chicharro M 1997 DNA electrochemical biosensors for environmental monitoring *Anal. Chim. Acta* **347** 1–8

[161] Bergveld P 1996 The future of biosensors *Sensors Actuators* A **56** 65–73

[162] Tvarozek V, Novotny I, Rehacek V, Ivanic R and Mika F 1998 Thin film electrode chips for microelectrochemical sensors *Nexus Res. News* **1** 15–7

[163] Pfeiffer D, Möller B, Klimes N, Szeponik J and Fischer S 1997 Amperometric lactate oxidase catheter for real-time lactate monitoring based on thin film technology *Biosens. Bioelectron.* **12** 539–50

[164] Lakard B, Herlem G, de Labachelerie M, Daniau W, Martin G, Jeannot J-C, Robert L and Fahys B 2004 Miniaturized pH biosensors based on electrochemically modified electrodes with biocompatible polymers *Biosens. Bioelectron.* **19** 595–606

[165] Senillou A, Jaffrezic N, Martelet C and Cosnier S 1999 A laponite clay-poly (pyrrole–pyridinium) matrix for the fabrication of conductimetric microbiosensors *Anal. Chim. Acta* **401** 117–24

[166] Finot E, Bourillot E, Meunier-Prest R, Lacroute Y, Legay G, Cherkaoui-Malki M, Latruffe N, Siri O, Braunstein P and Dereux A 2003 Performance of interdigitated nanoelectrodes for electrochemical DNA biosensor *Ultramicroscopy* **97** 441–9

[167] Van Hal R, Eijkel J and Bergveld P 1995 A novel description of ISFET sensitivity with the buffer capacity and double-layer capacitance as key parameters *Sensors Actuators* B **24** 201–5

[168] Pijanowska D G and Torbicz W 1997 pH-ISFET based urea biosensor *Sensors Actuators* B **44** 370–6

[169] Sergeyeva T, Soldatkin A, Rachkov A, Tereschenko M, Piletsky S and Elskaya A 1999 β-Lactamase label-based potentiometric biosensor for α-2 interferon detection *Anal. Chim. Acta* **390** 73–81

[170] Yang Y, Chen Y, Tang H, Zong N and Jiang X 2020 Microfluidics for biomedical analysis *Small Methods* **4** 1900451

[171] Koo K M, Dey S and Trau M 2018 A sample-to-targeted gene analysis biochip for nanofluidic manipulation of solid-phase circulating tumor nucleic acid amplification in liquid biopsies *ACS Sens.* **3** 2597–603

[172] Pu Z, Wang R, Wu J, Yu H, Xu K and Li D 2016 A flexible electrochemical glucose sensor with composite nanostructured surface of the working electrode *Sensors Actuators* B **230** 801–9

[173] Pu Z, Zou C, Wang R, Lai X, Yu H, Xu K and Li D 2016 A continuous glucose monitoring device by graphene modified electrochemical sensor in microfluidic system *Biomicrofluidics* **10** 011910

[174] Xu J, Xu K, Han Y, Wang D, Li X, Hu T, Yi H and Ni Z 2020 3D porous graphene aerogel@ GOx based microfluidic biosensor for electrochemical glucose detection *Analyst* **145** 5141–7

[175] Cao L, Han G-C, Xiao H, Chen Z and Fang C 2020 A novel 3D paper-based microfluidic electrochemical glucose biosensor based on rGO-TEPA/PB sensitive film *Anal. Chim. Acta* **1096** 34–43

[176] Tang C K, Vaze A, Shen M and Rusling J F 2016 High-throughput electrochemical microfluidic immunoarray for multiplexed detection of cancer biomarker proteins *ACS Sens.* **1** 1036–43

[177] Pursey J P, Chen Y, Stulz E, Park M K and Kongsuphol P 2017 Microfluidic electrochemical multiplex detection of bladder cancer DNA markers *Sensors Actuators* B **251** 34–9

[178] Uliana C V, Peverari C R, Afonso A S, Cominetti M R and Faria R C 2018 Fully disposable microfluidic electrochemical device for detection of estrogen receptor alpha breast cancer biomarker *Biosens. Bioelectron.* **99** 156–62

[179] De Oliveira R A, Nicoliche C Y, Pasqualeti A M, Shimizu F M, Ribeiro I R, Melendez M E, Carvalho A L, Gobbi A L, Faria R C and Lima R S 2018 Low-cost and rapid-production microfluidic electrochemical double-layer capacitors for fast and sensitive breast cancer diagnosis *Anal. Chem.* **90** 12377–84

Chapter 3

UV–visible spectroscopy in biomedical nanotechnology

Syed S Razi, Vivek Kumar Nautiyal and Gaurav Hitkari

In this chapter, we discuss the detailed description of the ultraviolet–visible (UV-Vis) spectroscopy technique and its applications with a special focus on nanotechnology. The UV–Vis technique is one of the most crucial methods for the study of nanomaterials. The optical properties of the materials can unfold the various applications in the biomedical field.

3.1 Introduction

Nanoparticles (NPs) (<100 nm) have a wide surface to volume ratio and contain varying physical and chemical properties [1]. NPs including quantum dots [2], upconverting nanophosphors [3], polymeric [4], metallic, and magnetic [5] have gathered significant attention in several current and emerging fields. A large number of research interests have focused on evaluating their optical, electronic, magnetic, catalytic properties, and applications (biological sensing [6], drug delivery [7], cancer therapy [8], and molecular imaging abilities [9]) have been performed. These applications primarily rely on the shape, size, and synthesis route of the NPs [10]. The requirement of different analytical tools to study metal NPs, metal oxide NPs, and their potential biomedical application has been growing tremendously. Normally, metal NPs and metal oxide NPs are characterized by various techniques like transmission electron microscopy (TEM), scanning electron microscopy (SEM), atomic force microscopy (AFM), dynamic light scattering (DLS), x-ray diffraction (XRD), Fourier transform infrared spectroscopy (FTIR), and ultraviolet–visible spectroscopy (UV–Vis) [11–14]. Each of these techniques has its advantages and disadvantages. It is difficult to compare them, as each of them has a unique purpose and provides specific information. UV–Vis spectroscopy is a facile, simple, sensitive, reliable, and low-cost method among all the mentioned techniques. It can be used for the kinetic study of the catalytic performance of NPs, swelling/deswelling of polymer and hybrid microgels with smaller particle sizes [15, 16]. Photoluminescence spectroscopy is an effective optical method for measuring the electronic structure of materials that is contactless, flexible, and non-destructive [17]. Light is transmitted to a sample, where it is absorbed and imparts excess energy into the material in a process called photo-excitation [17]. One way this excess energy can be dissipated by the sample is through the emission of light, or luminescence. In the case of photoexcitation, this luminescence is called photoluminescence [18]. Thus photoluminescence is the spontaneous emission of light from the material under optical excitation. The intensity and spectral content of this photoluminescence is a direct measure of various important material properties. UV–Vis absorption spectroscopy is the most widely used method for characterizing the optical properties, electronic structure, and determination of band gaps of all types of NPs obtained by various stabilizing agents such as surfactants [19], dendrimers [20] block copolymers [21], and microgels [22]. Catalytic activity and progress of the catalytic reaction can also be studied by using UV–Vis spectroscopy. For example, Espinosa *et al* applied UV–Vis spectroscopy for the evaluation of gold nanoparticles (AuNPs) fabricated with different concentrations of bovine serum albumin (BSA) at different concentrations (0.25, 0.5, 0.75 and 1% M/V), and constant temperature (25 °C) [23]. Volden *et al* studied temperature-dependent optical properties of gold nanoparticles (AuNPs), impregnated P(NIPAM) microgels by UV–Vis spectroscopy [24]. Liu *et al* measured the photocatalytic activity of nanodot-carbon nitride (C_3N_4) catalyst and determine the bandgap energy (2.74–2.77 eV) for water splitting [25]. Haiss *et al* have published a very high profile study on the utility of UV–Vis spectra to determine the size and concentration of Au NPs [26].

Recently, Nwankwo *et al* studied the absorption spectrum, bandgap energy, and photocatalytic degradation study for methyl blue dye (MB) of chemically synthesized rutile TiO_2 by using an advanced version of UV–Vis NIR spectroscopy [27]. Nasrollahzadeh *et al* reported a reduction of 4-nitrophenol on the surface of catalyst Ag/MgO NPs in reducing medium ($NaBH_4$) and monitored the reaction process by UV–Vis spectroscopy [28]. The different parameters of UV–Vis spectroscopy for evaluation and applications are shown in figure 3.1. Moreover, the evaluation of catalytic reactions occurring in the presence of NPs/composite samples and the

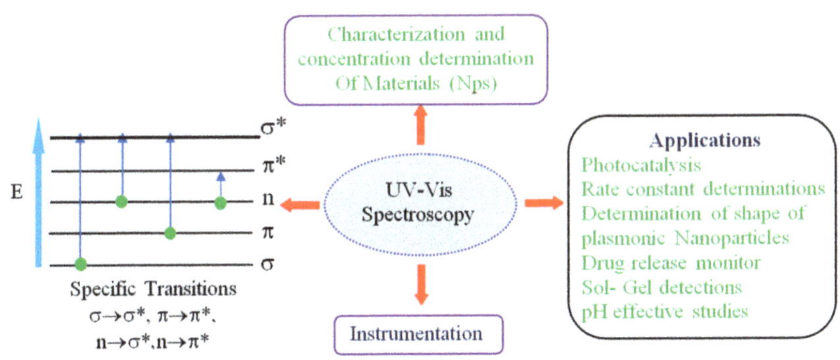

Figure 3.1. Different parameters of UV–Vis spectroscopy.

determination of various kinetic parameters of these catalytic reactions using UV–Vis spectroscopy has also been described in detail [28].

3.1.1 UV–Vis spectroscopy

Light is quantized into tiny packets called photons whose energy can be passed to an electron in the event of a collision. However, only when the photon's energy level is equal to the energy required for the electron to be transferred to the next energy state, e.g., from the ground to the first excitation state. The absorption spectroscopy is based on this principle. UV–Vis spectroscopy is an absorption or reflectance-based analytical technique. It is primarily employed for recognizing functional groups (based on transitions) in organic molecules and most importantly for determining the content and strength of a substance. UV–Vis spectroscopy is frequently used in chemical and biochemical laboratories for the evaluation of nanostructured materials. It can also give very valuable information to determine small quantities like trace metal content in alloys or the small number of assured drugs in various parts of the body. UV–Vis spectroscopy is used in solution or as a solid to obtain the absorption spectra. The UV–Vis energy area for the electromagnetic spectrum covers 1.5–6.2 eV corresponding to a wavelength range of 800–200 nm [29].

3.2 Visible spectrum

The transitions that result in the absorption of electromagnetic radiation in this region of the spectrum occurs often between electronic energy levels (figure 3.2). Generally, the most probable transition is from the highest occupied molecular orbital (HOMO) to the lowest occupied molecular orbital (LUMO). The standard energy difference between the ground and the first excited numbers of several molecules refers to the ultraviolet (UV) electromagnetic waves and visible electromagnetic spectrum regions (figure 3.3).

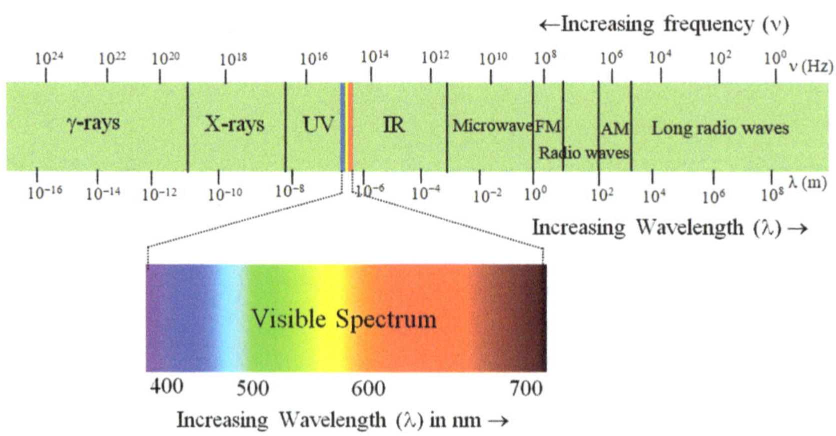

Figure 3.2. The electromagnetic spectrum. Reprinted from [29].

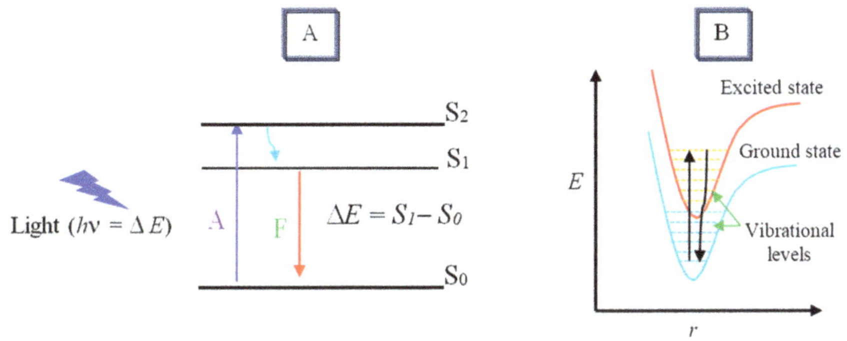

Figure 3.3. (A) Electronic transitions (A = absorption, F = fluorescence). (B) Spectrum of transition.

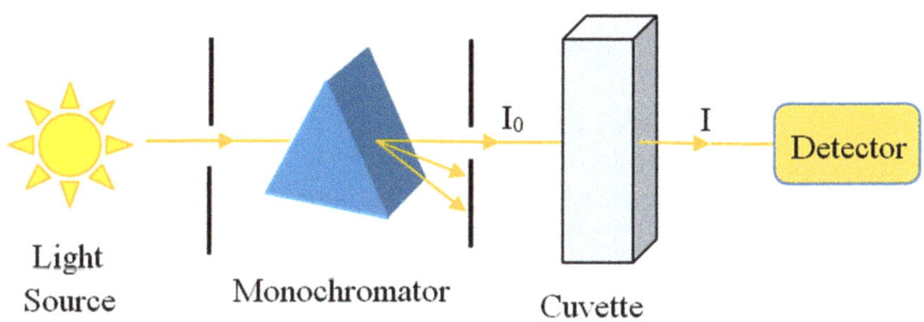

Figure 3.4. Experimental setup for Beer–Lambert law.

3.2.1 Basic principle

The energy of the light transmitted from the sample afterward is measured using a photodetector, which registers the absorbance of the sample. A spectrum is a graphical representation of the amount of light that the object absorbs or transmits as a function of the wavelength.

The absorption of light by molecules in a solution is governed by the Beer–Lambert law (figure 3.4). The following relationship is formed when light with intensity I_0 is directed towards a material and light is transmitted with the intensity I,

$$A = I/I_0 = \varepsilon bc$$

where, I_0 is the intensity of the reference beam and I is the intensity of the sample beam, ε is the molar absorptivity with units of l mol^{-1} cm^{-1}, b = path length of the sample in centimeters and c = concentration of the given solution represented in mol l^{-1} [30].

If the optical path is 1 cm and the target part concentration is 1 mol l^{-1}, the proportionality constant is called the molar absorption coefficient and is represented by the symbol ε. Under other unique conditions, the molar absorption coefficient is a characteristic value of a material. Consequently, absorption spectroscopy is often called 'electronic spectroscopy' in the UV–Vis spectral region. From the magnitude of A (λ), one can obtain information about sample composition or the probability of

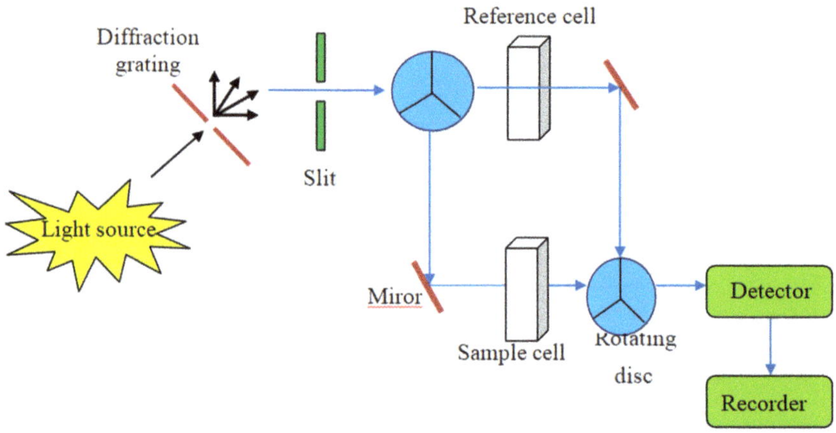

Figure 3.5. Schematic diagram of a double-beam UV–Vis spectrophotometer.

an electronic transition. Depending on the nature of the ground and excited-state orbital's this probability can be very different.

Two primary types of absorbance instruments are used to collect UV–Vis spectra. The first one is a single-beam spectrometer and the second is a double-beam spectrometer. These instruments have a light source (usually a deuterium or tungsten lamp), a sample holder, and a detector. The single-beam instrument has a filter or a monochromator between the source and the sample to analyze one wavelength at a time. The second type of spectrometers is called a double-beam instrument. Along with a light source and a monochromator, they have a beam-splitter and series of mirrors to direct the beam to the reference and the sample to be analyzed. It has a diode array detector that allows the instrument to simultaneously detect the absorbance at all wavelengths. The double-beam instruments are usually faster and more efficient (figure 3.5).

3.3 Instrumentation

The typical UV–Vis spectrophotometer consists of the following components.

1. light sources
2. source of visible radiation
3. the monochromator (wavelength selector)
4. sample cell
5. detectors
6. photomultiplier tube detector
7. the photodiode detector.

3.3.1 Light sources

The source of radiation must be consistent across the spectrum of wavelengths. Light is the key source of UV radiation. It is important to remember that the intensity of the source of the radiation does not suddenly shift across the wavelength spectrum [31]. Deuterium or hydrogen electrical excitation at low pressure results in a continuous UV spectrum. The mechanism behind this involves the formation of an excited molecular species, which splits to give two atomic species and an ultraviolet photon. This can be shown

$$D_2 + \text{ electrical energy} \rightarrow D_2^{*} + D' + D'' + hv$$

Both deuterium and hydrogen lamps can emit radiation in the range of 160–375 nm. Quartz windows and cuvettes must be used as glass absorbs radiation of wavelengths less than 350 nm.

3.3.2 Sources of visible radiation

The tungsten filament lamp is commonly employed as a source of visible light. This type of lamp emits light in the wavelength range of 350–2500 nm [31]. The energy emitted by a tungsten filament lamp is proportional to the fourth power of the operating voltage [31]. This means that for the energy output to be steady the voltage of the lamp should be very stable. Electronic voltage regulators or constant-voltage transformers are often used to ensure this stability.

3.3.3 The monochromator (wavelength selector)

All the monochromatic contain the following components:

- an entrance slit
- a collimating lens
- a dispersing device (usually a prism or a grating)
- a focusing lens
- an exit slit.

Polychromatic radiation (radiation of more than one wavelength) enters the monochromator chamber through the entrance slit. The beam is collimated and then strikes the dispersing element at an angle. The beam is decomposed into its component wavelengths by a grating or prism. By moving the dispersing element or the exit slit, radiation of only a particular wavelength leaves the monochromator through the exit slit [31].

3.3.4 Sample cell

The containers for the sample and reference solution must be transparent to the radiation. Quartz or fused silica cuvettes are required for spectroscopy in the UV region. These are also transparent in the visible region. Silicate glasses can be used for the cuvettes to be used between 350 and 2000 nm [31].

3.3.5 Detectors

The detector converts the light into an electrical signal. It should give a linear response over a wide range of low noise and high sensitivity. These are of two types

1. photomultiplier tube detector
2. photodiode detector.

3.3.6 Photomultiplier tube detector

The photomultiplier tube is a commonly used detector in UV–Vis spectroscopy. It consists of a photoemissive cathode (emits electrons upon excitation) and anodes (emits electrons for each electron striking them). A photon of radiation entering the tube strikes the cathode, causing the emission of several electrons. These electrons are accelerated towards the first anode (which is 90 V more positive than the cathode). The electrons strike the first anode, causing the emission of several electrons for each incident electron. These electrons are then accelerated towards the second anode, to produce more electrons which are accelerated towards the last anode. The electrons are collected at the anode. By this time, each original photon has produced 10^6–10^7 electrons. The resulting current is amplified and measured. Photomultipliers are very sensitive to UV–Vis radiation. They have a fast response time. However, strong light can damage photomultipliers. Therefore, they are limited to measuring low power radiation [31].

3.3.7 The photodiode detector

This is an example of a multichannel photon detector. These detectors are capable of measuring all the elements of a beam of dispersed radiation simultaneously. A linear photodiode array comprises many small silicon photodiodes over a single silicon chip. There can be any number between 64 and 4096 but the most common is 1024 photodiodes [31]. For each diode, there is also a storage capacitor and a switch. The individual diode–capacitor circuits can be sequentially scanned. During use, the photodiode array is positioned at the focal plane of the monochromator (after the dispersing element) in a manner that the spectrum falls on the diode array. They are useful for recording UV–Vis absorption spectra of samples that are rapidly passing through a sample flow cell, such as in an HPLC (high-performance liquid chromatography) detector [31].

3.4 Applications of UV–Vis spectroscopy

Nanomaterials are very useful due to their unique properties and have the potential to be employed in the field of biomedical sciences for different applications [32]. They have a wide range of applicability in improving human life and its environment. Nanoparticles of Au, Ag, and Pt, etc are mainly used in products which directly come in contact with our bodies like soaps, detergent, shoes, cosmetic products, shampoo, and toothpaste alongside medical and pharmaceutical applications [33]. These nanostructure materials can network with the living cells and are very useful in pharmaceuticals. Precisely they can be used to study the interaction of various antitumor drugs with living tissues, the detection of genes that are closely related to some types of cancer, as well as the detection of protein biomarkers for diseases [34]. The synthesis of ultrafine nanomaterial and their characterization using UV–Vis spectroscopy plays an essential role in biomedical application. Currently, many nanomaterials are reported which are characterized by using UV–Vis and use for various diseases in the medical field. It helps to understand the interaction mechanism on nanoparticles with the biomolecules for possible drug delivery applications.

3.4.1 Interaction of ZnO nanoparticles with sucrose and honey molecules for biomedical applications

Due to their unique properties nanoparticles are at the forefront of research in different fields ranging from optoelectronics to medical technology [35]. A large amount of research has been undertaken to find a unique way by which the drugs can be attached to the nanoparticles for precise delivery and targeting [36]. Before that, it is very important to understand the interaction of nanoparticles with blood, plasma, and other biological cells. It is also essential to understand the interaction of nanoparticles with the absorbed sucrose in the cell [36]. Samanta *et al* synthesized ultrafine ZnO nanoparticle and observed the interaction ZnO nanoparticle with sucrose and honey sugar with the help of UV–Vis spectroscopy [37]. The crystallite size of the ZnO nanoparticle was 38 nm, which interacts with sucrose and honey molecules and develops a corona. This study shows that how UV–Vis spectroscopy can be useful to understand the interaction mechanism of nanoparticles with the biomolecules for possible drug delivery applications.

3.4.2 Preparation of aluminum oxide nanoparticles by laser ablation and a study of their applications as antibacterial and wound healing agents

Aluminum oxide commonly exists in three forms, of which Al_2O_3 is commonly used in different applications [38, 39]. Jwad *et al* synthesized aluminum oxide by using liquid particles with the help of laser technology for medical applications such as antibacterial and for stimulation wound healing. Further, they tested the antimicrobial activity of synthesized Al_2O_3 nanoparticles by a well diffusion method against three types of bacteria: *Escherichia coli*, *Pseudomonas aeruginosa*, and *Staphylococcus aureus*. They concluded that aluminum oxide nanoparticles have antioxidant effects and can be useful in wound healing activity [40].

3.4.3 Silver nanoparticles for biomedical application using green synthesis

The preparation of metal nanoparticles (Ag, Au, Pt, etc) by the reduction of the biological compounds is an eco-friendly, cost-effective, and potentially applicable approach [41]. Silver nanoparticles (AgNPs) have worthy antimicrobial and anticancerous activities that can be used for air purifiers, imaging, sensors, and textiles. It is also used for disease diagnostics and drug delivery treatments [42, 43]. The biomolecules present in plant extracts have a significant role in nanoparticle synthesis [44]. The synthesis of nanoparticles through a green method is a good approach as it is free from chemical use. Sathiyamoorthi *et al* prepared the silver nanoparticle using gallnut extract and explored its biomedical applications. The absorption spectra of UV–Vis absorption spectrum depends on many factors including shape, size, and contact between particles. Gallnut-extract-synthesized AgNPs are confirmed by UV–Vis spectroscopy at different pH values showed characteristic UV–Vis absorption spectra at 428 nm. The biosynthesized

Ag-nanoparticle prepared from gallnut extract demonstrated 81% more antioxidant activity than chemically prepared Ag-nanoparticles using sodium borohydride. AgNPs prepared in this way can play an important role in the antioxidant function and have been shown to have powerful anticancer activity on cervical cancer lines such as ME180, SiHa, HeLa, and CaSki [45].

3.4.4 Synthesis of gold nanoparticles using the green approach for biomedical applications

Among the metal nanoparticles, AuNPs have attracted lots of attention because of their applications in catalysis, biosensors, bio-imaging, and drug delivery and are also applicable in the treatment of certain cancers [12, 14, 32–35]. AuNPs have some inimitable optical properties due to the free-electron oscillation of the surface plasmon [46]. AuNPs are used as immuno staining indicator particles for electron microscopy, and as chromophores for immuno reactions and nucleic acid hybridization in the field of biomedical sciences [47–50]. It is also used as marker proteins or DNA for recognition of biological targets with improved sensitivity and primarily utilized in imaging, and molecular diagnostic applications [51]. First-time Dhanasekar *et al* have reported that the AuNPs (isotropic and anisotropic) synthesis using the culture filtrate of the filamentous fungus *Alternaria* species by non-toxic and non-hazardous green synthesis [52]. The gold ions were reduced to Au^0, which lead to the formation of stable gold nanoparticles of different shapes and sizes. UV–Vis absorption spectroscopy is one of the most commonly used methods for characterizing the optical properties and electronic structure of nanoparticles, as the absorption bands are related to the diameter and aspect ratio of metal nanoparticles. AuNPs were prepared by both chemical and biosynthetic methods, and the changes in the UV–Vis spectra of the resultant colloids were measured to study the size effect of metal nanoparticles on the surface plasmon resonance [53]. The formation of AuNPs was confirmed by the UV–Vis spectroscopy by a decrease of Au^{3+} to Au^0 [52]. Spectroscopic analysis forms a basic and ideal technique to understand the optical properties of metal nanoparticles. The change in color was observed in the narrowed flask which contains the $AuCl_3$ (gold chloride) solution.

3.5 Conclusions

UV–Vis spectroscopy is one of the most useful techniques to extract the necessary information from the nanoparticles. All the materials have distinct properties of absorbance. The varying degrees of absorbance can help to identify the optical properties of materials for different applications. The UV–Vis technique is the preferred method to estimate the bandgap of organic or semiconductor nanomaterials. During the synthesis of appropriate nanostructures/nanocomposites for biomedical purposes, UV–Vis spectroscopy plays a very effective and significant role as a characterization technique. In the modern era, UV–Vis spectroscopy is more challenging and beneficial in some specific studies like examining structural protein changes and estimating battery composition, both of which can benefit from tracking changes in the wavelength corresponding to the peak absorbance. Shifts in peak absorbance wavelengths can also help with more current applications and characterization of very small nanoparticles. This approach has a wide range of applications that appear to be limitless.

Acknowledgment

Author (SSR) thankfully acknowledges financial support from University grant commission, New Delhi, Government of India through its UGC-BSR Research Start-Up-Grant award (No. F.30440/2018(BSR)).

References

[1] Cobley C M, Chen J, Cho E C, Wang L V and Xia Y 2011 Gold nanostructures: a class of multifunctional materials for biomedical applications *Chem. Soc. Rev.* **40** 44–56

[2] Michalet X, Pinaud F F, Bentolila L A, Tsay J M, Doose S, Li J J, Sundaresan G, Wu A M, Gambhir S S and Weiss S 2005 Quantum dots for live cells, *in vivo* imaging, and diagnostics *Science* **307** 538–44

[3] Liu X and Swihart M T 2014 Heavily-doped colloidal semiconductor and metal oxide nanocrystals: an emerging new class of plasmonic nanomaterials *Chem. Soc. Rev.* **43** 3908–20

[4] Trofymchuk K, Reisch A, Shulov I, Mély Y and Klymchenko A S 2014 Tuning the color and photostability of perylenediimides inside polymer nanoparticles: towards biodegradable substitutes of quantum dots *Nanoscale* **6** 12934–42

[5] Kim J *et al* 2006 Designed fabrication of multifunctional magnetic gold nanoshells and their application to magnetic resonance imaging and photothermal therapy *Angew. Chem. Int. Ed.* **45** 7754–8

[6] Li Y, Jing C, Zhang L and Long Y-T 2012 Resonance scattering particles as biological nanosensors *in vitro* and *in vivo Chem. Soc. Rev.* **41** 632–42

[7] Dreher M R, Liu W G, Michelich C R, Dewhirst M W, Yuan F and Chilkoti A 2006 Tumor vascular permeability, accumulation, and penetration of macromolecular drug carriers *J. Natl. Cancer Inst* **98** 335–44

[8] Bardhan R, LaL S, Joshi A and Halas N J 2011 Theranosticnanoshells: from probe design to imaging and treatment of cancer *Acc. Chem. Res.* **44** 936–46

[9] Louie A Y 2010 Multimodality imaging probes: design and challenges *Chem. Rev.* **110** 3146–95

[10] Hong Y N, Lam J W Y and Tang B Z 2011 *Chem. Soc. Rev.* **40** 5361–88

[11] Haldar K K, Kundu S and Patra A 2014 Core-size-dependent catalytic properties of bimetallic Au/Ag core–shell nanoparticles *ACS Appl. Mater. Interfaces* **6** 21946–53

[12] Jiang N, Zhuo X and Wang J 2018 Active plasmonics: principles, structures, and applications *Chem. Rev.* **118** 3054–99

[13] Moehrke J and Vana P 2015 Termination kinetics of surface-initiated radical polymerization measured by time-resolved ESR spectroscopy after laser-pulse initiation *Macromolecules* **48** 3190–6

[14] Chaudhuri R G and Paria S 2012 Core/shell nanoparticles: classes, properties, synthesis mechanisms, characterization, and applications *Chem. Rev.* **112** 2373–433

[15] Wang Q, Zhao Y, Xu H, Yang X and Yang Y 2009 Thermosensitive phase transition kinetics of poly(*N*-isopropylacryl amide-co-acrylamide) microgel aqueous dispersions *J. Appl. Polym. Sci.* **113** 321–6

[16] Tanaka T and Fillmore D J 1979 Kinetics of swelling of gels *J. Chem. Phys.* **70** 1214

[17] Swinehart D F 1962 The Beer–Lambert law *J. Chem. Educ.* **39** 333

[18] Chan G C-Y and Chan W T 2001 Beer's law measurements using non-monochromatic light sources—a computer simulation *J. Chem. Educ.* **78** 1285

[19] Pandey G, Dixit S and Shrivastava A 2014 Role of additives; sodium dodecyl sulphate and manganese chloride on morphology of $Zn_{1-x}Mn_xO$ nanoparticles and their photoluminescence properties *Mater. Chem. Phys.* **147** 423–32

[20] Niu Y and Crooks R M 2003 Dendrimer-encapsulated metal nanoparticles and their applications to catalysis *C. R. Chim.* **6** 1049–59

[21] Kumar D, Kumar P and Pandey J 2018 Binary grafted chitosan film: synthesis, characterization, antibacterial activity and prospects for food packaging *Int. J. Biol. Macromol* **115** 341–8

[22] Chen G Y, Qiu H, Prasad P N and Chen X 2014 Upconversion nanoparticles: design, nanochemistry, and applications in theranostics *Chem. Rev.* **114** 5161–214

[23] Espinosa J C M, Ramírez N A C, Oliva L E F, Fraga T C, Alvarado J B, Pablo A R and Anita R E N 2014 Coating of gold nanoparticles for medical application: UV–Vis *AIP Conf. Proc.* **1626** 147–50

[24] Volden S, Eilertsen J L, Singh G, Wang W, Zhu K, Nyström B and Glomm W R 2012 Effect of charge density matching on the temperature response of PNIPAAM block copolymer–gold nanoparticles *J. Phys. Chem.* C **116** 12844–53

[25] Liu J, Liu Y, Liu N, Han Y, Zhang X, Huang H, Lifshitz Y, Lee S-T, Zhong J and Kang Z 2015 Metal-free efficient photocatalyst for stable visible water splitting via a two-electron pathway *Science* **347** 970–74

[26] Haiss W, Thanh N T, Aveyard J and Fernig D G 2007 Determination of size and concentration of gold nanoparticles from UV–vis spectra *Anal. Chem.* **79** 4215–21

[27] Appasamy J S, Kurnia J C and Assadi M K 2020 Synthesis and evaluation of nitrogen-doped titanium dioxide/single walled carbon nanotube-based hydrophilic self-cleaning coating layer for solar photovoltaic panel surface *Sol. Energy* **196** 80–91

[28] Nasrollahzadeh M, Akbari R, Issaabadi Z and Sajadi S M 2020 Biosynthesis and characterization of Ag/MgO nanocomposite and its catalytic performance in the rapid treatment of environmental contaminants *Ceram. Int.* **46** 2093–101

[29] Picollo M, Aceto M and Vitorino T 2018 UV–Vis spectroscopy *Phy. Sci. Rev.* **4** 20180008

[30] Levinson R 2001 *More Modern Chemical Techniques* (London: Royal Society of Chemistry)

[31] Atkins P W and de Paula J 2013 *Physikalische Chemie* 5th edn (Weinheim: Wiley-VCH)

[32] Dreaden E C, Alkilany A M, Huang X H, Murphy C J and El-Sayed M A 2012 The golden age: gold nanoparticles for biomedicine *Chem. Soc. Rev.* **41** 2740–79

[33] Jain P K, Huang X, El-Sayed I H and El-Sayed M A 2008 Noble metals on the nanoscale: optical and photothermal properties and some applications in imaging, sensing, biology, and medicine *Acc. Chem. Res.* **41** 1578–86

[34] Zhou J, Liu Z and Li F Y 2012 Upconversion nanophosphors for small-animal imaging *Chem. Soc. Rev.* **41** 1323–49

[35] Xu Z C, Hou Y L and Sun S H 2007 Magnetic core/shell Fe_3O_4/Au and Fe_3O_4/Au/Ag nanoparticles with tunable plasmonic properties *J. Am. Chem. Soc.* **129** 8698–9

[36] Howes P D, Rana S and Stevens M M 2014 Plasmonic nanomaterials for biodiagnostics *Chem. Soc. Rev.* **43** 3835–53

[37] Samanta P K, Kamilya T and Pahari D 2019 Study of time-dependent interaction of ZnO nanoparticles with sucrose and honey molecules for biomedical applications *Curr. Nanomater.* **4** 216–22
[38] Ueda W, Sadakane M and Ogihara H 2008 Nano-structuring of complex metal oxides for catalytic oxidation *Catal. Today* **132** 2–8
[39] Pria P D 2007 Evolution and new application of the alumina ceramics in joint replacement *Eur. J. Orthop. Surg. Traumatol.* **17** 253–6
[40] Jwad K H, Saleh T H and Abd-Alhamza B 2019 Preparation of aluminum oxide nanoparticles by laser ablation and a study of their applications as antibacterial and wounds healing agent *Nanobiomed. Eng* **11** 313–19
[41] Salunke B K, Sawant S S and Kim B S 2016 Enhancement of antibacterial effect by biosynthesized silver nanoparticles with antibiotics *J. Nanosci. Nanotechnol.* **16** 7191–4
[42] Salunke B K, Sathiyamoorthi E, Tran T K and Kim B S 2017 Phyto-synthesized silver nanoparticles for biological applications *Korean J. Chem. Eng.* **34** 943–51
[43] Dar M A, Ingle A and Rai M 2013 Enhanced antimicrobial activity of silver nanoparticles synthesized by *Cryphonectria* sp. evaluated singly and in combination with antibiotics *Nanomedicine* **9** 105–10
[44] Song J Y and Kim B S 2009 Rapid biological synthesis of silver nanoparticles using plant leaf extracts *Bioprocess Biosyst. Eng.* **32** 79–84
[45] Sathiyamoorthi E, Iskandarani B, Salunke B K and Kim B S 2018 Biomedical potential of silver nanoparticles biosynthesized using gallnut extract *Green Mater.* **6** 48–57
[46] Anker J N, Hall W P, Lyandres O, Shan N C, Zhao J and Van Duyne R P 2008 Biosensing with plasmonic nanosensors *Nat. Mater.* **7** 442–53
[47] Tian Z Q, Ren B and Wu D Y 2002 Surface-enhanced Raman scattering: from noble to transition metals and from rough surfaces to ordered nanostructures *J. Phys. Chem.* B **106** 9463–83
[48] Kamat P V 2002 Photophysical, photochemical and photocatalytic aspects of metal nanoparticles *J. Phys. Chem.* B **106** 7729–44
[49] Shipway A N, Eugenii K and Itamar W 2000 Nanoparticle arrays on surfaces for electronic, optical, and sensor applications *Chem. Phys. Chem.* **1** 18–52
[50] Mirkin C A, Letsinger R L, Mucic R C and Storhoff J J 1996 A DNA-based method for rationally assembling nanoparticles into macroscopic materials *Nature* **382** 607–9
[51] Wilson R 2008 The use of gold nanoparticles in diagnostics and detection *Chem. Soc. Rev.* **37** 2028–45
[52] Dhanasekar N N, Rahul G R, Narayanan K B, Raman G and Sakthivel N 2015 Green chemistry approach for the synthesis of gold nanoparticles using the fungus *Alternaria* sp *J. Microbiol. Biotechnol.* **25** 1129–35
[53] Abdelhalim M A K, Mady M M and Ghannam M M 2012 Physical properties of different gold nanoparticles: ultraviolet–visible and fluorescence measurements *J. Nanomed. Nanotechol* **3** 3

Chapter 4

FTIR spectroscopy and microscopy in biomedical nanotechnology

Yash Thakare, Swapnil Dharaskar and Ritesh Palkar

Fourier transform infrared (FTIR) spectroscopy is one of the promising functional characterization tools used to confirm the available functional groups, drug functional characterization in pharmaceutical science, materials' characterization, tissues analysis including functional and morphological assessment, and confirmation of bindings between two active moieties. This approach is one of the potential methods to develop efficient optical sensors to detect a target analytic selectively. This chapter will cover the fundamental understanding of FTIR along with advanced biomedical applications.

4.1 Introduction

Human life has always been lived on the edge of a precipice. Thus the supervision of human health has been of major importance through the ages. It is one of the most crucial factors influencing the overall growth of a human being. Technological developments have led the way in the astonishing changes in the health sector, saving numerous patients and also ceaselessly enriching the quality of life. It is now known that as we move ahead into the era of technology, the number of benefits would rise. This is exactly where the concept of nanotechnology comes into the picture.

Nanotechnology is being referred as the most useful experimental technology in the 21st century providing immense opportunities in each discipline (Singh 2014). Indeed, figure 4.1 highlights the applications of nanotechnology in various fields. Nanotechnology has several definitions however, all the definitions focus on the development and design of bottom-up nanostructured materials that provide specific responses when they are exposed to definite stimuli. Nanotechnologies range from 10^{-9} m to 10^{-7} m in linear dimension (1–100 nm). For a perception of the size they are 80 million times smaller than an apple and 5 million times smaller than an ant. The idiosyncratic properties which are difficult for the bulk material to manifest are

doi:10.1088/978-0-7503-3379-5ch4

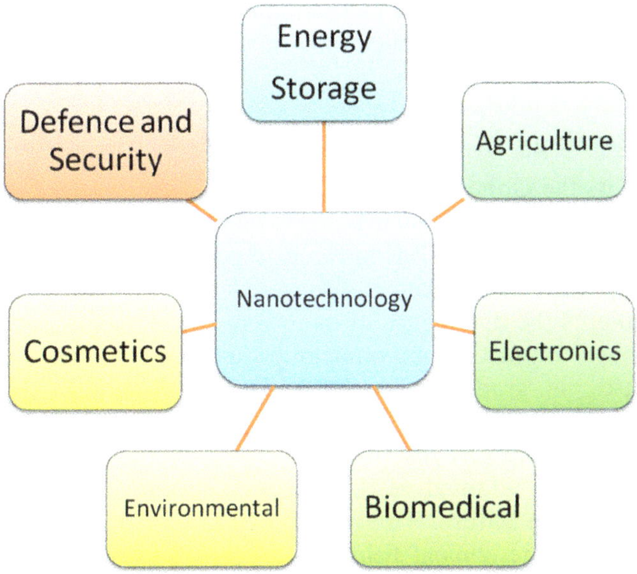

Figure 4.1. Application of nanotechnology in various fields.

the ability to achieve multiple functions from a single platform. It allows biologic barriers to be overcome that in the past restricted medical efforts for therapy and diagnosis (Pope-Harman *et al* 2007). Nanotechnology can permit the localization of therapeutic interruption to diseased areas inside the body and better control over temporal variables. Nanotechnology is thus a way to looking for transformation in biomedical sectors providing more sensitive and specific imaging techniques, nano-robotics (Gorjikhah *et al* 2016) and nano-devices for advanced detection of targeted and less toxic drug treatments, biochemical changes, tissue implantation as well as enhanced support for regenerative medicine thereby offering valuable and rewarding advantages to healthcare workers, patients, and society (Nalwa 2014). Thus biomedical nanotechnology is devoted to the exploration of nanotechnology for healthcare eventually attaining the goal of personalized health management thereby providing doctors and scientists with abilities they might never have dreamt of.

Despite the tremendous boons biomedical nanotechnology holds for healthcare, there is concern about its safety and the possibility of harmful effects (Polizu *et al* 2006). The apprehension that nanotechnology may have serious health and environmental risks has disrupted the field for many years (Ramos *et al* 2017). There was a huge need to develop methods to characterize nanomaterials in order to monitor the health and environmental hazard possessed by the nanotechnology since there is a lack of consensus about the morphology, size of the particle, surface charge after their interaction with the tissues and correlations with toxicity (Kaushik 2019). Thus, sophisticated instruments such as Fourier transform infrared (FTIR), scanning electron microscope (SEM), transmission electron microscope (TEM), x-ray diffraction (XRD) etc came into the limelight, which allowed evaluation of the nano-biomaterials and their interfaces (Saji *et al* 2010).

Thus this chapter will specifically focus on the FTIR characterization technique in detail along with its use and applications in various biomedical nanotechnology fields.

4.2 Nanotechnology in biomedical science

Researchers across the globe have discovered the significance of nanotechnology in the field of biological science. Thus with the evolution in nanotechnology, numerous research is being carried out in various areas especially in the biomedical field and many novel applications are being discovered day by day (Leso *et al* 2019). Figure 4.2 highlights the divergence of nanotechnology from its origin.

It has also been found that nanomachines and nanomaterials can be used for detecting disease, its grade and state and also the bio-molecular reactions. Nanosensors can also be employed to acquire biochemical reactions and processes taking place in the cell at any instant in time with the help of an image or video. Nanoparticles are also adopted as drug delivery agents targeting specific tissues being more selective in nature. Thus the breakthroughs of nanotechnology have paved the way from the clinical field with improvements in nanocoating, nano-fabrication and many more molecular nanotechnologies which helps in the

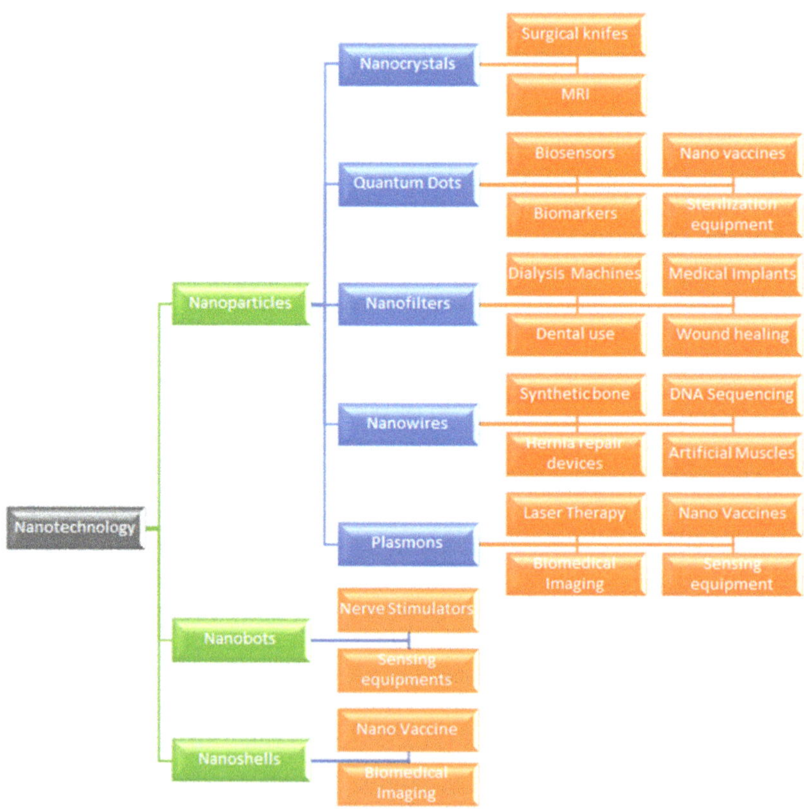

Figure 4.2. Divergence of nanotechnology from its origin.

management, detection, study, and treatment of numerous diseases (Whitman *et al* 2008). Treatment of these diseases incorporates the modification of the cellular activities, repair of the biological tissues and the substitution of diseased tissues with healthy tissue. Nanotechnology can also be used in the field of corrective surgery, termed nanosurgery, and also has potential in the field of regenerative medicines.

4.3 Methods of FTIR spectroscopy and microscopy

Depending on the type or amount of the sample to be examined, various methods of analysis by FTIR microscopy and spectroscopy is achieved and this is shown in figure 4.3.

4.3.1 FTIR spectroscopy

When the sample is irradiated with infrared radiation, FTIR scrutiny of the sample is carried out and results in more sensitive and accurate results. The samples to be

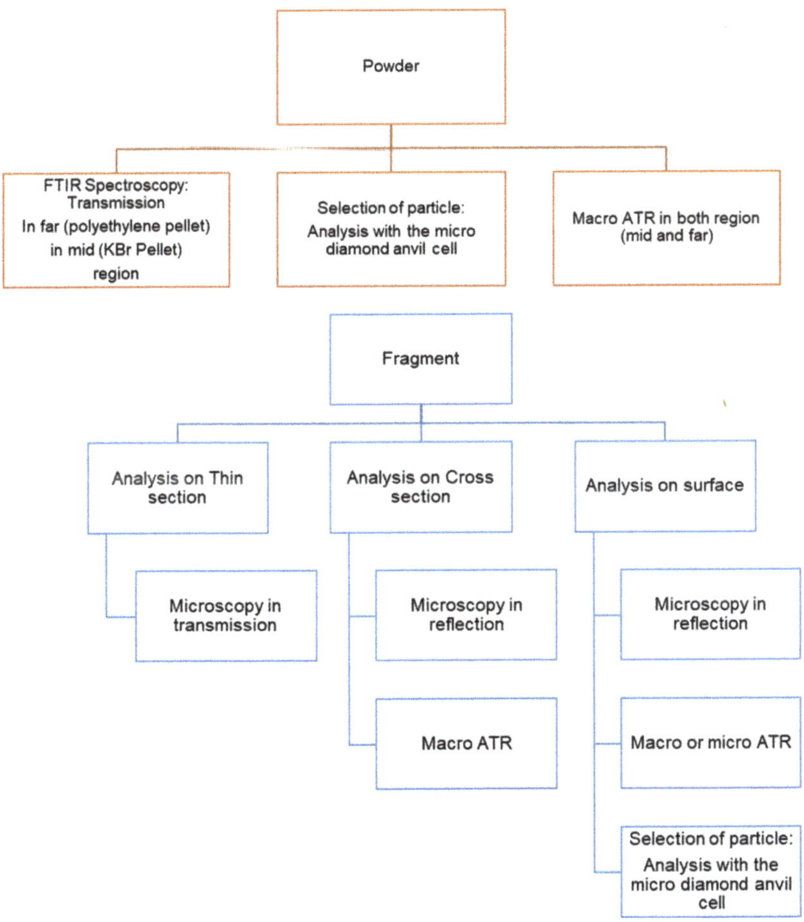

Figure 4.3. Several ways of analysis by FTIR spectroscopy and microscopy.

inspected are formulated as very fine and narrow films in between the infrared crystal clear aperture and are disseminated in the inactive infrared powdered substance whereas the non-transparent samples are just inspected in reflectance without any formulation (Prati *et al* 2010).

The principle for this technique is that whenever the radiation is passed through two separate media, the radiation is split into dissimilar fractions in transmitted and reflected beams based on the ratio of refractive index of two different materials. When the inspected surface of the sample is not reflecting completely there is the existence of scattering, refraction and dispersed reflection which results in the difficulty of elucidating the spectra thus macro attenuated total reflection (ATR) is used to acquire a spectra similar to that of the spectra acquired in the transmission. The sample to be examined is placed in proximity with a crystal also known as internal reflection element (IRE) having more refractive index than that of the sample, so when the radiation irradiates the crystal and passes to the sample at critical angle, the total reflection is generated but then the angle of incidence is more than that of the critical angle, the result is attenuated in which a disappearing wave is produced on the surface of the crystal which is capable of penetrating the sample.

4.3.2 FTIR microscopy

The instrument being used for the FTIR microscopy is a FTIR microscope which is a combination of an optical microscope and a FTIR spectrometer. The most critical component of this method is the spatial resolution of the microscope in order to characterize the tiny and nanoparticles or the fine and narrow layers (Prati *et al* 2010). In order to obtain good signal-to-noise ratio (S/N ratio) a minimum of a 20×20 μm infrared beam opening is required in the case of a single element mercury cadmium telluride (MCT) detector. In this technique the diamond anvil cell, an easy device which is mounted directly on the FTIR microscope stage is used for the analysis of micro or nanoparticles. The micro ATR technique is diversely utilized in this microscopy since it permits the scrutiny of narrow areas keeping the aperture constant due to the magnification element present in the internal reflection element.

Due to the enhanced potential of FTIR microscopy with the development of imaging techniques, enormous FTIR spectra are being accumulated and it also enables the collection of the patterns that shows the distribution of various compounds. A FTIR microscope incorporated with the combination of FTIR spectrometer and the microscope is the advance in this technique which is capable of enhancing the spatial resolution of the system thereby maintaining an adequate standard of spectra. This technique also provides more energy in comparison to that of the traditional techniques being used.

4.4 FTIR spectroscopy in biomedical applications

4.4.1 Cancer study, diagnosis, and treatment

Cancer is one of the primary diseases responsible for many deaths and occurs extensively across the globe. Worldwide nearly one in three individuals are diagnosed with cancer in their lifetime and one in six die as a result of cancer.

The primary objective in cancer research is to innovate a rapid, accurate, and economical technique for the detection of cancer in order to increase the likelihood of survival. Cancer is a stepwise disease that counts in the existence of epigenetic disparity in susceptible cells and addition of absolute as well as transmittable genetic irregularities as the first event and second event being the modification of the biomolecules in both molecular structure aspects and composition. It also takes into account an array of mutations and also alters the response to the microenvironment of the cell, seizure of the responses of the hosts immune and metastasis cancer cell phenotypes that eventually add to chemotherapy. Methods of vibrational spectroscopy that are sensitive to the chemical alteration at molecular scale are employed to detect the presence of cancer (Yano *et al* 2003).

FTIR has attracted huge interest in cancer research because of its ability to explicate quantitative as well as qualitative data of biochemical content. FTIR spectroscopy, as an efficient technique for the investigation of chemical alteration and the composition at the molecular level, has been adopted to detect carcinomas (Su and Lee 2020). The detection of a disease thus depends on biochemical changes instead of morphological changes in tissues. On the basis of the vibrational transitions obtained from the interaction with the IR light of the chemical bond in the sample, the molecular fingerprint is obtained for the biological samples. This method is indeed capable of early detection of the cancer before the abnormalities are obtained from the morphological studies by detecting biomolecular changes (Kumari *et al* 2018). FTIR microscopy and the spectroscopy techniques are capable of detecting the alteration of the chemical content during carcinogenesis progression. Somewhere in the middle of the 20th century these techniques were marked as highly sensitive, label-free, specific, and non-invasive for the tissues of various types of cancer such as colon, breast, skin, stomach, prostate, ovary, cervix etc. The spectrum of the FTIR for the biological sample is the combination of the absorption bands of all lipids, carbohydrates, nucleic acid and proteins, see figure 4.4 which depicts the general bands of FTIR for the biomolecules but specifically for oral epithelium (Wang and Wang 2021). Recent advances in modifications in the chips of integrators, waveguide, detectors, infrared sources, and software development boost the clinical translation of FTIR technique as a rapid, fruitful, cost effective, and automated diagnostic technique.

Biomarkers are defined as molecular changes that are related to the disease present in the body tissues or fluids that are necessary for diagnosing and screening in order to start clinical interventions rather than studying the morphological changes as in present histopathology methods. FTIR can be used directly for tissue analysis, which not only allows early detection but also enhances the accuracy thereby minimizing the discrepancies in the pathologist's interpretation (Levin and Bhargava 2005).

The leading areas where FTIR spectroscopy can be used:

- Differentiation of mormal and infected tissues in organs (liver, breast, cervix, colon).
- Keeping track of unusual growth of cells in tissues (body fluids and thyroid)
- Contrast between cancer and other pathologic conditions which have similar clinical manifestation (colon cancer and IBD)
- Supervision of the effect of the chemotherapy and the grading of the tumor.

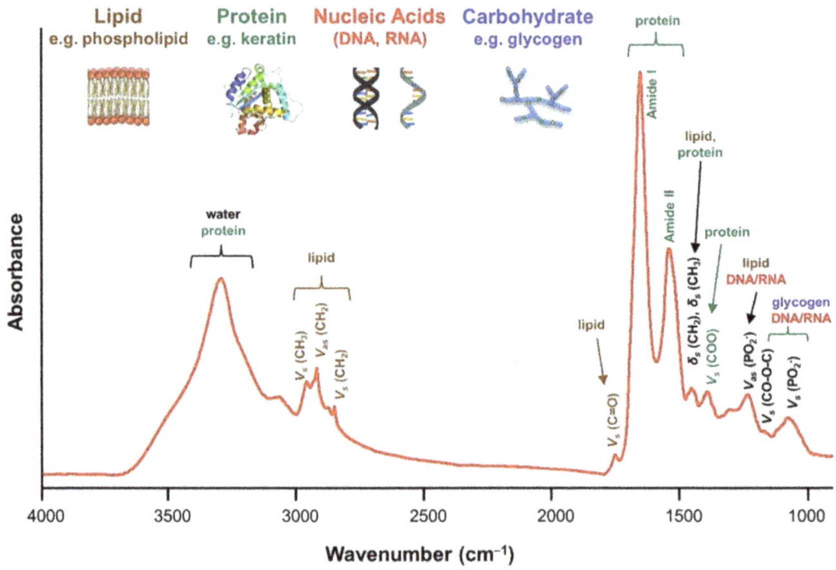

Figure 4.4. Common FTIR bands for biomolecules in oral epithelium. Reproduced from Wang and Wang (2021). CC BY 4.0.

Steps in cancer diagnosis using FTIR spectroscopy:

- Preparation of the sample.
- Collection of the data.
- Analysis of the data.
- Computational methods.
- Prediction or diagnosis.

Diagnosis using FTIR spectroscopy

The dried homogeneous samples (blood components, plasma, body fluids, and whole blood), which are mounted on transparent window materials are used for the collection of the biological sample which is collected by simple IR spectrometers. For frozen, fresh, or fixed tissues, FTIR microscopy is utilized where sections of microtome tissue are present. Colon or cervix-like tissues is easier to estimate since they have zones of proliferation which are defined. Usually, identical tissue sections which are of continuous nature are stained histochemically in order to get a direct comparison between the two methods so as to confirm the diagnosis. Imaging techniques use the data output, thereby allowing huge arrays of spectral quantification with the use of focal plane area detectors (Khanmohammadi *et al* 2011). The details of the spectra obtained for every point is then subjected to numerous mathematical analyses and the information is utilized for the generation of a color code for every point. The intensities of the colors are then reassembled to acquire a pseudo-colored image. In such cases, the malignant tissues have different colors to the normal tissue. Even though this type of examination takes a longer time, it maps the complete area simultaneously, identifying malignancies at each point if any. In the case of microscopic study there are chances of missing a few areas during the

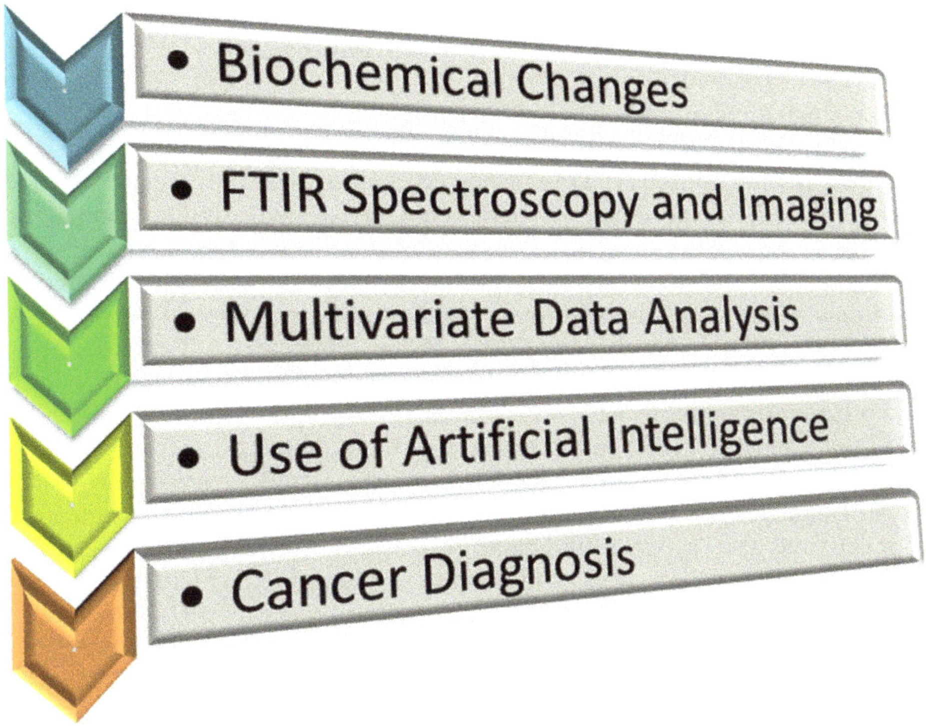

Figure 4.5. The general process for cancer diagnosis.

arbitrary sampling for the cancer. The general process for cancer diagnosis can be viewed in figure 4.5.

Different types of body materials which include tissue, bladder wash, blood, extracellular vesicles septum, urine etc are studied using FTIR spectroscopy in order to develop efficient alternatives for the management and diagnosis of cancer. Since every molecule has its own, unique spectrum which depends on the amount of IR and the wavelength absorbed, FTIR results in the formation of a unique fingerprint of the absorbance peaks of the various parameters that are present in the sample to be examined (Sahu and Mordechai 2005). These biochemical fingerprints are distinguished and are unique for the alteration of molecules in every disease thus provide the exact status for the patient's health.

In order achieve accurate results and distinguish between healthy people and those suffering from cancer, the technique utilized must have high sensitivity, accuracy, and specificity. FTIR spectroscopy does possess all the above characteristics. It has also been discovered that FTIR has the ability to distinguish between cancer and other diseases like hepatitis, heart disease, and many others. It also has applications in the rapid diagnosis of tumors which helps in to assist surgery. It is also found that coupling the ATR-FTIR with optical fiber helps in the evaluation of the surgical resection margin in the colorectal cancer surgery(Li *et al* 2005). FTIR with PCA-LDA helps to detect the difference in the spectrum of a healthy colon and a diseased colon, and cancer in a post- and pre-chemotherapy colon, which means that it is easier to monitor the efficacy of chemotherapy. Additionally, it also defines the tumor margin even of a mono cell of cancer before resectioning which helps to increase the chances of survival of patients.

When attenuated total reflectance Fourier transform infrared (ATR-FTIR) micro-spectroscopy was utilized for colon cancer detection as per the spectral data using the linear discriminate analysis (LDA) technique classification 100% sensitivity, 95.8% accuracy, and 93.1% specificity was achieved. Ovarian cancer is diagnosed by using ATR-FTIR spectroscopy in combination with (GA-LDA) genetic algorithm with linear discriminant analysis and when combined with (PC-DFA) principal component discriminant function analysis, formalin-fixed archival prostate cancer tissues were analyzed (Khanmohammadi *et al* 2007). When FTIR was utilized for the oral, pharyngeal, and laryngeal cancer, biochemical changes in the sputum was detected which was used as a non-invasive way to monitor the progression of the disease. In the case of skin cancer, FTIR spectroscopy is used to differentiate normal samples from those of the melanoma and non-melanoma samples with better accuracy (Menzies *et al* 2014, Shakya *et al* 2020). It has the ability to forecast the drug effectiveness on the tumor cells and also recognize and measure different subpopulations of tumor cells, which a prime factor that can aid fruitful immunotherapy, either with the addition of an antibody or without it. It is also found that high accuracy, up to 97%, is achieved for lung cancer annotation. Accuracy of 95% has also been achieved in the identification of subtypes of the prognostic adenocarcinoma using automated FTIR by reduction of manual errors during spectrum processing and the sample preparation. In general approximately 40 min are required for the pathological examination whereas FTIR only takes up to three minutes for the same evaluation. FTIR spectroscopy also has application in the grading, classification, and staging of cancer wherein up to 100% of specificity and sensitivity is achieved (Andrus and Strickland 1998).

Taken all together, FTIR spectroscopy carries potential to be used as the pioneer clinical technique for the study, diagnosis, and treatment of cancer. Moreover from the many examples and applications discussed in this section, it is proved that this techniques can be used extensively on multiple types of cancer. This indeed offers extreme results for the accuracy, specificity, and sensitivity for cancer detection when compared to the conventional methods being used. In addition, this technique validates the accurate grading, classification, and staging of cancer. When an automated process is used, the need for complex and time consuming processes is also removed. This technique is also employed for the follow up and monitoring of cancer patients. Healthy people can easily be differentiated from those with disease with greater accuracy. Therefore, FTIR spectroscopy is a boon for the transformation in the diagnosis and treatment of cancer.

4.4.2 Nanoscale imaging

Fourier transform infrared spectroscopic imaging and Fourier transform infrared microscopic imaging are comparatively modern techniques which have attracted considerable attention. The leading advantages of these techniques are their high molecular responsiveness in combination with a computative resolution at molecular scale. Another benefit of these techniques is their potential to examine samples under indigenous conditions, due to which it is easy to have insight of the sample without the requirement of stains, additional marker or fixation (Steiner and Koch 2009). This imaging technique is chemical distinct, readily apparent, non-destructive, and label-free with a vast scope for application.

Advances in the field of instrumentation has made FTIR imaging a versatile technique for a wide range of applications. The morphology of various samples can be examined using Fourier transform infrared microscopy imaging. This technique enables us to track down the high resolution spectral images having applications in medical and biochemical fields. High resolution and quantitative data is obtained from the FTIR microscopy which highlights the chemical distribution in the sample. In comparison with conventional histology, FTIR microscopy is particularly quantitative following the principle of Beer–Lambert's law which states that absorbance is directly proportional to the molecular absorbance (Andrew Chan and Kazarian 2016, Kazarian and Chan 2009). Infrared nano-spectroscopy permits innovative potentiality for chemical and structural evaluation of nano-composites, biomaterials, optoelectronic devices and many more. With the evaluation of far FTIR absorbance spectra, the organic material's FTIR spectrum at nanoscale is analyzed thereby permitting the identification and characterization in reference with standard IR data available (Amenabar *et al* 2017).

It is important to follow the proper workflow to obtain the image which helps to proceed further towards diagnosis and treatment, a typical workflow is shown in figure 4.6. Using traditional methods it was not possible to observe the local alteration of biochemical content past discectomy which is now possible with the use of FTIR microscopy. The collagen and proteoglycan content in the IVD is

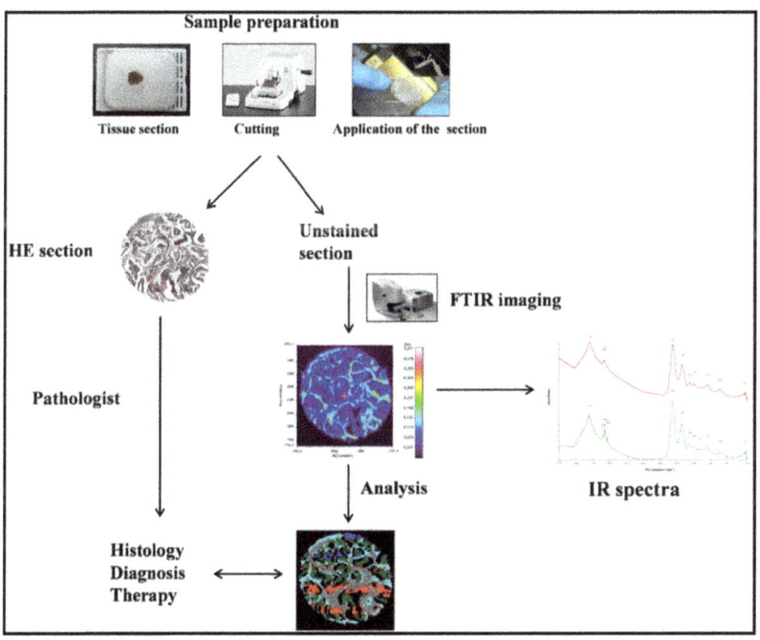

Figure 4.6. Typical workflow of sample preparation, infrared spectroscopic analysis, spectral diagnosis and image building. Reproduced from Pezzei *et al* (2013) with permission of The Royal Society of Chemistry].

quantified and it was found that there is some robust correlation with the Pfirrmann category of degradation (Sloan *et al* 2020). FTIR, a combination of the Fisher discriminant analysis (FDA) and principal component analysis (PCA), was utilized for sample identification of healthy and deteriorated articular cartilage. Imaging of the cartilage and the infrared spectrum of the sample is achieved as the result of FTIR which depicts the concentration of the sample where every pixel is illustrated with false color corresponding to the IR spectrum. Following the strict procedure for sample collection of articular cartilage, the sample was examined thoroughly and the report was generated (Mao *et al* 2015). Results have shown that this technique has an accuracy of approximately 95% and on comparison it was found that the prediction groups were identified accurately.

Tissues of the central nervous system are analyzed in order to understand the structural and biochemical changes linked with the neural degradation diseases including brain tumors, Alzheimer's, transmissible spongiform encephalopathy, Parkinson's, and multiple sclerosis by using this technique in combination with x-ray fluorescence microscopy (XRF) which is indeed a powerful approach for the identification of the chemical composition of a tissue along its trace element distribution. The results obtained are specific, highly accurate, and rapid. Various sections of the central nervous system (CNS) are also comfortably differentiated on the basis of existence or non-existence of myelin as healthy CNS tissue stores a greater amount of myelin in white matter than in gray matter (Caine *et al* 2012).

This practice was extended for the comparison of coronal brain tissue sections of a C6 glioblastoma multiform tumor-bearing rat to sections from a healthy animal by adapting the multiple least square (MLS) fitting procedure for the evaluation of the relative absorbance percentages of pure brain protein, lipid and nucleic acid compounds in FTIR images. The results obtained display the distribution of protein and lipids in the spectroscopic image extracted. Due to the intrinsic packaging property of tissues, augmented dissimilarity was noticed in the IR bright field in comparison with that obtained from the visible microscopic images. The graph of vibrational peak ratio of lipid-protein shows the gradients in the concentration (Levin and Bhargava 2005). Thus it was concluded that this technique is of importance in terms of its adaptability as an insight into the formation of tumors and extending it to the favorable results of numerous therapy processes.

FTIR imaging was further studied for pathological changes in bone by studying the healing process of fractured bones in availability and non-availability of therapy wherein the treated samples had more mineral content per matrix. Even the crystals had enhanced size for the same treated samples and also cellular activities were examined at the place of fracture with the help of fatty acids present in the cell membrane.

In breast implants, which are common for women in the western world, the leakage of silicone gel has become a primary concern. The shells of silicon elastomers being used for the enhancement of the breast are filled with silica gel which can leak from the implant either due to failure of the material or due to damage leading to tissue disorders. In order to evaluate the histopathological difference, the presence of the gel in the tissue is important and would easily be recognized by the FTIR imaging. Thus the chemical difference can be observed between the silicone gel and the tissue and the further treatment can proceed.

FTIR being a highly efficient technique is thus also adopted for application in the field of pharmaceuticals. This is well suited for kinetic study for the dissolution of polymers. Dissolution rate and polymer and solvent diffusion are monitored in this as a function of time with knowledge of the initial conditions. Thus the FTIR image is obtained as a result of the chemical change in the infrared spectra. Since the dissolution, structural properties, and drug release profiles are affected by the various component distributions, the FTIR imaging is also fruitful in this pharmaceutical area.

FTIR is also being applied for the diagnosis and treatment of various diseases in skin tissue, prostate tissue, esophageal tissue, etc. The results obtained have had high accuracy and sensitivity compared with the tradition methods and are rapid. When FTIR-guided LCM (laser capture microdissection) was used, an exemplary potential biomarker in bladder cancer was discovered, as shown in figure 4.7. Thus this

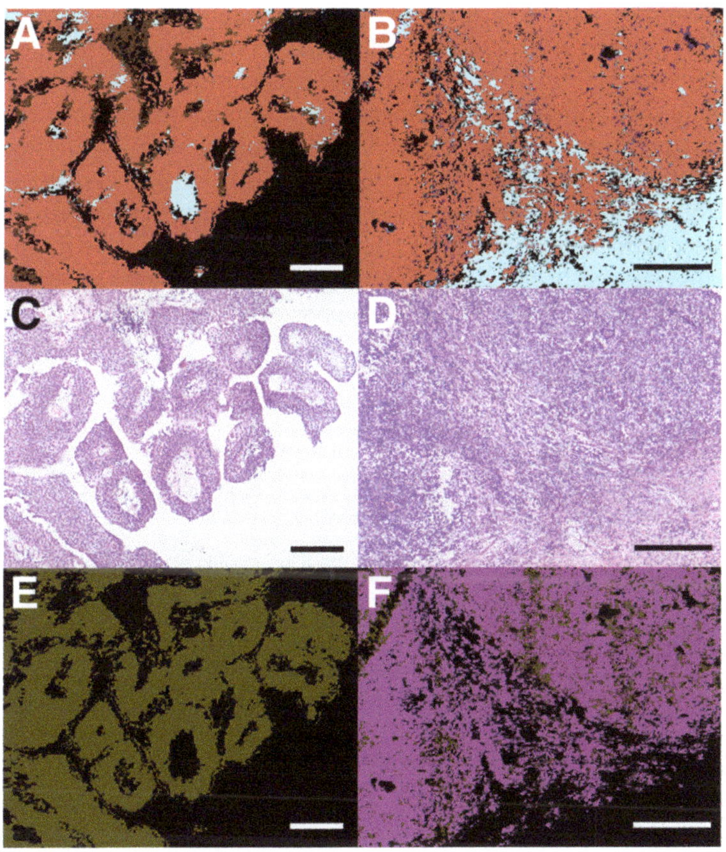

Figure 4.7. Fourier transform infrared (FTIR) imaging index color images obtained label-free before hematoxylin and eosin (H&E) staining of bladder cancer tissue. A and B: low-grade and invasive high-grade carcinoma (red, bladder cancer; cyan, connective tissue; brown, inflammation; purple, urothelial cells). C and D: corresponding H&E staining after FTIR imaging. The label-free classification matches the cancerous regions. E and F: results of the second random forest, which classified the cancer as invasive high-grade (purple) or low-grade (olive) carcinoma. E: no invasive high-grade carcinoma is observed. Scale bars *Z* 200 mm. Reproduced from Witzke *et al* (2019), with permission from Elsevier.

method enabled label-free spatial categorization with great accuracy and no interobserver variability, in addition to the molecular resolution of the proteomic analysis.

4.4.3 Drug release and drug delivery

Explication of the drug release mechanism and assessment of the effectiveness of the drugs in a biological specimen is essential in order to formulate the drug and control its quality. This is affected by numerous factors of synthesis like microstructure polymorphism and the drug delivery system. Proper development and the application of FTIR can be seen in figure 4.8. For the improvement of pharmaceutical tablets, proper knowledge of the tablet mechanism and the drug release process are prerequisites. Thus the application of FTIR imaging and nano-FTIR technique in biological specimens sets a base for proper understanding of the mechanism and process of drug release. Conventional methods of detection are slow, complex, and have less relevance globally, thus FTIR since it has more advantages over conventional techniques is applicable for a wide range of applications specifically in the field of pharmaceuticals for drug release and drug delivery applications (Song *et al* 2020).

In order to study and investigate the dissolution of tablets and the drug release, attenuated total reflection Fourier transform infrared spectroscopy (ATR-FTIR) has been used with the mono reflection accessory of ATR with the crystal of diamond. This allowed *in situ* FTIR imaging of the dissolution of tablets that yield more specificity toward chemicals and also provide spatial resolution at rapid speed.

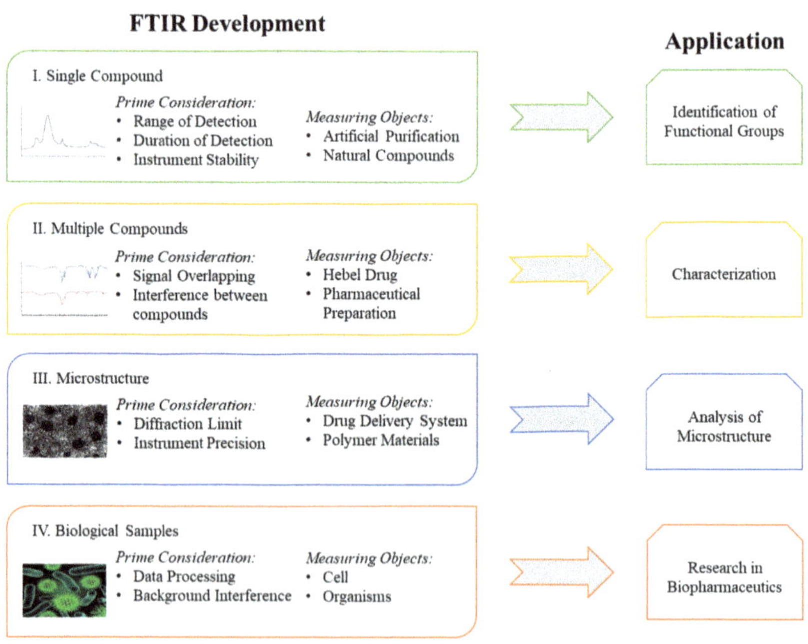

Figure 4.8. FTIR development and its application.

For example, the ATR-FTIR spectroscopic imaging technique was used to study the actions of drugs like ibuprofen and methylprednisolone on dissolution. The advantage of ATR mode is that it requires much less sample preparation whereas in the FTIR it provides information about the functional group present in the sample. Thus the chemical snapshots of the pharmaceutical tablet can be collected as a function of time in order to sort out the profiles of water, drug, and excipient to provide an understanding of drug release after the dissolution of the tablet (Kazarian and Ewing 2013).

Combining the mathematical models with the ATR-FTIR spectroscopic imaging enables a superior prognosis of the drug release and drug delivery thereby improving the particulars of novel systems. Combining ATR-FTIR and nano-FTIR techniques along with the chemometrics becomes a prospective tool for overcoming the inadequacy of traditional IR detection techniques. Nano-FTIR and ATR-FTIR enablesresolution far from the limit of optical diffraction to be acquired and to attain more effectiveness of the drug release mechanism. Structural details of drugs, their characterization and nano-structure scrutiny for can be analyzed in great detail using the FTIR technique. FTIR is used for the characterization of nanoparticles synthesized for anti-HIV drug delivery application. It shows well resolved peaks (Dev *et al* 2010). Peaks shown at various wavelength ranges represent the presence of various chemical bonds or linkage and some peaks are also the result of the interaction between the drug and the polymer.

The innovative approach of surface enhanced ATR-FTIR spectroscopy will permit recognition of the materials even at minute concentrations of the sample which would make it possible to study the nanoparticles for the drug delivery applications and will also feature the manifestation of drug particles which are nano-crystalline in nature. Further growth is based on ATR-FTIR (Tian *et al* 2016) imaging in microfluidic devices for the study of fluid flows. The primary benefit of using this combination is the speed of quantification, which provides a tremendous amount of chemical data which is crucial for the dynamic systems looking into the release of drugs in the pharmaceutical field (Chan and Kazarian 2005).

Contrasting the standard tests of dissolution, FTIR spectroscopic imaging provides insight and accurate data regarding the changes in the tablet during the course of dissolution. Experiments on real tablets can also be done with the help of ATR-FTIR spectroscopy imaging due to its very low sample preparation and thickness independency of the sample.

Various types of nanoparticle and modified nanoparticles have also been used for the enhancement of drug delivery by the improvement of the efficiency of the drug, reducing the dosage and also minimizing its side effects. Thus FTIR as a characterization technique is utilized.

To sum up, the ATR-FTIR imaging technique has tremendous benefits over traditional techniques of dissolution. Thus to differentiate the bio-molecular structures of the drugs, FTIR spectroscopy is a superior technique to adopt. The proper understanding of the mechanism and the process of drug release can be easily realized and studied with the use of FTIR spectroscopy.

4.4.4 Bioinformatics

Bioinformatics is an interesting field in the domain of life sciences. It is comprised of interdisciplinary work ranging from analysis of molecular sequence and genomics data, genome annotation, building biological networks, development of database along with data management systems. Apart from regular biological studies bioinformatics facilitates the development of methodologies and analysis of data using a wide range of tools; it includes storing large volumes of biological data, and organizing this data to make it user friendly. Bioinformatics helps to understand the complex data easily with the help of sophisticated computing facilities. Specially designed computer programmes consist of cloud computing along with a combination of statistics and mathematics. The well-known approaches are pattern recognition, reconstruction, machine learning, simulation, molecular modeling, etc (Ibrokhim 2016, Mount 2001). FTIR has showed significant use in pattern finding, biomarker identification, imaging, and diagnosis in extracting biological information. Figure 4.9 shows the possible contributions of FTIR in bioinformatics.

Computational molecular biology is also a most popular approach which is nevertheless similar to bioinformatics. In the several biomedical applications it is

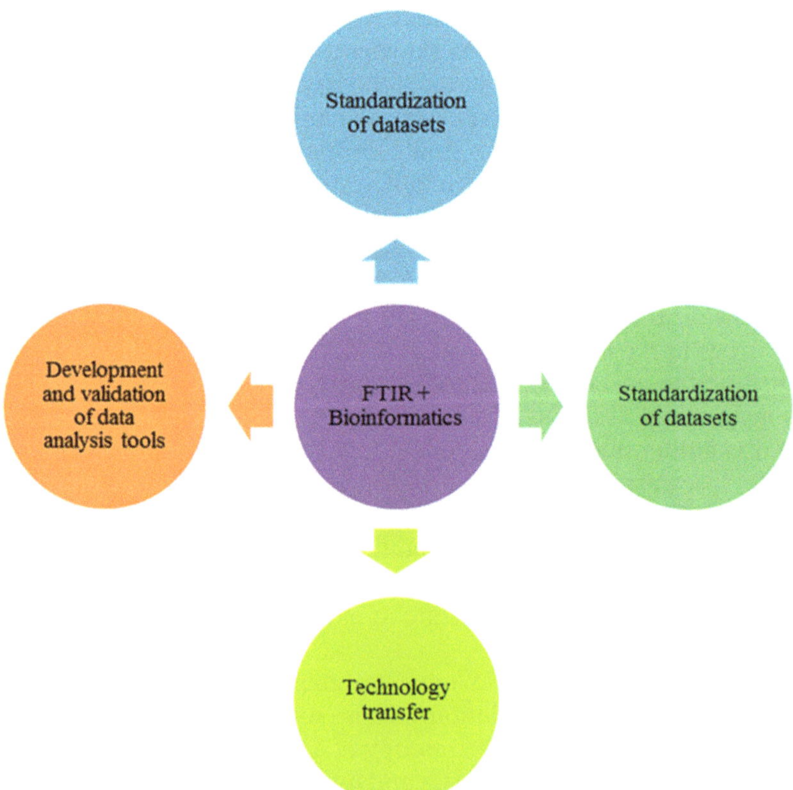

Figure 4.9. Combined approach highlighting the role of FTIR in bioinformatics.

very tedious task to store the data and identify the appropriate molecule within a stipulated time, FTIR has helped to overcome such restrictions.

4.4.5 Microbial cell identification and differentiation

The biomedical samples do not show inherent characteristics such as absorbance, transmission or reflection that is considered a prerequisite for FTIR analysis. Microbial cells need appropriate analysis since they have structural and biological diversity. In order to obtain useful information of structure as well as composition of whole cells FTIR plays an important role. In many biomedical applications the microbial cells occupy a wide range of characteristics thus FTIR is suitable to identify them accordingly. In this analysis scheme pattern recognition is used as it consists of a number of vibrational bands. As FTIR provides adequate qualities of cell structures it is preferred over the available classical microbiological techniques. In this analysis FTIR provides valuable information about total composition, structure of all structures present; these parameters show significant variation in the properties along with time, temperature of growth, and nutrient conditions. FT-Raman spectra have been used to characterize a number of microorganisms to date. The prime advantages of this technique are to provide quick support for estimation of gross composition of microbial cell samples and its behavioral change with respect to time, temperature, as well as growth.

4.4.6 Microbial microcolonies

Figure 4.10 shows the essential steps to be taken in the primary analysis phase of any microbiological sample analysis. These steps may be carried out using different

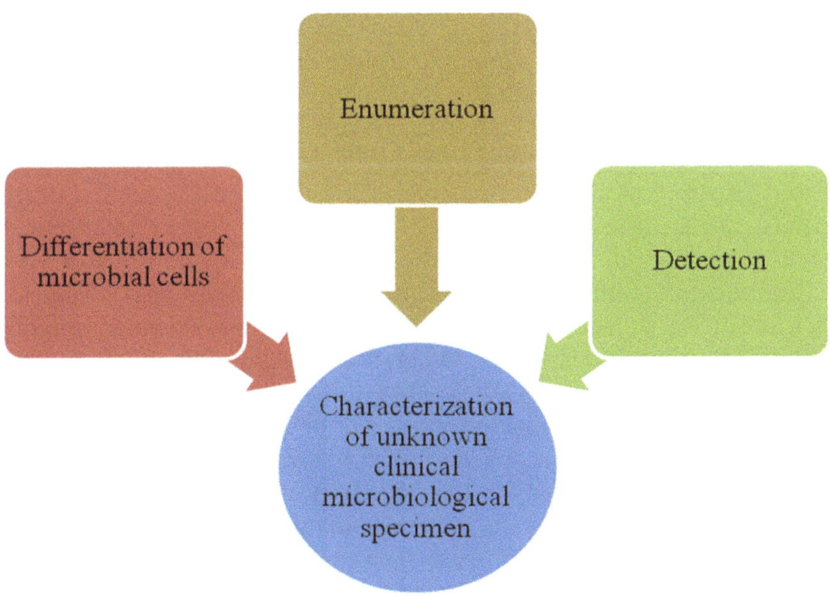

Figure 4.10. Essential steps in the characterization of unknown clinical microbiological specimen.

analysis techniques which may then be followed by the counting of colony-forming units, optical density analysis, etc. In view of these essential steps it would be beneficial to combine many of them to obtain faster and more efficient responses. FTIR is an important analysis tool in this scenario as well, before using FTIR for such systems the following prerequisites may be studied:

1. Is there any limitation in terms of real detection limit for microorganisms?
2. Do you have adequate sampling facilities?
3. Reproducibility of the sample.
4. Whether the sample which is to be analyzed will react in affirmative way in terms of absorbance, reflectance etc.

4.4.7 Identification and diagnosis of disease states

In addition to the identification of microbiological cells, FTIR is also applicable for analysis of human cells, tissues, biofluids, etc. The variation in the spectrum provides a wide range of data in terms of structural change along with compositional change due to any unwanted strain or disease. FTIR is used to analyze the biofluids (such as synovial fluids, to diagnose arthritic disorders in joints), blood and serum (clinical diagnosis), the characterization of disease states in tissues, such as a particular type of cancer (skin, breast or colon cancer); Alzheimer's disease—abnormalities in the central nervous system; analysis of normal leukemic or lymphocytes cells.

4.5 Conclusion

Nanotechnology in the field of biomedical science is a promising area of research having potential to improve the health of patients suffering from serious diseases. This chapter primarily highlights the applications of sophisticated characterization and diagnostic techniques like Fourier transformed infrared (FTIR) spectroscopy and microscopy in the diversified field of nanobiotechnology. Detailed applications in the field of pharmaceuticals like drug release and delivery along with cancer treatment and diagnosis, Nanoscale imaging, bioinformatics, microbial cell identification and differentiation, microbial microcolonies, identification and diagnosis of disease states are discussed. FTIR analysis signifies the presence of chemical bonds and functional groups in biological tissues. Moreover on the basis of absorption spectra obtained as a result of FTIR, the grade of cancer can be determined. FTIR imaging is proven to be fruitful since it is helpful in the easy identification of surface morphology. Microscopy enables the direct visualization of the biomolecules. It has potential for studying dynamic systems like drug delivery and release. From the unique absorption spectra obtained as a result of FTIR analysis, spatial distribution of the various bio-chemicals can be studied thoroughly.

FTIR thus can be referred as an advanced characterization technique for histopathological studies owing to its lower requirement with regard to sample preparation, low cost, high speed and less time consuming results, zero damage, high sensitivity, accuracy and specificity towards the discrimination and detection of complex biological tissues, cells and tissue sections.

References

Amenabar I *et al* 2017 Hyperspectral infrared nanoimaging of organic samples based on Fourier transform infrared nanospectroscopy. *Nat. Commun.* **8** 14402

Andrew Chan K L and Kazarian S G 2016 Attenuated total reflection Fourier-transform infrared (ATR-FTIR) imaging of tissues and live cells. *Chem. Soc. Rev.* **45** 1850–64

Andrus P G L and Strickland R D 1998 Cancer grading by Fourier transform infrared spectroscopy. *Biospectroscopy* **4** 37–46

Caine S *et al* 2012 The application of Fourier transform infrared microspectroscopy for the study of diseased central nervous system tissue. *Neuroimage* **59** 3624–40

Chan K L A and Kazarian S G 2005 Fourier transform infrared imaging for high-throughput analysis of pharmaceutical formulations. *J. Comb. Chem.* **7** 185–9

Dev A *et al* 2010 Preparation of poly(lactic acid)/chitosan nanoparticles for anti-HIV drug delivery applications. *Carbohydr. Polym.* **80** 833–8

Gorjikhah F *et al* 2016 Improving 'lab-on-a-chip' techniques using biomedical nanotechnology: a review. *Artif. Cells Nanomed. Biotechnol.* **44** 1609–14

Ibrokhim Y A 2016 *Bioinformatics – Updated Features and Applications* (Rijeka: InTech)

Kaushik A 2019 Biomedical nanotechnology related grand challenges and perspectives. *Front. Nanotechnol.* **1** 1–4

Kazarian S G and Ewing A V 2013 Applications of Fourier transform infrared spectroscopic imaging to tablet dissolution and drug release. *Expert Opin. Drug Deliv.* **10** 1207–21

Khanmohammadi M *et al* 2007 Cancer diagnosis by discrimination between normal and malignant human blood samples using attenuated total reflectance-Fourier transform infrared spectroscopy. *Cancer Investig.* **25** 397–404

Khanmohammadi M *et al* 2011 Application of linear discriminant analysis and attenuated total reflectance Fourier transform infrared microspectroscopy for diagnosis of colon cancer. *Pathol. Oncol. Res.* **17** 435–41

Kumari A, Jasmeet K and Bhattacharyya S 2018 Application of Fourier transform-infrared spectroscopy as a tool for early cancer detection. *Am. J. Biomed. Sci.* **10** 139–48

Leso V, Fontana L and Iavicoli I 2019 Biomedical nanotechnology: occupational views. *Nano Today* **24** 10–4

Levin I W and Bhargava R 2005 Fourier transform infrared vibrational spectroscopic imaging: integrating microscopy and molecular recognition. *Annu. Rev. Phys. Chem.* **56** 429–74

Li Q B *et al* 2005 In vivo and *in situ* detection of colorectal cancer using Fourier transform infrared spectroscopy. *World J. Gastroenterol.* **11** 327–30

Mao Z H *et al* 2015 Fourier transform infrared microscopic imaging and Fisher discriminant analysis for identification of healthy and degenerated articular cartilage. *Chin. J. Anal. Chem.* **43** 518–22

Menzies G E *et al* 2014 Fourier transform infrared for noninvasive optical diagnosis of oral, oropharyngeal, and laryngeal cancer. *Transl. Res.* **163** 19–26

Mount D W 2001 *Bioinformatics: Sequence and Genome Analysis* 2nd edn (New York: Cold Spring Harbor Laboratory Press)

Nalwa H S 2014 A special issue on reviews in biomedical applications of nanomaterials, tissue engineering, stem cells, bioimaging, and toxicity. *J. Biomed. Nanotechnol.* **10** 2421–3

Pezzei C, Brunner A, Bonn G K and Huck C W 2013 Fourier transform infrared imaging analysis in discrimination studies of bladder cancer. *Analyst* **138** 5719–25

Polizu S, Savadogo O, Poulin P and Yahia L-H 2006 Applications of carbon nanotubes-based biomaterials in biomedical nanotechnology. *J. Nanosci. Nanotechnol.* **6** 1883–904

Pope-Harman A *et al* 2007 Biomedical nanotechnology for cancer. *Med. Clin. North Am.* **91** 899–927

Prati S, Joseph E, Sciutto G and Mazzeo R 2010 New advances in the application of FTIR microscopy and spectroscopy for the characterization of artistic materials. *Acc. Chem. Res.* **43** 792–801

Ramos A P, Cruz M A E, Tovani C B and Ciancaglini P 2017 Biomedical applications of nanotechnology. *Biophys. Rev.* **9** 79–89

Sahu R K and Mordechai S 2005 Fourier transform infrared spectroscopy in cancer detection. *Future Oncol.* **1** 635–47

Saji V S, Choe H C and Yeung K W K 2010 Nanotechnology in biomedical applications: a review. *Int. J. Nano Biomater.* **3** 119–39

Kazarian S G and Andrew Chan K L 2009 Micro- and macro-attenuated total reflection Fourier transform infrared spectroscopic imaging. *Appl. Spectrosc.* **64** 135A–52A

Shakya B R, Shrestha P, Teppo H R and Rieppo L 2020 The use of Fourier transform infrared (FTIR) spectroscopy in skin cancer research: a systematic review. *Appl. Spectrosc. Rev.* **56** 1–33

Singh Y 2014 Trends in biomedical nanotechnology. *J. Nanomed. Biother. Discovery* **4** 4172

Sloan S R *et al* 2020 Imaging the local biochemical content of native and injured intervertebral disc using Fourier transform infrared microscopy. *JOR Spine* **3** 1–11

Song Y, Cong Y, Wang B and Zhang N 2020 Applications of Fourier transform infrared spectroscopy to pharmaceutical preparations. *Expert Opin. Drug Deliv.* **17** 551–71

Steiner G and Koch E 2009 Trends in Fourier transform infrared spectroscopic imaging. *Anal. Bioanal.Chem.* **394** 671–8

Su K Y and Lee W L 2020 Fourier transform infrared spectroscopy as a cancer screening and diagnostic tool: a review and prospects. *Cancers* **12** 115

Tian F *et al* 2016 Gold nanostars for efficient *in vitro* and *in vivo* real-time SERS detection and drug delivery via plasmonic-tunable Raman/FTIR imaging. *Biomaterials* **106** 87–97

Wang R and Wang Y 2021 Fourier Transform infrared spectroscopy in oral cancer diagnosis. *Int. J. Mol. Sci.* **22** 1–21

Whitman A G, Lambert P J, Dyson O F and Akula S M 2008 Applications of nanotechnology in the biomedical sciences: small materials, big impacts, and unknown consequences. *Philos. Med.* **101** 117–30

Witzke K E *et al* 2019 Integrated Fourier transform infrared imaging and proteomics for identification of a candidate histochemical biomarker in bladder cancer. *Am. J. Pathol.* **189** 619–31

Yano K *et al* 2003 Applications of Fourier transform infrared spectroscopy, Fourier transform infrared microscopy and near-infrared spectroscopy to cancer research. *Spectroscopy* **17** 315–21

Chapter 5

Raman spectroscopy and microscopy in biomedical nanotechnology

Zohreh Shahnavaz, Muhammad J A Shiddiky, Kamelia Saremi, Guanjun Qiao and Nam-Young Kim

Raman spectroscopy (RS) is an established technique based on inelastic scattering of light by vibrating molecules that allows the chemical fingerprinting and imaging of molecules based on their chemical constitution and structure. Due to high chemical specificity, minimal or lack of sample preparation, and the ability to use advanced optical technologies in the visible or near-infrared (NIR) spectral range, applications of RS to study clinically relevant biological species, disease pathogenesis, and diagnosis have been rapidly increasing since the last decade. RS is an analytical tool that can detect and quantify the molecular changes in cells, tissues, or biofluids that are the cause or the effect of diseases. Raman spectra have shown the potential to provide multivariate calibration and classification models to develop large training datasets to obtain a quantitative and objective diagnosis. The growing new Raman strategies (non-linear optical effects, metallic nanoparticles, optimized fibreoptic Raman probes) and multimodal integration with other optical techniques have enabled the rapid and accurate screening of disease susceptibility and onset, compatible with clinical use. This chapter outlines the fundamental principles of conventional Raman and advanced Raman spectroscopies, multi-directional approaches for biomedical applications, and improvements in performance using a combinational approach involving spectroscopy and microscopy.

5.1 Introduction

In 1923, Smekal [1] predicted Raman scattering of light by molecules using classical quantum theory, and it was observed experimentally by Raman and Krishnan in 1928 [2]. Raman spectroscopy (RS) is an experimental method to provide information regarding molecular vibrations for elucidating the structure, composition, coordination, and bonding of sample molecules by changes in energies of scattered

doi:10.1088/978-0-7503-3379-5ch5

monochromatic radiations and enables qualitative and quantitative analyses of sample materials [3]. This method is based on inelastic scattering of light (Raman scattering) and can be used to fine-tune structural data obtained by other methods, such as x-ray diffraction, because of Raman scattering's sensitivity to local structure. About two decades after the development of Raman scattering theory in crystals in 1947 [4], the study of small biomolecules and biopolymers was possible using laser-excited RS [5–9].

Raman and infrared (IR) spectroscopy techniques are complementary and have a broad range of applications to provide characteristic fundamental vibrations that are used for elucidating structural and chemical components of a compound. Measurement of vibrational and vibrational–rotational (the two modes of energy) are needed in both techniques. Generally, Raman and IR spectroscopy are the best symmetric vibrations of non-polar groups and asymmetric vibrations of polar groups, respectively. However, some vibrational modes are both Raman and IR active and arise from different selection rules. Vibrational mode symmetry and molecule symmetry are the essential factors for the activity of a certain vibrational mode. IR spectroscopy depends on the dipole moment of a molecule changes, but in RS, changes in a molecule's polarizability are determinative. Consequently, highly polar bonds are strong in IR and weak in Raman. Furthermore, the IR region of the electromagnetic spectrum absorbs water strongly, which is a drawback for the analysis of aqueous solutions or tissue with high water content using IR spectroscopy; however, RS is not only an ideal tool for *in vivo* tissue interrogation due to weak water signal but also provides a rapid molecular characterization of tissue *in vivo* or *in vitro* for biopsy, laboratory use, margin assessment, and therapeutic evaluation since it is a non-destructive, reagentless, and vibrational spectroscopic technique.

RS techniques can link the fundamental structural biology and its medical applications in cancer, cardiovascular, neurodegenerative, atherosclerotic, and other diseases. In structure-based drug design technologies, RS, with the help of coherent anti-Stokes Raman scattering (CARS), plays an important role in detecting and imaging membrane protein microcrystals. RS is a promising technique to distinguish between normal tissue and cancer tumor [10]. Both fast and accurate non-invasive cancer diagnostics and monitoring cancer cell response for therapy are approachable using this powerful tool [11, 16]. Food safety monitoring and clinical diagnostics are mainly based on the detection of nucleic acids [17, 18]. Binding agents or environmental factors cause changes in nucleic acids, and Raman difference spectroscopy (subtraction of spectra) enables characterization of nucleic acid conformational changes quantitatively [19–21]. Understanding ribonucleic acid (RNA) functions and chemical properties requires an efficient analytical tool for RNA identification and characterization. Surface-enhanced Raman spectroscopy (SERS) provides advanced analysis of ribonucleic acids at the ultrasensitive level [22]. Recently, the SERS technique has achieved a high precision detection of specific genes in the genomic deoxyribonucleic acid (DNA) sample [23].

Raman microscopy, a hybrid technique between Raman spectroscopy and microscopy, is applied to record Raman maps. The point mapping method shows the spatial distribution of different chemical components/information within the sample; as a result, the investigation of any minor changes in composition, orientation, crystallinity, inclusions, and stress is allowed. This review will cover the principles of RS, including theoretical and experimental considerations, advanced Raman scattering techniques, and technologies. Finally, their potential and contributions to biomedical technology will be discussed.

5.2 Raman spectroscopy

Principals The Raman spectroscopy technique typically uses a laser as the excitation source to measure Raman scattered radiation and provides information about chemical bonding and molecular structure by detecting photons that are scattered inelastically. The induced dipole moment after the interaction of light with the material can be expressed as [24, 25]:

$$\mathrm{p} = \alpha \bar{E} \tag{5.1}$$

where the polarizability factor is defined by α and the electric field of the incident light [24, 25].

$$\bar{E} = E_o \cos(2\pi v_o t) \tag{5.2}$$

where E_o is the field strength and v_o is the frequency of oscillation.

Substituting (5.2) in (5.1) gives the time-dependent induced dipole moment,

$$p = \alpha E_o \cos(2\pi v_o t) \tag{5.3}$$

The polarizability factor which depends on the instantaneous position of the individual atoms is determined by the capability of the electron cloud to interact with the electromagnetic wave. The molecular bonds in chemical compounds are associated with the vibrational modes and vibrational energies are described as [26]:

$$E_{\mathrm{vib}} = (j + (1/2)hv_{\mathrm{vib}}) \tag{5.4}$$

where j is the vibrational state, h is Plancks constant and v_{vib} is the vibrational frequency.

The displacement of atoms about their equilibrium position due to a particular vibrational mode can be defined by [24, 25]:

$$Q = Q_o \cos(2\pi v_{\mathrm{vib}} t) \tag{5.5}$$

where Q_o is the maximum displacement from the mean position.

Polarizability of small displacements (typical diatomic molecules), can be approximated as a Taylor series expansion in normal coordinates [24, 25]:

$$\alpha = \alpha_o + (\partial\alpha/\partial Q)_o Q \tag{5.6}$$

where α_o is the polarizability of the molecule when constituent atoms are at equilibrium positions.

The polarizability has a static term and a sinusoidal oscillating term. For Raman scattering to occur, the polarizability needs to change with vibration, $(\partial\alpha/\partial Q)_o \neq 0$. Here, the subscript 0 indicates that the parameters α_o and $(\partial\alpha/\partial Q)_o$ are evaluated at the equilibrium position of the atoms. Substituting equations (5.2), (5.5), and (5.6) into equation (5.1) yields [24, 25]:

$$\mathrm{p} = \alpha_o E_o \cos(2\pi v_o t) + \left[\left(\partial\alpha/\partial Q\right)\left(Q_o E_o/2\right)\right]\{\cos[2\pi(v_o - v_{\mathrm{vib}})t] + [2\pi(v_o + v_{\mathrm{vib}})t]\} \tag{5.7}$$

The incident photons can be absorbed, scattered, and/or pass through the material without interaction. The inelastic scattering occurs with a change in photon energy, whereas the elastic scattering occurs with no change in photon energy. The majority of the photons in the incident radiation are scattered without any change in energy, known as Rayleigh/elastic scattering. A small fraction of photons scatter inelastically, and energy transfer (lost or gained by the molecule) occurs, either from the photon to the molecule or vice versa. This process is named Raman scattering and that can be further categorized into two subtypes: Stokes scattering and anti-Stokes scattering. If the molecule loses vibrational energy to the incident photons and the energy of scattered photons will be higher than the incident photons, the scattering is called anti-Stokes scattering; if it is lower it is called Stokes Raman scattering (figure 5.1) [27]. At room temperatures, Stokes Raman scattering has a higher probability of occurrence than anti-Stokes Raman scattering, and therefore usually only recorded in typical RS measurements. The excited vibrational bond frequency is equivalent to the difference in energy between the incident light and the Raman scattered light. The sample spectrum can be obtained by plotting the intensity of Raman scattered light detected against these frequencies (typically as Raman shift in cm^{-1}). Every molecule has a unique spectrum, also known as a vibrational fingerprint. Geometry evaluation can be studied by applying a polarizer (polarized RS) in the optical path of the scattered light to only detect a single polarization component. Unpolarized RS means a simple evaluation of the intensities.

Instrumentation Figure 5.2(A) [28] shows the configuration of a typical laboratory Raman system. Spontaneous Raman scattering is induced using a laser to irradiate the sample. Raman scattered photons are collected into a spectrometer (at 90° or 180° to the sample) and are analyzed to obtain a Raman spectrum from a sample. Rayleigh scattering can be removed using a filter. The grating of the spectrometer disperses the light and splits it into individual frequencies, and then the light is converted into electrons by a charge-coupled device (CCD). Detailed information on biological Raman bands cannot be achieved without a spectrograph (coupled to the Raman probe and the CCD) owing to a spectral resolution of 8–10 cm^{-1}. The spectral resolution depends on spectrograph optical parameters, the diffraction grating, and the CCD pixel size. A Raman spectrometer can be coupled to a microscope that enables the focusing of light onto an object. Since the Raman signal is very weak, the choice of laser is essential to enhance Raman signal. Lasers can be applied at various visible-light and near-infrared (NIR) wavelengths to excite a sample. Power, integration time, and laser wavelength are essential factors to optimize the Raman system for *in vivo* biomedical applications. Fluorescence is a major interference in RS measurements, and fluorophore-generated signals can cover a weak Raman signal. Fluorescence background can be limited by lower

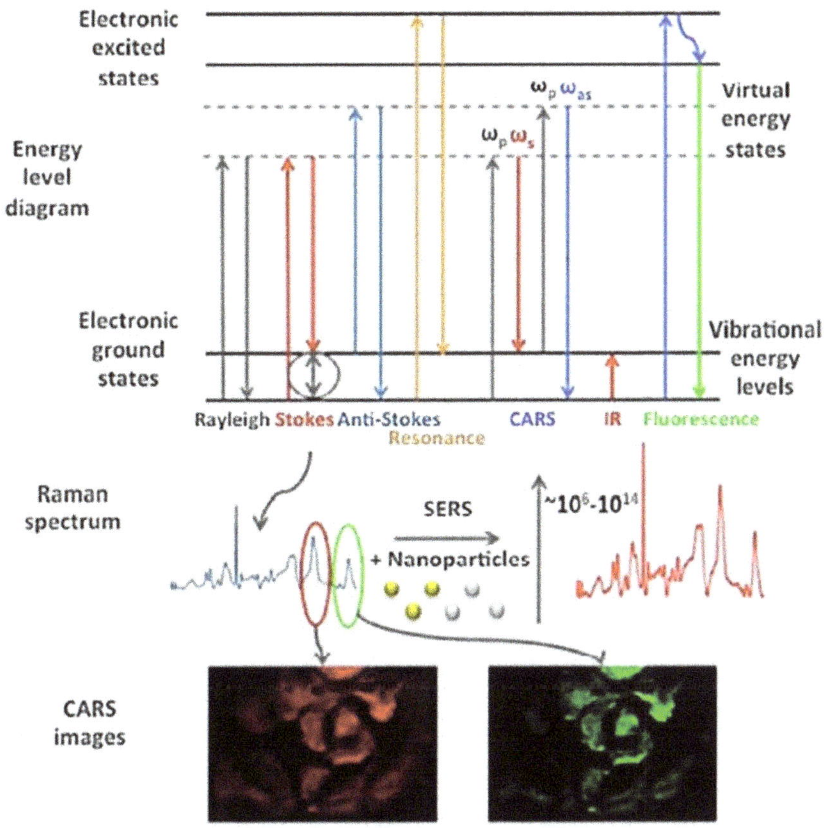

Figure 5.1. Energy level diagram depicting (from left to right): Rayleigh scattering, Stokes scattering, anti-Stokes scattering, resonance Raman, coherent anti-Stokes Raman spectroscopy (CARS), infrared absorption and fluorescence. Each process is explained further in the main text. Reproduced with permission from reference [27]. Copyright (2018) American Chemical Society.

energy NIR lasers [29]. For example, in skin diagnosis, a 785 nm diode laser is applied as the excitation source to generate low fluorescence to penetrate deep into human tissue. Most biological fluorophores are free of peak emission in this region of the spectrum, resulting in a lower fluorescence background than visible or UV excitation. However, assessing biological material at low physiological concentrations, such as proteins, lipids and DNA, could be a challenge due to the signal to noise ratio of NIR lasers. For instance, compared to a 785 nm laser, a 488 nm laser will produce a 6.7 times higher signal. Also, by decreasing the sensitivity of typical silicon-based CCD detectors at NIR wavelengths >900 nm [30], detection of Stokes Raman signals of vibrational frequencies >2000 cm^{-1} is an issue.

Resonance Raman spectroscopy shows improvement in the strength of Raman signal. Most organic molecules have electronic excitation energies in the UV region, so UV resonance Raman spectroscopy has been broadly employed for studying proteins and their conformations, while this technique is unsuitable for *in vivo* applications [31–35].

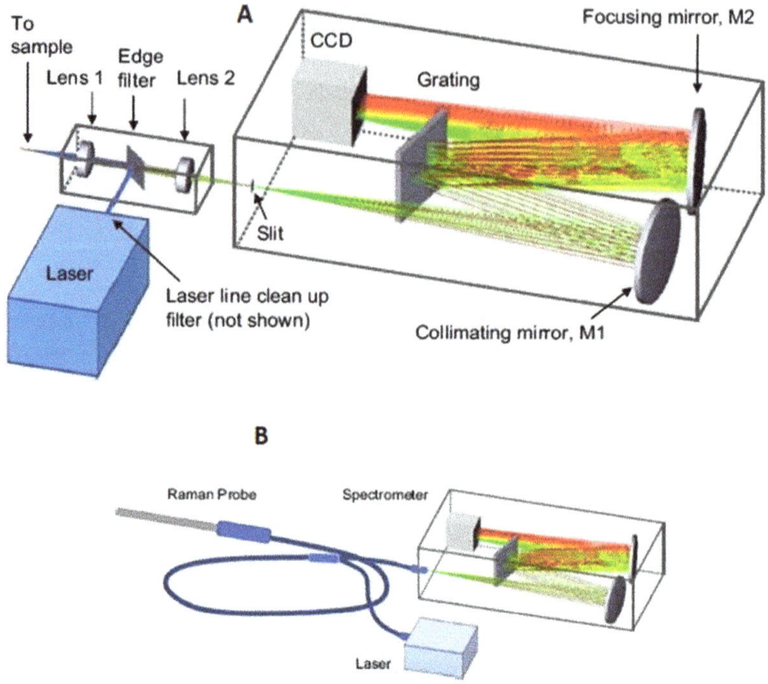

Figure 5.2. Configuration of a typical laboratory Raman system (A), Raman probe assembly (B). Reproduced from reference [28]. CC BY 4.0.

Spectral analysis A variety of methods are exploited to correlate Raman spectroscopic data with tissue type for diagnostic evaluation. Statistical models or classification algorithms containing great strength and low classification error can be used extensively to develop automated tissue classification schemes. Univariate analysis and multivariate analysis are two major approaches to inferential statistical analysis. Univariate analysis, the simplest form of data analysis, deals with only one variable at a time. It helps describe the data using one particular variable and can either be inferential or descriptive. Mean, median, mode, standard deviation, and variance are examples of this method [36]. In spectroscopy, a single variable means wavenumber and intensities of each band can be calculated by curve fitting or obtaining ratios. A Raman spectrum contains thousands of variables, and in most cases, molecular information is not entirely represented by one or two Raman bands, but univariate analysis suffers significant limitations in understanding the relationships between variables. Moreover, Raman hyperspectral imaging of biological samples records large volumes of data, and the differences among spectra are subtle. Hence, multivariate analysis is effective where multiple variables are considered simultaneously to extract complete chemical information. Multivariate analysis is divided into unsupervised and supervised learning. In unsupervised methods, no labels are provided, and the learning algorithm focuses only on detecting structure in unlabeled input data. They are used as a precursor to supervised methods when working on massive datasets. In biomedical applications of vibrational spectroscopy, this method can separate disease-related samples into a different class even when the relationship is not initially apparent.

Principle component analysis (PCA) is an unsupervised method that reduces complex datasets into a small number of principal components (PCs). These PCs are orthogonal (statistically independent), and only a small number of PCs may be required to capture all of the significant variations between the datasets. They represent the coefficient of each wavenumber used to transform the original data into the component scores in the new data space. Further analysis enables the determination of the biological/chemical source of variation between different conditions [37]. In contrast, supervised multivariate analysis methods are presented with labeled example inputs, where the labels indicate the desired output. Unlike unsupervised methods, there are two important phases. The training phase (passive modeling stage) uses labeled training datasets to find the patterns in the data and the prediction phase (active stage) where the unseen data (the data which were not part of the training set) are validated using the model parameters learned in the first phase. Discriminant analysis (DA), multiple linear regression (MLR), principal component regression (PCR), partial least squares (PLS), and support vector machine (SVM) are examples of supervised methods [37].

PLS is a supervised method and maximizes the separation of classes instead of the overall variance, making PLS useful for smaller datasets. Classification models such as linear discriminant analysis (LDA) can also be applied to maximize the separation of classes. In combination with multivariate statistical models, RS can be employed for both classification and diagnosis. Between group analysis (BGA), another supervised method, is for sample discrimination and class prediction. However, the supervised methods are dependent on labeling data, and it is very burdensome to label a large number of observations. Therefore, unsupervised methods are often used in conjunction with supervised methods to solve this problem [37]. To omit unwanted signals (fluorescence or other additive features) which intervene in the elucidation of Raman spectra of biological samples by generating the baseline noise in the raw spectra, spectral preprocessing is utilized. Two basic preprocessing methodologies include baseline corrections to remove spectral contributions due to fluorescence and normalization to remove focusing effects and effects that can arise from laser intensity fluctuations.

Raman probe Rapid measurement is ideal for *in vivo* clinical application and can be achieved by applying a small footprint high-resolution system. A Raman fibreoptic probe provides access to organs. However, compared to a laboratory research-grade instrument, the smaller footprint can interpret to lower resolution or smaller spectral range of measurement, which means information may be lost and spectral features may not be differentiated. Besides, shorter measurement times can lead to a lower signal-to-noise ratio (SNR). Therefore, improvement of sensitivity, reducing size and cost, and signal enhancement strategies in instrumentation are important parameters in promoting the feasibility of RS for clinical use. Figure 5.2(B) [28] shows a schematic of a Raman probe. Laser light is transmitted over optical fibers and a laser line cleanup filter (curbs unwanted signals) that is internal to the probe. The laser light is then focused onto the sample with an internal lens, and the lens collects backscattered light to direct through an edge filter (internal in the probe) specified for Raman signals. The Raman scattered light is then coupled into a second fiber (or assumedly of fibers) connected to the spectrometer at the slit.

5.3 Advanced Raman scattering techniques

5.3.1 Surface-enhanced Raman spectroscopy

5.3.1.1 Tip-enhanced Raman spectroscopy

Surface-enhanced methods Spontaneous Raman spectroscopy enables spontaneous Raman signals to be obtained from biological samples; however, detection of low concentration analytes is a challenge and requires enhancement. The Raman signal can be enhanced when the frequency of excitation laser and emitted Raman photons are resonant with the localized surface plasmon resonance (LSPR) of a nanostructure, and these improvements are associated with typically gold and silver nanoparticles [38, 39]. The following are the two complementary approaches that have been pursued to improve the sensitivity of Raman for biomedical applications. The weakness of signals in RS is a limitation for characterizing low concentrations of materials. Moreover, this technique is not suitable for rapid imaging. In 1974 Fleischmann and coworkers observed the adsorption of a monolayer of pyridine onto roughened Ag electrodes caused an intense increase in Raman signals [40]. This discovery, the SERS effect, was thought to be a combined effect of the large surface area of Ag electrodes and increased local concentration of adsorbed pyridine molecules. However, a few years later, it was concluded that this observation was caused by roughened Ag electrodes that induce enhanced electric fields and the cross-section increases [41]. Raman scattering signals by placing Raman active molecules near a surface of appropriate nanostructured electrically conducting surfaces can be tremendously enhanced by several (up to $>10^{12}$) orders of magnitude, which allows even single-molecule detection [42].

Two proposed theories for the SERS phenomenon show the total enhancement results from *electromagnetic enhancement* and *chemical enhancement*. In electromagnetic (EM) theory, the enhancement involves the optical excitation of electric fields created by collective oscillations of electrons on the surface of nanoparticles (surface plasmons). This interaction results in surface plasmon resonance (SPR) [43]. The enhancements observed in SERS are assigned to the excited SPR on nanoscale materials resulting in high local fields. If the plasmon frequency is in accordance with the frequency of the incident light, the resulting enhancement is most significant. In EM theory [44], the intensity (I) and the local electromagnetic field strength (E) are directly proportional, while E varies inversely to the distance (d) between the analyte and NP surface ($E \propto (1/d)^{12}$). Therefore, the electromagnetic theory is distance-dependent, and small modifications in d and E result in exponential changes in intensity. Signals in SERS are surface selective. Silver and gold nanoparticles are ideal for enhancing the Raman signal as their surface plasmon resonance frequencies fall within the visible and near-IR. To obtain the SERS optimum enhancement, the optimal number of analytes should be within regions of strong SPR and nanoparticles [45]. Chemical enhancement (CE), the second theory, is proposed to be involved in the electronic excitation of covalently chemical bonds formed between the molecule and surface of nanoparticles to increase the polarizability of adsorbed molecules [43]. The EM effect is more dominant and is independent of molecule type. Although SERS has an advantage over standard Raman, the required additional steps can be a disadvantage. To enhance tissue analysis, a nanoprobe molecule is needed [46].

SERS broadly used in biological and biomedical applications. Label-based and label-free measurements are the two available types of methodologies for these applications. In SERS label-free detection, vibrational spectroscopic information of biomolecules is gained by the interaction of the desired molecule with the SERS substrate providing intrinsic fingerprint information for the qualitative and quantitative detection of various analytes. This methodology employs physical parameters such as optical, acoustic, or electrical signals for ultrasensitive detection purposes. Compared with other detection methods, it possesses the advantages of simplicity, high sensitivity, and specific signals, thus gaining significant attraction [47, 48]. Label-based detection usually exploits Raman reporter molecules with strong and distinct Raman signals to label the SERS tags attached to metal nanostructures such as gold or silver for ultrasensitive detection, imaging, or sensing of biological and biomedical samples [49]. A biocompatible coating encapsulates the metal substrate and the Raman label to minimize any non-specific binding of the tags. Large Raman cross-section, affinity towards the metal substrate, and possessing fewer Raman peaks are the essential factors for the selection of Raman reporters. Furthermore, functionalizing SERS tags with specific antibodies, peptides, or aptamer sequences enables specific detection of biological targets. However, the labeling process is tedious, time-consuming, and can affect the native conformation of the analytes under study due to toxicity issues [47, 48]. The other applications of SERS technique including chemical and biological sensing applications, chemical analysis of food materials (additives and contaminants), probing the properties of graphene surface, monitoring the electroreduction of analytes, quantitative determination of proteins and their interactions (direct and indirect), and biotechnology and pharmaceutical manufacturing [50].

Tip-enhanced Raman scattering (TERS) is similar to the SERS phenomenon where enhancement records by focusing incident light onto a nanometer-scale metal-coated tip (Si or Si_3N_4 base coated by a thin evaporation deposit of Ag or Au) of a scanning probe [51, 52]. TERS improves lateral spatial resolution to as low as 10 nm [53] and provides a unique opportunity to assign spectral characteristics to topographical locations and correlate to mechanical properties. However, it is unsuitable for the surgical suite since robust sample preparation and data interpretation are sensitive to ambient conditions [54].

5.3.2 Coherent anti-Stokes Raman spectroscopy

5.3.2.1 Stimulated Raman spectroscopy

Coherent Raman scattering (non-linear methods) In spontaneous Raman scattering, the molecular vibrations in a sample are not correlated; therefore, coherent Raman spectroscopy is an incoherent phenomenon. In coherent Raman spectroscopy techniques, non-linear effects are used to improve the speed and spatial resolution of RS by inducing coherent molecular vibrations in the sample. The additional light beam in this method can produce an equal frequency to the frequency of the transition between vibrational and virtual levels to scan over the studied spectral region. Moreover, the scattered light can be separated from red-shifted fluorescence (unlike the spontaneous Raman) due to a blue-shift relative to the excitation light. The following two methods are the two major forms of this technique. While spontaneous RS uses a continuous wave laser, in non-linear Raman methods, two NIR pulsed lasers are applied to probe the third-order polarizability of a molecule. Coherent anti-Stokes Raman spectroscopy (CARS), a widespread biomedical tool, allows for a multimodal approach to simultaneously acquire second harmonic generation and two-photon excited fluorescence measurements, gaining more chemical and morphological information from biological samples [55–58].

When tuned to a molecular vibration, stimulated Raman spectroscopy (SRS) measures the energy loss and gain in the incident lasers and provides high-resolution images and chemical information equivalent to spontaneous Raman [59–61]. Although both CARS and SRS are sensitive to the same vibrational signatures as RS, they use multiple lasers of different wavelengths to excite the sample and can enhance signals up to 105 times over normal RS. SRS detects an enhanced Stokes spectral component and the excited vibrational population, while CARS detects an enhanced anti-Stokes spectral component and the vibrational coherence. Analogous to CARS, SRS uses a pump beam (ω_p) and a second laser beam, Stokes (ω_S), to stimulate the molecule to a virtual state and set up a coherence targeting the desired direction vibrational mode When the difference between the laser frequencies matches the vibrational frequency of the targeted bond vibration ($\upsilon_{vib} = \upsilon_p - \upsilon_S$), the molecules oscillate coherently, resulting in an enhanced Stokes signal. Another detection methodology in SRS is measuring the pump energy loss or energy gain in Stokes photons to measure the Raman scattered signals [56, 58].

In CARS, a strong anti-Stokes signal is generated at $\omega_{AS} = 2\omega_p - \omega_S$. Since the SRS and Raman spectra are identical, Raman spectroscopic data for SRS imaging applications have more efficiency than CARS [62, 63]. Despite CARS, SRS is free of the non-resonant background [64]. CARS has been mainly applied to image cells and tissues by exciting the CH stretching vibrations (2600–3000 cm^{-1}) in lipids and proteins [65]. In broadband CARS techniques, multiple Raman transitions are probed simultaneously to extend the fingerprint region resulting in imaging of biological tissues with improved molecular contrast [66]. Moreover, the SERS technique can enhance the signal of both CARS [67, 68] and SRS [69, 70].

5.3.3 Resonance Raman spectroscopy

5.3.3.1 Surface-enhanced resonance Raman spectroscopy

Signal enhancement with resonance Raman spectroscopy (RRS) is obtained when the frequency of incident radiation occurs simultaneously with the frequency of an electronic transition of a molecule to excite electrons to a higher electronic state. As a result, the intensity of signals enhances by several (up to $>10^6$) orders of magnitude

[71]. Since only Raman modes are resonantly enhanced within the RRS spectrum, the complexity of RRS is less than non-resonant spectra. RRS provides more selective molecular information but requires a tunable laser to selectively isolate the contributions from different chromophores [71]. One of the drawbacks of this technique is photo-degradation processes within the sample assigned to the excitation with laser light in electronic resonance. The sample should move faster under the illuminating beam to overcome this issue. However, combining RRS with microscopy to perform imaging of biological samples is challenging. RRS often suffers from a fluorescence background, and the larger cross-section of fluorescence can obscure the Raman signals. This issue occurs for small Stokes shifts while a large Stokes shift remains unaffected because the resonance Raman scattered light and the fluorescence signal are well separated. A useful technique, UV resonance Raman (UVRR) spectroscopy [72], to separate the RRS fingerprint information from fluorescence is applying deep UV wavelengths (<250 nm) to excite high-lying electronic states [72, 73]. In this technique by choosing an appropriate UV wavelength, the signal of individual species in complex samples can be selectively enhanced. The potential of UVRR spectroscopy to monitor residual DNA and RNA directly during biopharmaceutical manufacture is a specific advantage [73]. Another strategy to avoid fluorescence background is using the different time scales of RRS and fluorescence. A time window of 5–10 femtosecond for RRS and nanosecond scale for fluorescence processes after the electronic excitation can be employed [73]. By using molecules are in contact or in close vicinity with the surface of metallic nanostructures, SERS is achieved to enhance the Raman scattering signals by several orders of magnitude.

The Raman signal can be further amplified by tuning a laser corresponding to an adsorbed molecule's internal electronic transition to introduce the surface-enhanced resonance Raman spectroscopy (SERRS) method. The method is essentially the development of RRS and SERS. Although SERS and SERRS are not differentiated in many articles, they show different properties once applied in applications. Both enhancements from the plasmon resonance and molecular resonance from the analyte contribute to giving very intense scattering [74]. It is hard to achieve precisely the same frequency for both plasmon resonance and electronic transition in the analyte in SERRS, but it has been found that SERRS operates well with about a 250 nm separation between the maximum resonance frequencies of the two [75]. The findings show that in the presence of unaggregated colloid as a substrate and well separated resonances, the maximum scattering intensity was yielded close to the frequency of the electronic transition maximum rather than the plasmon maximum confirming the difference between SERS and SERRS. SERRS demonstrated tremendous enhancement compared to SERS; for instance, the recorded SERS enhancement for pyridine is at 106, while the SERRS enhancement factor for rhodamine is calculated at between 1013 and 1015, which is a major difference between SERS and SERRS [76, 77]. In SERRS, fluorescence is quenched on the active surface, and excellent Raman scattering can be obtained from fluorescent molecules. A very wide range of fluorescent and non-fluorescent dyes can be used as labels. However, this quenching is only effective for surface-bound species [78].

5.3.4 Spatially offset Raman spectroscopy

5.3.4.1 Surface-enhanced spatially offset Raman spectroscopy

5.3.4.1.1 Transmission Raman spectroscopy

Deep Raman spectroscopy techniques Spatially offset Raman spectroscopy (SORS), introduced by Matousek *et al* [79], is a non-invasive method used to investigate tissue samples at depth by offsetting the point of collection from the point of laser excitation typically in the region of a few mm [80, 81]. SORS consists of two main categories: a central illumination point and a collection ring and inverse SORS with an illumination ring and a central collection area. Unlike confocal techniques that provide spectral information at a particular depth by focusing the laser to a given distance on the z-axis, SORS utilizes a spatial offset to probe through the barrier/analyte system [80]. The spatial offset is between the laser illumination and collection areas on the surface of a sample. The offset distance determines the relative contribution of each layer to the measured spectrum. By increasing the spatial offset of the collection and the illumination points, measurements deeper in the tissue are possible. A two-layer sample requires at least two SORS spectra at different spatial offsets for recovery of the Raman spectra of individual layers. One spectrum would be a zero spatially offset spectrum, and one acquired at a non-zero spatial offset. For a multilayer sample with n-layers, n-SORS spectra at different spatial offsets to retrieve individual layer contributions are needed [79]. The optimum magnitude of the spatial offset is either determined empirically (trial and error) or numerically (Monte Carlo simulations) [81]. In SORS, larger offsets mainly detect photons that have traveled deeper into the tissue via multiple scattering, while smaller offsets mainly probe the superficial layer. SORS has been exploited in many clinical applications [82–84]. However, the applicability of SORS is challenging or impossible for samples which are highly absorbing at the laser or Raman signal wavelengths due to photon propagation distances and penetration depths decrement. Micro-spatially offset Raman spectroscopy (micro-SORS) is a newly developed technique that combines conventional macroscale SORS [85] with microscopy to resolve the limitation of intact very thin turbid layer investigation [86–90]. Micro-SORS can be applied for the analysis of artworks [88], stratified polymers, paper, and wheat seeds [91] with enhanced penetration depth by two orders of magnitude larger than confocal Raman microscopy [92]. Portable micro-SORS instruments can provide *in situ* non-invasive analysis of artworks without size restrictions [93–95]. This method consists of collecting spectra with varying degrees of the sublayer Raman signal compared with that from the surface layer to apply effectively in studying art objects, the biomedical field [96–100], heritage sciences [101, 102], biological samples, and polymers [103, 104]

The combination of SERS and SORS techniques, known as SESORS, enables the extension of sensitivity and specificity of SERS to the subsurface analysis of medical tissues. This powerful method was revealed by Stone *et al* [105], and further studies [106] confirmed its applicability for non-invasive multiplexed imaging of buried structures deep within the tissue (up to 45–50 mm) with high chemical specificity.

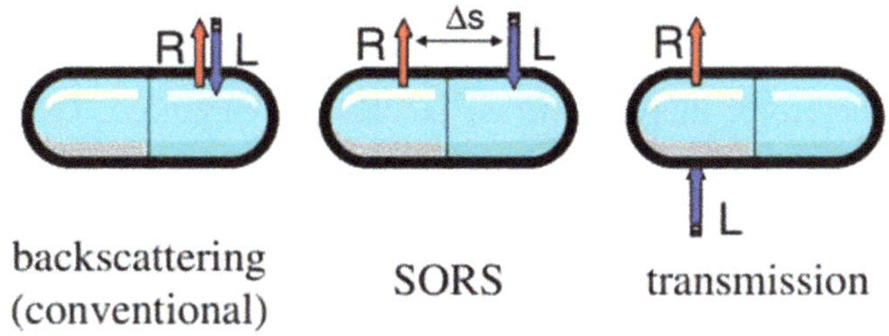

Figure 5.3. Basic types of Raman spectroscopy geometries with respect to the sample: conventional backscattering Raman, SORS and Raman transmission geometries. R Raman light, L laser beam. Reproduced from [108]. CC BY 4.0.

Recently, a new highly sensitive optical method has been developed for sensing and imaging [107]. This unique technique, spatially offset resonance Raman spectroscopy (SESORRS), was utilized by combining SERRS with SORS, demonstrating the benefit of using a resonant Raman reporter for superior levels of depth penetration.

Transmission Raman spectroscopy (TRS) can be considered a special form of SORS, where the laser beam and the Raman collection point are on the opposite sides of the sample (figure 5.3) [108]. In this technique, photons penetrate the sample, follow a random path through the material, and are scattered many times. There is always a probability of photon demolition and a new Raman-scattered photon creation at each scattering occurrence. Since the initial orientation of the photons is straight through the sample, a notable portion of them penetrate downward and are gathered at the sample's side. With TRS, bulk analysis of opaque or turbid materials is possible [109]. Contrary to SORS, TRS is incapable of providing the signatures of individual layers within the sample but can give the volumetric information of the sample to search for a specific signal at an unknown location in a large volume of the sample [110]. Although TRS was represented a few decades ago [111], its advantages for the non-invasive probing of biological and pharmaceutical samples have only been known recently [112].

5.3.5 Raman microscopy

Raman microscopy is a non-destructive and non-contact method to generate 3D Raman images of the studied object. In this method, a Raman spectrometer and a standard optical microscope are integrated to allow laser light to enter through a small pinhole, reach the objective lens, and focus on the sample, the scattered light from the sample is collected by the objective, passes through the dichroic mirror, and is directed toward the pinhole. The pinhole acts as a spatial filter that provides the analysis of the controlled sampling volumes of micrometer size, individual particles, or a few micrometer thick layers. The spatial resolution is determined by the laser source, the wavelength λ, the quality of the image formation, and the type of selected microscope for analyses. The optimum spatial resolution is achieved using a correctly matched high-magnification objective and visible laser. Typical spatial resolution is of the order of 0.5–1 mm. The pinhole allows only generated photons of the central part (not focal plane) to pass through the pinhole and transmit toward the detector. Therefore, image contrast is strongly enhanced. Great spatial resolution, clear image quality, the ability to perform 3D mapping of bulk samples, no sample preparation, and outstanding chemical differentiation are advantages of this non-invasive technique [113, 114]. After observing the Raman spectra of a tissue sample using an optical microscope in 1979 [115], Raman microscopy has been used for biomedical microscopy. This powerful analytical technique can be applied in polymeric and ceramic materials, chromosomes and tissue studies, pharmaceutical development, mineralogy, petrography, carbon nanotubes, graphene technology, and biological applications for cells [116–121].

5.4 Applications

5.4.1 Disease diagnostics

5.4.1.1 Diabetes

Diabetes is a common metabolic disease caused by impaired carbohydrate metabolism where the person suffers from high blood glucose levels. The number of diabetes patients has increased considerably in the past 40 years [122–124], and is expected to double by 2030 compared to 2015 [125]. Therefore, the measurement of blood glucose levels is essential for diagnosing and monitoring diabetes [126, 127]. Colorimetry, electrochemistry, and fluorescence techniques [127–129] have been developed to measure blood glucose levels. However, they can be inconvenient, painful, and even have the potential risk of cross-contamination. RS, one of the most promising optical approaches, is an accurate and painless means of blood glucose detection. The surface-enhanced method has been widely applied due to weak signals of spontaneous RS. Many researchers have illustrated the diagnostic potential of RS for the non-invasive detection of blood glucose using various body fluids, including tear fluid, salivary, sweat, and blood [130–136].

The SERS technique using silver nanoparticles (AgNPs) was employed to detect type II diabetes mellitus. Multivariate statistical methods of PCA analyzed the SERS spectra. Excess of adenine in patients' samples results in the intensity of Raman signal (probably originated from DNA (RNA) damage), which can be used as an important fingerprint in order to discriminate between diabetic patients and healthy subjects [137]. A similar study showed satisfying discrimination of normal samples from diabetic urine samples with a sensitivity of 85% and a specificity of 90.5%. Detection was based on a portable Raman spectrometer [138]. A recent publication presented the first direct observation of glucose Raman peaks from *in vivo* skin [139]. The experiments were carried out in a wide range of glucose concentrations and long integration times to obtain Raman spectra with a high optical throughput Raman system using oblique angle laser illumination, controlled by infusing dextrose solution and insulin into the swine subjects. RS results showed glucose signal and linearity between intensities of the glucose Raman peaks and the reference glucose concentrations. Deep Raman spectroscopy has been under investigation for several potential medical uses. The results indicate the potential of these techniques for clinical applications.

The first quantitative, *in vivo* transcutaneous glucose measurements using a combination of SERS and SORS, were studied to monitor glucose concentration in the interstitial fluid [140]. Silver film over nanosphere (AgFON) surfaces was functionalized with a mixed self-assembled monolayer and implanted subcutaneously in a Sprague–Dawley rat. SER spectra were collected from the sensor chip through the skin using SORS. However, experiments need more modifications to improve the current level of reproducibility and longevity of the SERS sensor chip and new partition/capture surface layers' developments to grow biological targets accessible to *in vivo* SERS.

TRS was applied to directly monitor glucose levels non-invasively without recourse to labeling [141]. Using a novel high-collection efficiency optical system based on non-imaging optics (compound hyperbolic concentrator) and incorporated within a portable system, the glucose levels were sampled *in vivo* through thenar skin fold in human subjects and results were obtained successfully. The use of the SESORS techniques has been demonstrated to potentially also be very promising.

5.4.1.2 Cancer

Cancer is the second leading cause of death worldwide, sometimes a genetic disease. The development of new techniques for cancer screening and diagnosis is essential. Cell and molecular biology are very important factors in cancer research. Raman-based methods have high resolution to investigate a single cell and organelles. Therefore, Raman scattering, as a powerful tool, enables the label-free detection of any changes of molecular signatures in a cell, tissue, and bodily fluids caused by diseases.

The Raman scattering signal level can also be tremendously enhanced using coherent Raman scattering (CRS) microscopy and surface-enhanced methods. Over the last three decades, various reviews have illustrated Raman scattering-based techniques' achievements, advantages, and limitations to differentiate between normal and cancerous tissues [142–146]. The ability of RS to probe the entire biochemical composition of a sample, thus producing a spectroscopic signature for different disease states based on the simultaneous integration of multiple biomarkers. A non-destructive multimodal system is required to fully analyze subcellular components and the ensemble effects identification. This system provides comprehensive analysis to explore viable live cells with little or no confounding interactive ligands or chemicals. A quantitative molecular and chemical analysis would be directly coordinated with cellular and subcellular imaging. The following studies have capitalized on the advantages of RS for the purpose of diagnosing various cancers through analysis of either *tissue*, *cells*, or *bodily fluids.*

5.4.1.3 Tissue analysis

Tissue analysis is common in disease diagnostic studies, especially cancer diagnosis, indicating the presence of cancer in the body and is available for *in vitro* Raman spectroscopic analysis.

Breast cancer represents the most common cancer among women. Traditional breast cancer screening is a triple assessment using images, clinical examination, and histological assessment. After detecting a cancerous tumor, a core biopsy, including needle technique sampling or surgical biopsy is required. However, both methods have their limitations and possible complications. Then a microscopic evaluation assessment helps to decide the treatment approach. However, this histopathological assessment also presents limitations. Minimally invasive optical imaging and spectroscopy techniques can improve breast cancer diagnosis, especially with the ability to distinguish benign from malignant breast tissues. Breast tissue is a very heterogeneous turbid medium where light scattering poses a great challenge because of the severe loss of the transmitted light and the effect on the directionality of the received signal due to random scattering events.

RS can analyze biopsy samples of solid tumors to differentiate between the Raman spectra of normal and malignant tissues. The integration of confocal microscopy to Raman systems has permitted the analysis of small volumes, in particular depth profiling of biological samples. The biochemical fingerprint of breast tissues has been described in many studies. Normal and malignant breast tissues are different in their lipid and protein contents resulting in differences in the 2800–3000 cm^{-1} region of the Raman spectrum. Therefore, lipids in normal tissue and proteins in malignant lesions dominate the Raman bands [147]. Some studies have reported protein dominance of abnormal tissue, both benign and malignant [148–150].

One of the first cases studied using RS included 123 spectra from 41 specimens from 12 patients, in a range of 1654–1439 cm^{-1} bands of the spectrum in 180° backscattered geometry and 784 nm laser wavelength [151]. Both bands are sensitive to histopathological abnormality, and findings showed the most obvious changes between the Raman spectra of normal and cancerous specimens. Since the chemical content of microcalcifications associated with benign and malignant calcifications was found to be significantly different [152], RS was used to analyze the chemical composition of microcalcifications occurring in benign and malignant ducts with a sensitivity of 88% and a specificity of 93%. This is a significant improvement over current x-ray mammography techniques, which are unable to reliably differentiate microcalcifications in benign and malignant breast lesions.

NIR Raman microimages of human breast tissue using a confocal microscope were acquired to develop a model of breast tissue Raman spectra [153]. Later, the authors applied this model to demonstrate the ability of RS to *ex vivo* diagnose benign and malignant breast lesions based on chemical/morphological changes with 94% sensitivity and 96% specificity [154].

A Raman optical fiber probe designed for medical applications in previous studies [155] was optimized to collect high SNR data from tissue in clinically relevant times in 1 s. Further studies by this research group have led to *in vivo* intraoperative tumor margin assessment [156]. Using their model, the data from nine patients undergoing partial mastectomy procedures were fitted resulting in the characterization of tissue in 1 s. The proposed grossly invisible cancer detection was validated later by pathology review. After these achievements, *in vitro* fresh-frozen tissues in a laboratory setting using normal breast tissue, fibrocystic change, fibroadenoma, and invasive carcinoma were examined in 126 sites from 58 patients [157]. The fit coefficients of Raman spectrum modeling for fat and collagen were found to be the key diagnostic parameters in distinguishing pathologies and were used to form the basis of a binary diagnostic algorithm. The resulting diagnostic algorithm achieved a sensitivity of 94%, a specificity of 96%, and total test efficiency of 95% for cancer diagnosis. This model was also employed in another work [158] for the real-time identification of microcalcifications as an early sign of breast cancer during stereotactic breast core needle biopsies. The results showed the possibility of RS to evaluate types of microcalcifications based on the presence or absence of vibrational bands characteristic of calcium oxalate at 912 and 1477 cm^{-1}. In another work [159], the sensitivity and specificity of RS in differentiating between cancer and normal breast tissue in a mouse model were studied. The data were processed first with principal component analysis to reduce the dimensionality. Secondly, discriminant function analysis was used for sample classification. As a result, 91% of tumor spectra were classified correctly.

RS not only distinguishes tumors from normal breast tissue but also detects early neoplastic changes prior to the definite morphologic alteration. By applying micro-Raman spectra to compare normal and malignant human breast tissues, spectral changes were observed in cancerous tissue, indicating decreased lipid content, increased nucleic acid content with conformation changes, and increased protein content with conformation changes and structural disorders such as broken molecular hydrogen bonds to confirm practicability of Raman microspectroscopy for biochemical study and *vivo* diagnosis of human breast cancers [160].

The first Raman 'optical biopsy' images (532 nm excitation source) of the normal and cancerous breast tissue of the same patient showed [161] the composition (including lipid, carotenoids, and fatty acid) of cancerous and non-cancerous breast tissue were noticeably different, and they were rich with metabolic products of arachidonic acid and monounsaturated oleic acid, respectively. These findings proved the ability of label-free Raman imaging for breast cancer tissue characterization precisely.

Deep Raman spectroscopy, TRS, for the first time, was used to recover Raman spectra of calcified materials buried within a chicken breast tissue slab 16 mm thick [112]. Calcium hydroxyapatite and calcium oxalate monohydrate spectrum were chemically identified. The experimental geometry and gross insensitivity of the Raman signal to the depth of the calcified lesion were in good agreement with probing human female breasts. The same authors [162] also showed the facility of advanced TRS to detect and identify the chemical composition of calcified material within a clinically relevant depth of 27 mm within mammalian tissue. The identification of HAP at 20 mm with an approximate volume ratio of around 1.25×10^{-3} was achieved with this technique. This successful demonstration of the proof of principle led to the next stage of instrumental development with the main goal to achieve a clinically relevant detection sensitivity of microcalcifications inside biological tissue of 40 mm thickness which is around double the penetration depth achieved with their previous instrument design [162] and around two orders of magnitude higher than that possible when using conventional RS [163].

The feasibility of SORS to determine cancer margins under a layer of normal breast tissue was studied [164]. This technique successfully detected breast cancer spectral signatures of tumors as small as 1–2 mm thick beneath up to 2 mm thick normal breast tissue. Subsequently, the authors enhanced the sensitivity and specificity of this approach to 95% and 100%, respectively [165] but the carbonate Raman band overlapped at 1070 cm^{-1} with Raman collagen bands from the tissue, which was a problem to differentiate type II microcalcifications as benign or malignant. This problem was solved by directly monitoring the position and bandwidth of the intense 960 cm^{-1} phosphate Raman band alone to determine carbonate content and thus differentiated type II microcalcifications as either benign or malignant to a depth of 5.6 mm using an 830 nm excitation source [166]. This approach is promising for non-invasive breast cancer screening.

The work progressed into the SESORRS technique for the first time [107]. This method enabled the detection of live breast cancer 3D MTS containing SERRS active nanoparticles (NPs) through 15 mm of tissue. False-color 2D heat intensity maps determined tumor model location. In addition, the authors displayed the tracking of SERRS active NPs through porcine tissue to depths of up to 25 mm. This novel performance is due to the use of red-shifted chalcogenpyrylium-based Raman reporters, which offered significant promise for the translation of NPs into clinical applications for non-invasive disease diagnostics based on this new chemical principle of measurement. Later [167], the depth penetration capabilities of SESORS was utilized and reported multiplexed imaging and classification of three singleplex nanotags and a triplex of nanotags within breast cancer tumor models through depths of 10 mm using a handheld SORS instrument for the first time. Although simultaneous detection of multiple targets *in vivo* is a significant challenge, this novel work was a significant step forward in detecting and classifying multiple vibrational fingerprints *in vivo*.

Brain cancer originates from brain neoplasm cells, and the metastatic cancerous cells (secondary origin) travel from other organs through the blood. The first studies on RS utilization in brain tumor research were performed within two years [168]. Near-infrared Fourier transform (NIR-FT) Raman spectroscopy was applied to the brain tissues of a male eight week old Wistar rat removed from the skull under pentobarbital anesthesia *in situ*. The spectrum was obtained from the cerebral cortex, white matter of the cerebrum, caudate-putamen, thalamus, synaptosomal fraction, and myelin fraction. In the 400–2940 cm^{-1} no interference of autofluorescence was observed. The ratios of the intensity at 1664 (amide I), 1442 (CH_2 deformation), 2885 (CH_2 asymmetric stretching), and 2938 cm^{-1} (CH_3 symmetric stretching) could be used for differentiation between the gray and white matter. By further investigations [169], the Raman spectra of various types of brain tumor showed characteristic bands as diagnostic markers. The brain tumor was diagnosed histologically as glioma grade II and grade III, neurinoma, and neurocytoma of the choroid. Histological examination of glioma grade III exposed a band at 856 cm^{-1} due to polysaccharides; one of the neurinomas containing a carotenoid exhibited two resonance Raman peaks at 1157 and 1524 cm^{-1}. However, another neurinoma was a free-carotenoid. The appearance of a strong Raman peak at 960 cm^{-1} suggested that the central neurocytoma of the choroid plexus was calcified.

Confocal micro-RS (an excitation wavelength of 532 nm over a spectral scan region of 500–4000 cm^{-1}) was employed to study the potential of resonance Raman for distinguishing between normal brain tissues and malignant brain tissues *in vitro* [170]. Resonance Raman spectra from six types of brain tissue were obtained. The ratio of the intensities of the spectral peaks of 2935 to 2880 cm^{-1} from the meningeal cancer tissues may be used as a distinct marker to differentiate between cancerous tissues and normal tissues since these peaks are lower compared to spectral peaks from normal, and benign tissues. The collected resonance Raman spectral data from meningeal cancer tissues were analyzed by the statistical methods of principal component analysis and the support vector machine resulting in a diagnostic sensitivity of 90.9% and specificity of 100%.

The first major study of normal, necrotic, and glioblastoma multiforme (GBM) tissue was investigated by RS using individual peaks to develop a diagnostic algorithm using detrended fluctuation analysis (DFA) [171]. Homogenous regions of normal gray matter, necrosis, and GBM tissue were distinguished with 99.5% and 97.8% accuracy in the primary training and validation groups, using a combination of 37 peaks input to DFA. In contrast with other methods, data compression and black box diagnostic algorithms are not used in this technique. Interpretation of the results presented an increased lipid content of normal brain tissue and protein and nucleic acid content of necrosis.

Lung cancer is one of the most common cancers in humans. However, the long-term survival rate remains low (15% at 5 years) [172]. This low survival rate is due to late-stage disease in patients (~75%), which makes effective treatment unsuccessful. Early detection is urgently required to allow appropriate treatment and reduce mortality rates [173].

Early *ex vivo* and *in vivo* Raman studies revealed this technique's potential to precisely differentiate tumors from healthy tissues [174, 175]. The possibility of distinguishing between normal and malignant lung tissues by using near-infrared Raman spectroscopy (NIR-RS) was discovered in a few studies [176, 177]. An early study employed RS to distinguish tumors from normal bronchial tissue specimens, squamous cell carcinoma, and adenocarcinoma. Nucleic acids, tryptophan, and phenylalanine showed higher intensity bands, while, phospholipids, proline and valine indicated lower signals in malignant tumors than normal tissue. Raman band intensity at 1445 cm^{-1} and 1655 cm^{-1} reveal the most discrimination power between normal and tumor tissues [177].

CARS imaging was also applied to discriminate between normal, benign, and malignant lung tissues [178–180]. Shifted subtracted RS has also been explored as a diagnostic technique for evaluating lung tissue samples [174]. To understand mutations of the epidermal growth factor receptor (EGFR), its relation to lung Adenocarcinoma (lung AC), and its potential to be used in future diagnostic studies, RS was employed to analyze 156 lung AC tissues using PCA-SVM with leave-one-out cross-validation (LOO-CV). The L858R and E19del mutation groups were differentiated from wild type EGFR tissue with 87.8% accuracy. This study provides significant evidence for a novel lung cancer screening method based on RS analysis of EGFR mutations [181]. RS, together with multivariable analysis, allowed differentiation of high-grade dysplasia and malignant lung lesions from tumor tissue and benign lung lesions with high sensitivity and good specificity for 280 tissue sites of 80 patients [182]. The analysis of this vibrational band allowed the discrimination of tumors from normal tissue with a sensitivity of 90% and specificity of 65%, respectively. It was further shown that the low specificity could be improved when RS was combined with autofluorescence and white-light bronchoscopy [183]. A very recent study used RS as a potential diagnostic tool for probing biomolecular changes in lung cancer [184]. The levels of saturated and unsaturated lipids and the protein-to-lipid, nucleic acid-to-lipid, and protein-to-nucleic acid ratios were significantly altered among malignant tissues compared to normal lung tissue, which has profound implications in the biochemical landscape of lung cancer progression and cytopathological classification. Classification methods including k-nearest neighbor (k-NN) and SVM were successfully applied to cytopathologically diagnose lung cancer with an accuracy approaching 99%. The present results indicate that RS is an excellent tool to biochemically interrogate and diagnose lung cancer.

Skin cancer can be divided into three subtypes: melanoma, basal cell carcinoma (BCC), and squamous cell carcinoma (SCC), with melanom, the most common fatal form of skin cancer, accounting for less than 2% of all skin cancer cases. Melanoma is preferably diagnosed at an early stage because it is a metastatic disease. The Breslow thickness is mainly associated with metastatic propensity and prognosis. Melanomas of <1 mm thickness can be treated surgically with a high cure rate without reducing life expectancy. The Breslow thickness >4 mm is diagnosed at an invasive stage with a survival rate of approximately 40%, while surgery and/or immunotherapy are needed with thick melanomas and signs of distant metastasis [185–187]. BCC and SCC are referred to as keratinocytic cancers or non-melanoma and are associated with low mortality rates but can demolish surrounding tissue, recur and (or) metastasize. SCC is associated with a 0.5%–5% risk of metastasis [188].

The applicability of RS *in vivo* and *in vitro*, plus its rapidity in examination and results, along with the good sensibility and specificity, make this technique one of the most valuable optical diagnostic methods in differentiating benign, premalignant, and malignant skin lesions with a good chance to enter common medical practice. BCC diagnosis has been addressed in many studies; in a few articles the analysis of the Raman spectra was performed with various methods such as PLS regression, DA, artificial neural networks (ANN), LOO-CV, etc [189–195]. The utility of RS (1064 nm excitation laser) for BCC diagnosis was carried out to distinguish the spectral features of BCC and normal skin biopsies [194]. BCC spectra showed a decrease at 1270 cm^{-1} (amide III-protein) and 1650 cm^{-1} (amide I-protein) due to disturbances in the α-helix secondary structure of the skin along with changes in protein and lipid structures. The ANN analysis technique separated BCC and normal tissues by spectral changes in the regions of 830–900 cm^{-1}, 900–990 cm^{-1}, and 1220–1360 cm^{-1}. Later [195], the authors again used this neural network system to automatically classify Raman spectra to differentiate melanoma from other clinically similar skin tumors. Based on their findings, melanoma showed a decrease in the intensity of the amide I-protein band around 1660 cm^{-1} as well as an increase in the intensity of the lipid-specific band peaks around 1310 cm^{-1}. These band alterations are also independently identified by ANN showing a sensitivity of 85% and specificity of 99% for melanoma diagnosis.

A logistic regression model was used to differentiate BCC from the surrounding normal, healthy epidermis [196]. The analysis system showed 100% sensitivity and 93% selectivity for BCC diagnosis. Further [197], the ability of high-wavenumber (2800–3125 cm^{-1}) RS to distinguish between BCC and surrounding healthy tissue was examined, revealing 100% and 99% prediction accuracies for BCC and healthy tissue, respectively. Fused silica-based optical fibers produced background signals in the fingerprint region which can be eliminated by high-wavenumber analysis to improve the feasibility of a fibreoptic probe to diagnose tumor borders in BCC.

Most of the articles relied on more than one analyzing technique to obtain reliable results, demonstrating that complex analysis is far superior to limited ones because changes in the spectra are rarely punctual. Multimodal imaging consisting of CARS microscopy, second harmonic generation (SHG), and two-photon excited fluorescence (TPF) were explored to investigate the morphochemistry of basal cell carcinoma [198]. This strategy established an unsupervised tissue classification method based on multimodal imaging and discriminating BCC from non-diseased tissue using chemometrics. Results revealed that BCC tumor cells could be distinguished due to the appearance of large storage cells or reservoirs of lipids, which is corroborated by additional Raman microspectroscopic experiments. Melanoma and non-melanoma have also been able to be distinguished from each other [199–202].

A fibreoptic Raman probe showed high-diagnosis accuracy for non-melanoma skin cancers with 100% sensitivity and 91% specificity for discriminating tumors from normal skin [199]. The real-time RS system was evaluated to diagnose skin cancer *in vivo* [200]. A total of 518 benign and malignant lesions from 453 patients were measured at one second per lesion. Malignant melanoma from non-melanoma pigmented lesions and seborrheic keratosis were differentiated with sensitivities ranging from 95% to 99% and specificities ranging from 15% to 54%. An integrated optical technique was demonstrated for BCC based on autofluorescence imaging and Raman scattering [203], where automated segmentation of autofluorescence images selected and prioritized sparse sampling points for RS, resulting in classification models with 100% sensitivity and 92% specificity. This technique provides a faster diagnosis compared to frozen section histopathology, FTIR spectroscopy alone, and Raman imaging alone. The approach was applied to diagnosing mammary ductal carcinoma [204] and basal cell carcinoma in skin tissue samples [204].

A selective sampling Raman microscopy method was used to collect Raman spectra of tissue samples from individuals with BCC and healthy volunteers, indicating 100% sensitivity and 92.9% specificity for correctly classifying an independent set of skin tissue samples [205]. Wavenumber selection based analysis in combination with multivariate techniques PCA-general discriminant analysis (GDA) and PLS with LOO-CV was used to diagnose skin cancer. 645 lesions (including skin cancer, pre-cancer, and benign skin lesions) from 573 patients with skin cancer were classified [206].

Skin cancer is not well studied using biological fluids or cell samples, suggesting the greatest success for diagnosing skin cancer is through tissue analysis.

Prostate cancer is one of the most common cancer types in men, accounting for approximately a quarter of all new cancer cases. The potential of RS for prostate cancer diagnosis was investigated to study benign epithelial (BE), prostatic intra-epithelial neoplasia (PIN), adenocarcinoma, and different Gleason scores in the human prostate bulk tissues. Raman spectral features of BE, PIN, and cancerous tissues showed two main differences, including strong variations in intensities of certain bands and shifts in certain band positions, which was further analyzed using PCA and DFA. This chemometric method separated the data into three main distinct pathological groups representing BE, PIN, and cancerous state in tissue. Likewise, the analysis of the Raman data of tissues with different Gleason scores showed that the data could be categorized into three distinct groups representing Gleason scores 6, 7, and 8, indicating the potential of RS for diagnosis of different stages of the prostate cancer based on their differences in biochemical compositions.

Immuno-SECARS microscopy tissue was applied for the selective, sensitive, and rapid localization of the basal cell protein p63 in normal prostate by SERS-labeled p63 antibodies in conjunction with coherent Raman microscopy for read-out [208]. To confirm the selective binding of the target-specific metal nanoprobes and to disentangle the role of plasmonic (metal) and molecular (Raman reporter) resonances in this plasmon-assisted four-wave mixing technique, negative control experiments were carried out. This combined plasmonic/non-linear vibrational imaging technique may serve as a promising method for more precise investigations.

RS imaging in combination with SERRS nanostars (a new generation of SERRS) due to their low limit of detection (1.5 fM using parameters amenable to *in vivo* imaging) enabled the visualization of the full tumor extent in state-of-the-art transgenic mouse models of prostate cancer without requiring a dedicated targeting moiety with microscopic precision [209]. Raman scans were performed using a Raman microscope (Renishaw) equipped with a 785 nm diode laser, and the statistical significance (level was set at $P < 0.05$) was determined based on the Student's t-test. The results revealed SERRS nanostars as a promising imaging agent for more precise cancer imaging.

Most recently, for the first time, Raman enhancement effects of hollow copper sulfide nanoparticles (CuSNPs) were identified as a SERS probe for Raman imaging of residual tumor lesions [210]. Contrary to the non-degradable property of Au or Ag nanostructures, which prevent their usage *in vivo* applications, CuS SERS probes are degradable and are cleared well from imaged tissues. This photodegradable CuS SERS probe can be applied in numerous biomedical applications.

Cervical cancer the second commonest gynecological cancer is not a communicable disease, but its cause is contagious. RS diagnostic potential has been investigated in the context of cervical cancer [211–213]. However, normal tissue spectral variations were a hindrance in accurately identifying cervical cancer lesions.

Raman microscopy, in combination with NIR-RS also have been employed for cervical cancer tissue diagnosis [214–220]. For this purpose, Raman spectra were acquired *in vivo* from 172 patients and classified into five tissue categories: true normal, previous disease normal, current normal diagnosis, adjacent normal, low grade, and high grade [211]. The inclusion of these subcategories led to a classification accuracy of 97%. Findings indicated the influence of abnormal changes on Raman spectra. The sensitivity of RS to subtle biochemical differences must be considered to successfully implement it in a clinical setting for diagnosing cervical dysplasia and cancer. Cervical pre-cancer detection was verified using RS *in vivo* [212]. 105 spectra from 29 patients (65 normal and 40 precancerous spectra) were analyzed using genetic algorithm-partial least squares-discriminant analysis (GAPLS-DA), yielding 82.9% diagnostic accuracy (72.5% sensitivity and 89.2% specificity). The possibility of using vaginal tissue to find normal baseline tissue, as well as internal control for spectroscopic assessment of the cervical tissue, was explored [213].

Since the Raman spectral features of normal vaginal and cervical tissues were very similar, cervical cancer diagnoses based on RS are very useful in conditions where normal cervical tissue is unavailable. By analyzing *in vivo* Raman spectra from 93 subjects under clinical supervision, the authors revealed abundant collagen in the normal cervix and prominent DNA in tumors. PCL-DA analysis yielded 97% efficiency to differentiate normal and tumor groups. The previous research [212] was expanded to examine the cervical Raman spectra's fingerprint and high-wave-number spectral bands [214]. Combining the data from both spectral domains into their analysis, the diagnostic accuracy of 82.6% was discerned for the 476 spectra (356 normal and 120 precancerous) collected from 44 patients.

Later, the use of confocal RS against near-infrared autofluorescence (NIR-AF) spectroscopy alone as well as composite NIR-AF/RS was evaluated [215]. Confocal RS yielded diagnostic accuracy of 84.1%, showing an increase over the composite approach (82.3%) and NIR-AF spectroscopy alone (59.6%). RS analysis of tissue samples is not the most optimal method for diagnosing breast cancer, and results are enhanced by analysis of cells instead.

5.4.1.4 Cells analysis

Cytology has been broadly applied for diagnosing cancer since the preparation of cytology specimens is easier, creates less discomfort, is low-cost, and is less complicated compared to biopsied tissue samples.

Breast cancer Non-invasive single-cell RS (785 nm excitation source) and PCA was utilized to analyze and correlate radiation-induced biochemical changes in a panel of human tumor cell lines that vary by the tissue of origin, p53 status, and intrinsic radiosensitivity [221]. The collected RS signatures were aroused from radiation-induced changes in cellular concentrations of aromatic amino acids, conformational protein structures, and certain nucleic acid and lipid functional groups and were detected from live, unfixed, single cells analyzed 1–3 days post-irradiation. The relationship between the RS radiation response signatures and intrinsic radiosensitivity enables RS for detecting radiation resistance or sensitivity in clinical practice.

Live non-malignant (MCF-10A), mildly malignant (MCF-7), and malignant (MDA-MB-231) breast cancer cells were studied [222] to demonstrate the first application of Raman imaging and spectroscopy in diagnosing the role of lipid droplets in cell line cultures that closely mimic an *in vivo* environment of various stages in human breast cancer tissue. Lipid droplets are potential bodies for localizing enzymes responsible for forming eicosanoids produced from arachidonic acid, a polyunsaturated 20-carbon fatty acid. Duraipandian et al [223] continued further studies and specifically targeted epigenetic modifications-acetylation or methylation of lysine in cell nucleoli within the nucleus and lipid droplets in the cytoplasm. An increase in histone acetylation in the nucleoli of the cells parallel with an increase in the aggressiveness of epithelial breast cancer cells was observed. The stretching vibration of the methyl group blue-shifted in cancer cells from 2933 cm^{-1} for non-malignant cells of MCF-10A to 2936 cm^{-1} for mildly malignant cells of MCF-7 and 2939 cm^{-1} for the aggressively malignant cells of MDA-MB-231 in this work. Dietary antioxidant isoflavone daidzein (DAID), a component of soybean, has a similar structure and functions to the endogenous hormone estrogen. Owing to its high antioxidant properties, DAID could inhibit cancer cell growth or trigger cell death. The impact of DAID on human breast cancer cells, MCF-7 (estrogen-dependent, ER+), and MDA-MB-231 (estrogen-independent, ER−) using RS (785 nm excitation source) were studied [224]. Both under investigation cells showed a decrease in cell growth and proliferation in a dose-dependent manner. In MDA-MB-231 cells, cellular protein content was affected, and in MCF-7 cells, DNA and lipids were affected compared to control cells.

Recently, SERS was employed for the early detection of metastatic cancers [225]. Surface sialic acid in metastatic cancer cell lines (MDA-MB-231) and on non-metastatic cancer cell lines (MCF-7) was measured using phenylboronic acid-installed PEGylated gold nanoparticles was coupled with Toluidine Blue O (T/BA-GNP) as SERS probe. Metastatic cancer cell lines produced strong SERS signals to prove the ability of SERS technique to distinguish the metastatic cells based on the surface Neu5Ac density. Moreover, it is very obvious to differentiate between hypersialylated tumor tissues and healthy tissues using T/BA-GNP–based SERS due to plasmon coupling between the specifically aggregated functionalized GNPs. Human epidermal growth factor receptor 2 (HER2) overexpression is associated with increased breast cancer recurrence and a worse prognosis. Lapatinib, the tyrosine kinase inhibitor, blocks HER2 signaling, but its activity is limited due to acquired drug resistance. HER2 amplification and drug resistance of lapatinib were studied using RS in BT474 (HER2+ breast cancer cell), MCF-10A (HER2− control), and HER2+ MCF-10A (HER2+ control) cell lines [226]. HER2 overexpression showed 99% sensitivity and specificity. In Her2+ cells, lipid content was enhanced, and proteome was decreased. Lapatinib-resistant breast cancer cells retained lipogenesis even after lapatinib treatment.

Differential effects of four polyphenols (epigallocatechin gallate (EGCG), gallic acid, resveratrol, and tannic acid) on MCF-7 breast cancer cells using a 532 nm excitation source were examined in 2017 [227]. Raman spectra from each polyphenol-treated (for 24 h) MCF-7 cell indicated an increase in lipid accumulation as well as an increase in cytochrome c into the cytosol in EGCG-treated due to caspase activation and the onset of apoptotic progress. Talari's group [150] reported two studies on breast cancer cell lines analysis. In the first one, two different breast cancer cell lines and one normal cell line were differentiated using a combination of PCA and LDA models with 100% sensitivity and 91% specificity. In a later study, normal proliferating, hypoxic, and necrotic regions of a T-47D human breast cancer spheroid model were analyzed by RS to identify chemical changes that occur as the regions progress to necrosis. PCA found these three regions to be very dissimilar in lipid, amide I, amide III, and nucleic acid content, resulting in a better understanding of the progression of cells to necrosis [228].

The metabolic changes required for metastasis progression of two triple-negative breast cancer cell lines, MDA-MB 231 and MDA-MB 435, were studied [229], and the obtained Raman spectra (532 nm excitation source) were analyzed using a multivariate curve resolution (MCR) method. It was determined that increased levels of amino acids and lower levels of mitochondrial signals are attributes of metastatic bone cells, while lung metastasis tropism is caused by high lipid and mitochondria levels. The authors proposed a method based on the MCR algorithm to achieve unique biochemical insights into the molecular progression of cancer cells using RS. Organ-specific isogenic metastatic breast cancer cell lines were demonstrated [230]. PLS-DA with LOO-CV was employed to categorize the different cell lines with 96.8% accuracy in similarity with obtained results by the support vector machine.

Brain cancer A handheld contact RS probe technique for live, local detection of cancer cells in the human brain was developed [231]. This probe intraoperatively enabled accurate differentiation of normal brain from dense cancer and normal brain invaded by cancer cells, with a sensitivity of 93% and a specificity of 91% in patients with grade 2–4 gliomas. By employing artificial neural network methods, the authors improved previous detection results [232]. They compared the efficacy of RS-MRI, which is considered a standard imaging modality. Further, the authors [233] compared the Raman findings of the previous intraoperative study with both T1-contrast-enhanced and T2-weighted MRI sequences resulting in cancer detection up to ~3.7 cm for T1-contrast enhanced and ~2.4 cm for T2 MRI boundary.

Lung cancer The feasibility of RS in clinical practice needs more improvements in identifying cancer cells from both their normal counterparts and the array of cells present in human tissues. This technique was evaluated to differentiate between lung cancer cells, lung epithelial cells, and lung fibroblasts [234]. Furthermore, the authors studied the reason for these differences and their location in the cell. Cell cytoplasm, cell nucleus, and isolated whole cell nuclei were used. Raman microspectroscopy could differentiate between lung cancer, lung epithelial cells, and lung fibroblasts as well as differentiate between two cells from the same lineage; however, one of them showed increased proliferative activity. The data introduced cells' nuclei are the main source of Raman spectral data that could lead to the application of this technique in cancer diagnosis.

Raman imaging was combined with multivariate classification (PLS-DA) to quantify the spatial distribution of oxide nanoparticles inside living lung epithelial cells (A549) [235]. Cells were exposed to TiO_2 (titania) and/or α-FeO(OH) (goethite) nanoparticles at various incubation times (4 or 48 h). A large fraction of spectra (up to 40%), classified as belonging to the cell nucleus, indicated Raman bands associated with nanoparticles. The conclusions are qualitatively supported by complementary transmission electron microscopy (TEM) data for thin cell sections.

A novel class of biocompatible, highly sensitive SERS nanotags based on chitosan-coated silver nanotriangles labeled with para-aminothiophenol (p-ATP) was designed to assay inside lung cancer cells (A549) [236]. These SERS nanotags showed low *in vitro* toxicity, detectability inside cells under a wide window of excitation wavelengths (from visible to NIR) without any cell proliferation interference which made them a promising candidate for intracellular SERS sensing and imaging.

Skin cancer RS was applied for the first time to discriminate the skin carcinoma model cell lines, the non-tumourigenic HaCaT and the cancerous A5RT3 cells using fixed-cell droplets (or adherent fixed), and living cells to provide molecular information about biochemical differences between healthy and cancerous cells [237]. The obtained information was rather reproducible and rapidly determined such changes. The Raman spectra show differences in the relative intensity ratios at 1656 cm^{-1} (amide I-protein), 1250 cm^{-1} (amide III), 1003.6 cm^{-1} (phenylalanine ring mode), and at 1448 cm^{-1} (CH_2 deformation) which were considerably greater for HaCaT cells than A5RT3 cells. The severe and consistent changes in the amide III region and the collagen marker region around 936 cm^{-1} revealed protein degradation along with changes in the essential amino acid phenylalanine and lipid components of tumourigenic A5RT3 cells. HaCaT cells presented higher lipid content and mainly proteins in α-helical conformation, but the tumourigenic A5RT3 cells have more disordered proteins, partially deregulated and degraded. There was a linear dependence of the tumourigenic changes on the passage number of the HaCaT cells, indicating a correlation of tumourigenic transformation with primarily genetic instabilities in HaCaT cells. The late pass HaCaT cells were more likely to acquire benign to premalignant capabilities.

Raman microscopy was also employed to study HaCaT cells, melanocytes (MC), and their malignant counterparts, SCC and melanoma (MM) cells. Reflectance confocal imaging is used to guide spectral measurements [238]. Significant differences were observed between the spectra of HaCaT cells and SCC cells, MC cells, MM cells, and all normal cells (HaCaT and MC) and all tumor cells (SCC and MM) with approximately 90% sensitivity and specificity. The capability of Raman microscopy in separating different cell lines was proved.

A label-free tumor imaging using Raman microspectroscopy exploits the intrinsic vibrational contrast of endogenous biomolecular species [239]. Normal human skin cells (keratinocytes and fibroblasts), the human HaCaT *in vitro* skin carcinogenesis model, and the tumor-derived mesenchymal -epithelial transition (MET) *in vivo* skin cancer progression model were monitored. Direct visualization of the distributions representative of tryptophan-rich proteins and nucleic acids with subcellular spatial resolution became possible by mapping the amplitudes of two spectrally well-isolated Raman bands at 752 cm^{-1} and 785 cm^{-1}. Normal human epidermal keratinocytes (NHEK) and dermal fibroblasts (NHDF) as well as all tumourigenic cells from both the NHEK and NHDF were differentiated using these Raman markers. An organotypic cutaneous squamous cell carcinomas (cSCC) model allowed the identification of tumor cells and their surrounding stroma in the tissue context, which showed the successful application of the proposed intracellular nucleic acid and tryptophan Raman signatures for skin cancer diagnosis. Unlike the previously reported distinction between normal and tumourigenic HaCaT cells [240], this group proposed a well-defined Raman peak amplitude ratio as a straightforward Raman signature for skin tumor diagnosis, corresponding to the abundance of nucleic acids relative to tryptophan-rich proteins. Moreover, this study expanded to the metastatic HaCaT-RAS A5RT3 cells grown in a 3D organotypic culture, suggesting more general applicability of this signature also in the tissue context.

Prostate cancer RS has successfully been used to distinguish normal and malignant cultured cell lines in cancer. Contrary to early studies of cells in culture, which used one measurement per cell, developed techniques comprehensive mapping of individual cells to visualize cell structure and biological processes in real-time. A SERRS-biotag approach was applied [241] to distinguish between cancerous and non-cancerous epithelial prostate cells *in vitro* using cell-specific peptides. SERRS spectra were collected from two sets of biotags simultaneously bound to the cells. One of the two sets of biotags (infused with a unique Raman reporter molecule) was functionalized to target cancer cells, and the other functions as a positive control (PC) and binds to both non-cancerous and cancer cells. Each was infused with a unique Raman reporter molecule. The authors employed a very low laser intensity to provide a good signal to noise and a single wavelength to excite all biotags. Obtained SERRS spectra were analyzed with subcellular resolution, extracting ratios of neuropilin-1/positive control (NRP/PC) that functioned as a statistically robust quantitative measure of the overexpression of neuropilin-1 by the cancer cell line. The results showed the two cell populations were well separated both visually and numerically as well as highly distinct ($P < 0.001$, the *t*-test). By applying proper tags and peptides, non-cancerous and cancerous cell discrimination is easily possible. The focal plane location, the local cell concentration, and turbidity did not affect the indicative ratio.

A label-free Raman microspectroscopy and biomolecular component analysis were utilized to investigate the role of lipogenesis in prostate cancer progression and the evaluation of prostate cancer biomarkers [242]. Increased lipid accumulation in late-stage transgenic adenocarcinoma of mouse prostate (TRAMP) tumors compared to early-stage TRAMP and normal prostate tissues were observed. Raman microscopy results were validated by direct quantitation of lipid content in TRAMP tumor tissues by estimating free faty acids (FFA) and cholesterol content. The overall genetic alterations add up to only 17% of patients within the Cancer Genome Atlas Prostate Adenocarcinoma dataset. Even this small number is sufficient to predict the overall survival of patients which may play an implemental role in prostate cancer diagnosis, but not a significant role in poorly differentiated neuroendocrine a disease.

RS in a combination of PCA/LDA was another technique to investigate biochemical changes in androgen-independent prostate cancer cells (DU145) concerning normal immortalized prostate cells (PNT2) [243]. The advanced principal component analysis method (APCA) analyzed collected Raman spectra from the two cell lines (sensitivity 95%; specificity 88%). DU145 cells showed greater phenylalanine, tyrosine, DNA, Amide III, and PNT2 cells contained L-arginine and B conformation DNA. PCA/LDA determined higher glycogen, phenylalanine, DNA and nucleic acid content were decisive for assigning cells to the DU145 class and greater L-arginine levels for attributing cells to the PNT2 class. RS as a diagnostic and detection (biomolecular changes) technique in androgen-independent prostate cancer cells was proved. The effect of the pesticide Aldrin on human prostate cancer cells was studied [244]. Aldrin increases the risk of developing prostate cancer in men exposed to it. Therefore, a portion of prostate cancer cells was exposed to Aldrin to analyze the differences between normal and treated prostate cell populations using PLS-DA with cross-validation (CV) identified biomarkers associated with pollutant stress. The best classifier built achieved 91.3% specificity and 80.0% sensitivity for distinguishing the two cell classes.

Most recently, deep-ultraviolet Raman spectroscopy (UVRS) also showed the powerful diagnostic capability of RS to differentiate normal human primary prostate epithelial cells and grade IV adenocarcinoma PC-3 prostate cancer successfully [245].

Cervical cancer There are relatively fewer studies on cervical cytology using RS [11, 246–251], most probably due to confounding parameters. The potential of RS for cervical cancer screening using routine cervical cytology samples from a cervical screening program was evaluated [250]. Both the cervical intraepithelial neoplasia (CIN) and the squamous intraepithelial lesion (SIL) terminology systems were used to classify cervical cancer cells. Good quality Raman spectra were recorded from unstained single cervical cells on glass slides. PCA-LDA analysis was employed to build classification models based on either CIN or SIL terminology. Excellent sensitivity and specificity values were obtained, particularly when CIN rather than SIL terminology was used to classify the samples. This suggests that the HSIL category is quite heterogeneous with CIN2 cases being biochemically different from CIN3 cases. High-grade squamous intraepithelial cells (HSIL) were detected by investigating HSIL associated biochemical changes in morphologically normal-appearing intermediate and superficial cells using RS [251]. 755 Raman spectra were measured from intermediate and superficial cells from negative cytology ThinPrep specimens and from morphologically normal-appearing intermediate and superficial cells from HSIL cytology ThinPrep specimens. The Raman data were subjected to multivariate algorithms, including PCA-LDA and PLS-DA with random subsets cross-validation for discriminating negative cytology from HSIL. The PCA-LDA method yielded sensitivities of 74.9%, 72.8%, and 75.6% and specificities of 89.9%, 81.9%, and 84.5%, for HSIL diagnosis based on the dataset obtained from intermediate, superficial and mixed intermediate/superficial cells, respectively. The PLS-DA method improved sensitivities of 95.5%, 95.2%, and 96.1% and specificities of 92.7%, 94.7%, and 93.5% compared to the PCA-LDA method. This study brings the translation of RS to cervical cancer screening closer by eliminating the difficulty of finding the rare morphologically abnormal cells on the unstained slides.

Most recently, a novel non-invasive and label-free approach with high accuracy was offered using a liquid-based cytology Pap smear. CARS and SHG/TPF imaging were performed at one wavenumber on the Pap smears from normal, low-grade

(LSIL), and high-grade (HSIL) squamous intraepithelial lesions, which were selected based on the ratio of the nucleus to the cytoplasm and cell morphology [11]. Raman spectral imaging of single cells from the same smears was obtained. Deep convolutional neural networks (DCNNs) were trained independently with CARS, SHG/TPF, and Raman images, taking both morphotextural and spectral information into account. DCNNs based on CARS, SHG/TPF, or Raman images have discriminated between normal and cancerous Pap smears with 100% accuracy, demonstrating the prospective use of CARS/SHG/TPF microscopy as a label-free imaging technique for the fast screening of a large number of cells in cytopathological samples.

5.4.1.5 Body fluids

Biofluids (blood, urine, or saliva) are considered perfect biological specimens for diagnostic tests since their collection is simple, non-invasive, less costly, and can be collected without harming the patient. Moreover, biofluid components such as DNA, hormones, proteins, and metabolites can provide biochemical information. These advantages have led to extensive research on the utility of advanced Raman techniques by analyzing biofluids for cancer detection and cancer stage determination.

Breast cancer Conventional RS coupled with BGA for breast cancer diagnosis by blood serum analysis was studied [252]. Samples were obtained from 11 clinically diagnosed patients with breast cancer and 12 healthy volunteer controls. These samples were frozen and solid residues were removed for spectral analysis to acquire Raman signal. Multivariate analysis revealed seven Raman band ratios involving the amino acids phenylalanine, tryptophan, and tyrosine as well as polysaccharides and β-carotene that led to the discrimination between cancerous and non-cancerous samples with 97% sensitivity and 78% specificity.

The possibility of using urine as a sample platform to detect breast cancer was examined [253]. Samples of unprocessed urine were collected from control and breast tumor-bearing rats and were evaluated using RS and Raman spectrum. Bands associated with urea (1006 cm^{-1} and 1161 cm^{-1}) and creatinine (680 cm^{-1} and 850 cm^{-1}) were obtained to show the greatest change between control and tumor-bearing rats. The results remained unchanged even with urine concentration increment and additional spectral features. PCA-LDA spectral analysis revealed efficiencies of 72% (unprocessed urine samples) and 91% (concentrated urine samples).

As a biological specimen, saliva was evaluated to diagnose breast cancer based on SERS [254]. After samples were collected from three groups, including 33 healthy subjects, 33 patients with benign breast tumors, and 31 patients with malignant breast tumors, 97 SERS spectra were acquired. Multiclass partial least squares-discriminant analysis displayed the saliva protein SERS spectra from healthy subjects, benign breast tumor patients, and malignant breast tumor patients, yielding diagnostic sensitivities of 75.75% (healthy subjects), 72.73% (benign breast tumor), and 74.19% (malignant breast tumor) as well as specificities of 93.75%, 81.25%, and 86.36%, respectively. The results confirmed the great potential of SERS as a non-invasive and label-free method for the detection of breast cancer.

Recently, SERS was applied for urine analysis samples from 53 patients and 22 controls to discriminate between the two groups using PCA-LDA. Silver nanoparticles were synthesized by reduction with hydroxylamine hydrochloride and activated with Ca^{2+} 10^{-4} M to promote the specific adsorption of anionic purine metabolites (uric acid, xanthine, and hypoxanthine) on the metal surface. The SERS spectra were acquired without any filtering or processing step for removing protein traces and other contaminants and classified with a sensitivity of 81%, a specificity of 95%, and an overall accuracy of 88%. Conclusion: the results of this preliminary study contribute to the translation of SERS in the clinical setting and highlight the potential of SERS as a novel screening strategy for breast cancer [255].

Due to cancer incidence and mortality rate, a simple and affordable treatment monitoring technique to facilitate tailored treatment protocols for better survival is an urgent need. A study based on a combination of RS techniques and statistical analysis was conducted to compare the Raman spectra of liquid blood plasma of biopsy proved 19 breast cancer patients under pre- and post-treatment conditions with the control group [256]. The results indicated a statistical significance in the spectral signatures between the normal and breast cancer patient's blood plasma as well as between pre-treated and post-treated plasma, possibly attributed to the changes in the vibrational characteristics of some of the key biomolecules. Also, the spectral signatures of post- treated plasma and normal subjects were almost matched. The characteristic vibration of the key biomolecules present in the fingerprint region of 700–1800 cm^{-1} could differentiate cancer from normal as well as pre-treated from post-treated cancer samples with high sensitivity and specificity resulting in survival improvement and therapeutic efficacy assessment.

SERS as a promising technique in providing specific molecular information requires the presence of a suitable plasmonic substrate that can generate enhanced and reproducible diagnostic relevant spectra. A very recent approach was presented for the synthesis of a plasmonic substrate [257]. Concentrated silver nanoparticles were purified by the tangential flow filtration method and employed to generate reproducibly and enhanced Raman signals. A combination of multivariate analysis (MVA) and SERS was used to test blood plasma samples collected from 35 healthy donors and 29 breast cancer patients. Analysis of all the spectra showed the great discrimination between healthy donors and breast cancer patients with 90% sensitivity, 89% specificity, and 89% accuracy indicating the ability of the substrate to generate diagnostic relevant spectral information. The utilization of this solid substrate type could be feasible for other types of cancer or disease diagnosis.

Lung cancer Blood serum was used in two different studies to successfully diagnose lung cancer, suggesting the advantage of blood serum over other body fluids for this purpose. Varieties of modeling techniques were studied to distinguish collected blood serum from 29 healthy donors and 68 donors with lung cancer [258]. Using uncorrelated linear discriminant analysis (ULDA) and LDA combined with multiple scatter correction (MSC) pretreatment, a distinction with 100% sensitivity and specificity was achieved. However, MSC combined with PLS-DA was unsuccessful in achieving the goal and further demonstrated the significance of chemometric technique selection. Analysis of 91 blood serum samples from healthy individuals and patients in different non-small cell lung cancer stages (stages I–IV) using LDA with CV was carried out [259]. Five different groups with an overall accuracy of 92% were obtained.

SERS as a good candidate for the easy-to-use diagnostic tool was applied to detect non-small cell lung cancer (NSCLC) [260]. A label-free serum test based on SERS spectroscopy was utilized to analyze human serum to diagnose of NSCLC. Highly-branched gold nanoparticle (HGNP) substrates were used. Spectral serum data were collected from healthy subjects, lung adenocarcinoma patients, lung squamous carcinoma patients, and large cell lung cancer patients and analyzed using PCA. The results revealed their intrinsic differences in type and the content of nucleic acids, proteins, carbohydrates, amino acids, and lipids. The advantages of this SERS-based approach, are that it is label-free, time efficient, and senstive suggesting that it is a promising method for mass screening of NSCLC, detecting, and preventing other diseases.

Prostate cancer Many prostate cancer diagnoses from blood serum and urine using SERS have been reported [261–266]. In 2003, one of the first immunoassays that utilized SERS to detect prostate-specific antigen (PSA) in human serum was made [261]. Raman probes were functionalized by 30 nm gold nanoparticles (AuNPs) with an anti-human PSA antibody and the Raman reporter 5,5′-dithio-bix(succinimidyl-2-nitrobenzoate) (DSNB). Covalently linking the PSA antibodies to the Raman reporter and, in turn, AuNPs increased performance over physisorption techniques. PSA was detected in human serum at very low levels (~1 pg ml^{-1}). SERS was also coupled with SVM analysis to evaluate blood serum from 93 prostate cancer patients and 68 healthy volunteers [262]. Three SVM classifier models, including linear, polynomial, and radial basis function (RBF) kernel functions, were built and evaluated with measured serum SERS spectra. PCA-LDA was also applied to classify the same datasets. The diagnostic accuracy of three SVM diagnostic models (98.1%) was higher than that of PCA-LDA algorithms (91.3%), and the maximum diagnostic accuracy of 98.8% was acquired with RBF kernel SVM classifier model. These discrepancies can be reconciled by the PCA technique losing a part of the effective diagnostic information during processing the SERS spectra, or PCA-LDA (linear algorithms) could not distinguish the non-linear boundary between normal and prostate cancer serum SERS spectra.

A high-throughput (HT) RS technique was developed to test peripheral blood plasma from 10 patients and 10 healthy volunteers using a Horiba (Jobin Yvon LabRAM HR 800) setup equipped with 785, 660, 532, and 473 nm lasers collecting spectra from each sample in a range of 400–1800 cm^{-1} [263]. Spectra were pre-processed and classified by PCA-LDA and revealed significant differences between Raman spectra of prostate cancer patients and non-cancer controls. The (HT) classification resulted in 96.5% and 95% sensitivity and specificity, respectively. The HT-Raman spectroscopy method used in this study overcame some limitations associated with the clinical translation of RS, suggesting the rapid and accurate diagnosis of prostate cancer using liquid plasma samples.

Cervical cancer Blood serum and urine were both studied in an attempt to diagnose cervical cancer. The feasibility of using AgNPs as a SERS substrate was evaluated along with multivariate statistical techniques to discriminate cervical cancer patients from healthy subjects using the blood plasma. This potential SERS-based label-free blood test examined human blood plasma with optimum diagnostic accuracy [267]. PCA was utilized to distinguish serum samples from 19 cervical cancer patients, 3 pre-cancer individuals, and 20 healthy controls [268]. Differences in Raman spectra indicated a high amount of carotenoids and intense protein in the control serum and higher concentrations of glutathione and tryptophan in the disease serum. Using a leave-one-participant-out cross-validation (LOPO-CV) technique, 100% sensitivity and specificity was achieved. The investigation of 27 urine samples collected from healthy volunteers and patients with cancer was accomplished [269]. Using an LDA diagnostic algorithm, 100% accuracy was achieved for discrimination. These two studies [268, 269] suggested that successfully obtained results for diagnosing cervical cancer were independent of body fluid type. In the future, this technique may be used for mass screening.

5.4.1.6 Other cancers

Colorectal cancer is the second most common cancer in males and the third most common cancer in females worldwide. Efficient diagnostic tools and effective therapy are essential due to the high mortality rate. RS, mainly SERS (blood analysis), has been comprehensively investigated by many studies using PCA-LDA, PLS-DA, SVM, MLR, etc [270–277] for fast and non-destructive detection of colorectal cancer patients, which can also surveil the treatment effects of receiving chemotherapy for long-term follow up when compared with tissue samples.

Most recently, electronic published article databases using the fixed-effect model and random effect model to calculate the pooled sensitivity, specificity, diagnostic accuracy, positive likelihood ratio (PLR), negative likelihood ratio (NLR), diagnostic odds ratio (DOR), and positive posttest probability (PPP) of colorectal cancer were systematically investigated [278]. The potential source of heterogeneity and risk of publication bias was assessed using meta-regression and subgroup analysis and Egger linear regression tests, respectively. This diagnosis accuracy was included in 13 studies (679 patients: 186 with premalignant lesions and 493 with malignant lesions). Based on the results, RS showed many capabilities regarding colorectal cancer, including using broadly in clinical practice rather than tentative research, early-stage diagnosis with high diagnostic authenticity and reliability, determination of the range of resection, and SERS might also be used to monitor the therapeutic effects of patients after receiving chemotherapy treatment. However, improvements in diagnostic authenticity and reliability of premalignant lesions of the colorectal are imperative.

Ovarian cancer is the fifth leading cause of cancer among women. The 5-year relative survival rate for women treated for cancer at stages IA and IB is 92%. However, only 15% of all ovarian cancers are found at this early stage [279]. Advances in identifying precursor lesions to ovarian cancer may enhance the ability to detect early-stage disease. RS along with multivariate analysis has been employed previously in ovarian cancer diagnosis from normal tissue [280–283], from patient serum [284–288], and cell lines [289–291].

In a recent study [292], both RS and SERS using silver nanoparticles in combination with the SVM algorithm were employed to identify signatures linked to cancer. Blood plasma samples were collected from 27 patients with ovarian cancer and 28 with benign gynecological conditions (the majority had a prolapse). For the detection of ovarian cancer, Raman achieved 94% sensitivity and 96% specificity, SERS 87% sensitivity and 89% specificity. Raman achieved sensitivity and specificity of 93% and 97% for early ovarian cancer, respectively, while SERS had 80% sensitivity and 94% specificity. Both techniques detected five spectral biomarkers. This minimally invasive test may provide an alternative diagnostic and screening tool for ovarian cancer superior to other established blood-based biomarkers.

Pancreatic cancer is the third leading cause of cancer-related death in the USA, and the survival rate of people treated for exocrine pancreatic cancer at stage IA is 12%, stage IIA 5%, stage III 3%, and stage IV 1% [293, 294].

Researchers at many cancer research centers investigated the potential of RS combined with multivariate analysis in early-stage diagnoses such as Raman microscopy [295, 296], RS and SRS microscopy [297], SERS and SERRS [298–301]. A new method based on serum RS for the first time was proposed [302] to distinguish patients with benign and malignant tumors of the pancreas using PLS to extract the Raman spectrum information. The cumulative variance of the first six PLS components reached 97.045% and then was classified. This experiment used three classification algorithms: LDA, SVM, and k-NN. SVM achieved the best classification effect with an accuracy of 96.4%. The experimental results show that serum RS may become a new auxiliary method for the clinical diagnosis of pancreatic cancer.

Bladder cancer is the ninth most frequently diagnosed epithelial cancer worldwide. Its histopathological diagnosis is based on the stage and grade of the tumor, where the stage refers to tumor invasion into the bladder wall and grade to the aggressiveness of the cells.

A bladder cancer diagnosis has been studied using a Raman fiber probe [303, 304], a combination of autofluorescence with RS [305–307], and Raman microspectroscopy [308, 309]. The first *in vivo* Raman probe used in the bladder was an Emvision® probe with a filtered six-around-one fiber configuration to collect raman spectra of bladder upper urothelium surface and deeper layers from suspicious and non-suspicious. Bladder cancer was distinguished from the normal bladder with a sensitivity of 85% and a specificity of 79%. The authors suggested a Raman probe that collects a shallower signal from the urothelium surface of the bladder would be ideal for early diagnosis [303].

Head and neck cancer include cancer of the oral cavity, nasopharynx, oropharynx, hypopharynx, and larynx. The most frequent type of cancer in the head and neck region is oral cavity squamous cell carcinoma (OCSCC). An *in vivo* multi-fiber Raman probe system was used [310, 311] to measure oral diseases. The results indicated that RS is a promising diagnostic tool.

5.4.1.7 Cardiovascular diseases

The leading cause of death worldwide with an even greater mortality rate than cancer are cardiovascular diseases [312]. Atherosclerosis (AT), one of the leading causes of cardiovascular events, reduces the blood flow and affects the nutritional supply of organs. The severity of an atherosclerotic plaque and its stability is strongly correlated with its biochemical composition [313], which can be analyzed by lipid cores, thin fibrous caps infiltrated by macrophages, proteoglycan matrices in a smooth muscle cell-rich environment, intraplaque hemorrhage, or calcified nodules protruding into the vessel lumen [314].

Various Raman-based sensing [315], spectroscopy [316–328], and microscopy [329–335] methods used in cardiac disease management either *ex vivo* [336] or *in vivo* [316–322, 336] are mostly cost-efficient, rapid, and practical for use in clinical applications. These techniques can be utilized in molecular and cellular level investigation [329–331] as well as tissue level anomalies [332–334].

SERS was applied for both *ex vivo* and *in vivo* models to diagnose and identify plaques. RRS examined the molecular signatures inside blocked arteries to find the inflammatory markers which cause the manifestation of rupture-thrombosis [336]. A protein, intercellular adhesion molecule-1 (ICAM-1), was utilized attached to gold NPs to detect ICAM-1 expression in aortic sinus tissues obtained from atherosclerotic-prone apolipoprotein E-deficient (apoe$^{-/-}$) mice for *in vivo* study [336].

Recently, label-free RS was applied to evaluate the viability of ischemic myocardial tissue in patients undergoing cardiac surgery. The four signature peaks of cardiomyocytes corresponding to heme proteins exhibited both myocardial infarction region (MI) and non-infarcted (non-MI). Since the non-MI tissues consisted mostly of cardiomyocytes, they showed higher peak intensities as they mainly consisted of cardiomyocytes. Peaks from collagen, suggesting the presence of fibrosis in the MI tissue. Cytochrome c, cytochrome b5, myoglobin, and hemoglobin bands were found in both MI and non-MI. The results showed that Raman bands in close proximity are difficult to identify due to high SNR. Therefore, multivariate spectral analysis was used for infarcted from the non-infarcted myocardial tissue differentiation to acquire a prediction model using PLS-DA in the Raman spectrum data [333]. A cardiovascular calcification study based on RS revealed that the concentrations of apatite, triglyceride and cholesterol increased, and the concentration of β-carotene decreased in atherosclerotic plaque [327]. Despite numerous studies on the biochemical applications of RS, cardiovascular Raman research is still considered to be a novel field that requires further studies.

5.4.1.8 Neurodegenerative diseases

These diseases, such as Alzheimer's disease (AD), Parkinson's disease (PD), prion diseases, Huntington's disease, amyotrophic lateral sclerosis (ALS), motor neuron disease, and dementia are caused by the degeneration and loss of function of neurons in the brain and peripheral nervous system. Not only is the diagnosis of these diseases in the early stages difficult but also there are currently no treatments available to slow disease progression or cure these diseases. Normal RS is applied to characterize and diagnose neurodegenerative diseases.

AD is characterized by widespread neuronal death leading to memory loss and cognitive decline with disease progression. Amyloid-β (Aβ) and tau are two main pathological markers for AD that aggregate into extracellular amyloid plaques and intracellular neurofibrillary tangles. The selective passage of several substances between the brain and blood systems is controlled by the blood–brain barrier. AD biomarkers can be transported into the vascular system across the blood–brain barrier, while the blood–brain barrier is not able to clear Aβ and tau protein from the brain leading to the development of AD [337]. These biomarkers can rejoin the vascularization of other body districts, like the retina, lens, and lacrimal regions, affecting the composition of tears. Also, they can be found in blood serum and saliva [338, 339].

Vibrational spectroscopic technique characterizations such as fast, reliable, cost-effective, non-destructive, smaller sample amount required, minimal sample preparation, providing both sample chemical composition information and the molecular structure, make them ideal for clinical practice use. Moreover, the simultaneous study of all molecules present in the sample and not individually is allowed for the diagnostics of complex and multifactorial diseases which can be used to efficiently and reliably discriminate spectra.

RS combined with multivariate statistical methods has been used to identify AD biomarkers in blood serum [340–343], saliva [344], and tears [345] to investigate the basic aggregation mechanisms of amyloids [346]. Through two-dimensional correlation spectroscopy, characteristic spectral features of peripheral blood plasma from AD patients that can be useful to sensitively and specifically diagnose AD were investigated. The authors studied the capability of Raman and IR spectroscopy of blood plasma for differentiating AD from normal ageing of healthy controls. Blood plasma samples were collected from 8 mild AD, 16 moderate AD, 11 severe AD, and 12 normal elderly control persons using Fourier transform spectrometers and a NIR laser beam as an excitation source for RS. Spectra were processed employing discriminant analysis to determine whether band areas and frequency–intensity relationships might reveal biochemical differences associated with AD. Seven spectral biomarkers were identified in the Raman regions of 1700–1600 cm^{-1} (protein secondary structure), 980–910 cm^{-1} (protein α-helices), 790–730 cm^{-1} (protein tertiary structure), and 440–390 cm^{-1} (protein backbone) and in the IR regions of 1700–1600 cm^{-1} (protein secondary structure) and 1150–1000 cm^{-1} (oxidative stress). DA differentiated AD from normal aging of elderly control persons with a sensitivity of 89% and specificity of 92%. Moreover, specificity increases to 100% to detect mild AD, indicating the possibility of using this spectroscopic approach for early accurate diagnosis of AD [340]. In another work [341], RS of blood serum was evaluated combined with ANN classification models for the differential diagnosis of AD from patients with other types of dementia and healthy elderly volunteers with an overall accuracy of 95%. The neural network algorithm showed limited significance for interpreting the spectra from a biochemical point of view and could not determine the Raman spectra's regions. To overcome this issue, a genetic algorithm was employed to find the most significant spectral regions for the discrimination of the measured spectra.

The development of SERS overcame some limits of conventional RS [341] and affectively improved the sensitivity [343]. A significant improvement in human serum analysis for AD diagnosis was highlighted [343]. Blood serum from AD patients was examined by SERS-AgNPs coupled with ANNs. The obtained spectra were compared with spectra from healthy controls (HC) from patients with other neurodegenerative dementias (OD). Diagnostic sensitivity is around 96% for differentiating AD samples HC samples in a binary model and 98% for differentiating AD, HC, and OD samples in a tertiary model. Also, SERS coupled with PCA and interval PCA generated the spectra acquired from human tears collected from AD subjects compared to samples from healthy subjects and subjects with ascertained mild-cognitive symptoms [345]. The results are very encouraging, with interesting perspectives for medical applications supporting clinical diagnosis and discrimination of AD from other forms of dementia.

Parkinson's disease is diagnosed by the death of dopaminergic neurons within the substantia nigra (SN), causing a breakdown of effective muscular control. Patients face memory and behavioral abnormalities with low life expectancy. Alpha-synuclein (α-syn) is one of the main pathological markers for PD, containing a toxic element that leads to neurodegeneration. Monomeric α-syn exists in a natively unfolded conformation which this secondary structure has a strong propensity for α-helical structure (N-terminal region).

RS was utilized to determine the contribution of secondary structure components to the overall structure of monomeric α-syn through deconvolution of the Amide I region of α-syn by fitting three-component bands (α-helix ~1650–1656 cm^{-1}, β-sheet ~1664–1670 cm^{-1} and unordered ~1680 cm^{-1}), as well as bands corresponding to aromatic amino acids [347]. Results confirmed the ability of RS to characterize the ensemble of secondary structures present in natively unfolded proteins. Augmented oxidative stress (OS) has been implicated in both neural and peripheral PD tissues.

Raman scattering and NIR spectroscopy were utilized to diagnose and quantify oxidative substrate modifications in blood plasma samples from PD and normal elderly control (NEC) subjects [348]. Hypothesis-driven preselection of OS-sensitive bandwidths differentiated PD from NEC subjects with approximately 75% sensitivity and specificity using both complementary spectroscopic techniques.

RS is not sensitive enough to detect physiological concentrations of α-syn and SERS can be employed. However, SERS has not been applied to detect α-synuclein. Dopamine level decreases during PD progression with striatal dopaminergic neuronal loss reported between 30%–70% before the onset of motor symptoms, suggesting dopamine levels as a biomarker for PD. A few studies have applied SERS to the detection of dopamine [349–353]. Magnetite-O-carboxymethyl chitosan–silver nanocomposite with Fe-NTA as a dopamine-selective compound (m@cmCH@Ag@Fe-NTA) was developed. O-carboxymethyl chitosan acts as an *in situ* reducing agent for silver ions to form a linker of both magnetite and silver NPs and enables good dispersity of the nanocomposite. Since all amino groups are involved in silver NPs binding, they did not affect the sorption of unwanted interferences on the polymer. Dopamine can be analyzed at a concentration level from units to thousands of femtomoles using a novel approach of purifying the sample with magnetic separation and consequent detection [350].

A few researchers have utilized RS to diagnose Huntington's disease (HD) [354–356] and SERS to diagnose prion diseases [357–360]. However, there are rare studies to date that have tested the diagnostic potential of RS for prion disease, specifically in sheep that are naturally susceptible to scrapie infection [361].

5.4.1.9 Inflammatory diseases

These are linked to a vast array of disorders characterized by inflammation, including allergic asthma, auto-immune disease, hepatitis, and inflammatory bowel disease (IBD), among others. The early diagnosis and treatment of auto-immune infections and metastatic diseases need inflammatory changes diagnosis [362].

Ex vivo Raman-based diagnostics of asthma and hepatitis were investigated by analyzing serum and blood plasma samples of patients with asthma and hepatitis [363, 364]. Ulcerative colitis (UC) and Crohn's (CC) disease are two distinct types of IBD. Detection of molecular alterations in UC and CC has already been studied using RS [365], a colonoscopy-coupled Raman fiber probe [366], and a sparse multinomial logistic regression algorithm based on a Bayesian machine learning framework of statistical pattern recognition [367] with a classification accuracy of 95%. A pilot *in vivo* Raman study to discriminate between IBD and normal colon was examined, but optimal sensitivity and specificity were not achieved. However, enough information to discriminate between IBD and normal colon was obtained, demonstrating the potential of RS as a diagnostic tool for IBD [368].

5.4.1.10 Bone diseases

Bone protein chemistry may undergo changes to cause many bone diseases invisible to conventional techniques. However, RS, as a powerful tool, can detect these molecular changes leading to the diagnosis of osteoarthritis and fragility fractures. Frequency shifts and the extracellular matrix provide bone tissue composition information. Osteoarthritis, a debilitating disease, is responsible for the degeneration of cartilage and bone in the synovial joints. The molecular structure of the subchondral bone matrix undergoes changes in both the medial and lateral (beneath intact cartilage) compartments of osteoarthritis knees which is difficult to detect by conventional techniques but RS can enhance the diagnosis of these changes [369]. Fragility fractures are associated with ageing, disease, or injury, and evaluating bone composition alterations by RS has acquired a facile diagnosis of these issues [370].

SORS was applied in the non-invasive characterization of bone through soft tissue *in vivo* [371–373]. The application of SORS for transcutaneous characterizing bones was first revealed by Schulmerich *et al* [374] and rapidly enhanced penetration depths to above 4 mm [373, 375]. The development of a multiple-fibreoptic Raman probe increased the accuracy of recovered bone spectra for more changes monitoring in composition [376]. Direct comparison of *in vivo* transcutaneous data with *in vivo* exposed bone in surgery on the same patient [377] using a commercially available Raman spectrograph and optical probe operating at 785 nm excitation indicates good correspondence between the exposed and transcutaneous data. Inverse SORS was applied to the non-invasive diagnosis of osteogenesis imperfect condition *in vivo* [378], and the obtained spectra were consistent with *ex vivo* results. Later authors [379] showed (building on earlier advances [373]) that bone fragments from the necks of fractured femora measured *ex vivo* is more mineralized than non-fractured controls, while the mineralization distributions of the two cohorts largely overlap. Many recent studies [380–383] revealed that SORS holds considerable promise for diagnosing bone diseases.

5.4.1.11 Malaria

Malaria, a widespread mosquito-borne disease, is a serious threat to human health. There were an estimated 216 million cases of infection in 2016, while the number of cases of death due to malaria infection reached 445 000 globally [384]. A parasite protozoan infects the blood cells of the host, and hemozoin biocrystals are disposed as byproducts after the ingestion of hemoglobin [385]. The early detection of hemozoin at low concentrations in infected blood cells is very important since malaria disease can aggravate a fatal illness within hours of the development of the first symptom [386].

RRS amplified the Raman signal of hemozoin in malaria parasite-infected blood cells by the close Raman shift matching between the laser source and the electronic transition of hemozoin [387, 388].

TERS enhanced the Raman spectrum of hemozoin in infected cells via the augmented electromagnetic coupling between hematin and gold/silver nanoparticles [389].

Further augmentation can be achieved by combining RRS and SERS, known as SERRS. The SERRS signal could be further enhanced by using a magnetic field to improve the hemozoin concentration. Magnetic purification has been employed in a similar strategy [390, 391]. Moreover, hemozoin is paramagnetic NPs and desires to attach magnetic nanoparticles (such as iron oxide) due to the effective magnetic property of NPs at room temperature [390, 392], which is similar to the used strategy for capturing and enriching bacteria [393]. Detection of β-hematin crystals using magnetic field-enriched SERRS was enabled by Fe_3O_4@Ag nanoparticles [394]. An external magnetic field intensified the capability of SERRS to increase augmentation in the Raman signal of β-hematin crystals. A parasitemia level of 30 parasites/μl in blood in the early stages of infection can be achieved using this method, demonstrating the potential of employing magnetic field-enriched SERRS in early malaria diagnosis.

Most recently, an antibody-free (gold nanostructure) AuNS-SERS was developed to investigate the time, sensitivity, and capacity for performing malaria diagnosis from blood samples of patients infected with malaria *Plasmodium falciparum* and *Plasmodium vivax*. The results revealed that sensitive malaria detection using AuNS-SERS is a practical direction for rapid in-field diagnosis of malaria infection [395].

5.4.1.12 Pathogen detection

Bacterial infections are a leading cause of death in both developed and developing nations. Current diagnostic methods are slow processes that require sample preparation. Therefore, a rapid and low-cost diagnosis method with the advantages of minimum sample pretreatment, high sensitivity, onsite interpretation, and main detection of the lower concentration of the sample is urgently needed.

RS is capable of classifying the species of bacteria and antibiotic resistance. Raman spectroscopy [396–399] and Raman microscopy [400–402] are feasible techniques for rapid pathogen identification. Clinically relevant single bacterial cells from cerebrospinal fluid (CSF) during bacterial meningitis were directly analyzed by Raman microscopy [401]. Also, a decontamination protocol for handling live pathogenic bacteria was established, not affecting identification and viability testing. The novelty of the work is the demonstration of simultaneous identification and viability assessment of bacteria using tuberculosis (TB)-causing bacteria, *Mycobacterium tuberculosis* at a single bacterial level for pathogenic bacteria by Raman microscopy [402]. The identification of *Mycobacterium tuberculosis* complex strains [396], *Staphylococci* [397], *Staphylococcus aureus* [398], and methicillin-resistant and -susceptible isolates of *S. aureus* (MRSA and MSSA), as well as 30 common bacterial pathogens [399], were carried out using RS.

Since Raman signals in SERS are significantly enhanced using a variety of substrates, this advanced technique is a great tool for identifying and detecting targets; such as the detection and quantification of three types of bacterial meningitis pathogens in the cerebral spinal fluid [403]. The SERS-based detection of bacteria has been performed by using different SERS substrates, e.g., bimetallic surfaces and membranes [404, 405], silver colloids [406] and *in situ* fabricated AgNPs [407–409]. The combination of SERS with microfluidic elements may lead to future automated detection schemes [410].

Monitoring viral pathogens is very important to prevent a pandemic (e.g., ebola hemorrhagic fever). The desirable suitability of RS for virus detection and identification has been verified [411]. However, the origin of a difference in Raman spectra remains a challenging question. Hence, it is essential to detect oncogenic viral infections in the early stage, which needs the development of practical methods.

Label-free SERS as a direct method is an attractive approach to screening patient samples across a broad range of potential pathogens. This technique can be used in the diagnosis of bacterial infections (blood or urinary tract infections) among many bacterial species and strains as well as diagnosis of viral infection [412–414], helping to distinguish between multiple viruses (no viral extraction of nucleic acids from patient samples). This direct method with potential in bioanalytical detection schemes was also illustrated by the identification of bacterial strains of urinary tract infection clinical samples as well as by combining SERS with ISO preparation procedures to identify foodborne pathogens [415]. Although, the complex nature of the infectious disease agent's spectra causes challenges with distinguishing and interpreting Raman spectra.

Advanced data analysis and prediction algorithms are very useful in interpreting and classifying spectra. For instance, determination of unknown features in Raman/SERS spectral data (by PCA), facilitation of species, and strain discrimination (by DA/SVM/ANN). Raman and SERS paired with PCA were implemented to interpret spectral data in infectious bacteria [416–419] and diagnose viral infections [420–422]. Respiratory human viruses in real-time were investigated at trace levels using SERS (silver nanorod arrays substrates).

Most recently, RS was applied to detect the infection with adenovirus in a single live human cell without staining or labeling [423]. Partial least-square regression discriminant analysis (PLSR-DA) was applied to extract variations that strongly correlated with the independent variable. Virus infection was successfully determined only 3 h after invagination by RS, even in its dormant state or during slow replication. Contrary to conventional methods, this approach did not require the expression of viral genes. However, SERS-based techniques suffer a lack of ability in virus titer determination due to the non-linear SERS enhancement at high analyte concentrations and non-uniform adsorption of molecules on the nanoparticle surface. Irregular 'hot spot' formation leads to signal intensity reduction [424].

Labeled-SERS provides rapid, sensitive, and specific detection from complex samples without further washing or amplification steps. This approach allows multiplexed detection of several biomarkers and uses affinity agents such as antibodies, aptamers, and polymers [425–427]. Reporters such as resonant fluorescent dyes or aromatic thiols enhance SERS signals further to facilitate detection and quantification of the pathogen with low concentrations by incorporation either onto the SERS substrate or into the affinity agent [428]. Au particle-on-wire system employing probe, target, and reporter DNAs was used as a specific, sensitive, and multiplex DNA sensor, providing reproducible SERS signals only in the presence of target DNAs in proportion to the DNA concentration spanning from 10 pM to 10 nM. This developed SERS system has the potential to be employed in various biosensing applications for the successful diagnosis of clinical pathogens [428]. However, cross-reactivity resulting from conjugation with affinity agents can lead to false-positive results [429].

The feasibility of TERS in combination with chemometrics to discriminate two pathogenic viruses (*Varicella-zoster* and *porcine teschovirus*) was investigated [430]. Chemometric methods transformed the spectral data with rapid visual discrimination of the two viruses. Further, these methods were utilized to perform an automatic quality rating of the measured spectra to select the best spectra for a classification model calculation. TERS spectra achieved a classification accuracy of 91%.

5.4.2 Biomolecule detection

Biomolecules play essential roles in life processes and carry out important metabolic reactions to maintain the overall biochemistry of living organisms, including (i) small molecules having low-molecular-weight (monomers: nucleotides, amino acids, fatty acids) and (ii) macromolecules (biopolymers: proteins, nucleic acids, carbohydrates, lipids). Biological materials (cell, tissue, etc) are made up of different compositions of various biomolecules. Thus, biomolecule analysis is important in various application fields, such as clinical diagnostics, food safety analysis, environmental monitoring, and pharmaceutical development [431–434], to understand their structure and properties. Common detection methods to determine the biomolecules *in vitro* or *in vivo* include chromatography-mass spectroscopy (GC-MS) [435], enzyme-linked immunosorbent assay (ELISA) [436], colorimetric, fluorescence detection [437, 438], and PCR [439, 440]. RS is a powerful and widely-used technique in structural biology and cell biophysics investigations due to the distinct chemical identities of biomolecules and their unique molecular structures [291, 441]. Although the Raman spectra of these biomolecules are quite complex, unique bands can be identified to differentiate these biomolecules.

5.4.2.1 Lipids

Lipids (fats) play a remarkable role in biochemical functions, including molecules trafficking, energy transfer, receptor recognition, and biosynthesis. These biomolecule structures are essential elements for membrane protein structural studies. Nucleic acids are enclosed within a membrane separated from the external environment. The cell membrane of living cells is mainly composed of two lipid molecules due to the amphiphilic nature of lipids.

Raman scattering investigation on lipids and lipid structures can estimate various structural properties of lipids, such as unsaturation degree, level of *E*, and *Z* unsaturation [442], along with developing different membrane-mimicking systems for structural studies of membrane proteins in close to native conditions. Early detection of several diseases, monitoring nanotoxicity, and drug resistance can be achieved by investigations of the dynamic characteristics of the cell membrane. The observed distinct stretching vibrations in lipids at around 1749 cm^{-1}, at 1430 cm^{-1}, 1443 cm^{-1}, and 1453 cm^{-1} are quite distinct.

RS has been used in cancer diagnostics by characterizing the lipid phenotype of breast cancer cells [443] and the utility of the protein-to-lipid ratio as a prospective spectral and biochemical marker for oral cancer diagnosis [444].

Raman microspectroscopy was applied to determine the degree of unsaturation for fungal lipids directly inside intact hyphae without elaborate sample handling [445]. Later in another approach [446], the authors demonstrated the feasibility of RS for direct measurement of lipid vesicles inside intact mycelia. RS was successfully applied to study lipid droplets in skeletal myocytes [447] and special lipid vesicles in algae [448].

SERS was also exploited in detecting biomolecules for providing valuable spectral information to get insights into the structural and functional state. The dynamic activities of a self-assembled PL membrane were verified on a SERS platform [449]. Another SERS study based on single-cell lipid profiling of algae was performed to identify produced saturated and unsaturated fatty acids by these algae, collected data can be developed to produce biodiesel [450].

A CARS method was similarly employed to study thermodynamic properties of lipid membranes [451, 452], lipid vesicles, liposomes, and even in living cells experiments [453], investigating lipid phase transitions and detecting the lipid main phase transition for unilateral lipid dimyristoylphosphatidylcholine (DMPC) vesicles [454]. Identification of lipids by advanced RS possesses the dominant potential to establish novel detection and treatment strategies in biomedicine and diagnostics.

5.4.2.2 Proteins

Many essential reactions in living organisms function by proteins such as electron flow in reactions, the transmission of information between specific cells, the passage of molecules around the cell membrane, filamentous architecture within cells, cell division, and metabolism. These large and complex molecules replicate and transcribe DNA and play the main roles in regulating processes in cells, tissues, and organs but do not function in isolation. Proteins possess 3D architecture acquired by the precise sequence of amino acids and their function is directly dependent on this unique structure [455]. Proteins interact with other proteins or bind to other molecules. 'Protein interaction' can be either used to describe the physical contact between proteins and their interacting partners to generate macromolecular structures of various complexities and heterogeneities or used to describe metabolic or genetic correlations, and even co-localization [456, 457]. Understanding the function of cells requires the understanding of protein functions. Deficiency, imbalance, or structural variation of proteins make them biologically inactive and lead to diseases. Alzheimer's disease and Parkinson's disease [458, 459] are associated with such denaturation of proteins. Therefore, proteins serve as important biomarkers of disease diagnosis. There are many techniques to detect, isolate, purify, and characterize the structure of proteins.

RS is one of the emerging techniques for diagnosis and prognosis. Structural investigation of proteins by Raman scattering is an excellent achievement in image microcrystals to study protein–protein interactions, their conformational and functional changes inside organelles, living cells, and tissues. The most characteristic Raman bands of proteins are associated with amide group (-CONH-) called the peptide bonds, i.e., amide A (NH stretching, about 3500 cm^{-1}), amide B (NH stretching, about 3100 cm^{-1}), amide I (1600–1700 cm^{-1}), originating mainly from C = O stretching which is very sensitive to the backbone conformation and not affected by the side chains. Amide II (1480–1580 cm^{-1}) and amide III (1230–1300 cm^{-1}), which are both associated with C–N stretching coupled to N–H bending [460]. The frequencies of these bands are sensitive to protein secondary structural elements; predominantly α-helical structures show amide I and amide III bands at 1655–1662 cm^{-1} and 1264–1272 cm^{-1}, and β-sheet structures at 1672–1674 cm^{-1} and 1227–1250 cm^{-1} [461]. A proposed empirical relation between Amide III frequency and dihedral angle F was suggested [462], which effectively analyses the conformation of proteins using amide III band of Raman spectra. Trp, Tyr, Phe, and Cys are specific amino acids having characteristic bands at: Trp doublet at 1340/1360 cm^{-1}, Phe ring breathing mode at 1004 cm^{-1}, Tyr band at 1270 cm^{-1}, and doublet at 833/860 cm^{-1}. Sulfur-containing amino acid residues have specific bands at 510–750 cm^{-1} and at 2530–2580 cm^{-1} (S–H stretching, sensitive to H bonding).

Apart from the secondary structure, characteristic Raman bands of various side chains and disulfide regions can be identified [463]. The SERS technique can monitor the structure, the orientation toward the metallic surface, the chemical environment of proteins, and protein interactions [464]. SERS detection of biomolecules relies on the measurement of Raman spectra of the targeted species upon spontaneous adsorption onto a plasmonic substrate. The molecular specificity of SERS, combined with simple sample preparation, makes the direct detection of proteins. The appearance of Ag–N vibration modes in the low wavenumber confirms the chemisorption of proteins on the metallic surface [465].

A label-free SERS-AgNPs (direct) approach could successfully be employed for detection of prostate-specific antigen within serum in the presence of other proteins [466], detection of the Aβ-40 oligomer, as a biomarker for the early-stage diagnosis of Alzheimer [467], and Myoglobin protein, a biomarker for acute myocardial infarction [468]. To avoid conformational changes of studied proteins due to the chemisorption on the metal, AgNPs were modified with iodine to improve the accuracy [469]. SERS fingerprint spectra for five proteins were recorded with high quality and reproducibility since the protein was studied in its native structure with no direct interaction of proteins with the metal surface. A further improvement to examine proteins in their native configuration was carried out using silver nanocubes coated with polyvinylpyrrolidone (PVP) to minimize protein-cube faces interaction and force the preferential interaction via the corners [470].

Label-based SERS (indirect), constructed with Raman reporter, plasmonically active-metal substrate, a biocompatible coating, is a promising platform for studying proteins at the single-molecule level. Indirect SERS showed its potential in detection of biomarkers of prostate [471, 472], pancreatic cancer [299, 473] as well as intercellular activity [474], protein interactions [475], and structure [476]. Heme proteins, containing a heme prosthetic group, are very large class of metalloproteins including hemoglobin, myoglobin, and cytochromes. The heme moiety consists of a substituted protoporphyrin ring containing a liganded iron atom.

Various RS studies have been done for the investigation of these proteins *in vitro*, *in vivo*, and *in situ* conditions. Hemeprotein can absorb the excitation laser light to make resonance Raman conditions which generate the intensive Raman scattering of heme molecules without interferences of amino acids of hemeprotein or other cell components. The detection potential of RRS was proved for the quantitative study of the oxyhemoglobin amount in vessels of the tongue, skin, mucosa, muscles, liver, and brain of anesthetized intubated rats or mice [477–480] and in blood samples of patients or rats with various cardiovascular pathologies or healthy donors under the application of chemicals [481–484], monitoring of blood oxygenation in tissue vessels of neonates [485].

For the first time, spatially resolved RRS was used to visualize blood oxygenation in the vascular networks (*in vivo* monitoring) [480]. RRS measurements of Hb oxygenation (laser 532 nm) caused by the modulation of O_2 fraction in the inspired gas were compared with clinical estimations. The appearance of deoxyhemoglobin (dHb) peaks in the RRS spectra of blood were assigned to the gradual decrease of pO_2. The most intensive peaks in the RRS spectrum of oxygenated blood are at 1375, 1585 and 1638 cm^{-1}, corresponding to symmetric vibrations of pyrrole rings (pyrrole breathing) and methine bridges (CaCm bonds) that decreased due to pO_2 reduction and shift to lower frequencies under Hb deoxygenation to generate the peaks at 1355, 1552, and 1602 cm^{-1}, respectively. Raman spectra of blood with various oxygenation levels demonstrated a combination of peaks of oxy and deoxyhemoglobin. Information about understanding the mechanical properties of heme proteins and enzymes can be obtained in the high-frequency region. The redox and spin state and coordination pattern of the heme iron, which is made by complex vibrations of porphyrin macrocycle, produce RRS spectra 'so-called' core-size marker bands (designated as ν_4, ν_3, ν_2 and ν_{10}), in the high-frequency (1300–1700 cm^{-1}) region. These parameters govern reactivity, molecular interactions and redox behavior of heme proteins and enzymes [486–488]. On the other hand, the low-frequency (200–600 cm^{-1}) region can provide RRS spectra to identify the physiological ligand, or monitoring substrate binding, and information on transient catalytic intermediate species [489, 490]. Unmatched information on heme group structure, geometry, and binding of small diatomic ligands (acting as substrates or inhibitors of functionally distinct heme proteins) has been acquired by RRS [489]. Characterization of oxy and deoxy forms of Hb and Mb, allosteric transitions in hemoglobin (Hb), and physiological ligands of periplasmic heme sensory domains in chemotaxis bacteria can be studied with the help of RRS [489, 491]. RRS has played a particularly important role in understanding conformational states of cytochrome complex (cyt c) [492]. His/Met ligated 6cLS state of cyt c adopts when it shuttles electrons between respiratory chain complexes, and 5cHS state of cyt c acquires peroxidase activity, becomes the key component of mitochondrial apoptotic pathways and therefore responsible for cell death. RRS can differentiate these states for the understanding and control of apoptosis [493]. For the assessment of structural and mechanistic properties of multihaemic oxidoreductases, S has played a crucial role in disentangling the active site structures and catalytic mechanisms of diverse heme copper oxygen reductases (HCOs) [490]. Nature and formation kinetics of the catalytic intermediates contributed to the overall description and understanding of mechanical properties of HCOs can be assessed from low-frequency time-resolved (TR) RRS spectra [490].

Development of RRS and SERS resulted in the SERRS method. SERRS offers a unique advantage of probing the structural features of metalloproteins which exert their function in the immobilized state, at natural interfaces or at electrode interfaces as well as an alternative to RRS for characterization of catalytic intermediates in heme peroxidases when fluorescence prevents RRS measurements in solution [494]. As further advantages, SERRS requires only small (submicromolar) amounts of protein, the detection of intermediates is possible at ambient temperature and applies to the EPR-silent species. Contrary to electrochemical methods, SERRS simultaneously probes the nature and structural features of the immobilized molecules to distinguish the native solution structure or structural changes upon immobilization. SERR spectroelectrochemistry has provided extensive information on novel insights into mechanistic features of complex membrane metalloenzymes, biological electron transfer, structural/functional properties of membrane heme proteins, and immobilized enzymes that function as biocatalysts in bioelectronic devices [487, 495–505]. SERRS studies of cyt c, immobilized under different orientations, and variable electric fields that the protein senses at electrode interface, highly contributed to our understanding of kinetics, dynamics and thermodynamics of heterogeneous biological electron transfer [486, 495, 497–499, 501, 502, 504, 506, 507].

Confocal resonance Raman microscopy was also used to study the dynamics and location of hemoproteins in cells (monitor exit of cytochrome c from mitochondria of cultured cells under apoptosis) [508] and visualize the distribution of the reduced cytochrome b558 in neutrophils and eosinophil peroxidase in eosinophils under stimulation of the innate immune response [509].

CARS is another approach used to analyze protein–lipid interactions using TEM and scanning electron microscopy (SEM) for characterizing protein lysozyme distribution in solid lipid microparticles [510]. In the presence of a reference or spectra database (for comparison), RS can investigate proteins that possess neither specific cofactors nor ligands [291, 511]. RRS was used to analyze non-metallic chromophores (flavins), visual pigments (rhodopsin, photosynthetic pigments), and photoreceptors [512–514] to reveal sensitive information on their structures. RR and TR RRS can describe conformations and interactions of chlorophyll and carotenoids along with excited states [513].

Raman crystallography is a new technique based on integrating a microscope in a Raman spectrometer to study protein crystals [515] including identifying and following intermediate conformations in single crystals. Protein structure in a crystal and solution may be different due to the influences of crystal packing on proteins, which causes one of the important issues for protein crystallography. Detection of different protein conformations [516], qualitative detection of lysozymes structural in crystal and solution [517], and the phase transition in lysozyme crystals [518] was carried out. The RS technique can use the small-angle scattering (SAS) method to detect proteins in solution [519–524]. The specificities of the surrounding protein crystals are the barrier of the probe, especially in the case of membrane proteins.

Polarized coherent anti-Stokes Raman scattering (P-CARS) [331], the third-order non-linear technique, can be used for membrane protein sub-microcrystal imaging and 3D characterization, resolving protein crystals up to less than 1 μm size in the presence of lipid cubic phase (LCP) and salt crystals in the probe, characterize their 3D shape, revealing twinning of the crystals and their disordered parts, and provide information of the protein's state in the crystals. P-CARS [525] is a beneficial technique for studying proteins in crystals and is extremely useful in the case of membrane protein crystals. Disordered and ordered parts of protein crystals, even non-chiral crystals, can be detected by P-CARS. The submicron resolution of this technique is used for the high-throughput detection of protein microcrystals for European x-ray free-electron laser (XFEL) experiments (figure 5.4). However, the measurement time for one crystallization probe is about 5–10 min. This limitation forces CARS imaging of microcrystals to be complementarily used with more high-throughput imaging techniques.

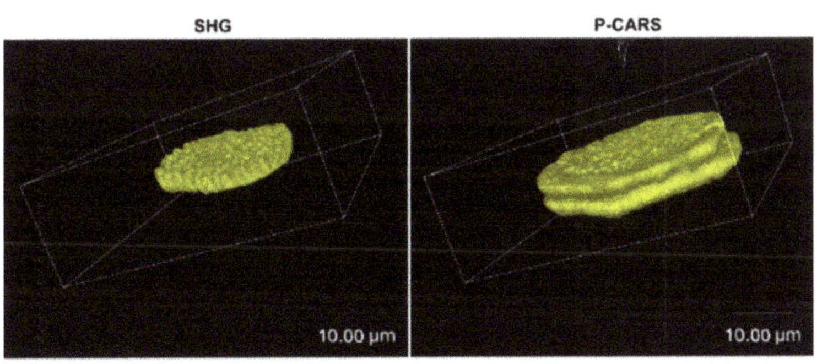

Figure 5.4. Comparison of second harmonic generation (3D SHG) and polarized coherent anti-Stokes Raman scattering (3D P-CARS). Detection of hexagonal bacteriorhodopsin crystal with twinning and contouring disordered part. Box size: 48 × 48 × 24 μm. Images were acquired with 6 ps laser source. Reprinted with permission from [525]. Copyright (2016) American Chemical Society.

5.4.2.3 Nucleic acids

The most characteristic bands of DNA and RNA are ring breathing modes at approximately 680 cm^{-1} (G), 730 cm^{-1} (A), 740–785 cm^{-1} (C, T, U), 1087–1100 cm^{-1} (PO_2-symmetric stretching). Several pronounced bands are found at higher frequencies: 1230–1250 cm^{-1} (C, T, U), 1290–1380 cm^{-1} (A, C, T), 1530–1590 cm^{-1} (A, C, G), and 1655 cm^{-1} (T) [460, 526]. During cell division and proliferation, the DNA is in a more uncondensed state and DNA Raman bands are more intense although the DNA content is identical. RS detects changes in a few bases in gene sequences that are associated with cancer or other diseases. RS is improbable since the human genome consists of more than 3 billion base pairs. Such spectral variations are simply too small. However, the genome determines the phenotype of bacteria, cells, and tissues, the proliferation rate, expression of proteins, or accumulation of lipids and metabolites which can be detected as Raman spectroscopic signatures for classification and disease recognition.

The first Raman spectra of various nucleic acid constituents were recorded in 1960 [527]. Constituent nucleosides (such as hydrogen bonding, base–protein interactions, base–drug interactions, and base–metal ion interactions), as well as conformations of the sugar-phosphate backbone of nucleic acids, are two groups of Raman markers for nucleic acids' structural studies [150, 239, 526, 528, 529]. Right-handed A-DNA, right-handed B-DNA, and left-handed Z-DNA forms are considered to be possible conformations of DNA, which can be distinguished by the appearance of specific bands in Raman spectra. Moreover, specific bands' intensity enables the calculation of the proportion of different DNA forms [530–532]. B-DNA's relatively large deviations reflect the structural complexity and dependency upon AT and GC base pair content [533]. RS for investigating DNA structure in both crystals and solutions are feasible. Detection of nucleic acids such as DNA and RNA is significant for disease diagnosis and gene therapy [534–536].

Nucleic acid conformational changes induced by the addition of binding agents (ions, proteins, drugs, etc) or induced by altering environmental factors (temperature, pH, salinity, etc) can be described quantitatively by Raman difference spectroscopy. This method is an appropriate tool for demonstrating localized interactions in nucleic acid complexes combined with site-specific labeling [537], residue-specific labeling, and single-site mutagenesis [538]. Polarized RS provides both general chemical identification (similar to unpolarized Raman scattering) and molecular orientation and symmetry of bond vibrations data [526, 539, 540]. Polarized RS can determine the relative spatial orientation of DNA residues, drug molecules [541], analysis of DNA quadruplexes, and telomeres identification and characterization [542].

SERS detection method used in the nucleic acid analysis is based on two major strategies; Label-free strategy is based on the distinctive SERS signals from four bases of DNA/RNA, and the second one, which has more extensive applications than the label-free strategy is modifying nucleic acid with extrinsic Raman labels or constructing SERS nanotags. Ingenious methods such as the classical 'sandwich' method [543], the hairpin DNA-assisted method [544], and the signal amplification method [545] are based on the properties of complementarity and amplification to detect a nucleic acid.

A label-based SERS technique was used to detect human immunodeficiency virus type 1 (HIV-1) DNA [546], indicating potential feasibility in POC self-diagnostics with LOD of 0.24 pg ml^{-1}. SERS nanotag significantly improves the sensitivity of biosensors used in DNA amplification method [547]. SERS analysis on the detection of nucleobases, essential parts of the DNA construction, showed distinctive SERS signals [548]. The concentration of adenine showed a good linear relationship with SERS intensity quantified by the peak area of SERS peak at 770 cm^{-1} (the ring breathing band). Single nucleotide polymorphism in mitochondrial DNA can also be detected by SERS analysis utilizing the ion-mediated cascade amplification strategy [549]. A variety of SERS-active substrates were fabricated to enhance the Raman sensitivity, such as hollow Au nanoflowers substrates [550], silver nanorod array substrates [551], and SWNTs@AgNPs [552]. The SWNTs@AgNPs biosensor can sensitively quantify miRNA-21 with a detection limit of 5 pM. Sensitive and simultaneous detection of multiple microRNAs (miRNA-21, miRNA-141, and miRNA-203) were carried out [553] by a series of signal amplification methods (A dual functional DNA–linker–DNA-probe). Similarly, SERS-based detection of three Hepatic carcinoma related miRNAs [554] and multiple microRNAs (three miRNAs) [555] were reported.

Recently, label-free and modification-free nanotechnology based on SERS was employed for DNA analysis. Phosphate backbone as an internal standard is used for quantitative detection of nucleobases at a single-base level. The method was combined with PCA-LDA for real blood circulating DNA detection for the first time with an ideal diagnostic sensitivity of 83.3% and specificity of 82.5% to diagnose nasopharyngeal cancer. The method demonstrated promising potential as alternative nanotechnology for nasopharyngeal cancer screening based on liquid biopsy [556].

The SERRS technique provides a key advantage over fluorescent techniques due to the quantitative detection of multiplexed labeled DNA in one sample [557]. Labeled DNA detection also covers the application of fluorescent-labeled DNA-probe immobilized on the surface of nanoparticles. DNA duplex changes conformation when the target sequence is found and the Raman signal increases significantly. Prostate cancer antigen 3 mimic DNA was detected by hybridization reactions with the detection limit of 2.7 fM, which means that it has a higher sensitivity than conventional polymerase chain reaction [543].

The first TERS experiments on DNA base nanocrystals [558–560] and a study of the hydrogen bonding between adenine and thymine on a gold substrate [561] showed that a distinction of the respective nucleobases is possible, and this eventually led to successful TERS measurements on a single RNA strand of a cytosine homopolymer [562]. TERS successfully detected nanoparticles targeting antigens on the plasma membrane of cells, proposing a pathway in sensitivity and selectivity increment in intact membranes [563]. The research was based on cancer cells incubated with antibody-functionalized gold nanoparticles and increased scattering was observed when the nanoparticle probe interacts with a TERS tip indicating a method to simultaneously identify proteins of interest and obtain Raman scattering characteristics of the interaction. Micrometer dimensioned metal tips (μ-TERS) can selectively enhance residues in the cell membrane [564]. Other investigations include studying the protein osteopontin adsorption to kidney stones [565], nanooxidation sites on hemoglobin crystals [566], and hemozoin crystals associated with malaria infection from sectioned erythrocytes [389] were also employed TERS. One challenge in TERS is discriminating against the near-field from the far-field background. By synchronizing detection with the tapping mode frequency, it is possible to remove the far-field contribution [567]. Advances in AFM tips appropriate for biological samples will further facilitate biomedical TERS [568]. Silver tips are reported to give the largest enhancements, and a photochemical method for attaching silver to AFM cantilevers *in situ* has been reported [569]. DNA double-strand breaks were probed with TERS coupled with AFM and suggested that the O–C bond in the DNA backbone is most sensitive to UVC radiation, and its cleavage causes DSBs most of the time [570]. Bailo's group recorded the TERS spectra from an artificial DNA single-strand with alternating blocks of adenine and cytosine. These bases are placed at a distance of 2.1 nm by unique Raman spectral features proving that TERS can offer resolutions up to a single nucleobase level [571, 572].

5.4.2.4 Carbohydrates

Carbohydrates are naturally occurring compounds and essential constituents for living organisms. They have significant functions such as molecular agents in cellular recognition, the main source of energy, and the major constituent of cell walls, plants, and microorganisms. There are three major size classes of carbohydrates: monosaccharides, oligosaccharides, and polysaccharides. Structural investigations of different carbohydrates are difficult due to the similarity of the basic monomeric unit in the polymeric chains. Despite this, the different nature of H bonding or the ring configuration gives rise to several marker peaks for carbohydrates [573].

Raman and IR features of 14 carbohydrates in the solid-state were compiled [574]. Raman spectra of nine anomerically stable monosaccharides in solutions with concentrations of 10 mM and volumes of 15 ml were recorded [575].

For the first time, *in vivo* quantification of glucose in an animal model using SERS was presented [576]. The Raman spectra of carbohydrates show a large degree of variability because different monosaccharides as subunits are known, such as glucose, fructose, and galactose. Glycogen is a multi-branched polysaccharide of glucose that serves as a form of energy storage in organisms. The Raman spectrum of glycogen shows a number of broad bands with maxima near 481, 855, 940, 1044, 1084, 1127, 1337, 1383, and 1459 cm^{-1}.

RS also can identify and quantify (in some cases) small biomolecules, like urea, cholesterol, triglycerides, etc, in biofluids and other samples [497]. The analysis of the molecule possesses a Raman active group with isolated or characteristic bands is particularly straightforward when the molecule possesses a Raman active group with isolated, well-resolved characteristic bands, which can be used as markers (e.g., collagen fibers at 950 cm^{-1}, dipicolinic acid (DPA) at 1016 and 1395 cm^{-1}, ergosterol at 1602 cm^{-1}, etc).

5.4.3 Circulating tumor cell detection

When tumors are in a stable size and growth, some cancer cells, referred to as circulating tumor cells (CTCs), separate and enter the bloodstream of the patient [577–579]. Once CTCs are transported to a distal tissue and adapt to the new environment, metastasis is formed [580, 581]. Initial cancer research in 1869 discovered the existence of CTCs as well as the possible relationships between CTCs and metastasized cancer [582]. Through research, CTCs have indicated information about cancer type, cancer progression, and patient response before, during, and after treatment [578, 582, 583]. The fast and accurate detection of CTCs at an early stage can significantly improve the prognosis, therapeutic evaluation, and individualized treatment of patients [584–586]. Since the concentration of CTCs in blood could reflect the condition of cancer [587, 588]. Based on clinical research, CTCs are detectable in blood when the tumor size is only 1–2 mm, but conventional methods cannot detect these tumors [8]. During diagnosis, CTCs can assist in locating a cancer tumor by indicating cancer type. This is done by growing a new tumor in a xenograft and identifying the cancer [578]. The presence of CTCs is a viable independent prognostic indicator for breast, prostate, and colorectal cancer because the concentration of CTCs does indicate the actual size of an existing tumor [582, 590, 591]. However, the concentration of CTCs changes in the patient reflects changes in the cancer tumor throughout treatment including re-occurrence after treatment is concluded [578]. CTCs detection needs supersensitive methods because of extremely low CTCs concentration. In 1 ml blood, there are ~5.0 × 109 erythrocytes and 1.0 × 107 leukocytes, but only several CTCs. The methods need to employ an enrichment process prior to the quantification step, based on physical properties (size, density, deformability) or biological properties (protein expression). Antibody capture, using cancer-derived DNA, and cytopathology are currently the three main detection research paths for CTCs. The most common protocol uses antibody capture based on epithelial marker epithelial cell adhesion molecule (EpCAM) on the CTCs, due to the presumption that CTCs have not undergone epithelial-mesenchymal transition [578, 579]. Cancer-derived DNA does not require the whole cells, so it is free of cancer stem cells (CSC) and clinical and translational medicine (CTM). However, this method suffers from specificity and sensitivity issues and cannot be used routinely [579]. Cytopathology is not currently in use but is a proposed method. This approach has a higher specificity, but the lack of sensitivity makes it impractical. The multiple steps damaged or degraded the cells have made both density gradient separation and filtration unsuccessful enrichment methods due to low sensitivity and specificity [592].

RS could provide increased specificity and sensitivity compared to the mentioned techniques. It was demonstrated, for the first time, SERS-based detection of tumor cells in a homogeneous, no-wash whole blood assay with no sample preparation.

Using a combination of gold magnetic particles and nanoplex biotags, the detection limit was 10 cells ml^{-1} with 99.7% confidence in buffer solution. In a proof-of-concept experiment, the breast cancer cell line SKBR3, expressing high levels of her2 receptor on the cell surface [593], was used as a model target. Results proved the potential of RS in CTCs detection [594, 595].

In another approach, microscopic Raman spectroscopy identified CTCs in suspension to mimic a clinical test using spiked blood serum with a prediction accuracy of 92.4% and a false-positive of less than 0.5% (cytopathology above 1%–3%) [596].

SERS could also enable the presence of CTCs to be indicated before treatment and their absence following treatment appropriately [595, 597]. Recent approaches based on encoded plasmonic NPs and SERS enable the multiplex quantification of different CTCs [598, 599]. This methodology is a combination of ultrahigh analytical resolution with a virtually unlimited number of available codes and markers that can be studied simultaneously. However, this technique is unsuitable for real samples due to long SERS acquisition times (<10 ms) where a single CTC is diluted among massive numbers of other cells.

The combination of the acquisition speed of fluorescence (down to ns) for rapid screening and sorting with the analytical resolution of SERS applied to the smaller cell fraction resulted in a viable solution [600].

5.4.4 Raman imaging of cells and tissues

The Raman scattering process is weak in discriminating subtly different states of cells and tissues and limits the use of RS in high-resolution imaging, which is essential to biological research and clinical practice. The spectral and spatial information combination is used in Raman imaging, collecting in the point mapping mode. The sample's scattered light is registered and the focus is moved by a scanning mirror, or a motorized stage moves the sample to the next position. The number of spectra, the exposure time per spectrum, and moving the stage time determine the total exposure time of the laser onto the sample. Registration of spatial data on the detector on a line parallel to the entrance slit of the spectrometer is possible after laser line illumination of the sample, and then the spectral information is dispersed perpendicularly. Line-mapping registration mode is the second spatial dimension of an image recorded by scanning in the direction perpendicular to that line, and it is also fast since only one dimension has to be scanned in the point mapping mode. The parallel registration approach (direct or wide-field Raman imaging) applied intense, global sample illumination. Wide-field Raman (direct) imaging applies any dielectric/acousto-optic tunable/liquid-crystal tunable filters for the wavelength selection. Based on parameters such as acquisition times, image quality, spatial resolution, the intensity of profiles, spatial coordinates, and spectral signal to noise ratios, Raman imaging methodologies are compared.

The application of RS for biology can be divided into hyperspectral broadband imaging (BCARS) [66] and single-frequency CRS imaging. Spectral separation of different components in the range of 500–3500 cm^{-1} for simultaneous multicomponent imaging can be carried out using BCARS [66]. However, SNR and imaging speed are sacrificed (~3.5 ms pixel dwell time). This method is suitable for either tissue imaging or fixed sample studies due to its slow image acquisition of about 2 min. The pixel dwell time reduction to tens of microseconds utilizing the more constrained spectral window with multichannel data acquisition leads the way for RS to confocal laser scanning microscopy speeds [601]. CRS has gained in popularity for imaging applications.

CARS and SRS have the ability of video-rate imaging of single Raman bands [602, 603] but are inadequate in the breadth and speed of laser tuning rates. A non-resonant background as a barrier distorts the Raman signal in CARS. Multiplex techniques (multiplex SRS, BCARS) provide simultaneous probing of multiple Raman transitions. Single-frequency CRS imaging using a narrow-band laser is best for targeted imaging, in which the molecule bears an *a priori*–determined isolated Raman peak. Hyperspectral CRS is preferred, especially when signature peaks of molecules are not separated from the cellular background [604–606]. Overlapping spectra decomposition and recovery of underlying molecular composition are obtained by a combination of spectral imaging and chemometrics. Rapid imaging of the cells with pixel dwell times in nanoseconds is possible by single-frequency CARS or SRS, limiting to only specific bond vibrations, and by extension-specific molecules inside the cell, such as fatty acids/DNA/proteins.

Single-frequency CRS microscopy compared to usual fluorescent is highly selective and provides the incorporation of extremely small labels. Several small molecules, such as DNA, RNA, proteins, and phospholipids via alkyne were labeled metabolic precursors [607, 608].

Labeling with different isotopes was applied to the image *in vivo* degradation of protein by labeling phenylalanine with 13C [609] study deuterium-labeled choline metabolism [610], and deuterium-labeled fatty acids processing into lipid droplets [611]. Deuterium-labeled glucose is very useful for rapidly screening the effectiveness of new antibiotics. It determines differentiating metabolism in antibiotic-resistant and wild type bacteria during one cell cycle [612]. Also, SRS imaging of lipogenesis under antimicrobial treatment in *Candida albicans* fungi was employed for screening for antibiotic resistance in a matter of hours instead of days [613].

Label-free Raman imaging has been applied in many studies such as cell state and metabolism, cancer, diseases, ageing, drug treatments and interactions, infectious diseases, hard tissues, etc.

Raman imaging for analysis of cells and tissues needs the understanding of the origins of generated Raman signals. Comparing cell and tissue spectra to the spectra of individual cellular components is the simplest way, especially for samples with simple composition. However, for a large number of different molecular species contributing to the overall signal is challenging. Raman and fluorescence image comparison is one way to overcome this complexity for different cellular compartments and organelles [614]. Study distribution of c- and b-type cytochromes in cardiomyocytes [331, 615], cytochrome c release from mitochondria of cultured cells [508] were applied Raman imaging. Mitochondria in the periphery and the center of healthy rod-shaped cardiomyocytes possess a different amount of reduced b-type cytochromes versus reduced c-type cytochromes, unlike round-shaped transforms that have a lower relative amount of all reduced cytochromes [331]. Biochemical methods with the selective isolation of mitochondria from the peripheral and central cell regions were employed to study the heterogeneity of mitochondria in healthy cardiomyocytes but never non-invasively demonstrated on living cells.

Raman imaging was employed to identify nuclei and cytoplasm within the cells and the extracellular matrix between the cells [616], distinguish between different microorganisms [617] determine the activation state of B lymphocytes [618], assess the quality of human sperm [619], characterize the communication between different cell types [620], and monitor different states of a cell during normal cellular processes [621]. Hsu *et al* combined Raman measurements with autofluorescence imaging to follow the division of cells during cytokinesis and interphase [622].

Raman imaging reveals information on biochemical composition and spatial distribution, identifying the presence of different cell types within a tissue section in cancer investigations [623, 624]. Cancer and pre-cancer cells, erythrocytes, and lymphocytes were successfully assigned to colon cancer tissue sections by combining Raman imaging with histopathology (H&E staining) and immunohistochemistry [625]. The tumor protein p53 is normally highly expressed in cancer and pre-cancer cells because it is a tumor suppresser. Obtained false-color Raman maps with the images given by the anti-p53 immunohistochemical stained image were compared to show the sample autofluorescence matched the fluorescence from the anti-p53 stained tissue [625].

Raman imaging has been also used to study skin tissue damages [626], atherosclerosis [627], Alzheimer's disease [628], macrophage cells [629], malaria [630] as well as hair follicle [631], teeth [632, 633], and enamel [634]. Line scanning and improvements in detector sensitivity have increased the speed of Raman imaging performance; however, in comparison to many cellular processes, it is still slow.

A combination of Raman with other modalities with faster imaging capabilities to provide additional information on the nature of the sample can be one of the ways to recoup. Two or more combined techniques as a multimodal approach can simultaneously be applied to the sample for Raman measurement to provide easy information comparison between the different modes [635]. However, instrumental challenges are significant [636]. Fluorescent staining measured following Raman can be a very useful validation technique. One of the significant challenges with multimodal imaging is the image registration between different measurement techniques. This is particularly problematic where one modality is used to provide information on what another modality is measuring as differences in the z-resolution, and probed volume will mean that there will be differences in the morphological and, potentially, molecular species measured by each technique [636, 637].

5.5 Current challenges and future prospective

RS maintains its powerful extension as a broad field of research in a wide range of novel applications, providing sensitive photonic information at the molecular level. This technique is sensitive, delicate, and informative due to the number of properties and reasons: an excellent non-invasive *in situ* probe, a photonic probe of molecules and materials at nanostructured surfaces, disease diagnosis, clinical practices enhancement, advanced design of ultrafast lasers, enhanced Raman imagining instrumentation, developments of chemometric analysis of spectral data, and exo-laboratory applications. One of the growing applications in RS is biomedical applications. SERS as the largest and one of the most important advanced RS techniques has been an excellent tool for biomedical investigations due to its great sensitivity, compatibility, and non-invasive efficiency [638].

As an alternative for fluorescence-based biological and biomedical detection and imaging, there are still limitations due to the low intensity and poor reproducibility of SERS-active nanostructures. Therefore, discoveries for higher sensitivity and improved reproducibility continue. Several methods can improve the sensitivity including the instrument noise level decrement, throughput increment, the interfering species noise signals reduction, the design of the SERS-active nanostructure with appropriate size, shape, coupling modes, and LSPR properties. Encapsulating and impurity removal of surface refrain from adsorption of interfering species, leading to improved reproducibility. Employment of internal standards in designing SERS-active nanostructures improves quantitative analysis [639].

Raman scattering-based imaging is a very powerful optical tool for biomedical diagnostics. Distinct tissue structures generate different Raman signatures. Label-free SERS detection of tissue provides a rapid and facile way to differentiate tumors from normal tissues. Also, SERS labels presented their ability for developing detection and bioimaging platforms. Few studies have demonstrated that the SERS imaging of tumor tissues using SERS labels can be realized through the passive accumulation of enhanced permeability and retention (EPR) effect. The development of active targeting imaging of tumor tissues using controllable targeting ligands to reduce diagnostic errors is necessary. Challenges in the non-invasive detection of invisible tumors and metastatic sites due to the fast attenuation of SERS signal can be overcome by a combination of SERS nanoprobes with SESORS imaging techniques to attain deeper detection [84].

Recent findings revealed that the second optical window offers more efficient tissue penetration than the first biological optical window; as a result, investigation of plasmonic materials responsive in the second biological optical window and SERS performances and photothermal therapy should be considered in future studies. Nanostructure-based Raman techniques and rapid nanoscience developments will provide next-generation plasmonic substrates with significant sensitivity, reproducibility, and stability. Over the last decades, SERS has been demonstrated as a robust analytical technique coupled with various optical imaging or molecular imaging techniques. Multimodal imaging can provide us with multi-parameter results for an accurate diagnosis. SERS in combination with *in vivo* endoscopic techniques has great potential for applications in surgical treatment. In the development of SERS in clinical diagnosis, particularly, the rapid evaluation of drug levels, drug metabolites, or biomarkers in blood serum, portable Raman systems combined with simple cartridge systems are needed to assess the health status of the patient. Extended biomedical applications will be definitely in parallel with modern optical features [640].

Contrary to the analysis of linear Raman spectroscopic tissue data, which is quite established, the evaluation of hyperspectral non-linear Raman data has not yet been evaluated in detail. CRS microscopy as a new imaging modality has been employed in both fundamental research and clinical settings, resulting in new biology and medicine learning. The two most common CRS methods are CARS and SRS. The linear concentration dependence of SRS compared to the quadratic dependence of CARS has fostered the application of SRS tissue imaging. Hyperspectral coherent Raman imaging combined with data processing is suitable for tissue characterization. However, combining CARS and SRS hyperspectral data into a single data stack does not lead to clustering improvement results because of different concentration dependence and the spectral peak position. In multiplex CRS, primarily CARS has been applied, while SRS might be preferable in hyperspectral imaging [641, 642].

Label-free SRS microscopy imaging enables the study of cellular processes, lipid metabolism, and cell differentiation and most probably will be used in cancer biology. Owing to the high spatial resolution of SRS microscopy, the effects of different microenvironments can be studied using this method. Significant progress has been made to decrease image acquisition and hyperspectral data collection times. Implementation of real-time background subtraction techniques helps eliminate the parasitic background signal of SRS. Photo-damage and potential motion artifacts are generated during hyperspectral SRS imaging, which is a slow method; as a result, the amount of spectral information needed to resolve molecular species of interest is minimized by careful experimental design. Possessing both chemical specificity and non-perturbative nature, SRS microscopy has made significant biological insights possible in recent years in many important areas of biology such as cancer metabolism and antibiotic resistance. Based on recent advancements, regardless of the normal and inherent drawbacks of SRS microscopy technique, SRS imaging techniques will retain their main role in biological imaging in the future [641, 642].

CRS microscopy has presented unrivaled chemical information in biological functions for the global science community, which will continue. Physics, chemistry, engineering, biology, and mathematics are merged in this technique. Many of the advancements in CRS microscopies, such as improved laser technology, better detectors, breakthroughs in chemical engineering, and the development of new data analysis algorithms are inseparable from progress in other fields. New concepts and technologies in other fields will also continue to permeate CRS microscopy, leading to major changes. Although challenges continue to exist, particularly for higher detection sensitivity, an excellent future for CRS microscopy to become a staple analytical tool in biological, medical, and material sciences is predicted [641, 642].

Despite the impressive works in clinical fields and the various instrumentation considerations relevant to the clinical fulfillment of RS, clinical translation for Raman-based technologies remains a big challenge. One of the current challenges is a platform design that enables accurate, effective, and non-invasive clinical pathological analysis and diagnosis. Robust system design with consistent internal calibration is an urgent need to allow users to set up a system and collect repeatable data. For this purpose, many requirements should be implemented, such as high-performance fibreoptic probes. The transition from research instrument to clinical relevance requires reliable and consistent performance for interfacing the sample and system. Calibration of inter-system and large libraries of spectral data to be compared between instruments are pivotal to expand the utility of the devices for multiple medical targets. Clinical instrumentation generates Raman spectra that need to be condensed by standardized and reliable data analysis methods. These methods provide the salient features used for both clinical evaluation and easy communication with the user. While the preparative efforts of many of these aspects for clinical translation are in progress, the transition from benchtop to bedside is the next step. Since the target of developed technologies is to provide meaningful clinical information, collaboration and input from the medical community are preferable to direct Raman techniques research efforts at relevant needs in medicine and surgery. The added value of new optical technologies should be compared with existing medical devices in large cohort studies of patient outcomes and relative accepted gold standards. This demonstration is a major barrier to clinical translation [643].

The various RS-based applications were recognized to affect patient care. Few of these systems have been commercialized following regulatory approval. However, the adoption of this technology suffers from the limited size of the target market revenue caused by the prevention of potential industrial partners and investors. River Diagnostics has sold Raman instruments for skin assessment in the cosmetic industry (not for a clinical application), and Verisante Technology has released Raman-based devices for oral and skin cancer diagnosis. These successful commercial devices represent that the clinical implementation of RS is able to overcome hindrances in the widespread acceptance of this technology [643].

References

[1] Smekal A 1923 Zur quantentheorie der dispersion *Sci. Nat.* **11** 873–5

[2] Raman C V and Krishnan K S 1928 A new type of secondary radiation *Nature* **121** 501–2

[3] Colthup N B, Daly L H and Wiberley S E (ed) 1990 *Introduction to Infrared and Raman Spectroscopy* 3rd edn (San Diego, CA: Academic) pp 1–73

[4] Born M and Bradburn M 1947 The theory of the Raman effect in crystals, in particular rock-salt *Proc. Math. Phys. Eng. Sci.* **188** 161–78

[5] Kashima T, Watari T and Mikubo H 1961 Raman spectra and structure of molecular addition compound of aminopyrine and barbital in aqueous solution *Eisei Shikenjo Hokoku* **79** 59–63

[6] Tobin M C 1968 Raman spectra of crystalline lysozyme, pepsin, and alpha chymotrypsin *Science* **161** 68–9

[7] Lord R C and Yu N T 1970 Laser-excited Raman spectroscopy of biomolecules. II. Native ribonuclease and α-chymotrypsin *J. Mol. Biol.* **51** 203–13

[8] Rimai L, Kilponen R G and Gill D 1970 Resonance-enhanced Raman spectra of visual pigments in intact bovine retinas at low temperatures *Biochem. Biophys. Res. Commun.* **41** 492–7

[9] Long T V and Loehr T M 1970 Possible determination of iron coordination in nonheme iron proteins using laser-Raman spectroscopy. Rubredoxin *J. Am. Chem. Soc.* **92** 6384–6

[10] Singh N, Kumar P and Riaz U 2019 Applications of near infrared and surface enhanced Raman scattering techniques in tumor imaging: a short review *Spectrochim. Acta* A **222** 117279
[11] Aljakouch K, Hilal Z, Daho I, Schuler M, Krauß S D, Yosef H K, Dierks J, Mosig A, Gerwert K and El-Mashtoly S F 2019 Fast and noninvasive diagnosis of cervical cancer by coherent anti-Stokes Raman scattering *Anal. Chem.* **91** 13900–6
[12] Gniadecka M, Philipsen P A, Sigurdsson S, Wessel S, Nielsen O F, Christensen D H, Hercogova J, Rossen K, Thomsen H K and Gniadecki R 2004 Melanoma diagnosis by Raman spectroscopy and neural networks: structure alterations in proteins and lipids in intact cancer tissue *J. Investig. Dermatol* **122** 443–9
[13] Singh S and Jha H C 2019 *Machine Intelligence and Signal Analysis* vol 746 ed M Tanveer and R B Pachori (Berlin: Springer) pp 609–19
[14] Liang L, Huang D, Wang H, Li H, Xu S, Chang Y, Li H, Yang Y W, Liang C and Xu W 2015 In situ surface-enhanced Raman scattering spectroscopy exploring molecular changes of drug-treated cancer cell nucleus *Anal. Chem.* **87** 2504–10
[15] El-Mashtoly S F, Yosef H K, Petersen D, Mavarani L, Maghnouj A, Hahn S, Kötting C and Gerwert K 2015 Label-free Raman spectroscopic imaging monitors the integral physiologically relevant drug responses in cancer cells *Anal. Chem.* **87** 7297–304
[16] Deng R, Qu H, Liang L, Zhang J, Zhang B, Huang D, Xu S, Liang C and Xu W 2017 Tracing the therapeutic process of targeted aptamer/drug conjugate on cancer cells by surface-enhanced Raman scattering spectroscopy *Anal. Chem.* **89** 2844–51
[17] Prado E, Colin A, Servant L and Lecomte S 2014 SERS spectra of oligonucleotides as fingerprints to detect label-free RNA in microfluidic devices *J. Phys. Chem.* C **118** 13965–71
[18] Swierczewska M, Liu G, Lee S and Chen X 2012 High-sensitivity nanosensors for biomarker detection *Chem. Soc. Rev.* **41** 2641–55
[19] Kankia B I and Marky L A 2001 Folding of the thrombin aptamer into a G-quadruplex with Sr^{2+}: stability, heat, and hydration *J. Am. Chem. Soc.* **123** 10799–804
[20] Aubrey K L, Thomas G J and Casjens S R 1992 Secondary structure and interactions of the packaged dsDNA genome of bacteriophage P22 investigated by Raman difference spectroscopy *Biochemistry* **31** 11835–42
[21] Dong R, Yan X, Pang X and Liu S 2004 Temperature-dependent Raman spectra of collagen and DNA *Spectrochim. Acta* A **60** 557–61
[22] Morla-Folch J, Xie H, Alvarez-Puebla R A and Guerrini L 2016 Fast optical chemical and structural classification of RNA *ACS Nano* **10** 2834–42
[23] Garcia-Rico E, Alvarez-Puebla R A and Guerrini L 2018 Direct surface-enhanced Raman scattering (SERS) spectroscopy of nucleic acids: from fundamental studies to real-life applications *Chem. Soc. Rev.* **47** 4909–23
[24] Bernath P F (ed) 2005 *Spectra of Atoms and Molecules* 2nd edn (New York: Oxford University Press) pp 293–317
[25] Ferraro J R, Nakamoto K and Brown C W (ed) 2003 *Introductory Raman spectroscopy* 2nd edn (San Diego, CA: Academic) pp 1–94
[26] Abramczyk H 2005 *Introduction to Laser Spectroscopy* 1st edn (New York: Elsevier)
[27] Devitt G, Howard K, Mudher A and Mahajan S 2018 Raman spectroscopy: an emerging tool in neurodegenerative disease research and diagnosis *ACS Chem. Neurosci.* **9** 404–20
[28] Auner G W, Koya S K, Huang C, Broadbent B, Trexler M, Auner Z, Angela E, Katlyn C M and Brusatori M A 2018 Applications of Raman spectroscopy in cancer diagnosis *Cancer Metastasis Rev.* **37** 691–717

[29] Zhao J, Lui H, McLean D I and Zeng H 2010 *New Developments in Biomedical Engineering* ed D Campolo (London: IntechOpen) pp 455–74
[30] Yamamoto K, Sakamoto A, Nagano T and Fukumitsu K 2010 NIR sensitivity enhancement by laser treatment for Si detectors *Nucl. Instrum. Methods Phys. Res.* A **624** 520–3
[31] Mikhonin A V, Bykov S V, Myshakina N S and Asher S A 2006 Peptide secondary structure folding reaction coordinate: correlation between UV Raman amide III frequency, Psi Ramachandran angle, and hydrogen bonding *J. Phys. Chem.* B **110** 1928–43
[32] Ozdemir A, Lednev I K and Asher S A 2002 Comparison between UV Raman and circular dichroism detection of short alpha helices in Bombolitin III *Biochemistry* **41** 1893–6
[33] Asher S A, Ianoul A, Mix G, Boyden M N, Karnoup A, Diem M and Schweitzer- Stenner R 2001 Dihedral psi angle dependence of the amide III vibration: a uniquely sensitive UV resonance Raman secondary structural probe *J. Am. Chem. Soc.* **123** 11775–81
[34] Song S H and Asher S A 1989 UV resonance Raman studies of peptide conformation in poly (L-lysine), poly (L-glutamic acid), and model complexes – the basis for protein secondary structure determinations *J. Am. Chem. Soc.* **111** 4295–305
[35] Chi Z H, Chen X G, Holtz J S W and Asher S A 1998 UV resonance Raman-selective amide vibrational enhancement: quantitative methodology for determining protein secondary structure *Biochemistry* **37** 2854–64
[36] Canova S, Cortinovis D L and Ambrogi F 2017 How to describe univariate data *J. Thorac. Dis.* **9** 1741–3
[37] Gautam R, Vanga S, Ariese F and Umapathy S 2015 Review of multidimensional data processing approaches for Raman and infrared spectroscopy *EPJ Tech. Instrum* **2** 8
[38] Sharma B, Frontiera R R, Henry A I, Ringe E and Van Duyne R P 2012 SERS: materials, applications, and the future *Mater. Today* **15** 16–25
[39] Ando J and Fujita K (ed) 2013 *Current Pharmaceutical Biotechnology* vol 14 (Sharjaj: Bentham Science Publishers) pp 141–9
[40] Fleischmann M, Hendra P J and McQuillan A J 1974 Raman spectra of pyridine adsorbed at a silver electrode *Chem. Phys. Lett.* **26** 163–6
[41] Jeanmaire D L and Vanduyne R P 1977 Surface Raman spectro electrochemistry: part I. Heterocyclic, aromatic, and aliphatic amines adsorbed on anodized silver electrode *J. Electroanal. Chem.* **84** 1–20
[42] Albrecht M G and Creighton J A 1977 Anomalously intense Raman spectra of pyridine at a silver electrode *J. Am. Chem. Soc.* **99** 5215–7
[43] Kneipp K, Kneipp H, Itzkan I, Dasari R R and Feld M S 1999 Ultrasensitive chemical analysis by Raman spectroscopy *Chem. Rev.* **99** 2957–76
[44] Willets K A and Van Duyne R P 2007 Localized surface plasmon resonance spectroscopy and sensing *Annu. Rev. Phys. Chem.* **58** 267–97
[45] Stiles P L, Dieringer J A, Shah N C and Van Duyne R R 2008 Surface-enhanced Raman spectroscopy *Annu. Rev. Anal. Chem.* **1** 601–26
[46] Schlucker S 2014 Surface-enhanced Raman spectroscopy: concepts and chemical applications *Angew. Chem. Int. Ed.* **53** 4756–95
[47] Xie W and Schlucker S 2013 Medical applications of surface enhanced Raman scattering *Phys. Chem. Chem. Phys.* **15** 5329–44
[48] Manu M J, Nisha N, Jyothi B N, Varsha K, Adukkadan N R, Palasseri T S, Giridharan S, Jayadev S A, Vineeth M V and Kaustabh K M 2018 Exploring the margins of SERS in

practical domain: an emerging diagnostic modality for modern biomedical applications *Biomaterials* **181** 140–81
[49] Wang L *et al* 2015 Sea-urchin-like Au nanocluster with surface-enhanced Raman scattering in detecting epidermal growth factor receptor (EGFR) mutation status of malignant pleural effusion *ACS Appl. Mater. Interfaces* **7** 359–69
[50] He Y, Su S, Xu T, Zhong Y, Zapien J A, Li J, Fan C and Lee S T 2011 Silicon nanowires based highly-efficient SERS-active platform for ultrasensitive DNA detection *Nano Today* **6** 122–30
[51] Zhang Z, Sheng S, Wang R and Sun M 2016 Tip-enhanced Raman spectroscopy *Anal. Chem.* **88** 9328–46
[52] Sonntag M D, Pozzi E A, Jiang N, Hersam M C and Van Duyne R P 2014 Recent advances in tip-enhanced Raman spectroscopy *J. Phys. Chem. Lett.* **5** 3125–30
[53] Shao F and Zenobi R 2019 Tip-enhanced Raman spectroscopy: principles, practice, and applications to nanospectroscopic imaging of 2D materials *Anal. Bioanal. Chem.* **411** 37–61
[54] Deckert-Gaudig T, Taguchi A, Kawata S and Deckert V 2017 Tip-enhanced Raman spectroscopy—from early developments to recent advances *Chem. Soc. Rev.* **46** 4077–110
[55] Evans C L and Xie X S 2008 Coherent anti-Stokes Raman scattering microscopy: chemical imaging for biology and medicine *Annu. Rev. Anal. Chem.* **1** 883–909
[56] Min W, Freudiger C W, Lu S J and Xie X S 2011 *The Annual Review of Physical Chemistry* vol 62 ed S R Leone, P S Cremer, J T Groves and M A Johnson (San Mateo, CA: Annual Reviews) pp 507–30
[57] Chung C Y, Boik J and Potma E O 2013 *The Annual Review of Physical Chemistry* vol 64 ed M A Johnson and T J Martinez (San Mateo, CA: Annual Reviews) pp 77–99
[58] El-Diasty F 2011 Coherent anti-Stokes Raman scattering: spectroscopy and microscopy *Vib. Spectrosc.* **55** 1–37
[59] Freudiger C W, Min W, Saar B G, Lu S, Holtom G R, He C W, Tsai J C, Kang J X and Xie X S 2008 Label-free biomedical imaging with high sensitivity by stimulated Raman scattering microscopy *Science* **322** 1857–61
[60] Ploetz E, Laimgruber S, Berner S, Zinth W and Gilch P 2007 Femtosecond stimulated Raman microscopy *Appl. Phys.* B **87** 389–93
[61] Ferrara M A and Sirleto L 2019 *Nonlinear Optics: Novel Results in Theory and Application* ed B Lembrikov (London: IntechOpen) pp 127–43
[62] Min W, Freudiger C W, Lu S J and Xie X S 2011 Coherent nonlinear optical imaging: beyond fluorescence microscopy *Annu. Rev. Phys. Chem.* **62** 507–30
[63] Tipping W J, Lee M, Serrels A, Brunton V G and Hulme A N 2016 Stimulated Raman scattering microscopy: an emerging tool for drug discovery *Chem. Soc. Rev.* **45** 2075–89
[64] Saar B G, Freudiger C W, Reichman J, Stanley C M, Holtom G R and Xie X S 2010 Videorate molecular imaging *in vivo* with stimulated Raman scattering *Science* **330** 1368–70
[65] Evans C L, Potma E O, Puoris'haag M, Cote D, Lin C P and Xie X S 2005 Chemical imaging of tissue *in vivo* with video-rate coherent anti-Stokes Raman scattering microscopy *Proc. Natl Acad. Sci. USA* **102** 16807–12
[66] Camp C H Jr, Lee Y J, Heddleston J M, Hartshorn C M, Walker A R H, Rich J N, Lathia J D and Cicerone M T 2014 High-speed coherent Raman fingerprint imaging of biological tissues *Nat. Photonics* **8** 627–34

[67] Ichimura T, Hayazawa N, Hashimoto M, Inouye Y and Kawata S 2003 Local enhancement of coherent anti-Stokes Raman scattering by isolated gold nanoparticles *J. Raman Spectrosc.* **34** 651–4
[68] Steuwe C, Kaminski C F, Baumberg J J and Mahajan S 2011 Surface enhanced coherent anti-Stokes Raman scattering on nanostructured gold surfaces *Nano Lett.* **11** 5339–43
[69] Frontiera R R, Henry A I, Gruenke N L and Van Duyne R P 2011 Surface-enhanced femtosecond stimulated Raman spectroscopy *J. Phys. Chem. Lett.* **2** 1199–203
[70] Prince R C, Frontiera R R and Potma E O 2017 Stimulated Raman scattering: from bulk to nano *Chem. Rev.* **117** 5070–94
[71] Asher S A 1998 UV resonance Raman studies of molecular structure and dynamics: applications in physical and biophysical chemistry *Annu. Rev. Phys. Chem.* **39** 537–88
[72] Ashton L, Hogwood C E M, Tait A S, Kuligowski J, Smales C M, Bracewell D G, Dickson A J and Goodacre R 2015 UV resonance Raman spectroscopy: a process analytical tool for host cell DNA and RNA dynamics in mammalian cell lines *J. Chem. Technol. Biotechnol.* **90** 237–43
[73] Cialla-May D, Schmitt M and Popp J 2017 Theoretical principles of Raman spectroscopy *Phys. Sci. Rev.* **4** 20170040
[74] Stacy A M and Van Duyne R P 1983 Surface enhanced Raman and resonance Raman spectroscopy in a non-aqueous electrochemical environment: tris (2,2′-bipyridine) ruthenium (II) adsorbed on silver from acetonitrile *Chem. Phys. Lett.* **102** 365–70
[75] Cunningham D, Littleford R E, Smith W E, Lundahl P J, Khan I, McComb D W, Graham D and Laforest N 2006 Practical control of SERRS enhancement *Faraday Discuss.* **132** 135–45
[76] Kneipp K, Wang Y, Kneipp H, Perelman L T, Itzkan I, Dasari R R and Feld M S 1997 *Phys. Rev. Lett.* **78** 1667
[77] Nie S and Emory S R 1997 Probing single molecules and single nanoparticles by surface-enhanced Raman scattering *Science* **275** 1102–6
[78] McNay G, Eustace D, Smith W E, Faulds K and Graham D 2011 Surface-enhanced Raman scattering (SERS) and surface-enhanced resonance Raman scattering (SERRS): a review of applications *Appl. Spectrosc.* **65** 825–37
[79] Matousek P, Clark I P, Draper E R, Morris M D, Goodship A E, Everall N, Towrie M, Finney W F and Parker A W 2005 Subsurface probing in diffusely scattering media using spatially offset Raman spectroscopy *Appl. Spectrosc.* **59** 393–400
[80] Matousek P 2007 Deep non-invasive Raman spectroscopy of living tissue and powders *Chem. Soc. Rev.* **36** 1292–304
[81] Matousek P and Stone N 2016 Development of deep subsurface Raman spectroscopy for medical diagnosis and disease monitoring *Chem. Soc. Rev.* **45** 1794–802
[82] Baker R, Matousek P, Ronayne K L, Parker A W, Rogers K and Stone N 2007 Depth profiling of calcifications in breast tissue using picosecond Kerr-gated Raman spectroscopy *Analyst* **132** 48–53
[83] Matousek P and Stone N 2009 Emerging concepts in deep Raman spectroscopy of biological tissue *Analyst* **134** 1058–66
[84] Matousek P and Stone N 2013 Recent advances in the development of Raman spectroscopy for deep non-invasive medical diagnosis *J. Biophotonics* **6** 7–19
[85] Buckley K and Matousek P 2011 Non-invasive analysis of turbid samples using deep Raman spectroscopy *Analyst* **136** 3039–50

[86] Matousek P, Conti C, Realini M and Colombo C 2016 Micro-scale spatially offset Raman spectroscopy for non-invasive subsurface analysis of turbid materials *Analyst* **141** 731–9
[87] Conti C, Colombo C, Realini M, Zerbi G and Matousek P 2014 Subsurface Raman analysis of thin painted layers *Appl. Spectrosc.* **68** 686–91
[88] Conti C, Realini M, Colombo C and Matousek P 2015 Subsurface analysis of painted sculptures and plasters using micrometre-scale spatially offset Raman spectroscopy (micro-SORS) *J. Raman Spectrosc.* **46** 476–82
[89] Conti C, Colombo C, Realini M and Matousek P 2015 Comparison of key modalities of micro-scale spatially offset Raman spectroscopy *Analyst* **140** 8127–33
[90] Conti C, Colombo C, Realini M, Botteon A and Matousek P 2016 Contrasting confocal with defocusing microscale spatially offset Raman spectroscopy *J. Raman Spectrosc.* **47** 565–70
[91] Conti C, Realini M, Colombo C, Sowoidnich K, Afseth N K, Bertasa M, Botteon A and Matousek P 2015 Noninvasive analysis of thin turbid layers using microscale spatially offset Raman spectroscopy *Anal. Chem.* **87** 5810–5
[92] Matousek P, Conti C, Colombo C and Realini M 2015 Monte Carlo simulations of subsurface analysis of painted layers in micro-scale spatially offset Raman spectroscopy *Appl. Spectrosc.* **69** 1091–5
[93] Realini M, Botteon A, Conti C, Colombo C and Matousek P 2016 Development of portable defocusing micro-scale spatially offset Raman spectroscopy *Analyst* **141** 3012–9
[94] Realini M, Conti C, Botteon A, Colombo C and Matousek P 2017 Development of a full micro-scale spatially offset Raman spectroscopy prototype as a portable analytical tool *Analyst* **142** 351–5
[95] Vandenabeele P, Conti C, Rousaki A, Moens L, Realini M and Matousek P 2017 Development of a fiber-optics microspatially offset Raman spectroscopy sensor for probing layered materials *Anal. Chem.* **89** 9218–23
[96] Nicolson F, Kircher M F, Stone N and Matousek P 2020 Spatially offset Raman spectroscopy for biomedical applications *Chem. Soc. Rev.* **50** 556–68
[97] Gautam R, Oh J Y, Patel R P and Dluhy R A 2018 Non-invasive analysis of stored red blood cells using diffuse resonance Raman spectroscopy *Analyst* **143** 5950–8
[98] Di Z, Hokr B H, Cai H, Wang K, Yakovlev V V, Sokolov A V and Scully M O 2015 Spatially offset Raman microspectroscopy of highly scattering tissue: theory and experiment *J. Mod. Opt.* **62** 97–101
[99] Khan K M, Ghosh N and Majumder S K 2016 Off-confocal Raman spectroscopy (OCRS) for subsurface measurements in layered turbid samples *J. Opt.* **18** 095301
[100] Matthiae M and Kristensen A 2019 Hyperspectral spatially offset Raman spectroscopy in a microfluidic channel *Opt. Express* **27** 3782–90
[101] Rousaki A, Botteon A, Colombo C, Conti C, Matousek P and Moens L 2017 Development of defocusing micro-SORS mapping: a study of a 19th century porcelain card *Anal. Methods* **9** 6435–42
[102] Botteon A, Colombo C, Realini M, Bracci S, Magrini D and Matousek P 1652–9 Exploring street art paintings by microspatially offset Raman spectroscopy *J. Raman Spectrosc.* **49** 1652–9
[103] Buckley K, Atkins C G, Chen D, Schulze H G, Devine D V, Blades M W and Turner R F B 2016 Non-invasive spectroscopy of transfusable red blood cells stored inside sealed plastic blood-bags *Analyst* **141** 1678–85

[104] Conti C, Botteon A, Colombo C, Realini M and Matousek P 2019 *Raman Spectroscopy in Archaeology and Art History* vol 2 ed P Vandenabeele and H Edwards (London: Royal Society of Chemistry) pp 174–83
[105] Stone N, Faulds K, Graham D and Matousek P 2010 Prospects of deep Raman spectroscopy for noninvasive detection of conjugated surface enhanced resonance Raman scattering nanoparticles buried within 25 mm of mammalian tissue *Anal. Chem.* **82** 3969–73
[106] Stone N, Kerssens M, Lloyd G R, Faulds K, Graham D and Matousek P 2011 Surface enhanced spatially offset Raman spectroscopic (SESORS) imaging – the next dimension *Chem. Sci.* **2** 776–80
[107] Nicolson F, Jamieson L E, Mabbott S, Plakas K, Shand N C, Detty M R, Graham D and Faulds K 2018 Through tissue imaging of a live breast cancer tumour model using handheld surface enhanced spatially offset resonance Raman spectroscopy (SESORRS) *Chem. Sci.* **9** 3788–92
[108] Macleod N A and Matousek P 2008 Emerging non-invasive Raman methods in process control and forensic applications *Pharm. Res.* **25** 2205–15
[109] Matousek P and Parker A W 2006 Bulk Raman analysis of pharmaceutical tablets *Appl. Spectrosc.* **60** 1353–7
[110] Smith E and Dent G (ed) 2005 *Modern Raman Spectroscopy – A Practical Approach* (Chichester: Wiley) pp 210
[111] Schrader B and Bergmann G 1967 The intensity of the Raman spectrum of polycrystalline substances *Anal. Chem.* **225** 230–47
[112] Matousek P and Stone N 2007 Prospects for the diagnosis of breast cancer by noninvasive probing of calcifications using transmission Raman spectroscopy *J. Biomed. Opt.* **12** 024008
[113] Giridhar G, Manepalli R R K N and Apparao G 2017 *Spectroscopic Methods for Nanomaterials Characterization* vol 2 ed S Thomas, R Thomas, A K Zachariah and R Kumar (Amsterdam: Elsevier Science) pp 141–61
[114] John N and George S 2017 *Spectroscopic Methods for Nanomaterials Characterization* vol 2 ed S Thomas, R Thomas, A K Zachariah and R Kumar (Amsterdam: Elsevier Science) pp 95–127
[115] Abraham J L and Etz E S 1979 Molecular microanalysis of pathological specimens *in situ* with a laser-Raman microprobe *Science* **206** 716–8
[116] Romero G, Rojas E, Estrela-Lopis I, Donath E and Moyal S E 2011 Spontaneous confocal Raman microscopy – a tool to study the uptake of nanoparticles and carbon nanotubes into cells *Nanoscale Res. Lett.* **6** 429
[117] Kojima T, Onoue S, Murase N, Katoh F, Mano T and Matsuda Y 2006 Crystalline form information from multi-well plate salt screening by use of Raman microscopy *Pharm. Res.* **23** 806–12
[118] Breitenbach J, Schrof W and Neumann J 1999 Confocal Raman-spectroscopy: analytical approach to solid dispersions and mapping of drugs *Pharm. Res.* **16** 1109–13
[119] Chen Y, Dai J, Zhou X, Liu Y, Zhang W and Peng G 2014 Raman spectroscopy analysis of the biochemical characteristics of molecules associated with the malignant transformation of gastric mucosa *PLoS One* **9** e93906
[120] Bonnier F and Byrne H J 2012 Understanding the molecular information contained in principal component analysis of vibrational spectra of biological systems *Analyst* **137** 322–32

[121] Bonnier F, Knief P, Lim B, Meade A, Dorney J, Bhattacharya K, Lyng F and Byrne H 2010 Imaging live cells grown on a three dimensional collagen matrix using Raman micro spectroscopy *Analyst* **135** 3169–77

[122] Yonzon C R, Lyandres O, Shah N C, Dieringer J A and Van Duyne R P 2006 *Surface-Enhanced Raman Scattering* vol 103 ed K Kneipp, M Moskovits and H Kneipp (Berlin: Springer) pp 367–79

[123] Stanley S A 2018 Diabetes: peripheral nerve modulation to treat metabolic disease *Nat. Rev. Endocrinol.* **14** 193–4

[124] Collaboration N R F 2016 Worldwide trends in diabetes since 1980: a pooled analysis of 751 population-based studies with 4.4 million participants *Lancet* **387** 1513–30

[125] Bommer C, Sagalova V, Heesemann E, ManneGoehler J, Atun R, Bärnighausen T, Davies J and Vollmer S 2018 Global economic burden of diabetes in adults: projections from 2015 to 2030 *Diabetes Care* **41** 963–70

[126] Veiseh O, Tang B C, Whitehead K A, Anderson D G and Langer R 2015 Managing diabetes with nanomedicine: challenges and opportunities *Nat. Rev. Drug Discov.* **14** 45–57

[127] Song Y, Lu X, Li Y, Guo Q, Chen S, Mao L, Hou H and Wang L 2016 Nitrogen-doped carbon nanotubes supported by macroporous carbon as an efficient enzymatic biosensing platform for glucose *Anal. Chem.* **88** 1371–7

[128] Peng X, Wan G, Wu L, Zeng M, Lin S and Wang G 2018 Peroxidase-like activity of Au@ TiO_2 yolk-shell nanostructure and its application for colorimetric detection of H_2O_2 and glucose *Sens. Actuators* B **257** 166–77

[129] Liu Y, Zhu J, Xu Y, Qin Y and Jiang D 2015 Boronic acid functionalized aza-bodipy (azaBDPBA) based fluorescence optodes for the analysis of glucose in whole blood *ACS Appl. Mater. Interfaces* **7** 11141–5

[130] Iguchi S, Kudo H, Saito T, Ogawa M, Saito H, Otsuka K, Funakubo A and Mitsubayashi K 2007 A flexible and wearable biosensor for tear glucose measurement *Biomed. Microdevices* **9** 603–9

[131] Baca J T, Finegold D N and Asher S A 2007 Tear glucose analysis for the noninvasive detection and monitoring of diabetes mellitus *Ocul. Surf.* **5** 280–93

[132] Panchbhai A S 2012 Correlation of salivary glucose level with blood glucose level in diabetes mellitus *J. Oral Maxil. Res* **3** e3

[133] Munje R D, Muthukumar S and Prasad S 2017 Lancet-free and label-free diagnostics of glucose in sweat using zinc oxide based flexible bioelectronics *Sens. Actuators* B **238** 482–90

[134] Cengiz E and Tamborlane W V 2009 A tale of two compartments: interstitial versus blood glucose monitoring *Diabetes Technol. Therap* **11** S11

[135] Shao J, Lin M, Li Y, Li X, Liu J, Liang J and Yao H 2012 In vivo blood glucose quantification using Raman spectroscopy *PLoS One* **7** 1–6

[136] Pandey R, Paidi S K, Valdez T A, Zhang C, Spegazzini N, Dasari R R and Barman I 2017 Noninvasive monitoring of blood glucose with Raman spectroscopy *Acc. Chem. Res.* **50** 264–72

[137] Han H W, Yan X L, Dong R X, Ban G and Li K 2009 Analysis of serum from type II diabetes mellitus and diabetic complication using surface-enhanced Raman spectra (SERS) *Appl. Phys.* B **94** 667–72

[138] Zou Y, Huang M, Wang K, Song B, Wang Y, Chen J, Liu X, Li X, Lin L and Huang G 2016 Urine surface-enhanced Raman spectroscopy for non-invasive diabetic detection based on a portable Raman spectrometer *Laser Phys. Lett.* **13** 65604

[139] Kang J W *et al* 2020 Direct observation of glucose fingerprint using *in vivo* Raman spectroscopy *Sci. Adv.* **6** eaay520

[140] Yuen J M, Shah N C, Walsh J T, Glucksberg M R and Van Duyne R P 2010 Transcutaneous glucose sensing by surface-enhanced spatially offset Raman spectroscopy in a rat model *Anal. Chem.* **82** 8382–5

[141] Kong C R, Barman I, Dingari N C, Kang J W, Galindo L, Dasari R R and Feld M S 2011 A novel non-imaging optics based Raman spectroscopy device for transdermal blood analyte measurement *AIP Adv.* **1** 032175

[142] Mahadevan-Jansen A and Richards-Kortum R 1997 Raman spectroscopy for cancer detection: a review *Proc. 19th Annual Int. Conf. of the IEEE Engineering in Medicine and Biology Society. Magnificent Milestones and Emerging Opportunities in Medical Engineering vol 6 (Chicago, 30 Oct.–2 Nov. 1997)* pp 2722–8

[143] Liu C H *et al* 1992 Raman, fluorescence, and time-resolved light scattering as optical diagnostic techniques to separate diseased and normal biomedical media *J. Photochem. Photobiol.* B **16** 187–209

[144] Kallaway C, Almond L M, Barr H, Wood J, Hutchings J, Kendall C and Stone N 2013 Advances in the clinical application of Raman spectroscopy for cancer diagnostics *Photodiagn. Photodyn. Ther.* **10** 207–19

[145] Almond L M, Hutchings J, Shepherd N, Barr H, Stone N and Kendall C 2011 Raman spectroscopy: a potential tool for early objective diagnosis of neoplasia in the oesophagus *J. Biophotonics* **4** 685–95

[146] Old O J, Fullwood L M, Scott R, Lloyd G R, Almond L M, Shepherd N A, Stone N, Barr H and Kendall C 2014 Vibrational spectroscopy for cancer diagnostics *Anal. Methods* **6** 3901–17

[147] Manoharan R, Wang Y and Feld M S 1996 Histochemical analysis of biological tissues using Raman spectroscopy *Spectrochim. Acta* A **52** 215–49

[148] Frank C J, Redd D C B, Gansler T S and McCreery R L 1994 Characterization of human breast biopsy specimens with near-IR Raman spectroscopy *Anal. Chem.* **66** 319–26

[149] Marro M, Nieva C, Sanz-Pamplona R and Sierra A 2014 Molecular monitoring of epithelial-to-mesenchymal transition in breast cancer cells by means of Raman spectroscopy *Biochim. Biophys. Acta - Mol. Cell Res* **1843** 1785–95

[150] Talari A C S, Evans C A, Holen I, Coleman R E and Rehman I U 2015 Raman spectroscopic analysis differentiates between breast cancer cell lines *J. Raman Spectrosc.* **46** 421–7

[151] Frank C J, McCreery R L and Redd D C B 1995 Raman Spectroscopy of normal and diseased human breast tissues *Anal. Chem.* **67** 777–83

[152] Haka A S, Shafer-Peltier K E, Fitzmaurice M, Crowe J, Dasari R R and Feld M S 2002 Identifying microcalcifications in benign and malignant breast lesions by probing differences in their chemical composition using Raman spectroscopy *Cancer Res.* **62** 5375–80

[153] Shafer-Peltier K E, Haka A S, Fitzmaurice M, Crowe J, Myles J, Dasari R R and Feld M S 2002 Raman microspectroscopic model of human breast tissue: implications for breast cancer diagnosis *in vivo J. Raman Spectrosc.* **33** 552–63

[154] Haka A S, Shafer-Peltier K E, Fitzmaurice M, Crowe J, Dasari R R and Feld M S 2005 Diagnosing breast cancer by using Raman spectroscopy *Proc. Natl Acad. Sci. USA* **102** 12371–6

[155] Motz J T, Hunter M, Galindo L H, Gardecki J A, Kramer J R, Dasari R R and Feld M S 2004 Optical fiber probe for biomedical Raman spectroscopy *Appl. Opt.* **43** 542–54
[156] Haka A S, Volynskaya Z, Gardecki J A, Nazemi J, Lyons J, Hicks D, Fitzmaurice M, Dasari R R, Crowe J P and Feld M S 2006 In vivo margin assessment during partial mastectomy breast surgery using Raman spectroscopy *Cancer Res.* **66** 3317–22
[157] Haka A S, Volynskaya Z I, Gardecki J A, Nazemi J, Shenk R, Wang N, Dasari R R, Fitzmaurice M and Feld M S 2009 Diagnosing breast cancer using Raman spectroscopy: prospective analysis *J. Biomed. Opt.* **14** 054023
[158] Saha A *et al* 2011 Raman spectroscopy: a real-time tool for identifying microcalcifications during stereotactic breast core needle biopsies *Biomed. Opt. Express* **2** 2792–803
[159] Kast R E *et al* 2008 Raman spectroscopy can differentiate malignant tumors from normal breast tissue and detect early neoplastic changes in a mouse model *Biopolymers* **89** 235–41
[160] Yu G, Xu X X, Niu Y, Wang B, Song Z F and Zhang C P 2004 Studies on human breast cancer tissues with Raman microspectroscopy *Guang Pu Xue Yu Guang Pu Fen Xi* **24** 1359–62
[161] Abramczyk H, Brozek-Pluska B, Surmacki J, Jablonska- Gajewicz J and Kordek R 2012 Raman 'optical biopsy' of human breast cancer *Prog. Biophys. Mol. Biol.* **108** 74–81
[162] Stone N and Matousek P 2008 Advanced transmission Raman spectroscopy: a promising tool for breast disease diagnosis *Cancer Res.* **68** 4424–30
[163] Ghita A, Matousek P and Stone N 2017 High sensitivity non-invasive detection of calcifications deep inside biological tissue using transmission Raman spectroscopy *J. Biophotonics* **11** e201600260
[164] Keller M D, Majumder S K and Mahadevan-Jansen A 2009 Spatially offset Raman spectroscopy of layered soft tissues *Opt. Lett.* **3** 926–8
[165] Keller M D, Vargis E, de Matos Granja N, Wilson R H, Mycek M A and Kelley M C 2011 Development of a spatially offset Raman spectroscopy probe for breast tumor surgical margin evaluation *J. Biomed. Opt.* **16** 077006
[166] Kerssens M M, Matousek P, Rogers K and Stone N 2010 Towards a safe non-invasive method for evaluating the carbonate substitution levels of hydroxyapatite (HAP) in microcalcifications found in breast tissue *Analyst* **135** 3156–61
[167] Nicolson F, Jamieson L E, Mabbott S, Plakas K, Shand N C, Detty M R, Graham D and Faulds K 2018 Multiplex imaging of live breast cancer tumour models through tissue using handheld surface enhanced spatially offset resonance Raman spectroscopy (SESORRS) *Chem. Commun.* **54** 8530–3
[168] Mizuno A, Kitajima H, Kawauchi K, Muraishi S and Ozaki Y 1994 Near-infrared Fourier transform Raman spectroscopic study of human brain tissues and tumours *J. Raman Spectrosc.* **25** 25–9
[169] Mizuno A, Hayashi T, Tashibu K, Maraishi S, Kawauchi K and Ozaki Y 1992 Near-infrared FT-Raman spectra of the rat brain tissues *Neurosci. Lett.* **141** 47–52
[170] Zhou Y, Liu C H, Sun Y, Pu Y, Boydston-White S, Liu Y and Alfano R R 2012 Human brain cancer studied by resonance Raman spectroscopy *J. Biomed. Opt.* **17** 116021
[171] Kalkanis S N, Kast R E, Rosenblum M L, Mikkelsen T, Yurgelevic S M, Nelson K M and Auner G W 2014 Raman spectroscopy to distinguish grey matter, necrosis, and glioblastoma multiforme in frozen tissue sections *J. Neuro-Oncol* **116** 477–85
[172] Yang P 2009 Epidemiology of lung cancer prognosis: quantity and quality of life *Methods Mol. Biol.* **471** 469–86

[173] Oken M M 2011 Screening by chest radiograph and lung cancer mortality: the prostate, lung, colorectal, and ovarian (PLCO) randomized trial *JAMA* **306** 1865–73

[174] Magee N D, Villaumie J S, Marple E T, Ennis M, Elborn J S and McGarvey J J 2009 Ex vivo diagnosis of lung cancer using a Raman miniprobe *J. Phys. Chem.* B **113** 8137–41

[175] Zeng H, Short M A, McWilliams A and Lam S 2010 In vivo Raman spectroscopy for early lung cancer detection *Asia Communications and Photonics Conf. and Exhibition (Shanghai, Dec. 2010)* p 535

[176] Kaminaka S, Yamazaki H, Ito T, Kohda E and Hamaguchi H 2001 Near-infrared Raman spectroscopy of human lung tissues: possibility of molecular-level cancer diagnosis *J. Raman Spectrosc.* **32** 139–41

[177] Huang Z W, McWilliams A, Lui H, McLean D I, Lam S and Zeng H S 2003 Near-infrared Raman spectroscopy for optical diagnosis of lung cancer *Int. J. Cancer* **107** 1047–52

[178] Gao L, Wang Z, Li F, Hammoudi A A, Thrall M J, Cagle P T and Wong S T C 2012 Differential diagnosis of lung carcinoma with coherent anti-Stokes Raman scattering imaging *Arch. Pathol. Lab. Med* **136** 1502–10

[179] Gao L *et al* 2011 On-the-spot lung cancer differential diagnosis by label-free, molecular vibrational imaging and knowledge-based classification *J. Biomed. Opt.* **16** 096004–10

[180] Cheng J X and Xie X S 2004 Coherent anti-Stokes Raman scattering microscopy: instrumentation, theory, and applications *J. Phys. Chem.* B **108** 827–40

[181] Wang L *et al* 2014 Evaluation of Raman spectroscopy for diagnosing EGFR mutation status in lung adenocarcinoma *Analyst* **139** 455–63

[182] McGregor H C 2016 Real-time endoscopic Raman spectroscopy for *in vivo* early lung cancer detection *J. Biophotonics* **13** 98–110

[183] McGregor H C 2015 *In vivo* real-time endoscopic Raman spectroscopy for improving early lung cancer detection *Asia Communications and Photonics Conf.* ed C Lu, J Luo, Y Ji, K Kitayama, H Tam, K Xu, P Ghiggino and N Wada (OSA Technical Digest) (Washington, DC: Optical Society of America) paper AM4A.1

[184] Zheng Q, Li J, Yang L, Zheng B, Wang J, Lv N, Luo J, Martin F L, Liu D and He J 2020 Raman spectroscopy as a potential diagnostic tool to analyse biochemical alterations in lung cancer *Analyst* **145** 385–92

[185] Siegel R, Ma J, Zou Z and Jemal A 2014 Cancer statistics, 2014 *CA Cancer J. Clin.* **64** 9–29

[186] Balch C M 2009 Final version of 2009 AJCC melanoma staging and classification *J. Clin. Oncol.* **27** 6199–206

[187] Dickson P V and Gershenwald J E 2011 Staging and prognosis of cutaneous melanoma *Surg. Oncol. Clin. N. Am.* **20** 1–17

[188] Lewis K G and Weinstock M A 2004 Nonmelanoma skin cancer mortality (1988–2000) the Rhode Island follow-back study *Arch. Dermatol.* **140** 837–42

[189] Nunes L O, Martin A A, Silveira L Jr and Zampieri M 2003 FT-Raman spectroscopy study for skin cancer diagnosis *J. Spectrosc.* **17** 597–602

[190] Silveira L Jr, Silveira F L, Bodanese B, Zangaro R A, Tadeu M and Pacheco T 2012 Discriminating model for diagnosis of basal cell carcinoma and melanoma *in vitro* based on the Raman spectra of selected biochemicals *J. Biomed. Opt.* **17** 077003

[191] Larraona-Puy M, Ghita A, Zoladek A, Perkins W, Varma S, Leach I H, Koloydenko A A, Williams H and Notingher I 2009 Development of Raman microspectroscopy for automated detection and imaging of basal cell carcinoma *J. Biomed. Opt.* **14** 31–54

[192] Bodanese B, Silveira L Jr, Albertini R, Zangaro R A, Tavares and Pacheco M T 2010 Differentiating normal and basal cell carcinoma human skin tissues *in vitro* using dispersive Raman spectroscopy: a comparison between principal components analysis and simplified biochemical models *Photomed. Laser Surg* **28** S119–27

[193] Bodanese B, Silveira F L, Zangaro R A, Pacheco M T T, Pasqualucci C A and Silveira L Jr 2012 Discrimination of basal cell carcinoma and melanoma from normal skin biopsies *in vitro* through Raman spectroscopy and principal component analysis *Photomed. Laser Surg* **30** 381–7

[194] Gniadecka M, Wulf H, Mortensen N N, Nielsen O F and Christensen D H 1997 Diagnosis of basal cell carcinoma by Raman spectroscopy *J. Raman Spectrosc.* **28** 125–9

[195] Gniadecka M *et al* 2004 Melanoma diagnosis by Raman spectroscopy and neural networks: structure alterations in proteins and lipids in intact cancer tissue *J. Invest. Dermatol.* **122** 443–9

[196] Nijssen A, Schut T C B, Heule F, Caspers P J, Hayes D P, Neumann M H and Puppels G J 2002 Discriminating basal cell carcinoma from its surrounding tissue by Raman spectroscopy *J. Invest. Dermatol.* **119** 64–9

[197] Nijssen A, Maquelin K, Santos L F, Caspers P J, Bakker Schut T C, den Hollander J C, Neumann M H A and Puppels G J 2007 Discriminating basal cell carcinoma from perilesional skin using high wave-number Raman spectroscopy *J. Biomed. Opt.* **12** 034004–7

[198] Vogler N, Meyer T, Akimov D, Latka I, Krafft C, Bendsoe N, Svanberg K, Dietzek B and Popp J 2010 Multimodal imaging to study the morphochemistry of basal cell carcinoma *J. Biophotonics* **3** 728–36

[199] Lieber C A, Majumder S K, Ellis D L, Billheimer D D and Mahadevan-Jansen A 2008 In vivo nonmelanoma skin cancer diagnosis using Raman microspectroscopy *Lasers Surg. Med.* **40** 461–7

[200] Lui H, Zhao J, McLean D and Zeng H 2012 Real-time Raman spectroscopy for *in vivo* skin cancer diagnosis *Cancer Res.* **72** 2491–500

[201] Schleusener J, Gluszczynska P, Reble C, Gersonde I, Helfmann J, Fluhr J W, Lademann J, Röwert-Huber J, Patzelt A and Meinke M C 2015 In vivo study for the discrimination of cancerous and normal skin using fibre probe-based Raman spectroscopy *Exp. Dermatol.* **24** 767–72

[202] Santos I P, Doorn R V, Caspers P J, Schut T C B, Barroso E M, Nijsten T E C, Hegt V N, Koljenović S and Puppels G J 2018 Improving clinical diagnosis of early-stage cutaneous melanoma based on Raman spectroscopy *Br. J. Cancer* **119** 1339–46

[203] Kong K, Rowlands C J, Varma S, Perkins W, Leach I H, Koloydenko A A, Williams H C and Notingher I 2013 Diagnosis of tumors during tissue-conserving surgery with integrated autofluorescence and Raman scattering microscopy *Proc. Natl Acad. Sci. USA* **110** 15189–94

[204] Kong K, Zaabar F, Rakha E, Ellis I, Koloydenko A and Notingher I 2014 Towards intra-operative diagnosis of tumours during breast conserving surgery by selective-sampling Raman micro-spectroscopy *Phys. Med. Biol.* **59** 6141–52

[205] Kong K, Rowlands C J, Varma S, Perkins W, Leach I H, Koloydenko A A, Pitiot A, Williams H C and Notingher I 2014 Increasing the speed of tumour diagnosis during surgery with selective scanning Raman microscopy *J. Mol. Struct.* **1073** 58–65

[206] Zhao J, Zeng H, Kalia S and Lui H 2016 Wavenumber selection based analysis in Raman spectroscopy improves skin cancer diagnostic specificity *Analyst* **141** 1034–43

[207] Devpura S, Thakur J S, Sarkar F H, Sakr W A, Naik V M and Naik R 2010 Detection of benign epithelia, prostatic intraepithelial neoplasia, and cancer regions in radical prostatectomy tissues using Raman spectroscopy *Vib. Spectrosc.* **53** 227–32

[208] Schlucker S, Salehi M, Bergner G, Schutz M, Strobel P, Marx A, Petersen I, Dietzek B and Popp J 2011 Immuno-surface-enhanced coherent anti-Stokes Raman scattering microscopy: immunohistochemistry with target-specific metallic nanoprobes and nonlinear Raman microscopy *Anal. Chem.* **83** 7081–5

[209] Harmsen S *et al* 2015 Scattering nanostars for high-precision cancer imaging *Sci. Transl. Med.* **7** 271ra7

[210] Qiu Y *et al* 2019 Photodegradable CuS SERS probes for intraoperative residual tumor detection, ablation, and self-clearance *ACS Appl. Mater. Interfaces* **11** 23436–44

[211] Vargis E, Kanter E M, Majumder S K, Keller M D, Beaven R B, Rao G G and Mahadevan-Jansen A 2011 Effect of normal variations on disease classification of Raman spectra from cervical tissue *Analyst* **136** 2981–7

[212] Duraipandian S, Zheng W, Ng J, Low J J H, Ilancheran A and Huang Z 2011 In vivo diagnosis of cervical precancer using Raman spectroscopy and genetic algorithm techniques *Analyst* **136** 4328–36

[213] Shaikh R, Dora T K, Chopra S, Maheshwari A D, Kedar K, Bharat R and Krishna C M 2014 In vivo Raman spectroscopy of human uterine cervix: exploring the utility of vagina as an internal control *J. Biomed. Opt.* **19** 087001

[214] Duraipandian S, Zheng W, Ng J, Low J J H, Ilancheran A and Huang Z 2012 Simultaneous fingerprint and high-wavenumber confocal Raman spectroscopy enhances early detection of cervical precancer *in vivo Anal. Chem.* **84** 5913–9

[215] Duraipandian S, Zheng W, Ng J, Low J J H, Ilancheran A and Huang Z 2013 Near-infrared-excited confocal Raman spectroscopy advances *in vivo* diagnosis of cervical precancer *J. Biomed. Opt.* **18** 067007

[216] Rashid N, Nawaz H, Poon K W, Bonnier F, Bakhiet S, Martin C, O'Leary J J, Byrne H J and Lyng F M 2014 Raman microspectroscopy for the early detection of premalignant changes in cervical tissue *Exp. Mol. Pathol.* **97** 554–64

[217] Duraipandian S, Zheng W, Ng J, Low J J H, Ilancheran A and Huang Z 2013 Integrated fingerprint and high wavenumber confocal Raman spectroscopy for *in vivo* diagnosis of cervical precancer *Proc. SPIE* **8572** 85720Z–7

[218] Daniel A, Aruna P and Ganesan S 2018 Near-infrared Raman spectroscopy for estimating iochemical changes associated with different pathological conditions of cervix *Spectrochim. Acta* A **190** 409–16

[219] Duraipandian S, Mo J, Zheng W and Huang Z 2014 Near-infrared Raman spectroscopy for assessing biochemical changes of cervical tissue associated with precarcinogenic transformation *Analyst* **139** 5379–86

[220] Rubina S and Krishna C M 2015 Raman spectroscopy in cervical cancers: an update *J. Cancer Res. Ther* **139** 5379–86

[221] Matthews Q, Jirasek A, Lum J J and Brolo A G 2011 Biochemical signatures of *in vitro* radiation response in human lung, breast and prostate tumour cells observed with Raman spectroscopy *Phys. Med. Biol.* **56** 6839–55

[222] Abramczyk H, Surmacki J, Kopec M, Olejnik A K, Lubecka-Pietruszewska K and Fabianowska-Majewska K 2015 The role of lipid droplets and adipocytes in cancer.

Raman imaging of cell cultures: MCF10A, MCF7, and MDAMB-231 compared to adipocytes in cancerous human breast tissue *Analyst* **140** 2224–35

[223] Abramczyk H, Surmacki J, Kopec M, Olejnik A K, Kaufman-Szymczyk A and Fabianowska-Majewska K 2016 Epigenetic changes in cancer by Raman imaging, fluorescence imaging, AFM and scanning near-field optical microscopy (SNOM). Acetylation in normal and human cancer breast cells MCF10A, MCF7 and MDA-MB-231 *Analyst* **141** 5646–58

[224] Medeiros P S, Batista de Carvalho A L M, Ruano C, Otero J C and Marques M P 2016 Raman microspectroscopy for probing the impact of a dietary antioxidant on human breast cancer cells *Food Funct* **7** 2800–10

[225] Shashni B, Horiguchi Y, Kurosu K, Furusho H and Nagasaki Y 2017 Application of surface enhanced Raman spectroscopy as a diagnostic system for hypersialylated metastatic cancers *Biomaterials* **134** 143–53

[226] Bi X, Rexer B, Arteaga C L, Guo M and Mahadevan-Jansen A 2014 Evaluating HER2 amplification status and acquired drug resistance in breast cancer cells using Raman spectroscopy *J. Biomed. Opt.* **19** 025001

[227] Mignolet A, Wood B R and Goormaghtigh E 2017 Intracellular investigation on the differential effects of 4 polyphenols on MCF-7 breast cancer cells by Raman imaging *Analyst* **143** 258–69

[228] Talari A C S, Raza A, Rehman S and Rehman I U 2017 Analyzing normal proliferating, hypoxic and necrotic regions of T-47D human breast cancer spheroids using Raman spectroscopy *Appl. Spectrosc. Rev.* **52** 909–24

[229] Marro M, Nieva C, de Juan A and Sierra A 2018 Unravelling the metabolic progression of breast cancer cells to bone metastasis by coupling Raman spectroscopy and a novel use of MCR-ALS algorithm *Anal. Chem.* **90** 5594–602

[230] Winnard P T Jr, Zhang C, Vesuna F, Kang J W, Garry J, Dasari R R, Barman I and Raman V 2017 Organ-specific isogenic metastatic breast cancer cell lines exhibit distinct Raman spectral signatures and metabolomes *Oncotarget* **8** 20266–87

[231] Jermyn M, Mok K, Mercier J, Desroches J, Pichette J, Saint-Arnaud K and Leblond F 2015 Intraoperative brain cancer detection with Raman spectroscopy in humans *Sci. Transl. Med.* **7** 274ra19

[232] Jermyn M, Desroches J, Mercier J, Tremblay M A, St-Arnaud K, Guiot M C, Petrecca K and Leblond F 2016 Neural networks improve brain cancer detection with Raman spectroscopy in the presence of operating room light artifacts *J. Biomed. Opt.* **21** 094002

[233] Jermyn M, Desroches J, Mercier J, St-Arnaud K, Guiot M C, Leblond F and Petrecca K 2016 Raman spectroscopy detects distant invasive brain cancer cells centimeters beyond MRI capability in humans *Biomed. Opt. Express* **7** 5129–37

[234] Pijanka J K, Stone N, Rutter A V, Forsyth N, Sockalingum G D, Yang Y and Sule-Suso J 2013 Identification of different subsets of lung cells using Raman microspectroscopy and whole cell nucleus isolation *Analyst* **138** 5052–8

[235] Ahlinder L, Ekstrand-Hammarstrom B, Geladi P and Osterlund L 2013 Large uptake of titania and iron oxide nanoparticles in the nucleus of lung epithelial cells as measured by Raman imaging and multivariate classification *Biophys. J.* **105** 310–9

[236] Potara M, Boca S, Licarete E, Damert A, Alupei M C, Chiriac M T, Popescu O, Schmidt U and Astilean S 2013 Chitosan-coated triangular silver nanoparticles as a novel class of

biocompatible, highly sensitive plasmonic platforms for intracellular SERS sensing and imaging *Nanoscale* **5** 6013–22

[237] Donfack P, Rehders M, Brix K, Boukamp P and Materny A 2009 Micro Raman spectroscopy for monitoring alterations between human skin keratinocytes HaCaT and their tumorigenic derivatives A5RT3—toward a Raman characterization of a skin carcinoma model *J. Raman Spectrosc.* **41** 16–26

[238] Wang H, Tsai T, Zhao J, Lee A M D, Lo B K K, Yu M, Lui H, McLean D I and Zeng H 2012 Differentiation of HaCaT cell and melanocyte from their malignant counterparts using micro-Raman spectroscopy guided by confocal imaging *Photodermatol. Photoimmunol. Photomed.* **28** 147

[239] Piredda P, Berning M, Boukamp P and Volkmer A 2015 Subcellular Raman microspectroscopy imaging of nucleic acids and tryptophan for distinction of normal human skin cells and tumorigenic keratinocytes *Anal. Chem.* **87** 6778–85

[240] Pudlas M, Koch S, Bolwien C, Thude S, Jenne N, Hirth T, Walles H and Schenke-Layland K 2011 Raman spectroscopy: a noninvasive analysis tool for the discrimination of human skin cells *Tissue Eng.* **17** 1027–40

[241] Pallaoro A, Braun G B and Moskovits M 2011 Quantitative ratiometric discrimination between noncancerous and cancerous prostate cells based on neuropilin-1 overexpression *Proc. Natl Acad. Sci. USA* **108** 16559–64

[242] O'Malley J, Kumar R, Kuzmin A, Pliss A, Yadav N, Balachandar S, Wang J, Attwood K, Prasad P N and Chandra D 2017 Lipid quantification by Raman microspectroscopy as a potential biomarker in prostate cancer *Cancer Lett.* **397** 52–60

[243] Corsetti S, Rabl T, McGloin D and Nabi G 2018 Raman spectroscopy for accurately characterizing biomolecularchanges in androgen-independent prostate cancer cells *J. Biophotonics* **11** e201700166

[244] Olmos V, Bedia C, Tauler R and Juan A D 2018 Preprocessing tools applied to improve the assessment of Aldrin effects on prostate cancer cells using Raman spectroscopy *Appl. Spectrosc.* **72** 489–500

[245] Ralbovsky N M, Egorov V, Moskovets E, Dey P, Dey B K and Lednev I K 2019 Deep ultraviolet Raman spectroscopy for cancer diagnostics: a feasibility study with cell lines and tissues *Cancer Stud. Mol. Med. Open J.* **5** 1–10

[246] Vargis E, Tang Y W, Khabele D and Mahadevan-Jansen A 2012 Near-infrared Raman microspectroscopy detects high-risk human papillomaviruses *Transl. Oncol.* **5** 172–9

[247] Rubina S, Amita M, Kedar K D, Bharat R and Krishna C M 2013 Raman spectroscopic study on classification of cervical cell specimens *Vib. Spectrosc.* **68** 115–21

[248] Bonnier F, Traynor D, Kearney P, Clarke C, Knief P, Martin C, O'Leary J J, Byrne H J and Lyng F 2014 Processing ThinPrep cervical cytological samples for Raman spectroscopic analysis *Anal. Methods* **6** 7831–41

[249] Byrne H J, Baranska M, Puppels G J, Stone N, Wood B, Gough K M, Lasch P, Heraud P, Sulé-Suso J and Sockalingum G D 2015 Spectropathology for the next generation: quo vadis? *Analyst* **140** 2066–73

[250] Ramos I R, Meade A D, Ibrahim O, Byrne H J, McMenamin M, McKenna M, Malkin A and Lyng F M 2016 Raman spectroscopy for cytopathology of exfoliated cervical cells *Faraday Discuss.* **187** 187–98

[251] Duraipandian S, Traynor D, Kearney P, Martin C, O'Leary J J and Lyng F M 2018 Raman spectroscopic detection of high-grade cervical cytology: using morphologically normal appearing cells *Sci. Rep.* **8** 15048
[252] Pichardo-Molina J, Frausto-Reyes C, Barbosa-García O, Huerta-Franco R, González-Trujillo J, Ramírez-Alvarado C, Gutiérrez-Juárez G and Medina-Gutiérrez C 2007 Raman spectroscopy and multivariate analysis of serum samples from breast cancer patients *Lasers Med. Sci.* **22** 229–36
[253] Bhattacharjee T, Khan A, Maru G, Ingle A and Krishna C M 2015 A preliminary Raman spectroscopic study of urine: diagnosis of breast cancer in animal models *Analyst* **140** 456–66
[254] Feng S, Huang S, Lin D, Chen G, Xu Y, Li Y, Huang Z, Pan J, Chen R and Zeng H 2015 Surface-enhanced Raman spectroscopy of saliva proteins for the noninvasive differentiation of benign and malignant breast tumors *Int. J. Nanomed.* **10** 537–47
[255] Moisoiu V *et al* 2019 Breast cancer diagnosis by surface-enhanced Raman scattering (SERS) of urine *Appl. Sci.* **9** 806
[256] Chithraa K, Arunaa P, Vijayaraghavan S, Prasad G N S and Ganesan S 2019 Monitoring of breast cancer patients under pre and post treated conditions using Raman spectroscopic analysis of blood plasma *Vib. Spectrosc.* **105** 102982
[257] Ştiufiuc G F *et al* 2020 Solid plasmonic substrates for breast cancer detection by means of SERS analysis of blood plasma *Nanomaterials* **10** 1212
[258] Li Y, Jia M, Zeng X, Huang K and Bai Z 2017 Pattern recognition methods combined with Raman spectra applied to distinguish serums from lung cancer patients and healthy people *J. Biosci. Med* **5** 95–105
[259] Wang H, Zhang S, Wan L, Sun H, Tan J and Su Q 2018 Screening and staging for non-small cell lung cancer by serum laser Raman spectroscopy *Spectrochim. Acta* A **201** 34–8
[260] Cao X, Wang Z, Bi L and Zheng J 2018 Label-free detection of human serum using surface-enhanced Raman spectroscopy based on highly branched gold nanoparticle substrates for discrimination of non-small cell lung cancer *J. Chem.* **2018** 1–13
[261] Grubisha D S, Lipert R J, Park H Y, Driskell J and Porter M D 2003 Femtomolar detection of prostate-specific antigen: an immunoassay based on surface-enhanced Raman scattering and immunogold labels *Anal. Chem.* **75** 5936–43
[262] Li S, Zhang Y, Xu J, Li L, Zeng Q, Lin L, Guo Z, Liu Z, Xiong H and Liu S 2014 Noninvasive prostate cancer screening based on serum surface-enhanced Raman spectroscopy and support vector machine *Appl. Phys. Lett.* **105** 091104
[263] Medipally D K R, Maguire A, Bryant J, Armstrong J, Dunne M, Lyng F M and Meade A D 2017 Development of a high throughput (HT) Raman spectroscopy method for rapid screening of liquid blood plasma from prostate cancer patients *Analyst* **142** 1216–26
[264] Wang J, Koo K M, Wee E J H, Wang Y and Trau M 2017 A nanoplasmonic label-free surface-enhanced Raman scattering strategy for non-invasive cancer genetic subtyping in patient samples *Nanoscale* **9** 3496–503
[265] Shao X G *et al* 2017 Evaluation of expressed prostatic secretion and serum using surface-enhanced Raman spectroscopy for the noninvasive detection of prostate cancer, a preliminary study *Nanomedicine* **13** 1051–9
[266] Mistro G D, Cervo S, Mansutti E, Spizzo R, Colombatti A, Belmonte P, Zucconelli R, Steffan A, Sergo V and Bonifacio A 2015 Surface-enhanced Raman spectroscopy of urine for prostate cancer detection: a preliminary study *Anal. Bioanal. Chem.* **407** 3271–5

[267] Feng S *et al* 2013 Blood plasma surface-enhanced Raman spectroscopy for non-invasive optical detection of cervical cancer *Analyst* **138** 3967–74

[268] González-Solís J L, Martínez-Espinosa J C, Torres-González L A, Aguilar- Lemarroy A, Jave-Suárez L F and Palomares-Anda P 2014 Cervical cancer detection based on serum sample Raman spectroscopy *Lasers Med. Sci.* **29** 979–85

[269] Pappu R, Prakasarao A, Dornadula K and Singaravelu G 2017 Raman spectroscopic characterization of urine of normal and cervical cancer subjects *Proc. SPIE* **10054** 1005404

[270] Bergholt M S, Zheng W, Lin K, Wang J, Xu H, Ren J L, Ho K Y, Teh M, Yeoh K G and Huang Z 2014 Characterizing variability of *in vivo* Raman spectroscopic properties of different anatomical sites of normal colorectal tissue towards cancer diagnosis at colonoscopy *Anal. Chem.* **87** 960–6

[271] Synytsya A, Judexova M, Hoskovec D, Miskovicova M and Petruzelka L 2014 Raman spectroscopy at different excitation wavelengths (1064, 785 and 532 nm) as a tool for diagnosis of colon cancer *J. Raman Spectrosc.* **45** 903–11

[272] Li S, Chen G, Zhang Y, Guo Z, Liu Z, Xu J, Li X and Lin L 2014 Identification and characterization of colorectal cancer using Raman spectroscopy and feature selection techniques *Opt. Express* **22** 25895–908

[273] Liu W, Sun Z, Chen J and Jing C 2016 Raman spectroscopy in colorectal cancer diagnostics: comparison of PCA-LDA and PLS-DA models *J. Spectrosc.* **2016** 1603609

[274] Lin D, Feng S Y, Pan J J, Chen Y P, Lin J Q, Chen G N, Xie S S, Zeng H S and Chen R 2011 Colorectal cancer detection by gold nanoparticle based surface-enhanced Raman spectroscopy of blood serum and statistical analysis *Opt. Express* **19** 13565–77

[275] Jenkins C A, Lewis P D, Dunstan P R and Harris D A 2016 Label-free serum ribonucleic acid analysis for colorectal cancer detection by surface-enhanced Raman spectroscopy and multivariate analysis *World J. Gastrointest. Oncol.* **8** 427–38

[276] Chen Y *et al* 2012 Label-free serum ribonucleic acid analysis for colorectal cancer detection by surface-enhanced Raman spectroscopy and multivariate analysis *J. Biomed. Opt.* **17** 67003

[277] Li X, Yang T, Li C S, Song Y, Lou H, Guan D and Jin L 2018 Surface enhanced Raman spectroscopy (SERS) for the multiplex detection of BRAF, KRAS, and PIK3CA mutations in plasma of colorectal cancer patients *Theranostics* **8** 1678–89

[278] Zheng Q, Kang W, Chen C, Shi X, Yang Y and Yu C 2019 Diagnosis accuracy of Raman spectroscopy in colorectal cancer: a PRISMA-compliant systematic review and meta-analysis *Medicine (Baltimore)* **98** e16940

[279] The American Cancer Society medical and editorial content team *Survival rate for ovarian cancer, by stage. Resource document. American Cancer Society* https://cancer.org/cancer/ovarian-cancer/detection-diagnosis-staging/survival-rates.html (accessed March 2018)

[280] Maheedhar K, Brat R A, Malini R, Prathima N, Keerthi P, Kushtago P and Krishna C M 2008 Diagnosis of ovarian cancer by Raman spectroscopy: a pilot study *Photomed. Laser Surg.* **26** 83–90

[281] Parker F S 1983 *Applications of Infrared, Raman, and Resonance Raman Spectroscopy in Biochemistry* (New York: Plenum)

[282] Tonge P and Carey P 1993 *Advances in Spectroscopy* vol 20 ed R J H Clark and R E Hester (Chichester: Wiley) pp 129–61

[283] Oseledchyk A, Andreou C, Wall M A and Kircher M F 2017 Folate-targeted surface-enhanced resonance Raman scattering nanoprobe ratiometry for detection of microscopic ovarian cancer *ACS Nano* **11** 1488–97

[284] Jenkins A L, Larsen R A and Williams T B 2005 Characterization of amino acids using Raman spectroscopy *Spectrochim. Acta* A **61** 1585–94

[285] Li J, Dowdy S, Tipton T, Podratz K, Lu W G, Xie X and Jiang S W 2014 HE4 as a biomarker for ovarian and endometrial cancer management *Expert Rev. Mol. Diagn.* **9** 555–66

[286] Zhao C, Annamalai L, Guo C, Kothandaraman N, Koh S, Zhang H, Biswas A and Choolani M 2007 Circulating haptoglobin is an independent prognostic factor in the sera of patients with epithelial ovarian cancer *Neoplasia* **9** 1–7

[287] Schorge J O, Drake R D, Lee H, Skates S J, Rajanbabu R, Miller D S, Kim J H, Cramer D W, Berkowitz R S and Mok S C 2004 Osteopontin as an adjunct to CA125 in detecting recurrent ovarian cancer *Clin. Cancer Res.* **10** 3474–8

[288] Hassan R, Remaley A T, Sampson M L, Zhang J, Cox D D, Pingpank J, Alexander R, Willingham M, Pastan I and Onda M 2006 Detection and quantitation of serum mesothelin, a tumor marker for patients with mesothelioma and ovarian cancer *Clin. Cancer Res.* **12** 447–53

[289] Moradi H, Ahmad A, Sheperdson D, Vuong N H, Niedbala G, Libni E, Vanderhyden B, Nyiri B and Murugkar S 2017 Raman micro-spectroscopy applied to treatment resistant and sensitive human ovarian cancer cells *J. Biophotonics* **10** 1327–34

[290] Beier B D and Berger A J 2009 Method for automated background subtraction from Raman spectra containing known contaminants *Analyst* **134** 1198–202

[291] De Gelder J, De Gussem K, Vandenabeele P and Moens L 2007 Reference database of Raman spectra of biological molecules *J. Raman Spectrosc.* **38** 1133–47

[292] Paraskevaidi M, Ashton K M, Stringfellow H F, Wood N J, Keating P J, Rowbottom A W, Martin-Hirsch P L and Martin F L 2018 Raman spectroscopic techniques to detect ovarian cancer biomarkers in blood plasma *Talanta* **189** 281–8

[293] Key statistics for pancreatic cancer https://cancer.org/cancer/pancreatic-cancer/about/key-statistics.html (accessed 27 April 2018)

[294] Pancreatic cancer survival rate https://cancer.org/cancer/pancreatic-cancer/detection-diagnosis-staging/survivalrates.html (accessed 27 April 2018)

[295] Schie I W, Kiselev R, Krafft C and Poppa J 2016 Rapid acquisition of mean Raman spectra of eukaryotic cells for a robust single cell classification *Analyst* **141** 6387–95

[297] Li J *et al* 2016 Abrogating cholesterol esterification suppresses growth and metastasis of pancreatic cancer *Oncogene* **35** 6378–88

[296] Pandya A K *et al* 2008 Evaluation of pancreatic cancer with Raman spectroscopy in a mouse model *Pancreas* **36** e1–8

[298] Harmsen S *et al* 2015 Surface-enhanced resonance Raman scattering nanostars for high-precision cancer imaging *Sci. Transl. Med.* **7** 271ra7

[299] Wang G, Lipert R J, Jain M, Kaur S, Chakraboty S, Torres M P, Batra S K, Brand R E and Porter M D 2011 Detection of the potential pancreatic cancer marker MUC4 in serum using surface-enhanced Raman scattering *Anal. Chem.* **83** 2554–61

[300] Banaei N, Foley A, Houghton J M, Sun Y and Byung Kim B 2017 Multiplex detection of pancreatic cancer biomarkers using a SERS-based immunoassay *Nanotechnology* **28** 455101

[301] Huang H *et al* 2013 Silver nanoparticle based surface enhanced Raman scattering spectroscopy of diabetic and normal rat pancreatic tissue under near-infrared laser excitation *Laser Phys. Lett.* **10** 045603

[302] Yan Z, Ma C, Mo J, Han W, Lv X, Chen C, Cheng C and Nieb X 2020 Rapid identification of benign and malignant pancreatic tumors using serum Raman spectroscopy combined with classification algorithms *Optik* **208** 164473
[303] Grimbergen M C M, van Swol C F P, Draga R O P, van Diest P, Verdaasdonk R M, Stone N and Bosch J H L R 2009 Bladder cancer diagnosis during cystoscopy using Raman spectroscopy *Proc. SPIE* **7161** 716114
[304] Cordero E, Rüger J, Marti D, Mondol A S, Hasselager T, Mogensen K, Hermann G G, Popp J and Schie I W 2020 Bladder tissue characterization using probe-based Raman spectroscopy: evaluation of tissue heterogeneity and influence on the model prediction *J. Biophotonics* **13** e201960025
[305] Draga R O P, Grimbergen M C M, Vijverberg P L M, van Swol C F P, Jonges T G N, Kummer J A, Ruud and Bosch J L H 2010 In vivo bladder cancer diagnosis by high-volume Raman spectroscopy *Anal. Chem.* **82** 5993–9
[306] Grimbergen M C M, van Swol C F P, van Moorselaar R J A, Uff J, Mahadevan-Jansen A and Stone N 2009 Raman spectroscopy of bladder tissue in the presence of 5-aminolevulinic acid *J. Photochem. Photobiol.* B **95** 170–6
[307] Cicchi R, Cosci A, Rossari S, Kapsokalyvas D, Baria E, Maio V, Massi D, De Giorgi V, Pimpinelli N and Pavone F S 2014 Combined fluorescence-Raman spectroscopic setup for the diagnosis of melanocytic lesions *J. Biophotonics* **7** 86–95
[308] Koljenovic S, Schut T C B, Wolthuis R, de Jong B, Santos L, Caspers P J, Kros J M and Puppels G J 2005 Tissue characterization using high wave number Raman spectroscopy *J. Biomed. Opt.* **10** 031116
[309] Kerr L T, Lynn T M, Cullen I M, Daly P J, Shah N, O'Dea S, Malkin A and Hennelly B M 2016 Methodologies for bladder cancer detection with Raman based urine cytology *Anal. Methods* **8** 4991–5000
[310] Krishna H, Majumder S K, Chaturvedi P, Sidramesh M and Gupta P K 2014 In vivo Raman spectroscopy for detection of oral neoplasia: a pilot clinical study *J. Biophotonics* **7** 690–702
[311] Guze K, Pawluk H C, Short M, Zeng H, Lorch J, Norris C and Sonis S 2015 Pilot study: Raman spectroscopy in differentiating premalignant and malignant oral lesions from normal mucosa and benign lesions in humans *Head Neck* **37** 511–7
[312] World Health Organization Cardiovascular diseases (CVDs) https://who.int/news-room/fact-sheets/detail/cardiovascular-diseases-(cvds)#:~:text=Cardiovascular%20diseases%20(CVDs)%20are%20the,%2D%20and%20middle%2Dincome%20countries (accessed 11 June 2021)
[313] Moreno P R, Marshik B and Muller J E 2006 *The Vulnerable Atherosclerotic Plaque: Strategies for Diagnosis and Management* ed R Virmani, J Narula, M B Leon and J T Willerson (Oxford: Blackwell Publishing) pp 257–62
[314] Naghavi M *et al* 2003 From vulnerable plaque to vulnerable patient: a call for new definitions and risk assessment strategies: part II *Circulation* **108** 1772–8
[315] El-Said W A, Fouad D M and El-Safty S A 2016 Ultrasensitive label-free detection of cardiac biomarker myoglobin based on surface-enhanced Raman spectroscopy *Sensors Actuators* B **228** 401–9
[316] Buschman H P J, Marple E T, Wach M L, Bennett B, Bakker Schut T C, Bruining H A, Bruschke A V, van der Laarse A and Puppels G J 2000 In vivo determination of the molecular composition of artery wall by intravascular Raman spectroscopy *Anal. Chem.* **72** 3771–5

[317] Motz J T, Fitzmaurice M, Miller A, Gandhi S J, Haka A S, Galindo L, Dasari R R, Kramer J R Jr and Feld M S 2006 In vivo Raman spectral pathology of human atherosclerosis and vulnerable plaque *J. Biomed. Opt.* **11** 021003

[318] Sc´epanovic´ O R 2006 Detection of morphological markers of vulnerable atherosclerotic plaque using multimodal spectroscopy *J. Biomed. Opt.* **11** 021007

[319] Matthäus C, Dochow S, Bergner G, Lattermann A, Romeike B F M, Marple E T, Krafft C, Dietzek B, Brehm B R and Popp J 2012 In vivo characterization of atherosclerotic plaque depositions by Raman-probe spectroscopy and *in vitro* coherent anti-Stokes Raman scattering microscopic imaging on a rabbit model *Anal. Chem.* **84** 7845–51

[320] Matthäus C, Dochow S, Egodage K D, Romeike B F, Brehm B R and Popp J 2018 Detection and characterization of early plaque formations by Raman probe spectroscopy and optical coherence tomography: an *in vivo* study on a rabbit model *J. Biomed. Opt.* **23** 015004

[321] Dochow S, Fatakdawala H, Phipps J E, Ma D, Bocklitz T, Schmitt M, Bishop J W, Margulies K B, Marcu L and Popp J 2016 Comparing Raman and fluorescence lifetime spectroscopy from human atherosclerotic lesions using a bimodal probe *J. Biophotonics* **9** 958–66

[322] Huang X, Irmak S, Lu Y, Pipinos I, Casale G and Subbiah J 2015 Spontaneous and coherent anti-Stokes Raman spectroscopy of human gastrocnemius muscle biopsies in CH-stretching region for discrimination of peripheral artery disease *Biomed. Opt. Express* **6** 2766–77

[323] Salenius J P, Brennan J F, Miller A, Wang Y, Aretz T, Sacks B, Dasari R R and Feld M S 1989 Biochemical composition of human peripheral arteries examined with nearinfrared Raman spectroscopy *J. Vasc. Surg.* **27** 710–9

[324] Cluff K, Kelly A M, Koutakis P, He X N, Huang X, Lu Y F, Pipinos I I, Casale G P and Subbiah J 2014 Surface-enhanced Raman spectral biomarkers correlate with Ankle Brachial Index and characterize leg muscle biochemical composition of patients with peripheral arterial disease *Physiol. Rep.* **2** e12148

[325] Bonetti A, Bonifacio A, Della Mora A, Livi U, Marchini M and Ortolani F 2015 Carotenoids co-localize with hydroxyapatite, cholesterol, and other lipids in calcified stenotic aortic valves. Ex vivo Raman maps compared to histological patterns *Eur. J. Histochem.* **59** 2505

[326] Pilarczyk M, Czamara K, Baranska M, Natorska J, Kapusta P, Undas A and Kaczor A 2013 Calcification of aortic human valves studied *in situ* by Raman microimaging: following mineralization from small grains to big deposits *J. Raman Spectrosc.* **44** 1222–9

[327] You A Y, Bergholt M S, St-Pierre J P, Kit-Anan W, Pence I J, Chester A H, Yacoub M H, Bertazzo S and Stevens M M 2017 Raman spectroscopy imaging reveals interplay between atherosclerosis and medial calcification in the human aorta *Sci. Adv.* **3** e1701156

[328] Brazhe N A, Treiman M, Faricelli B, Vestergaard J H and Sosnovtseva O 2013 In situ Raman study of redox state changes of mitochondrial cytochromes in a perfused rat heart *PLoS One* **8** e70488

[329] Almohammedi A, Kapetanaki S, Wood B, Raven E L, Storey N and Hudson A J 2015 Spectroscopic analysis of myoglobin and cytochrome c dynamics in isolated cardiomyocytes during hypoxia and reoxygenation *J. R. Soc. Interface* **12** 20141339

[330] Pascut F C, Kalra S, George V, Welch N, Denning C and Notingher I 2013 Non-invasive label-free monitoring the cardiac differentiation of human embryonic stem cells in-vitro by Raman spectroscopy *Biochim. Biophys. Acta* **1830** 3517–24

[331] Brazhe N A, Treiman M, Brazhe A R, Maksimov G V and Sosnovtseva O V 2012 Mapping of redox state of mitochondrial cytochromes in live cardiomyocytes using Raman microspectroscopy *PLoS One* **7** e41990

[332] Ohira S, Tanaka H, Harada Y, Minamikawa T, Kumamoto Y, Matoba S, Yaku H and Takamatsu T 2017 Label-free detection of myocardial ischaemia in the perfused rat heart by spontaneous Raman spectroscopy *Sci. Rep.* **7** 42401

[333] Yamamoto T, Minamikawa T, Harada Y, Yamaoka Y, Tanaka H, Yaku H and Takamatsu T 2018 Label-free evaluation of myocardial infarct in surgically excised ventricular myocardium by Raman spectroscopy *Sci. Rep.* **8** 14671

[334] Nishiki-Muranishi N, Harada Y, Minamikawa T, Yamaoka Y, Dai P, Yaku H and Takamatsu T 2014 Label-free evaluation of myocardial infarction and its repair by spontaneous Raman spectroscopy *Anal. Chem.* **86** 6903–10

[335] Ogawa M, Harada Y, Yamaoka Y, Fujita K, Yaku H and Takamatsu T 2009 Label-free biochemical imaging of heart tissue with high-speed spontaneous Raman microscopy *Biochem. Biophys. Res. Commun.* **382** 370–4

[336] MacRitchie N, Grassia G, Noonan J, Garside P, Graham D and Maffia P 2018 Molecular imaging of atherosclerosis: spotlight on Raman spectroscopy and surface-enhanced Raman scattering *Heart* **104** 460–7

[337] Cockerill I, Oliver J, Huaxi X, Fu B M and Zhu D 2018 Blood–brain barrier integrity and clearance of amyloid-β from the BBB *Adv. Exp. Med. Biol* **1097** 261–78

[338] Koronyo Y, Salumbides B C, Black K L and Koronyo-Hamaoui M 2012 Alzheimer's disease in the retina: imaging retinal AβAβ plaques for early diagnosis and therapy assessment *Neurodegener Dis* **10** 285–93

[339] Moncaster J A *et al* 2010 Alzheimer's disease amyloid-ββ links lens and brain pathology in down syndrome *PLoS One* **5** e10659

[340] Carmona P, Molina M, Calero M, Bermejo-Pareja F, Martínez-Martín P and Toledano A 2013 Discrimination analysis of blood plasma associated with Alzheimer's disease using vibrational spectroscopy *J. Alzheimers Dis.* **34** 911–20

[341] Ryzhikova E, Kazakov O, Halámková L, Celmins D, Malone P, Molho E, Zimmerman E A and Lednev I K 2015 Raman spectroscopy of blood serum for Alzheimer's disease diagnostics: specificity relative to other types of dementia *J. Biophotonics* **8** 584–96

[342] Paraskevaidi M, Morais C L M, Halliwell D E, Mann D M A, Allsop D, Martin-Hirsch P L and Martin F L 2018 Raman spectroscopy to diagnose Alzheimer's disease and dementia with Lewy bodies in blood *ACS Chem. Neurosci.* **9** 2786–94

[343] Ryzhikova E, Ralbovsky N M, Halámková L, Celmins D, Malone P, Molho E, Quinn J, Zimmerman E A and Lednev I K 2019 Multivariate statistical analysis of surface enhanced Raman spectra of human serum for Alzheimer's disease diagnosis *Appl. Sci.* **9** 3256

[344] Ralbovsky N M, Halámková L, Wall K, Anderson-Hanley C and Lednev I K 2019 Screening for Alzheimer's disease using saliva: a new approach based on machine learning and Raman hyperspectroscopy *J. Alzheimer Dis* **71** 1351–9

[345] Cennamo G *et al* 2020 Surface-enhanced Raman spectroscopy of tears: toward a diagnostic tool for neurodegenerative disease identification *J. Biomed. Opt.* **25** 087002

[346] Miura T, Suzuki K and Takeuchi H 2001 Binding of iron(III) to the single tyrosine residue of amyloid β-peptide probed by Raman spectroscopy *J. Mol. Struct.* **598** 79–84

[347] Maiti N C, Apetri M M, Zagorski M G, Carey P R and Anderson V E 2004 Raman spectroscopic characterization of secondary structure in natively unfolded proteins: alphasynuclein *J. Am. Chem. Soc.* **126** 2399–408

[348] Schipper H M, Kwok C S, Rosendahl S M, Bandilla D, Maes O, Melmed C, Rabinovitch D and Burns D H 2008 Spectroscopy of human plasma for diagnosis of idiopathic Parkinson's disease *Biomark. Med.* **2** 229–38

[349] Palanisamy S, Yan L, Zhang X and He T 2015 Surface enhanced Raman scattering active worm-like Ag clusters for sensitive and selective detection of dopamine *Anal. Methods* **7** 3438–47

[350] Ranc V, Markova Z, Hajduch M, Prucek R, Kvitek L, Kaslik J, Safarova K and Zboril R 2014 Magnetically assisted surface-enhanced Raman scattering selective determination of dopamine in an artificial cerebrospinal fluid and a mouse striatum using Fe_3O_4/Ag nanocomposite *Anal. Chem.* **86** 2939–46

[351] Lim J W and Kang I J 2013 Chitosan gold nano composite for dopamine analysis using Raman scattering *Bull. Korean Chem. Soc.* **34** 237–42

[352] Lim J W and Kang I J 2014 Fabrication of chitosan-gold nanocomposites combined with optical fiber as SERS substrates to detect dopamine molecules *Bull. Korean Chem. Soc.* **35** 25–9

[353] An J H, El-Said W A, Yea C H, Kim T H and Choi J W 2011 Surface-enhanced Raman scattering of dopamine on self-assembled gold nanoparticles *J. Nanosci. Nanotechnol.* **11** 4424–9

[354] Tsikritsis D, Elfick A and Downes A 2016 Raman spectroscopy of fibroblast cells from a Huntington's disease patient *Spectrosc. Lett.* **49** 535–41

[355] Huefner A, Kuan W L, Mason S L, Mahajan S and Barker R A 2020 Serum Raman spectroscopy as a diagnostic tool in patients with Huntington's disease *Chem. Sci.* **11** 525–33

[356] Muratore M 2013 Raman spectroscopy and partial least squares analysis in discrimination of peripheral cells affected by Huntington's disease *Anal. Chim. Acta* **793** 1–10

[357] Manno D, Filippo E, Fiore R, Serra A, Urso E, Rizzello A and Maffia M 2010 Monitoring prion protein expression in complex biological samples by SERS for diagnostic applications *Nanotechnology* **21** 165502

[358] Serra A, Manno D, Filippo E, Buccolieri A, Urso E, Rizzello A and Maffia M 2011 SERS based optical sensor to detect prion protein in neurodegenerate living cells *Sensors Actuators* B **156** 479–85

[359] Croes E A *et al* 2004 Octapeptide repeat insertions in the prion protein gene and early onset dementia *J. Neurol. Neurosurg. Psychiatry* **75** 1166–70

[360] Stevens D J, Walter E D, Rodriguez A, Draper D, Davies P, Brown D R and Millhauser G L 2009 Early onset prion disease from octa repeat expansion correlates with copper binding properties *PLoS Pathog.* **5** e1000390

[361] Carmona P, Monleon E, Monzon M, Badiola J J and Monreal J 2004 Raman analysis of priori protein in blood cell membranes from naturally affected scrapie sheep *Chem. Biol* **11** 759–64

[362] McQueenie R, Stevenson R, Benson R, MacRitchie N, McInnes I, Maffia P, Faulds K, Graham D, Brewer J and Garside P 2012 Detection of inflammation *in vivo* by surface enhanced Raman scattering provides higher sensitivity than conventional fluorescence imaging *Anal. Chem.* **84** 5968–75

[363] Sahu A, Dalal K, Naglot S, Aggarwal P and Krishna C M 2013 Serum based diagnosis of asthma using Raman spectroscopy: an early phase pilot study *PLoS One* **8** e78921

[364] Nawaz H *et al* 2017 Prediction of viral loads for diagnosis of hepatitis C infection in human plasma samples using Raman spectroscopy coupled with partial least squares regression analysis *J. Raman Spectrosc.* **48** 697–704

[365] Bi X, Walsh A, Mahadevan-Jansen A and Herline A 2011 Development of spectral markers for the discrimination of ulcerative colitis and Crohn's disease using Raman spectroscopy *Dis. Colon Rectum* **54** 48–53

[366] Pence I J, Nguyen Q T, Bi X, Herline A J, Beaulieu D M, Horst S N, Schwartz D A and Mahadevan-Jansen A 2014 Endoscopy-coupled Raman spectroscopy for *in vivo* discrimination of inflammatory bowel disease *Proc. SPIE* **8939** 89390R

[367] Krishnapuram B, Carin L, Figueiredo M A T and Hartemink A J 2005 Sparse multinomial logistic regression: fast algorithms and generalization bounds *IEEE Trans. Pattern Anal. Mach. Intell.* **27** 957–68

[368] Pence I J, Beaulieu D B, Horst S N, Bi X, Herline A J, Schwartz D A and Mahadevan-Jansen A 2017 Clinical characterization of *in vivo* inflammatory bowel disease with Raman spectroscopy *Biomed. Opt. Express* **8** 524–35

[369] Kerns J G *et al* 2014 Evidence from Raman spectroscopy of a putative link between inherent bone matrix chemistry and degenerative joint disease *Arthritis Rheumatol.* **66** 1237–46

[370] Morris M D and Mandair G S 2011 Raman assessment of bone quality *Clin. Orthop. Relat. Res.* **469** 2160–9

[371] Carden A and Morris M D 2000 Application of vibrational spectroscopy to the study of mineralized tissues (review) *J. Biomed. Opt.* **5** 259–68

[372] Draper E R C, Morris M D, Camacho N P, Matousek P, Towrie M, Parker A W and Goodship A E 2005 Novel assessment of bone using time-resolved transcutaneous Raman spectroscopy *J. Bone Miner. Res.* **20** 1968–72

[373] McCreadie B R, Morris M D, Chen T, Rao D S, Finney W F, Widjaja E and Goldstein S A 2006 Bone tissue compositional differences in women with and without osteoporotic fracture *Bone* **39** 1190–5

[374] Schulmerich M V, Finney W F, Popescu V, Morris M D, Vanasse T M and Goldstein S A 2006 Transcutaneous fiber optic Raman spectroscopy of bone using annular illumination and a circular array of collection fibers *J. Biomed. Opt.* **11** 060502

[375] Mandair G S, Esmonde-White F W L, Akhter M P, Swift A M, Kreider J, Goldstein S A, Recker R R and Morris M D 2010 Potential of Raman spectroscopy for evaluation of bone quality in osteoporosis patients: results of a prospective study *Proc. SPIE* **7548** 754846

[376] Okagbare P I, Esmonde-White F W L, Goldstein S A and Morris M D 2010 Development of non-invasive Raman spectroscopy for *in vivo* evaluation of bone graft osseointegration in a rat model *Analyst* **135** 3142–6

[377] Esmonde-White F W L and Morris M D 2013 Validating *in vivo* Raman spectroscopy of bone in human subjects *Proc. SPIE* **8565** 85656K–1

[378] Gikas P D, Birch H L, Vinton J, Keen R, Parker A W, Matousek P and Goodship A E 2014 Measurement of abnormal bone composition *in vivo* using noninvasive Raman spectroscopy *IBMS BoneKEy* **11** 1–3

[379] Buckley K, Kerns J G, Vinton J, Gikas P D, Smith C, Parker A W, Matousek P and Goodship A E 2015 Towards the *in vivo* prediction of fragility fractures with Raman spectroscopy *J. Raman Spectrosc.* **46** 610–8

[380] Sowoidnich K, Churchwell J, Buckley K, Goodship A E, Parker A W and Matousek P 2016 Photon migration of Raman signal in bone as measured with spatially offset Raman spectroscopy *J. Raman Spectrosc.* **47** 240–7

[381] Feng G, Ochoa M, Maher J R, Awad H A and Berger A J 2017 Sensitivity of spatially offset Raman spectroscopy (SORS) to subcortical bone tissue *J. Biophotonics* **10** 990–6

[382] Liao Z, Sinjab F, Gibson G, Padgett M and Notingher I 2016 DMD-based software-configurable spatially-offset Raman spectroscopy for spectral depth-profiling of optically turbid samples *Opt. Express* **24** 12701–12

[383] Liao Z, Sinjab F, Nommeots-Nomm A, Jones J, Ruiz-Cantu L, Yang J, Rose F and Notingher I 2017 Feasibility of spatially offset Raman spectroscopy for *in vitro* and *in vivo* monitoring mineralization of bone tissue engineering scaffolds *Anal. Chem.* **89** 847–53

[384] World Health Organization Malaria https://who.int/malaria/publications/world-malaria-report-2017/en/ (accessed 5 November 2018)

[385] Weissbuch I and Leiserowitz L 2008 Interplay between malaria, crystalline hemozoin formation, and antimalarial drug action and design *Chem. Rev.* **108** 4899–914

[386] Crawley J, Chu C, Mtove G and Nosten F 2010 Malaria in children *Lancet* **375** 1468–81

[387] Froch T, Koncarevic S, Zedler L, Schmitt M, Schenzel K, Becker K and Popp J 2007 In situ localization and structural analysis of the malaria pigment hemozoin *J. Phys. Chem.* **B 111** 11047–56

[388] Wood B R, Hermelink A, Lasch P, Bambery K R, Webster G T, Khiavi M A, Cooke B M, Deed S, Naumann D and McNaughton D 2009 Resonance Raman microscopy in combination with partial dark-field microscoy lights up a new path in malaria diagnostics *Analyst* **134** 1119–25

[389] Wood B R *et al* 2011 Tip-enhanced Raman scattering (TERS) from hemozoin crystals within a sectioned erythrocyte *Nano Lett.* **11** 1868–73

[390] Newman D M, Heptinstall J, Matelon R J, Savage L, Wears M L, Beddow J, Cox M, Schallig H D F H and Mens P F 2008 A magneto-optic route toward the *in vivo* diagnosis of malaria: preliminary results and preclinical trial data *Biophys. J.* **95** 994–1000

[391] Kim C C, Wilson E B and DeRisi J L 2010 Improved methods for magnetic purification of malaria parasites and haemozoin *Malar. J.* **9** 17–21

[392] Kim J, Oh J and Choi B 2010 Magnetomotive laser speckle imaging *J. Biomed. Opt.* **15** 011110

[393] Gao J, Gu H and Xu B 2009 Multifunctional magnetic nanoparticles: design synthesis, and biomedical applications *Acc. Chem. Res.* **42** 1097–107

[394] Yuen C and Liu Q 2012 Magnetic field enriched surface enhanced resonance Raman spectroscopy for early malaria diagnosis *J. Biomed. Opt.* **17** 017005

[395] Wang W, Dong R L, Gu D, He J A, Yi P, Kong S K, Ho H P, Loo J F C, Wang W and Wang Q 2020 Antibody-free rapid diagnosis of malaria in whole blood with surface-enhanced Raman spectroscopy using nanostructured gold substrate *Adv. Med. Sci.* **65** 86–92

[396] Buijtels P C, Willemse-Erix H, Petit P, Endtz H P, Puppels G J, Verbrugh H A, van Belkum A, van Soolingen D and Maquelin K 2008 Rapid identification of mycobacteria by Raman spectroscopy *J. Clin. Microbiol.* **46** 961–5

[397] Rebrošová K, Šiler M, Samek O, Ruzicka F, Bernatova S, Hola V, Ježek J, Zemánek J, Sokolová J and Petráš P 2017 Rapid identification of staphylococci by Raman spectroscopy *Sci. Rep.* **7** 14846

[398] Große C, Bergner N, Dellith J, Heller R, Bauer M, Mellmann A, Popp J and Neugebauer U 2015 Label-free imaging and spectroscopic analysis of intracellular bacterial infections *Anal. Chem.* **87** 2137–42
[399] Ho C S, Jean N, Hogan C A, Blackmon L, Jeffrey S S, Holodniy M, Banaei N, Saleh A A E, Ermon S and Dionne J 2019 Rapid identification of pathogenic bacteria using Raman spectroscopy and deep learning *Nat. Commun.* **10** 4927
[400] Maquelin K, Choo-Smith L P, Endtz H P, Bruining H and Puppels G 2002 Rapid identification of *Candida* species by confocal Raman microspectroscopy *J. Clin. Microbiol.* **40** 594–600
[401] Harz M, Kiehntopf M, Stöckel S, Rösch P, Straube E, Deufel T and Popp J 2009 Direct analysis of clinical relevant single bacterial cells from cerebrospinal fluid during bacterial meningitis by means of micro-Raman spectroscopy *J. Biophotonics* **2** 70–80
[402] Kumar S, Gopinathan R, Kumar Chandra G, Umapathy S and Kumar Saini D Rapid detection of bacterial infection and viability assessment with high specificity and sensitivity using Raman micro-spectroscopy *Anal. Bioanal. Chem.* **412** 2505–16
[403] Gracie K, Correa E, Mabbott S, Dougan J A, Graham D, Goodacre R and Faulds K 2014 Simultaneous detection and quantification of three bacterial meningitis pathogens by SERS *Chem. Sci.* **5** 1030–40
[404] Sivanesan A, Witkowska E, Adamkiewicz W, Dziewit L, Kaminska A and Waluk J 2014 Nanostructured silver–gold bimetallic SERS substrates for selective identification of bacteria in human blood *Analyst* **139** 1037–43
[405] Kaminska A, Witkowska E, Kowalska A, Skoczynska A, Ronkiewicz P, Szymborski T and Waluk J 2016 Rapid detection and identification of bacterial meningitis pathogens in *ex vivo* clinical samples by SERS method and principal component analysis *Anal. Methods* **8** 4521–9
[406] Yang D T, Zhou H B, Haisch C, Niessner R and Ying Y B 2016 Reproducible *E. coli* detection based on label-free SERS and mapping *Talanta* **146** 457–63
[407] Zhou H B, Yang D T, Mircescu N, Ivleva N P, Schwarzmeier K, Wieser A, Schubert S, Niessner R and Haisch C 2015 Surface-enhanced Raman scattering detection of bacteria on microarrays at single cell levels using silver nanoparticles *Microchim. Acta* **182** 2259–66
[408] Zhou H B, Yang D T, Ivleva N P, Mircescu N E, Niessner R and Haisch C 2014 SERS detection of bacteria in water by *in situ* coating with Ag nanoparticles *Anal. Chem.* **86** 1525–33
[409] Dina N E, Zhou H, Colnita A, Leopold N, Szoke-Nagy T, Coman C and Haisch C 2017 Rapid single-cell detection and identification of pathogens by using surface-enhanced Raman spectroscopy *Analyst* **142** 1782–9
[410] Mühlig A *et al* 2016 LOC-SERS: a promising closed system for the identification of mycobacteria *Anal. Chem.* **88** 7998–8004
[411] Tong D, Chen C, Zhang J J, Lv G D, Zheng X, Zhang Z and Lv X 2019 Application of Raman spectroscopy in the detection of hepatitis B virus infection *Photodiagn. Photodyn. Ther.* **28** 248–52
[412] Shanmukh S, Jones L, Driskell J, Zhao Y, Dluhy R and Tripp R A 2006 Rapid and sensitive detection of respiratory virus molecular signatures using a silver nanorod array SERS substrate *Nano Lett.* **6** 2630–6
[413] Yeh Y T *et al* 2020 A rapid and label-free platform for virus capture and identification from clinical samples *Proc. Natl Acad. Sci. USA* **117** 895–901

[414] Park H J, Yang S C and Choo J 2016 Early diagnosis of influenza virus a, using surface-enhanced Raman scattering-based lateral flow assay *Bull. Korean Chem. Soc.* **37** 2019–24

[415] Witkowska E *et al* 2017 Surface-enhanced Raman spectroscopy introduced into the International Standard Organization (ISO) regulations as an alternative method for detection and identification of pathogens in the food industry *Anal. Bioanal. Chem.* **409** 1555–67

[416] Langer J *et al* 2020 Present and future of surface-enhanced Raman scattering *ACS Nano* **14** 28–117

[417] Wang P, Wang X, Sun Y, Gong G, Fan M and He L 2020 Rapid identification and quantification of the antibiotic susceptibility of lactic acid bacteria using surface enhanced Raman spectroscopy *Anal. Methods* **12** 376

[418] Akanny E, Bonhommé A, Commun C, Doleans-Jordheim A, Farre C, Bessueille F, Bourgeois S and Bordes C 2020 Surface-enhanced Raman spectroscopy using uncoated gold nanoparticles for bacteria discrimination *J. Raman Spectrosc.* **51** 619–29

[419] Prakash O, Sil S, Verma T and Umapathy S 2020 Direct detection of bacteria using positively charged Ag/Au bimetallic nanoparticles: a label-free surface-enhanced Raman scattering study coupled with multivariate analysis *J. Phys. Chem.* C **124** 861–9

[420] Sohail A, Khan S, Ullah R, Qureshi S A, Bilal M and Khan A 2018 Analysis of hepatitis C infection using Raman spectroscopy and proximity based classification in the transformed domain *Biomed. Opt. Express* **9** 2041–55

[421] Shanmukh S, Jones L, Zhao Y P, Driskell J D, Tripp R A and Dluhy R A 2008 Identification and classification of respiratory syncytial virus (RSV) strains by surface-enhanced Raman spectroscopy and multivariate statistical techniques *Anal. Bioanal. Chem.* **390** 1551–5

[422] Lim J Y, Nam J S, Shin H, Park J, Song H I, Kang M, Lim K I and Choi Y 2019 Identification of newly emerging influenza viruses by detecting the virally infected cells based on surface enhanced Raman spectroscopy and principal component analysis *Anal. Chem.* **91** 5677–84

[423] Moor K, Terada Y, Taketani A, Matsuyoshi H, Ohtani K and Sato H 2018 Early detection of virus infection in live human cells using Raman spectroscopy *J. Biomed. Opt.* **23** 1–7

[424] Ambartsumyan O, Gribanyov D, Kukushkin V, Kopylov A and Zavyalova E 2020 SERS-based biosensors for virus determination with oligonucleotides as recognition elements *Int. J. Mol. Sci.* **21** 3373

[425] Negri P, Chen G, Kage A, Nitsche A, Naumann D, Xu B and Dluhy R A 2012 Direct optical detection of viral nucleoprotein binding to an anti-influenza aptamer *Anal. Chem.* **84** 5501–8

[426] Negri P, Kage A, Nitsche A, Naumann D and Dluhy R A 2011 Detection of viral nucleoprotein binding to anti-influenza aptamers via SERS *Chem. Commun.* **47** 8635–7

[427] Kukushkin V I, Ivanov N M, Novoseltseva A A, Gambaryan A S, Yaminsky I V, Kopylov A M and Zavyalova E G 2019 Highly sensitive detection of influenza virus with SERS aptasensor *PLoS One* **14** e0216247

[428] Kang T, Yoo S M, Yoon I, Lee S Y and Kim B 2010 Patterned multiplex pathogen DNA detection by Au particle-on-wire SERS sensor *Nano Lett.* **10** 1189–93

[429] Tadesse L F, Safir F, Ho C S, Hasbach X, Khuri-Yakub B, Jeffrey S S, Saleh A A E and Dionne J 2020 Toward rapid infectious disease diagnosis with advances in surface-enhanced Raman spectroscopy *J. Chem. Phys.* **152** 240902

[430] Olschewski K, Kammer E, Stockel S, Bocklitz T, Deckert-Gaudig T, Zell R, Cialla-May D, Weber K, Deckert V and Popp J 2015 A manual and an automatic TERS based virus discrimination *Nanoscale* **7** 4545–52

[431] Li L, Yang H J, Liu D C, He H B, Wang C F, Zhong J F, Gao Y D and Zeng Y J 2012 Analysis of biofilms formation and associated genes detection in *Staphylococcus* isolates from bovine mastitis *Int. J. Appl. Res. Vet. Med.* **10** 62–8

[432] Xie S and Zhou J 2017 Harnessing plant biodiversity for the discovery of novel anticancer drugs targeting microtubules *Front. Plant Sci.* **8** 720

[433] Zhou L, Zhou J, Feng Z, Wang F Y, Xie S S and Bu S Z 2016 Immunoassay for tumor markers in human serum based on Si nanoparticles and SiC@Ag SERS-active substrate *Analyst* **141** 2534–41

[434] Zhang Z, Wang Q, Han L, Du S, Yu H and Zhang H 2018 Rapid and sensitive detection of *Salmonella typhimurium* based on the photothermal effect of magnetic nanomaterials *Sens. Actuators* B **268** 188–94

[435] Black D M, Robles G, Lopez P, Bach S B H, Alvarez M and Whetten R L 2018 Liquid chromatography separation and mass spectrometry detection of silver-lipoate $Ag_{29}(LA)_{12}$ nanoclusters: evidence of isomerism in the solution phase *Anal. Chem.* **90** 2010–7

[436] Sun Z, Lv J, Liu X, Tang Z, Wang X, Xu Y and Hammock B D 2018 Development of a nanobody-AviTag fusion protein and its application in a streptavidin–biotin-amplified enzyme-linked immunosorbent assay for ochratoxin A in cereal *Anal. Chem.* **90** 10628–34

[437] Deng Y Q, Feng Z T, Yuan F, Guo J R, Suo S S and Wang B S 2015 Identification and functional analysis of the autofluorescent substance in limonium bicolor salt glands *Plant Physiol. Biochem.* **97** 20–7

[438] Yuan F, Chen M, Leng B Y and Wang B S 2013 An efficient auto-fluorescence method for screening limonium bicolor mutants for abnormal salt gland density and salt secretion *S. Afr. J. Bot.* **88** 110–7

[439] Guo F D, Liu C L, Xia H, Bi Y P, Zhao C Z, Zhao S Z, Hou L, Li F G and Wang X J 2013 Induced expression of *AtLEC1* and *AtLEC2* differentially promotes somatic embryogenesis in transgenic tobacco plants *PLoS One* **8** e71714

[440] Li X Z, Yang T Y, Li C S, Jin L L, Lou H and Song Y T 2018 Prenatal detection of thalassemia by cell-free fetal DNA (cffDNA) in maternal plasma using surface enhanced Raman spectroscopy combined with PCR *Biomed. Opt. Express* **9** 3167–76

[441] Carey P R 1985 *Modern Physical Methods in Biochemistry* vol 11 ed A Neuberger and L L M van Deenen (New York: Academic) pp 27–64

[442] Czamara K, Majzner K, Pacia M Z, Kochan K, Kaczor A and Baranska M 2015 Raman spectroscopy of lipids: a review *J. Raman Spectrosc.* **46** 4–20

[443] Nieva C, Marro M, Santana-Codina N, Rao S, Petrov D and Sierr A 2012 The lipid phenotype of breast cancer cells characterized by Raman microspectroscopy: towards a stratification of malignancy *PLoS One* **7** e46456

[444] Singh S P and Krishna C M 2014 Raman spectroscopic studies of oral cancers: correlation of spectral and biochemical markers *Anal. Methods* **6** 8613–20

[445] Munchberg U, Wagner L, Rohrer C, Voigt K, Rosch P, Jahreis G and Popp J 2015 Quantitative assessment of the degree of lipid unsaturation in intact *Mortierella* by Raman microspectroscopy *Anal. Bioanal. Chem.* **407** 3303–11

[446] Münchberg U, Wagner L, Spielberg E T, Voigt K, Rösch P and Popp J 2013 Spatially resolved investigation of the oil composition in single intact hyphae of *Mortierella* spp. with micro-Raman spectroscopy *BBA Mol. Cell Biol. Lipids* **1831** 341–9

[447] Brazhe N A, Nikelshparg E I, Prats C, Dela F and Sosnovtseva O 2017 Raman probing of lipids, proteins, and mitochondria in skeletal myocytes: a case study on obesity *J. Raman Spectrosc.* **48** 1158–65

[448] Wu H, Volponi J V, Oliver A E, Parikh A N, Simmons B A and Singh S 2011 In vivo lipidomics using single-cell Raman spectroscopy *Proc. Natl Acad. Sci. USA* **108** 3809–14

[449] Suga K, Yoshida T, Ishii H, Okamoto Y, Nagao D, Konno M and Umakoshi H 2015 Membrane surface-enhanced Raman spectroscopy for sensitive detection of molecular behavior of lipid assemblies *Anal. Chem.* **87** 4772–80

[450] Ramya A N, Ambily P S, Sujitha B S, Arumugam M and Maiti K K 2017 Single cell lipid profiling of *Scenedesmus quadricauda* CASA-CC202 under nitrogen starved condition by surface enhanced Raman scattering (SERS) fingerprinting *Algal Res* **25** 200–6

[451] Müller M and Schins J M 2002 Imaging the thermodynamic state of lipid membranes with multiplex CARS microscopy *J. Phys. Chem.* B **106** 3715–23

[452] Wurpel G W H, Schins J M and Müller M 2004 Direct measurement of chain order in single phospholipid monoandbi layers with multiplex CARS *J. Phys. Chem.* B **108** 3400–3

[453] Cheng J X, Volkmer A, Book L D and Xie X S 2002 Multiplex coherent anti-Stokes Raman scattering microspectroscopy and study of lipid vesicles *J. Phys. Chem.* B **106** 8493–8

[454] Rinia H A, Bonn M, Müller M and Vartiainen E M 2007 Quantitative CARS spectroscopy using the maximum entropy method: the main lipid phase transition *ChemPhysChem.* **8** 279–87

[455] Schulz G E and Schirmer R H (ed) 1979 *Principles of Protein Structure* (New York: Springer)

[456] De Las Rivas J and de Luis A 2004 Interactome data and databases: different types of protein interaction *Comp. Funct. Genomics* **5** 173–8

[457] Gonzalez M W and Kann M G 2012 Protein interactions and disease *PLoS Comput. Biol.* **8** e1002819

[458] Chaudhuri T K and Paul S 2006 Protein-misfolding diseases and chaperone-based therapeutic approaches *FEBS J.* **273** 1331–49

[459] Hartl F U 2017 Protein misfolding diseases *Annu. Rev. Biochem.* **86** 21–6

[460] Niaura G 2014 *Encyclopedia of Analytical Chemistry* (Chichester: Wiley) pp 1–34

[461] Rygula A, Majzner K and Marzec K M 2013 Raman spectroscopy of proteins: a review *J. Raman Spectrosc.* **44** 1061–76

[462] Mikhonin A V, Bykov S V, Myshakina N S and Asher S A 2006 Peptide secondary structure folding reaction coordinate: correlation between UV Raman amide III frequency, Ψ Ramachandran angle, and hydrogen bonding *J. Phys. Chem.* B **110** 1928–43

[463] Thomas G J Jr 2002 New structural insights from Raman Spectroscopy of proteins and their assemblies *Biopolymers* **67** 214–25

[464] Zeinabad H A, Kachooei E, Saboury A A, Kostova I, Attar F, Vaezzadeh M and Falahati M 2016 Thermodynamic and conformational changes of protein toward interaction with nanoparticles: a spectroscopic overview *RSC Adv.* **6** 105903–19

[465] Reymond-Laruinaz S, Saviot L, Potin V and Marco de Lucas M D C 2016 Protein–nanoparticle interaction in bioconjugated silver nanoparticles: a transmission electron microscopy and surface enhanced Raman spectroscopy study *Appl. Surf. Sci.* **389** 17–24

[466] Panikkanvalappil S R and El-Sayed M A 2014 Gold-nanoparticle-decorated hybrid mesoflowers: an efficient surface-enhanced Raman scattering substrate for ultratrace detection of prostate specific antigen *J. Phys. Chem.* B **118** 14085–91

[467] Buividas R, Dzingelevicius N, Kubiliute R, Stoddart P R, Truong V K, Ivanova E P and Juodkazis S 2015 Statistically quantified measurement of an Alzheimer's marker by surface-enhanced Raman scattering *J. Biophotonics* **8** 567–74

[468] El-Said W A, Fouad D M and El-Safty S A 2016 Ultrasensitive label-free detection of cardiac biomarker myoglobin based on surface-enhanced Raman spectroscopy *Sensors Actuators* B **228** 401–9

[469] Xu L J, Zong C, Zheng X S, Hu P, Feng J M and Ren B 2014 Label-free detection of native proteins by surface-enhanced Raman spectroscopy using iodide-modified nanoparticles *Anal. Chem.* **86** 2238–45

[470] Matteini P, Cottat M, Tavanti F, Panfilova E, Scuderi M, Nicotra G, Menziani M C, Khlebtsov N, de Angelis M and Pini R 2017 Site-selective surface-enhanced Raman detection of proteins *ACS Nano* **11** 918–26

[471] Grubisha D S, Lipert R J, Park H, Driskell J and Porter M D 2003 Femtomolar detection of prostate-specific antigen: an immunoassay based on surface-enhanced Raman scattering and immunogold labels *Anal. Chem.* **75** 5936–43

[472] Ramya A N, Joseph M M, Nair J B, Karunakaran V, Narayanan N and Maiti K K 2016 New insight of tetraphenylethylene-based Raman signatures for targeted SERS nanoprobe construction toward prostate cancer cell detection *ACS Appl. Mater. Interfaces* **8** 10220–5

[473] Krasnoslobodtsev A V, Torres M P, Kaur S, Vlassiouk I V, Lipert R J, Jain M, Batra S K and Lyubchenko Y L 2015 Nano-immunoassay with improved performance for detection of cancer biomarkers *Nanomedicine* **11** 167–73

[474] Xu L, Zhao S, Ma W, Wu X, Li S, Kuang H, Wang L and Xu C 2016 Multigaps embedded nanoassemblies enhance *in situ* Raman spectroscopy for intracellular telomerase activity sensing *Adv. Funct. Mater.* **26** 1602–8

[475] Craig D, Simpson J, Faulds K and Graham D 2003 Formation of SERS active nanoparticle assemblies via specific carbohydrate–protein interactions *Chem. Commun.* **49** 30–2

[476] Robson A F, Hupp T R, Lickiss F, Ball K L, Faulds K and Graham D 2012 Nanosensing protein allostery using a bivalent mouse double minute (MDM2) assay *Proc. Natl Acad. Sci. USA* **109** 8073–8

[477] Torres Filho I P, Terner J, Pittman R N, Prott E and Ward K R 2008 Measurement of hemoglobin oxygen saturation using Raman microspectroscopy and 532-nm excitation *J. Appl. Physiol.* **104** 1809–17

[478] Torres Filho I P, Nguyen N M, Jivani R, Terner J, Romfh P, Vakhshoori D and Ward K R 2016 Oxygen saturation monitoring using resonance Raman spectroscopy *J. Surg. Res.* **201** 425–31

[479] Ward K R, Barbee R W, Reynolds P S, Torres Filho I P, Tiba M H, Torres L, Pittman R N and Terner J 2007 Oxygenation monitoring of tissue vasculature by resonance Raman spectroscopy *Anal. Chem.* **79** 1514–8

[480] Brazhe N A, Thomsen K, Lønstrup M, Brazhe A R, Nikelshparg E I, Maksimov G V, Lauritzen M and Sosnovtseva O 2018 Monitoring of blood oxygenation in brain by resonance Raman spectroscopy *J. Biophotonics* **11** e201700311

[481] Wood B R, Caspers P, Puppels G J, Pandiancherri S and McNaughton D 2007 Resonance Raman spectroscopy of red blood cells using near-infrared laser excitation *Anal. Bioanal. Chem.* **387** 1691–703

[482] Chowdhury A, Dasgupta R and Majumder S K 2017 Changes in hemoglobin–oxygen affinity with shape variations of red blood cells *J. Biomed. Opt.* **22** 1–9

[483] Rusciano G, De Luca A, Pesce G and Sasso A 2008 Raman Tweezers as a diagnostic tool of hemoglobin-related blood disorders *Sensors* **8** 7818–32

[484] Atkins C G, Buckley K, Blades M W and Turner R F B 2017 Raman spectroscopy of blood and blood components *Appl. Spectrosc.* **71** 767–93

[485] Lombardi J R and Birke R L A 2009 Unified view of surface-enhanced Raman scattering *Acc. Chem. Res.* **42** 734–42

[486] Murgida D H and Hildebrandt P 2004 Electron-transfer processes of cytochrome c at interfaces. New insights by surface-enhanced resonance Raman spectroscopy *Acc. Chem. Res.* **37** 854–61

[487] Sezer M, Genebra T, Mendes S, Martins L O and Todorovic S 2012 A DyP-type peroxidase at a bio-compatible interface: structural and mechanistic insights *Soft Matter* **8** 10314–21

[488] Siebert F and Hildebrandt P 2007 *Vibrational Spectroscopy in Life Science* (Weinheim: Wiley-VCH)

[489] Spiro T G and Li X Y 1988 *Resonance Raman Spectroscopy of Metalloproteins* vol 3 ed T G Spiro (New York: Wiley) pp 1–95

[490] Rousseau D L and Han S 2002 Time-resolved resonance Raman spectroscopy of intermediates in cytochrome oxidase *Methods Enzymol.* **354** 351–68

[491] Catarino T, Pessanha M, de Candia A G, Gouveia Z, Fernandes A P, Pokkuluri P R, Murgida D, Marti M A, Todorovic S and Salgueiro C A 2010 Probing the chemotaxis periplasmic sensor domains from *Geobacter sulfurreducens* by combined resonance Raman and molecular dynamic approaches: NO and CO sensing *J. Phys. Chem.* B **114** 11251–60

[492] Capdevila D A, Marmisolle W A, Tomasina F, Demicheli V, Portela M, Rafael R and Murgida D H 2015a Specific methionine oxidation of cytochrome c in complexes with zwitterionic lipids by hydrogen peroxide: potential implications for apoptosis *Chem. Sci.* **6** 705–13

[493] Capdevila D A, Rouco S O, Tomasina F, Tortora V, Demicheli V, Radi R and Murgida D H 2015b Active site structure and peroxidase activity of oxidatively modified cytochrome c species in complexes with cardiolipin *Biochemistry* **54** 7491–504

[494] Todorovic S, Hildebrandt P and Martins L O 2015 Surface enhanced resonance Raman detection of a catalytic intermediate of DyP-type peroxidase *Phys. Chem. Chem. Phys.* **17** 11954–7

[495] Todorovic S, Pereira M M, Bandeiras T M, Teixeira M, Hildebrandt P and Murgida D H 2005 Midpoint potentials of hemes a and a_3 in the quinol oxidase from *Acidianus ambivalens* are inverted *J. Am. Chem. Soc.* **127** 13561–6

[496] Todorovic S, Jung C, Hildebrandt P and Murgida D H 2006 Conformational transitions and redox potential shifts of cytochrome P450 induced by immobilization *J. Biol. Inorg. Chem.* **11** 119–27

[497] Todorovic S, Rodrigues M L, Matos D and Pereira I A C 2012 Redox properties of lysine- and methionine coordinated hemes ensure downhill electron transfer in $NrfH_2A_4$ nitrite reductase *J. Phys. Chem.* B **116** 5637–43

[498] Murgida D H and Hildebrandt P 2008 Disentangling interfacial redox processes of proteins by SERR spectroscopy *Chem. Soc. Rev.* **37** 937–45

[499] Sezer M, Spricigo R, Utesch T, Millo D, Leimkuehler S, Mroginski M A, Wollenberger U, Hildebrandt P and Weidinger I M 2010 Redox properties and catalytic activity of

surface-bound human sulfite oxidase studied by a combined surface enhanced resonance Raman spectroscopic and electrochemical approach *Phys. Chem. Chem. Phys.* **12** 7894–903

[500] Sezer M, Santos A, Kielb P, Pinto T, Martins L O and Todorovic S 2013 Distinct structural and redox properties of the heme active site in bacterial dye decolorizing peroxidase-type peroxidases from two subfamilies: resonance Raman and electrochemical study *Biochemistry* **52** 3074–84

[501] Sezer M, Kielb P, Kuhlmann U, Mohrmann H, Schulz C, Heinrich D, Schlesinger R, Heberle J and Weidinger I M 2015 Surface enhanced resonance Raman spectroscopy reveals potential induced redox and conformational changes of cytochrome c oxidase on electrodes *J. Phys. Chem.* B **119** 9586–91

[502] Silveira C M, Quintas P O, Moura I, Moura J J G, Hildebrandt P, Almeida M G and Todorovic S 2015 SERR spectro electrochemical study of cytochrome cd1 nitrite reductase co-immobilized with physiological redox partner cytochrome c552 on biocompatible metal electrodes *PLoS One* **10** e0129940

[503] Silveira C M, Castro M A, Dantas J M, Salgueiro C, Murgida D H and Todorovic S 2017 Structure, electrocatalysis and dynamics of immobilized cytochrome PccH and its micro-peroxidase *Phys. Chem. Chem. Phys.* **19** 8908–18

[504] Molinas M F, de Candia A, Szajnman S H, Rodríguez J B, Martí M, Pereira M, Teixeira M, Todorovic S and Murgida D H 2011 Electron transfer dynamics of *Rhodothermus marinus caa*$_3$ cytochrome *c* domains on biomimetic films *Phys. Chem. Chem. Phys.* **13** 18088–98

[505] Todorovic S and Murgida D H 2016 *Encyclopedia of Analytical Chemistry: Applications, Theory and Instrumentation* ed R A Meyers (Chichester: Wiley) pp 1–29

[506] Murgida D H and Hildebrandt P 2001 Active-site structure and dynamics of cytochrome c immobilized on self-assembled monolayers: a time-resolved surface enhanced resonance Raman spectroscopic study *Angew. Chem. Int. Ed.* **40** 728–31

[507] Todorovic S, Verissimo A, Wisitruangsakul N, Zebger I, Hildebrandt P, Pereira M M, Teixeira M and Murgida D H 2008 SERR-spectroelectrochemical study of a cbb3 oxygen reductase in a biomimetic construct *J. Phys. Chem.* B **112** 16952–9

[508] Okada M, Smith N I, Palonpon A F, Endo H, Kawata S, Sodeoka M and Fujita K 2012 Label-free Raman observation of cytochrome c dynamics during apoptosis *Proc. Natl Acad. Sci. USA* **109** 28–32

[509] Van Manen H J, Kraan Y M, Roos D and Otto C 2004 Intracellular chemical imaging of heme-containing enzymes involved in innate immunity using resonance Raman microscopy *J. Phys. Chem.* B **108** 18762–71

[510] Christophersen P C, Birch D, Saarinen J, Isomäki A, Nielsen H M, Yang M, Strachan C J and Mu H 2015 Investigation of protein distribution in solid lipid particles and its impact on protein release using coherent anti-Stokes Raman scattering microscopy *J. Control. Release* **197** 111–20

[511] Rygula A, Majzner K, Marzec K M, Kaczor A, Pilarczyk M and Baranska M 2013 Raman spectroscopy of proteins: a review *J. Raman Spectrosc.* **44** 1061–76

[512] Benecky M, Li T J, Schmidt J, Frerman F, Watters K L and McFarland J 1997 Resonance Raman study of flavins and the flavoprotein fatty acyl coenzyme A dehydrogenase *Biochemistry* **18** 3471–6

[513] Gall A, Pascal A A and Robert B 2015 Vibrational techniques applied to photosynthesis: resonance Raman and fluorescence line-narrowing *Biochim. Biophys. Acta* **1847** 12–8

[514] Tschirner N, Schenderlein M, Brose K, Schlodder E, Mroginski M A, Thomsena C and Hildebrandt P 2009 Resonance Raman spectra of beta-carotene in solution and in photosystems revisited: an experimental and theoretical study *Phys. Chem. Chem. Phys.* **11** 11471–8

[515] Carey P R 2006 Raman crystallography and other biochemical applications of Raman microscopy *Annu. Rev. Phys. Chem.* **57** 527–54

[516] Bandekar J 1992 Amide modes and protein conformation *Biochim. Biophys. Acta* **1120** 123–43

[517] Yu N T and Jo B H 1973 Comparison of protein structure in crystals and in solution by laser Raman scattering: I. Lysozyme *Arch. Biochem. Biophys.* **156** 469–74

[518] Frontzek A V, Paccou L, Guinet Y and Hédoux A 2016 Study of the phase transition in lysozyme crystals by Raman spectroscopy *Biochim. Biophys. Acta* **1860** 412–23

[519] Zabelskii D V 2018 Ambiguities and completeness of SAS data analysis: investigations of apoferritin by SAXS/SANS EID and SEC-SAXS methods *J. Phys.: Conf. Ser.* **994** 012017

[520] Vlasov A V *et al* 2014 Protein structure and structural ordering versus concentration dependence *FEBS J.* **281** 593–4

[521] Vlasov A V, Ryzhykau Y L, Gordeliy V I and Kuklin A I 2017 Spinach ATP-synthases form dimers in nanodiscs. Small-angle X-ray and neutron scattering investigations *FEBS J.* **284** 87

[522] Kuklin A I *et al* 2018 SANS investigations of biological objects on a YuMO spectrometer: results and possibilities *J. Bioenerg. Biomembr.* **50** 555

[523] Murugova T N *et al* 2015 Low resolution structural studies of apoferritin via SANS and SAXS: the effect of concentration *J. Optoelectron. Adv. Mater.* **17** 1397–402

[524] Kazantsev A S *et al* SAXS studies of apoferritin in diff erent pH with consideration of dimers *J. Bioenerg. Biomembr.* **50** 467–603

[525] Arzumanyan G, Doroshkevich N V, Mamatkulov K, Shashkov S, Zinovev E V, Vlasov A, Round E and Gordeliy V 2016 Highly sensitive coherent anti-Stokes Raman scattering imaging of protein crystals *J. Am. Chem. Soc.* **138** 13457–60

[526] Benevides J M, Overman S A and Thomas G J Jr 2005 Raman, polarized Raman and ultraviolet resonance Raman spectroscopy of nucleic acids and their complexes *J. Raman Spectrosc.* **36** 279–99

[527] Lord R C and Thomas G J Jr 1967 Raman studies of nucleic acids. II. Aqueous purine and pyrimidine mixtures *Biochim. Biophys. Acta* **142** 1–11

[528] Denbigh J L *et al* 2017 Probing the action of a novel anti-leukaemic drug therapy at the single cell level using modern vibrational spectroscopy techniques *Sci. Rep.* **7** 2649

[529] Dutta A, Gautam R, Chatterjee S, Ariese F, Sikdar S K and Umapathy S 2015 Ascorbate protects neurons against oxidative stress: a Raman microspectroscopic study *ACS Chem. Neurosci.* **6** 1794–801

[530] Benevides J M and Thomas G J 1983 Characterization of DNA structures by Raman spectroscopy: high-salt and low-salt forms of double helical poly(dG-dC) in H_2O and D_2O solutions and application to B, Z and A-DNA *Nucleic Acids Res.* **11** 5747–61

[531] Nishimura Y, Tsuboi M, Sato T and Aoki K 1986 Conformation-sensitive Raman lines of mononucleotides and their use in a structure analysis of polynucleotides: guanine and cytosine nucleotides *J. Mol. Struct.* **146** 123–53

[532] Serban D, Benevides J M and Thomas G J 2002 DNA secondary structure and Raman markers of supercoiling in *Escherichia coli* plasmid pUC19 *Biochemistry* **41** 847–53

[533] Deng H, Bloomfield V A, Benevides J M and Thomas G J 1999 Dependence of the Raman signature of genomic B-DNA on nucleotide base sequence *Biopolymers* **50** 656–66
[534] Wang X *et al* 2012 The relationship between the variants of the bovine MBL2 gene and milk production traits, mastitis, serum MBL-C levels and complement activity *Vet. Immunol. Immunopathol.* **148** 311–9
[535] Li H, Zhang F M, Guo H Y, Zhu Y Y, Yuan J D, Yang G W and An L G 2013 Molecular characterization of hepcidin gene in common carp (*Cyprinus carpio* L.) and its expression pattern responding to bacterial challenge *Fish Shellfish Immunol.* **35** 1030–8
[536] Shan S J, Liu D Z, Wang L, Zhu Y Y, Zhang F M, Li T, An L G and Yang G W 2015 Identification and expression analysis of irak1 gene in common carp *Cyprinus carpio* L.: Indications for a role of antibacterial and antiviral immunity *J. Fish Biol.* **87** 241–55
[537] Thorogood H, Waters T R, Parker A W, Wharton C W and Connolly B A 1996 Resonance Raman spectroscopy of 4-thiothymidine and oligodeoxynucleotides containing this base both free in solution and bound to the restriction endonuclease EcoRV *Biochemistry* **35** 8723–33
[538] Toyama A, Miyagawa Y, Yoshimura A, Fujimoto N and Takeuchi H 2001 Characterization of individual adenine residues in DNA by a combination of site-selective C8-deuteration and UV resonance Raman difference spectroscopy *J. Mol. Struct.* **598** 85–91
[539] Tsuboi M, Kubo Y, Ikeda T, Overman S A, Osman O and Thomas G J 2003 Protein and DNA residue orientations in the filamentous virus Pf1 determined by polarized Raman and polarized FTIR spectroscopy *Biochemistry* **42** 940–50
[540] Thomas G J, Benevides J M, Overman S A, Ueda T, Ushizawa K, Saitoh M and Tsuboi M 1995 Polarized Raman spectra of oriented fibers of A DNA and B DNA: anisotropic and isotropic local Raman tensors of base and backbone vibrations *Biophys. J.* **68** 1073–88
[541] Tsuboi M, Benevides J M and Thomas G J 2007 The complex of ethidium bromide with genomic DNA: structure analysis by polarized Raman spectroscopy *Biophys. J.* **92** 928–34
[542] Friedman S J and Terentis A C 2016 Analysis of G-quadruplex conformations using Raman and polarized Raman spectroscopy *J. Raman Spectrosc.* **47** 259–68
[543] Yu J, Jeon J, Choi N, Lee J O, Kim Y P and Choo J 2017 SERS-based genetic assay for amplification-free detection of prostate cancer specific PCA3 mimic DNA *Sens. Actuators* B **251** 302–9
[544] Wang R, Kim K, Choi N, Wang X, Lee J, Jeon J H, Rhie G E and Choo J 2018 Highly sensitive detection of high-risk bacterial pathogens using SERS-based lateral flow assay strips *Sens. Actuators* B **270** 72–9
[545] Qian Y, Fan T T, Yao Y, Shi X, Liao X J, Zhou F Y and Gao F L 2018 Label-free and Raman dyes-free surface-enhanced Raman spectroscopy for detection of DNA *Sens. Actuators* B **254** 483–9
[546] Han B *et al* 2018 Direct laser scribing of AGNPS@RGO biochip as a reusable SERS sensor for DNA detection *Sens. Actuators* B **270** 500–7
[547] Ye S J, Wu Y Y, Zhang W, Li N and Tang B 2014 A sensitive SERS assay for detecting proteins and nucleic acids using a triple-helix molecular switch for cascade signal amplification *Chem. Commun.* **50** 9409–12
[548] Kammer E, Olschewski K, Bocklitz T, Rosch P, Weber K, Cialla D and Popp J A new calibration concept for a reproducible quantitative detection based on SERS measurements in a microfluidic device demonstrated on the model analyte adenine *Phys. Chem. Chem. Phys.* **16** 9056–63

[549] Shi M L, Zheng J, Tan Y J, Tan G X, Li J S, Li Y H, Li X, Zhou Z G and Yang R H 2015 Ultrasensitive detection of single nucleotide polymorphism in human mitochondrial DNA utilizing ion-mediated cascade surface-enhanced Raman spectroscopy amplification *Anal. Chem.* **87** 2734–40

[550] Cao X W, Bao M, Shan Y B, Li W and Shi H C 2017 Rapid detection and identification of miRNAs by surface- enhanced Raman spectroscopy using hollow au nanoflowers substrates *J. Nanomater.* **2017** 1–11

[551] Driskell J D and Tripp R A 2010 Label-free SERS detection of microRNA based on affinity for an unmodified silver nanorod array substrate *Chem. Commun.* **46** 3298–300

[552] Zheng J, Bai J H, Zhou Q F, Li J S, Li Y H, Yang J F and Yang R H 2015 DNA-templated *in situ* growth of AgNPs on SWNTs: a new approach for highly sensitive SERS assay of microRNA *Chem. Commun.* **51** 6552–5

[553] Ye S, Wu Y, Zhai X and Tang B 2015 Asymmetric signal amplification for simultaneous SERS detection of multiple cancer markers with significantly different levels *Anal. Chem.* **87** 8242–9

[554] Zhou W, Tian Y F, Yin B C and Ye B C 2017 Simultaneous surface-enhanced Raman spectroscopy detection of multiplexed microRNA biomarkers *Anal. Chem.* **89** 6121–9

[555] Shin K, Choi J, Kim Y, Lee Y, Kim J, Lee S and Chung H 2018 Feasibility study for combination of field-flow fractionation (FFF)-based separation of size-coded particle probes with amplified surface enhanced Raman scattering (SERS) tagging for simultaneous detection of multiple miRNAs *J. Chromatogr.* A **1556** 97–102

[556] Lin D, Wu Q, Qiu S, Chen G, Feng S, Chen R and Zeng H 2019 Label-free liquid biopsy based on blood circulating DNA detection using SERS-based nanotechnology for nasopharyngeal cancer screening *Nanomed. Nanotechnol. Biol. Med.* **22** 102100

[557] Li X, Yang T, Li C S, Song Y, Lou H, Guan D and Jin L 2018 Surface enhanced Raman spectroscopy (SERS) for the multiplex detection of BRAF, KRAS, and PIK3CA mutations in plasma of colorectal cancer patients *Theranostics* **8** 1678–89

[558] Rasmussen A and Deckert V J 2006 Surface- and tip-enhanced Raman scattering of DNA components *Raman Spectrosc* **37** 311–7

[559] Watanabe H, Ishida Y, Hayazawa N, Inouye Y and Kawata S 2004 Tip-enhanced near-field Raman analysis of tip-pressurized adenine molecule *Phys. Rev.* B **69** 155418

[560] Domke K F, Zhang D and Pettinger B 2007 Tip-enhanced Raman spectra of picomole quantities of DNA nucleobases at Au (111) *J. Am. Chem. Soc.* **129** 6708–9

[561] Zhang D, Domke K F and Pettinger B 2010 Tip-enhanced Raman spectroscopic studies of the hydrogen bonding between adenine and thymine adsorbed on Au (111) *ChemPhysChem.* **11** 1662–5

[562] Bailo E and Deckert V 2008 Tip-enhanced Raman spectroscopy of single RNA strands: towards a novel direct-sequencing method *Angew. Chem. Int. Ed.* **47** 1658–61

[563] Alexander K D and Schultz Z D 2012 Tip-enhanced Raman detection of antibody conjugated nanoparticles on cellular membranes *Anal. Chem.* **84** 7408–14

[564] Naumenko D, Snitka V, Serviene E, Bruzaite I and Snopok B 2013 In vivo characterization of protein uptake by yeast cell envelope: single cell AFM imaging and μ-tip-enhanced Raman scattering study *Analyst* **138** 5371–83

[565] Kazemi-Zanjani N, Chen H, Goldberg H A, Hunter G K, Grohe B and Lagugne-Labarthet F 2012 Label-free mapping of osteopontin adsorption to calcium oxalate monohydrate crystals by tip-enhanced Raman spectroscopy *J. Am. Chem. Soc.* **134** 17076–82

[566] Wood B R, Asghari-Khiavi M, Bailo E, McNaughton D and Deckert V 2012 Detection of nano-oxidation sites on the surface of hemoglobin crystals using tip-enhanced Raman scattering *Nano Lett.* **12** 1555–60
[567] Yu J, Saito Y, Ichimura T, Kawata S and Verma P 2013 Far-field free tapping-mode tip-enhanced Raman microscopy *Appl. Phys. Lett.* **102** 123110
[568] Moretti M, Canale C, Canale C, Francardi M, Dante S, De Angelis F and Di Fabrizio E 2012 AFM characterization of biomolecules in physiological environment by an advanced nanofabricated probe *Microsc. Res. Tech.* **75** 1723–31
[569] Sinjab F, Lekprasert B, Woolley R A J, Roberts C J, Tendler S J B and Notingher I 2012 Near-field Raman spectroscopy of biological nanomaterials by *in situ* laser-induced synthesis of tip-enhanced Raman spectroscopy tips *Opt. Lett.* **37** 2256–8
[570] Lipiec E, Sekine R, Bielecki J, Kwiatek W M and Wood B R 2014 Molecular characterization of DNA double strand breaks with tip-enhanced Raman scattering *Angew. Chem. Int. Ed.* **53** 169–72
[571] Bailo E and Deckert V 2008 Tip-enhanced Raman spectroscopy of single RNA strands: towards a novel direct-sequencing method *Angew. Chem. Int. Ed.* **47** 1658–61
[572] Treffer R, Bohme R, Deckert-Gaudig T, Lau K, Tiede S, Lin X and Deckert V 2012 Advances in TERS (tip-enhanced Raman scattering) for biochemical applications *Biochem. Soc. Trans.* **40** 609–14
[573] Kuhar N, Sil S, Verma T and Umapathy S 2018 Challenges in application of Raman spectroscopy to biology and materials *RSC Adv.* **8** 25888–908
[574] Wiercigroch E, Szafraniec E, Czamara K, Pacia M Z, Majzner K, Kochan K, Kaczor A, Baranska M and Malek K 2017 Raman and infrared spectroscopy of carbohydrates: a review *Spectrochim. Acta* A **185** 317–35
[575] Arboleda P H and Loppnow G R 2000 Raman spectroscopy as a discovery tool in carbohydrate chemistry *Anal. Chem.* **72** 2093–8
[576] Stuart D A, Yuen J M, Shah N, Lyandres O, Yonzon C R, Glucksberg M R, Walsh J T and Van Duyne R P 2006 In vivo glucose measurement by surface-enhanced Raman spectroscopy *Anal. Chem.* **78** 7211–5
[577] Williams S C P 2013 Circulating tumor cells *Proc. Natl Acad. Sci. USA* **110** 4861–2
[578] Plaks V, Koopman C D and Werb Z 2013 Circulating tumor cells *Science* **341** 1186–8
[579] Yu M, Statt S, Toner M, Maheswaran S and Haber D A 2011 Circulating tumor cells: approaches to isolation and characterization *J. Cell Biol.* **192** 373–82
[580] Kim J H *et al* 2006 Nanoparticle probes with surface enhanced Raman spectroscopic tags for cellular cancer targeting *Anal. Chem.* **78** 6967–73
[581] Sun L *et al* 2007 Composite organic–inorganic nanoparticles as Raman labels for tissue analysis *Nano Lett.* **7** 351–6
[582] Cohen S J, Punt C J, Iannotti N, Saidman B H, Sabbath K D, Gabrail N Y and Meropol N J 2008 Relationship of circulating tumor cells to tumor response, progression-free survival, and overall survival in patients with metastatic colorectal cancer *J. Clin. Oncol.* **26** 3213–21
[583] Cristofanilli M, Budd G T, Ellis M J, Stopeck A, Matera J, Miller M C and Hayes D F 2004 Circulating tumor cells, disease progression, and survival in metastatic breast cancer *N. Engl. J. Med.* **351** 781–91
[584] Mulvaney S P, Musick M D, Keating C D and Natan M J 2003 Glass-coated, analyte-tagged nanoparticles: a new tagging system based on detection with surface-enhanced Raman scattering *Langmuir* **19** 4784–90

[585] Doering W E, Piotti M, Natan M J and Freeman R G 2007 SERS as a foundation for nanoscale, optically detected biological labels *Adv. Mater.* **19** 3100–8

[586] Sha M Y, Xu H, Penn S G and Cromer R 2007 SERS nanoparticles: a new optical detection modality for cancer diagnosis *Nanomedicine* **2** 725–34

[587] Yu K N *et al* 2007 Multiplex targeting, tracking, and imaging of apoptosis by fluorescent surface enhanced Raman spectroscopic dots *Bioconjugate Chem.* **18** 1155–62

[588] Zhang X, Yin H, Cooper J M and Haswell S J 2008 Characterization of cellular chemical dynamics using combined microfluidic and Raman techniques *Anal. Bioanal. Chem.* **390** 833–40

[590] de Bono J S, Scher H I, Montgomery R B, Parker C, Miller M C, Tissing H and Raghavan D 2008 Circulating tumor cells predict survival benefit from treatment in metastatic castration-resistant prostate cancer *Clin. Cancer Res.* **14** 6302–9

[591] Stott S, Hsu C H, Tsukrov D I, Yu M, Miyamoto D T, Waltman B and Toner M 2010 Isolation of circulating tumor cells using a microvortex-generating herringbone-chip *Proc. Natl Acad. Sci. USA* **107** 18392–7

[592] Paterlini-Brechot P and Benali N L 2007 Circulating tumor cells (CTC) detection: clinical impact and future directions *Cancer Lett.* **253** 180–204

[593] Hayes D F, Walker T M, Singh B, Vitetta E S, Uhr J W, Gross S, Rao C, Doyle G V and Terstappen L W 2002 Monitoring expression of HER-2 on circulating epithelial cells in patients with advanced breast cancer *Int. J. Oncol.* **21** 1111–7

[594] Sha M Y, Xu H, Natan M J and Cromer R 2008 Surface enhanced Raman scattering tags for rapid and homogeneous detection of circulating tumor cells in the presence of human whole blood *J. Am. Chem. Soc.* **130** 17214–5

[595] Vendrell M, Maiti K K, Dhaliwal K and Chang Y T 2013 Surface-enhanced Raman scattering in cancer detection and imaging *Trends Biotechnol.* **31** 249–59

[596] Neugebauer U, Bocklitz T, Clement J H, Krafft C and Popp J 2010 Towards detection and identification of circulating tumour cells using Raman spectroscopy *Analyst* **135** 3178–82

[597] Wang X, Qian X, Beitler J, Chen Z G, Khuri F R, Lewis M M and Shin D M 2011 Detection of circulating tumor cells in human peripheral blood using surface-enhanced Raman scattering nanoparticles *Cancer Res.* **71** 1526–32

[598] Pallaoro A, Hoonejani M R, Braun G B, Meinhart C D and Moskovits M 2015 Rapid identification by surface-enhanced Raman spectroscopy of cancer cells at low concentrations flowing in a microfluidic channel *ACS Nano* **9** 4328–36

[599] Wu X, Luo L, Yang S, Ma X, Li Y, Dong C, Tian Y, Zhang L, Shen Z and Wu A 2015 Improved SERS nanoparticles for direct detection of circulating tumor cells in the blood *ACS Appl. Mater. Interfaces* **7** 9965–71

[600] Garcia-Algar M, Fernandez-Carrascal A, Olano-Daza A, Guerrini L, Feliu N, Parak W J, Guimera R, Garcia-Rico E and Alvarez-Puebla R A 2018 Adaptive metabolic pattern biomarker for disease monitoring and staging of lung cancer with liquid biopsy *NPJ Precis. Oncol* **2** 16

[601] Liao C S, Slipchenko M N, Wang P, Li J, Lee S Y, Oglesbee R A and Cheng J X 2015 Microsecond scale vibrational spectroscopic imaging by multiplex stimulated Raman scattering microscopy *Light Sci. Appl.* **4** e265

[602] Evans C L, Potma E O, Puoris'haag M, Côté D, Lin C P and Xie X S 2005 Chemical imaging of tissue *in vivo* with video-rate coherent anti-Stokes Raman scattering microscopy *Proc. Natl Acad. Sci. USA* **102** 16807–12

[603] Saar B G, Freudiger C W, Reichman J, Stanley C M, Holtom G R and Xie X S 2010 Video-rate molecular imaging *in vivo* with stimulated Raman scattering *Science* **330** 1368–70
[604] Alfonso-García A, Pfisterer S G, Riezman H, Ikonen E and Potma E O 2016 D38-cholesterol as a Raman active probe for imaging intracellular cholesterol storage *J. Biomed. Opt.* **21** 61003
[605] Fu D and Xie X S 2014 Reliable cell segmentation based on spectral phasor analysis of hyperspectral stimulated Raman scattering imaging data *Anal. Chem.* **86** 4115–9
[606] Ozeki Y, Umemura W, Otsuka Y, Satoh S and Hashimoto H *et al* 2012 High-speed molecular spectral imaging of tissue with stimulated Raman scattering *Nat. Photon.* **6** 845–51
[607] Wei L, Hu F, Shen Y, Chen Z, Yu Y, Lin C C, Wang M C and Min W 2014 Live-cell imaging of alkyne-tagged small biomolecules by stimulated Raman scattering *Nat. Methods* **11** 410–2
[608] Hosokawa M, Ando M, Mukai S, Osada K, Yoshino T, Hamaguchi H O and Tanaka T 2014 In vivo live cell imaging for the quantitative monitoring of lipids by using Raman microspectroscopy *Anal. Chem.* **86** 8224–30
[609] Shen Y, Xu F, Wei L, Hu F and Min W 2014 Live-cell quantitative imaging of proteome degradation by stimulated Raman scattering *Angew. Chem. Int. Ed.* **53** 5596–9
[610] Hu F, Wei L, Zheng C, Shen Y and Min W 2014 Live-cell vibrational imaging of choline metabolites by stimulated Raman scattering coupled with isotope-based metabolic labeling *Analyst* **139** 2312–7
[611] Zhang D, Slipchenko M N and Cheng J X 2011 Highly sensitive vibrational imaging by femtosecond pulse stimulated Raman loss *J. Phys. Chem. Lett.* **2** 1248–53
[612] Hong W, Karanja C W, Abutaleb N S, Younis W, Zhang X, Seleem M N and Cheng J X 2018 Antibiotic susceptibility determination within one cell cycle at single-bacterium level by stimulated Raman metabolic imaging *Anal. Chem.* **90** 3737–43
[613] Karanja C W, Hong W, Younis W, Eldesouky H E, Seleem M N and Cheng J X 2017 Stimulated Raman imaging reveals aberrant lipogenesis as a metabolic marker for azole-resistant *Candida albicans Anal. Chem.* **89** 9822–9
[614] Klein K, Gigler A M, Aschenbrenner T, Monetti R, Bunk W, Jamitzky F, Morfill G, Stark R W and Schlegel J 2012 Label-free live cell imaging with confocal microscopy *Biophys. J.* **102** 360–8
[615] Brazhe N A, Treiman M, Brazhe A R, Find N L, Maksimov G V and Sosnovtseva O V 2012 Mapping of redox state of mitochondrial cytochromes in live cardiomyocytes using Raman microspectroscopy *PLoS One* **7** e41990
[616] Zuser E, Chernenko T, Newmark J, Miljković M and Diem M 2010 Confocal Raman microspectral imaging (CRMI) of murine stem cell colonies *Analyst* **135** 3030–3
[617] Ashton L, Lau K, Winder C L and Goodacre R 2011 Raman spectroscopy: lighting up the future of microbial identification *Future Microbiol.* **6** 991–7
[618] Mazur A I, Monahan J L, Miljkovic M, Laver N, Diem M and Bird B 2013 Vibrational spectroscopic changes of B-lymphocytes upon activation *J. Biophotonics* **6** 101–9
[619] Meister K, Schmidt D A, Bründermann E and Havenith M 2010 Confocal Raman microspectroscopy as an analytical tool to assess the mitochondrial status in human spermatozoa *Analyst* **135** 1370–4
[620] Zoladek A B, Johal R K, Garcia-Nieto S, Pascut F, Shakesheff K M, Ghaemmaghami A M and Notingher I 2010 Label free molecular imaging of the immunological synapse between dendritic and T-cells by Raman micro-spectroscopy *Analyst* **135** 3205–12

[621] Konorov S O, Schulze H G, Piret J M, Blades M W and Turner R F B 2013 Label-free determination of the cell cycle phase in human embryonic stem cells by Raman micro-spectroscopy *Anal. Chem.* **85** 8996–9002

[622] Hsu J F, Hsieh P Y, Hsu H Y and Shigeto S 2015 When cells divide: label-free multimodal spectral imaging for exploratory molecular investigation of living cells during cytokinesis *Sci. Rep.* **5** 17541

[623] Brozek-Pluska B, Kopec M and Abramczyk H 2016 Development of a new diagnostic Raman method for monitoring epigenetic modifications in the cancer cells of human breast tissue *Anal. Methods* **8** 8542–53

[624] Kumar P, Bhattacharjee T, Pandey M, Hole A, Ingle A and Krishna C M 2016 Raman spectroscopy in experimental oral carcinogenesis: investigation of abnormal changes in control tissues *J. Raman Spectrosc.* **47** 1318–26

[625] Mavarani L, Petersen D, El-Mashtoly S F, Mosig A, Tannapfel A, Kötting C and Gerwert K 2013 Spectral histopathology of colon cancer tissue sections by Raman imaging with 532 nm excitation provides label free annotation of lymphocytes, erythrocytes and proliferating nuclei of cancer cells *Analyst* **138** 4035–9

[626] Ali S M, Bonnier F, Ptasinski K, Lambkin H, Flynn K, Lyng F M and Byrne H J 2013 Raman spectroscopic mapping for the analysis of solar radiation induced skin damage *Analyst* **138** 3946–56

[627] Kochan K, Marzec K M, Chruszcz-Lipska K, Jasztal A, Maslak E, Musiolik H, Chłopicki S and Baranska M 2013 Pathological changes in the biochemical profile of the liver in atherosclerosis and diabetes assessed by Raman spectroscopy *Analyst* **138** 3885–90

[628] Michael R, Otto C, Lenferink A, Gelpi E, Montenegro G A, Rosandić J, Tresserra F, Barraquer R I and Vrensen G F J M 2014 Absence of amyloid beta in lenses of Alzheimer's patients: a confocal Raman study *Exp. Eye Res.* **119** 44–53

[629] Hobro A J, Pavillon N, Fujita K, Ozkan M, Coban C and Smith N I 2015 Label-free Raman imaging of the macrophage response to the malaria pigment hemozoin *Analyst* **140** 2350–9

[630] Hobro A J, Konishi A, Coban C and Smith N I 2013 Raman spectroscopic analysis of malaria disease progression via blood and plasma samples *Analyst* **138** 3927–33

[631] Franzen L, Mathes C, Hansen S and Windbergs M 2013 Advanced chemical imaging and comparisons of human and porcine hair follicles for drug delivery by confocal Raman microscopy *J. Biomed. Opt.* **18** 061210

[632] Toledano M, Aguilera F S, Osorio E, Cabello I and Osorio R 2014 Microanalysis of thermalinduced changes at the resin-dentin interface *Microsc. Microanal.* **20** 1218–33

[633] Toledano M, Cabello I, Aguilera F S, Osorio E and Osorio R 2015 Effect of *in vitro* chewing and bruxism events on remineralisation at the resin–dentin interface *J. Biomech.* **48** 14–21

[634] Fraser S J, Natarajan A K, Clark A S S, Drummond B K and Gordon K C 2015 A Raman spectroscopic study of teeth affected with molar–incisor hypomineralisation *J. Raman Spectrosc.* **46** 202–10

[635] Petibois C 2010 Imaging methods for elemental, chemical, molecular and morphological analysis of single cells *Anal. Bioanal. Chem.* **397** 2051–65

[636] Pavillon N and Smith N I 2015 Implementation of simultaneous quantitative phase with Raman imaging *EPJ Tech. Instrum.* **2** 1–11

[637] Krauß S D, Petersen D, Niedieker D, Fricke I, Freier E, El-Mashtoly S F, Gerwert K and Mosig A 2015 Colocalization of fluorescence and Raman microscopic images for the identification of subcellular compartments: a validation study *Analyst* **140** 2360–8
[638] Nafie L A 2014 Recent advances in linear and nonlinear Raman spectroscopy. Part XIII *J. Raman Spectrosc.* **45** 1326–46
[639] Zheng X S, Jahn I J, Weber K, Cialla-May D and Popp J 2018 Label-free SERS in biological and biomedical applications: recent progress, current challenges and opportunities *Spectrochim. Acta* A **197** 56–77
[640] Shan B, Pu Y, Chen Y, Liao M and Li M 2018 Novel SERS labels: rational design, functional integration and biomedical applications *Coord. Chem. Rev.* **371** 11–37
[641] Hill A H and Fu D 2019 Cellular imaging using stimulated Raman scattering microscopy *Anal. Chem.* **91** 9333–42
[642] Bocklitz T W, Meyer T, Schmitt M, Rimke I, Hoffmann F, von Eggeling F, Ernst G, Guntinas-Lichius O and Popp J 2018 Comparison of hyperspectral coherent Raman scattering microscopies for biomedical applications *APL Photonics* **3** 092404
[643] Pence I and Mahadevan-Jansen A 2016 Clinical instrumentation and applications of Raman spectroscopy *Chem. Soc. Rev.* **45** 1958–79

Chapter 6

Quartz crystal microbalance for biomedical nanotechnology

Kshitij RB Singh, Vanya Nayak and Ravindra Pratap Singh

The quartz crystal microbalance (QCM) has potential applications in the fields of biosensors, pertaining to the environmental, agricultural, and biomedical domains. The QCM is a very sensitive analytical instrument which estimates the nature of binding interactions in real time samples with good stability and sensitivity. The QCM biosensor is based on a mechanical transducer which converts the mass of target analytes into an electrical signal. The QCM in biosensing applications has label-free detection capability, and fast response at low cost. It is useful in the biomedical nanotechnology for use in nanovehicle detection and testing of micro-organisms, bacteria pathogen, environmental monitoring, and in the food industry. The aim of this chapter is to discuss the opportunities of QCM in the binding interaction in the biological environment to nanoconstruct (using nanoparticles) a design to enhance performance and also be utilized for the detection of potent chemicals and biomolecules.

6.1 Introduction

The use of the quartz crystal microbalance (QCM) is a technique for *in situ* interaction binding onto surfaces used in biosensing/nanobiosensing fields with label-free, high sensitivity, high stability, fast response, and low cost. In 1946 Cady reported QCM biosensors with a combination of nanoparticles (NPs) and bio-molecules, a new versatile detection method based on piezoelectricity [1]. In 1880 Curie and Curie reported piezoelectricity for the first time [2]. Lippman, in 1881, reported the converse piezoelectric effect, the deformation of a piezoelectric material by an applied electric field [3]. The quartz crystal microbalance (A-T cut quartz slide) using electrodes are used in various fields, such as food analysis, medicine, environmental protection, and biotechnology [4]. The QCM detection theory can be interpreted by the Sauerbrey equation that is based on the mass change that is

doi:10.1088/978-0-7503-3379-5ch6

proportional to the oscillation frequency shift of the piezoelectric quartz crystal [5]. Dirria *et al* [6] reported QCM sensors which are used in space missions to monitor the contaminants generated by the outgassing processes of materials. The QCM technique is a bioanalytical approach which monitors adsorption reactions onto a solid–liquid interface using piezoelectric quartz crystals and shows resonant shear oscillation frequency. The mass change is the dependence of the oscillation frequency on the total mass of the metal-coated crystal, calculated by the Sauerbrey equation. There are several sophisticated instruments used for the detection of various chemicals but their use is time consuming. To overcome this problem, the QCM technique is a solution which is non-toxic, label-free, real time, and has high sensitivity. Curie and Curie [2] reported mechanical stress using quartz and a voltage. Sauerbrey [7] reported quartz oscillation frequency change and mass change on a surface; he also coined the term quartz crystal microbalance. QCM is the mass balance that measures ng to mg level changes in mass per unit area using a quartz disc which is a piezoelectric material able to oscillate at a defined frequency when a voltage is applied via metal electrodes. The addition or removal of mass onto the electrode surface can produce an oscillation frequency change, this change of frequency provides information about molecular interactions or reactions on the electrode surface under vacuum, gas phase, and in liquid media. The change in mass in terms of oscillation frequency can be calculated by the Sauerbrey equation. In the vacuum or gas phase the Sauerbrey equation is valid; this is because molecular adsorption onto rigid films coupled with the oscillation of the electrode surface and change in mass of such films is linearly related to the change in the oscillation frequency. In the liquid environment, molecular adsorption cannotbe sustained due to hydration/solvation or entrapment within the adsorbed film and as a result dampening, or energy loss, of the oscillation and measurement of frequency change is not possible. The frequency change and energy loss as a dissipation change needs to be measured to determine the mass change of a viscoelastic film and this type of approach is known as quartz crystal microbalance with dissipation (QCM-D) [8]. Viscoelastic properties (i.e., viscosity, elasticity, and density) of the adsorbed film can be measured by QCM-D in liquid. QCM-D has a wide range of potential applications such as the study of protein–protein, molecule–surface, polymer films and their interactions with different constituents of liquid media, effect and biosensor etc [9]. The QCM is based on the piezoelectric effect of quartz crystals. The quartz crystal, due to its piezoelectric nature, has the ability to deform when a voltage is applied and this characteristic feature is used for the ultrasensitive devices. This crystal is found in nature and it is very simple to grow and process [10]. The quartz crystal resonator used in QCMs has specific orientations to the crystallographic axis, but quartz discs use the AT cut which provides thickness shear mode oscillation onto a pair of coinage metal electrodes, if alternating current is applied to the quartz disc, it will oscillate at its resonance frequency and resonance frequencies are inversely proportional to the crystal thickness [11, 12].

The quartz crystals act as sensitive mass balances, in which the frequency change of the oscillating quartz can be linearly related to its mass change. In 1963, Warner and Stockbridge demonstrated the measurement of a change in mass as small as

1 pg cm^{-2} that corresponded to about 0.1% of a monolayer of hydrogen [13]. Tje Sauerbrey equation has limitations. This equation is used in several industries for monitoring the rate and thickness of metal deposition under the vacuum or gas phase. Nomura and Hattori reported in 1980 that a quartz crystal stably oscillated in liquid media even when submerged [14]. In liquid media, QCM applications have potential applications in biology, biotechnology, nanotechnology, polymers, lipids, proteins, electrochemistry, environmental studies, etc. Viscoelastic films violate/fail or limit Sauerbrey's equation condition because of the generation of dissipation of oscillation energy due to mechanical losses in the flexible mass.

There are three approaches using the electrical circuit model for measuring energy dissipation (a) resistance analysis (QCM-R), (b) impedance analysis (QCM-Z) and (c) QCM-D. QCM-R is the resistance of the crystal which can be measured by introducing a small resistor into the circuit and measuring the voltage, this approach provides relative structural data. QCM-Z is a clear cut approach to measure energy losses based on impedance analysis using an equivalent circuit. The QCM-D approach is the quartz crystal excitation to its resonance frequency for a short period by applying a driving voltage. Wegener *et al* reported analysis of the composite response of shear wave resonators to the attachment of mammalian cells [15]. The film properties like density, thickness, viscosity and shear modulus or elasticity are mandatory for accurate calculation of the viscoelastic mass, i.e., product of density and thickness which can used to obtain the viscoelastic properties of the adsorbed film. Voinova *et al* reported the Voigt viscoelastic model which consists of the arrangement of a (viscous) dashpot and (elastic) spring in parallel. They have described the frequency and dissipation responses of the quartz crystal, upon adsorption of a viscoelastic film in liquid medium [16]. Cho *et al* reported a quartz crystal microbalance with dissipation monitoring of supported lipid bilayers on various substrates [17]. Reviakine *et al* interpreted quartz crystal microbalance data from solvated interfaces and suggested that a film can be considered rigid [18]. The QCM-D is a technique used to measure mass and viscosity at surfaces, in thin films in a liquid environment and is frequently used in the biomedical biotechnology such as in the study of cell behavior and cell surface interactions and also to design biomedical devices. Kanazawa and Gordon (1985) reported that the Sauerbrey equation is valid in air or in vacuum but in liquid environment the Sauerbery equation is not valid [19]. QCM-D is able to characterize the biological interactions of engineered surfaces of biosensors. It is equipped with a temperature-controlled system for the cell behavior or response study. Also it monitors cell phenomena and behavior on surfaces/cell interfaces in biomedical science.

The QCM consists of a quartz crystal with electrodes deposited on both the front and back sides, a crystal holder to secure the crystal and provide electrical connection, an oscillator which drives the crystal to its resonance frequency, and a controller or monitor that reads the frequency change and stores process parameters. Figure 6.1 shows a schematic representation of the QCM equipment.

Such an electrode design allows the QCM to oscillate only in the central area where electrodes are deposited. The motion wave generated as a result of crystal oscillation is focused in the center of the quartz crystal which makes it easier to

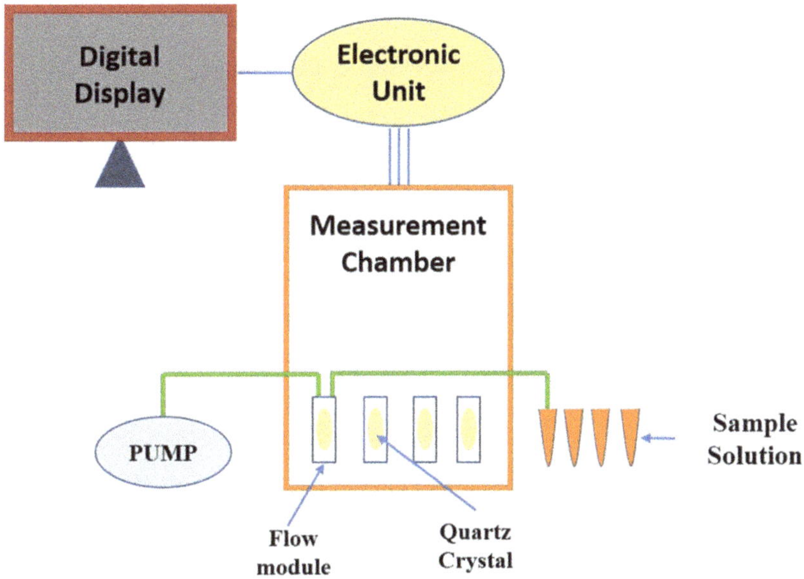

Figure 6.1. A schematic representation of QCM equipment.

mount the crystal at the edge without excessive dampening of oscillation. Since the oscillation frequency stability is affected by temperature changes, the quartz crystal holder is usually placed in an enclosed, temperature-controlled chamber.

A basic QCM-D instrument includes a quartz crystal with electrodes deposited on both the front and back side, a flow module that holds the quartz crystal and enables liquid media to flow across the top face of the crystal, a pump to flow the sample solution, a temperature-controlled chamber where the flow module is mounted and held at a set temperature, and an electronics unit that drives the crystal by applying appropriate voltage and recording the frequency and dissipation changes. Figure 6.2 shows a quartz crystal with electrodes in top view and bottom view.

Syariena *et al* (2008) reported QCM coated TiO_2–porphyrin nanocomposite thin film gas sensors to detect a few volatile organic compounds such as ethanol, acetone, 2-propanol, cyclohexane, toluene, and *o*-xylene [20]. Gas safety is very important in every area of life. Wang (2020) reported the detection and control of hazardous gases and humidity. A metal–organic framework (MOF) is a functional material with unique physical and chemical properties for the use in QCM gas sensing such as formaldehyde, toluene, acetone, etc and humidity also [21]. Chena *et al* (2016) reported QCM-D to study *in situ* interactions in liquids [22]. Chen *et al* (2018) reported the quartz crystal microbalance with a label-free biosensing system to monitor the cell–substrate adhesion control and regulation of cellular behavior such as cell morphology, cell mechanics, cell motility, cell signaling, and their impact on human health [23]. There are two types of external physical loading namely gravimetric and viscoelastic loading.

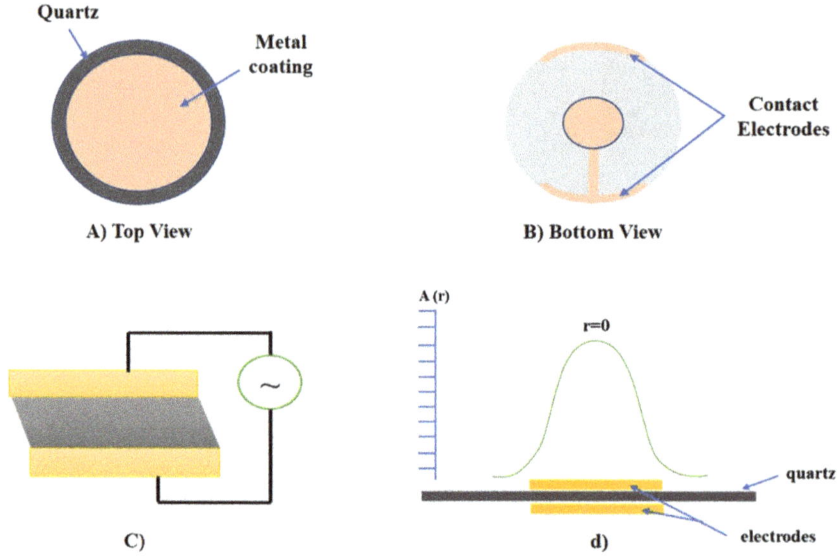

Figure 6.2. Quartz crystal with electrodes in top view and bottom view. Reprinted from [24], copyright 2011 John Wiley & Sons, Inc.

6.2 QCM biosensor

A biosensors consists of a biological macromolecule immobilized on the surface of a transducer which measures a physical change and finally converts it into an electrical signal. QCM is one of the most important transducers that is a piezoelectric mass-sensing device using a gold-plated quartz crystal. An immobilization of antibodies on the crystal surface based on passive adsorption leads to random functionally active orientation on the gold-coated QCM surface with free antigen binding sites for interaction of the desired antibody. The gold affinities with thiols are known for antibody binding via SAM, e.g., avidin/streptavidin-coated QCM gold-surface. Marx (2003) reported QCM biosensors with label-free detection of a variety of analytes [25]. Janshoff *et al* (2000) reported piezoelectric mass-sensing devices as biosensors which is an alternative to an optical biosensor [26]. Acoustic sensor technology is an optical technique which analyses molecular changes occurring in biochemical processes. Braunhut *et al* (2005) reported the QCM biosensor technique to detect taxanes in response to drug resistance of human breast cancer cells [27]. Kim *et al* (2009) reported a DNA aptamer-immobilized interdigitated array electrode chip for the detection of oxytetracycline [28]. Fang *et al* (2008) reported electrochemiluminescence based an aptasensor for the detection of thrombin using a thio-silanized ITO electrode [29]. Yao *et al* (2010) reported antibody-based QCM biosensors for the detection of immunoglobulin E [30]. Wu *et al* (2007) reported a DNA based QCM for the detection of *Escherichia coli* O157:H7 [31].

6.3 QCM biosensors and nanoparticles

Currently nanobiotechnology is a very hot topic and nanoparticles are use in DNA, protein and even cell sensing systems but potential risks and toxicity to human health cannot be ruled out. Despite that, the use of nanoparticles (1–100 nm) is growing in the energy and environment sector, healthcare, agriculture and in biosensing pertaing to clinical, and environmental [32, 33]. Nanoparticle based biosensors, i.e., nanobiosensors are utilizing functional nanoparticles or nanobiomaterials [34]. QCM biosensors using nanoparticles are remarkable achievements with high sensitivity and label-free detection. Chu *et al* reported a QCM biosensor using colloidal gold immunocomplex for the detection of human IgG [35]. Jin *et al* reported a QCM immunosensor using gold nanoparticles for the detection of Aflatoxin B1[36]. Recently, Chu *et al* reported a QCM immunosensor using gold nanoparticles for the detection of gliadin [37]. Kaewphinit *et al* reported a QCM biosensor using gold nanoparticle for the detection of *Mycobacterium tuberculosis* [38]. Willner *et al* reported a microgravimetric QCM for the detection of single-base mismatches in DNA [39].

Recently, Hao *et al* reported a DNA QCM biosensor using gold nanoparticle for the detection of *Bacillus anthracis* [40]. Chen *et al* reported a QCM DNA sensing system using layer-by-layer gold nanoparticles for the detection of dengue virus [41]. Scodeller *et al* reported a QCM using core–shell nanoparticles for the detection of glucose [42]. Reimhult *et al* (2008) reported a QCM sensor with surfaces coated with molecularly imprinted nanoparticles for sensing systems [43]. Kong *et al* (2014) reported a molecular imprinted polyners (MIPs) QCM sensor for the detection of ractopamine [44]. Uludag and Tothill (2010) reported an antibody modified QCM sensor and nanoparticle amplification system for the detection of cancer biomarkers prostate-specific antigen and PSA–alpha 1-antichymotrypsin complex [45].

Ma *et al* (2002) reported a QCM–AuNPs for the detection of human lung carcinoma cell *in vitro* [46]. Chen *et al* (2010) reported an aptamer-functionalized AuNPs QCM-D biosensor for protein adsorption [47]. Shan *et al* (2014) reported an aptamer-based QCM biosensor (aptamer/thrombin/Apt-GNPs on chip surface) for the detection of leukemia cells using human α-thrombin as the target protein [48]. Kaufman *et al* reported the adsorption of protein onto a self-assembled monolayer (SAM) of mercaptoundecanoic acid (MUA) on AuNPs surfaces [49]. Su *et al* reported a QCM (PPy/Ag/TiO_2 NPs) composite thin films-based humidity sensors [50]. Yang *et al* reported a QCM polymer poly (3,4-ethylenedioxythiophene) nanoparticles sensor system for the detection of ammonia gas [51]. Salam *et al* reported a QCM–AuNPs-antibody system for the detection of *Salmonella typhimurium* [52]. Guo *et al* reported a QCM immunosensor for the detection of pathogens [53]. Crooks and Ricco reported hyperbranch polymer monolayers and poly (amidoamine) dendrimer monolayers which can interact with small organic molecules [54]. Chen *et al* reported QCM–AuNP surface thin films for the study of interactions [55]. Shen *et al* reported AuNPs thin films for the study of interactions binding to the target [56]. Liu and Hu reported QCM and CV for the study of interaction binding of proteins [57]. Guleryuz *et al* reported QCM-D for the study of thin film growth using SiO_2 NPs on alumina [58].

6.4 Potential applications of QCM

Figure 6.3 shows the broad spectrum of applications of QCM in the biomedical field. We discuss some biomedical areas pertaining to QCM along with some of the most common advantages.

6.4.1 Detection of cell adhesion

QCM-D sensors can be used to study cell adhesion, cell attachment, and cell spreading. They are biophysicals tool used for the study of cell surface interactions to confirm the changes of cytoskeleton [59]. Tymchenko *et al* reported QCM-D for changes in cell morphology [60]. Westas *et al* reported QCM–hydroxyapatite NPs for the study of interaction of human gingival fibroblasts [61]. Kao *et al* reported QCM-D to study NIH3T3 mouse embryonic fibroblast adhesion [62]. Kushiro *et al* reported QCM-D using SAM surfaces for the study of protein–material interactions [63]. Furthermore, Chronaki *et al* reported QCM for the study of adhesion ability of normal and cancer human thyroid cells [64]. Reipa *et al* reported QCM for the study of biofilm growth and disinfection [65]. Olsson *et al* reported QCM for the study of bacterium–substratum bond maturation [66]. Furthermore, Olsson *et al* in their study reported QCM-D sensing of the bacterium–substratum interface [67]. Joshi *et al* reported QCM-D for the study of aminoglycoside activity of bacterial mimetic membranes [68]. Tonda-Turo *et al* reported QCM-D role in biomedical applications for the cell behavior/surface interactions [69]. Yao *et al* reported the point of care blood coagulation self-testing function monitoring using device based on new smartphone, i.e., parylene-C coated quartz crystal microbalance dissipation measuring and analysis. The parylene-C is an adhesive found in nature for capturing fibrin. The dissipation factor was obtained by measuring the frequency response of the sensor [70]. Proteins are biomaterials which mediate the interactions between the material and the environment, for instance, bovine serum albumin, fibronectin, and collagen type-I used in biomedical applications. Felgueiras *et al* reported a quartz crystal microbalance with dissipation to monitor the adsorption of proteins onto materials used in functional bone replacement, e.g., titanium alloy. They also

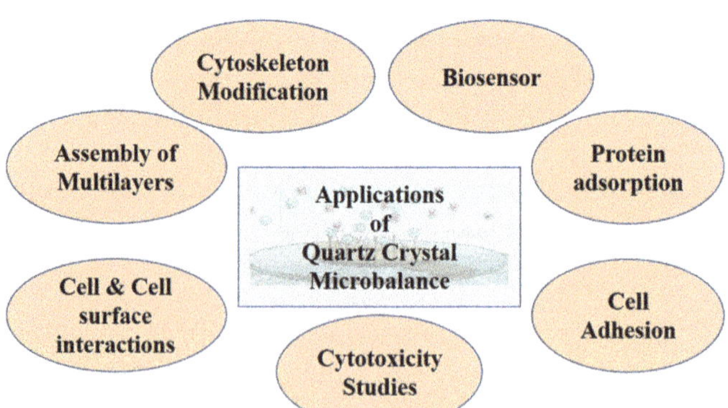

Figure 6.3. Broad spectrum of applications of QCM in biomedical field.

suggested that protein conformational changes induced by the adsorbing surfaces, protein–protein interactions, and the affinities of proteins [71].

Kompf *et al* reported real-time measurement of *Plasmodium falciparum*-infected erythrocyte cytoadhesion with a quartz crystal microbalance. Quartz crystal microbalances are sensitive to nanogram-scale changes in mass and to measure binding of *P. falciparum*-infected erythrocytes to two receptors: CD36 and chondroitin sulfate A [72]. Kojima reported QCM sensor for the study of molecule–substrate and molecule–molecule interactions [73]. Lin *et al* reported effective construction of a high-capacity boronic acid layer on a QCM chip for high-density antibody immobilization [74]. Kobayashi *et al* reported the thermoresponsive, dynamic behavior of serum protein adsorption/desorption using the QCM-D technique [75]. The biomarker of diabetes is acetone in breath. Tao *et al* reported QCM-ionic liquid sensing system for the detection of acetone which was coated on a quartz crystal microbalance for an applications in non-invasive early diabetic diagnosis [76]. Phan *et al* reported that combinatorial quartz crystal microbalance with dissipation and spectroscopic ellipsometry to evaluate attachment and detachment of adsorbed proteins in systems with environmental implications [77]. Rajaram *et al* reported real-time analysis of dual-display phage immobilization and autoantibody screening using quartz crystal microbalance with dissipation monitoring [78]. Nielson *et al* reported the peptide interaction with supported lipid model membranes using a combination of complementary surface sensitive techniques: neutron reflectometry, atomic force microscopy, and quartz crystal microbalance with dissipation monitoring [79]. Liu *et al* reported ultrathin two-dimensional transition metal dichalcogenides using in biomedicine, biosensing, bioimaging, drug delivery, and cancer therapy. However, interactions between metal dichalcogenides and mucin using quartz crystal microbalance with a dissipation monitor (QCM-D), spectroscopic probing and surface plasmon resonance [80]. Movilli *et al* reported the use of modified poly(L-lysine) (PLL) polymers with immobilized oligo(ethylene glycol) (OEG) and thiol-reactive maleimide (Mal) moieties (PLL-OEG-Mal) for DNA detection using quartz crystal microbalance frequency shifts of the binding of complementary DNA versus the density of Mal moieties grafted to the PLL, a linear relationship between probe density and PLL grafting density [81]. Miyake *et al* reported QCM coated dendrimer-triamine-coordinated Gd-MRI Contrast agents for biomedical diagnostic [82].

Alexander *et al* reported QCM-D for the investigations of bacterial adhesion in the formation of biofilms in real time [83]. Silva *et al* reported the pH-dependent properties of multilayered films made of chitosan and alginate and focused on their post-assembly response to different pH environments using a QCM-D, swelling studies, potential measurements, and dynamic mechanical analysis. It has also been suggested that surface functionalization using pH responsiveness endows several biomedical applications such as diagnostics, drug delivery, microfluidics, and biosensing [84]. Browning *et al* reported that high- and low-density lipoproteins play roles in the onset and development of atherosclerosis. A protocol for monitoring the *in situ* kinetics of lipoprotein deposition and lipid exchange/removal at model cellular membranes using the non-invasive, surface sensitive methods of QCM with dissipation [85]. Bahmanzadeh *et al* reported that gelatin is a biodegradable constituent making film with poor mechanical properties, its biodegradability was monitored by QCM-D [86]. Heath *et al* reported multilayer lipid membranes performing electrical isolation (myelination of axons), increased surface area for biocatalytic purposes (thylakoid grana and mitochondrial cristae), and sequential processing (golgi cisternae). The assembly process was monitored at the macroscale by quartz crystal microbalance with dissipation [87]. Peiris *et al* reported oncogenesis due to an alteration in protein glycosylation which affected cancer cell behavior perturbing to cell adhesion, favouring cell migration and metastasis. In this study they investigated the effect of N-linked glycosylation on the binding of herceptin to HER2 protein in breast cancer and on the sensitivity of cancer cells to the chemotherapeutic agent doxorubicin and growth factors which was assessed by QCM biosensor [88]. Lakshmanan *et al* reported the coagulation of blood plasma in response to activation with a range of tissue factor concentrations which was studied with a QCM [89]. Chouirfa *et al* reported grafting of bioactive polymers such as poly (sodium styrene sulfonate) onto titanium surfaces uses a modified dopamine as an anchor molecule which is characterized by QCM-D using human bone cells in cell culture for cell adhesion, proliferation, differentiation, and mineralization [90]. Dubacheva *et al* reported multivalent binding to the orientation of surface-bound molecules, for example, streptavidin binding on biotinylated surfaces such as supported lipid bilayers and self-assembled monolayers and their stability and kinetics of streptavidin binding are characterized by QCM with dissipation monitoring [91]. Dalgarno *et al* reported the solubilization of membranes by detergents to induce cell rupture, extract cell constituents. The thermodynamic details and kinetic aspects can be done by QCM with dissipation monitoring to access the real-time kinetics [92]. Geisler *et al* reported the coating deposition kinetics of the polyphenol tannic acid and the simple phenolic compound pyrogallol on titanium surfaces using a QCM with dissipation monitoring to evaluate coating, deposition kinetics and coating thickness [93].

6.4.2 Detection of cytotoxicity and cell viability

Cells are very viable and sensitive to the external environment. The monitoring of cell behavior on bioengineered surfaces of QCM is an easy way to detect cytoskeletal changes and which can check cytotoxicity/viability effects in a better way when compare with traditional methods of cytotoxicity and cell viability tests. Fatisson *et al* (2011) reported QCM sensor coated bovine aortic endothelial cells to study the cellular response [94]. Kandel *et al* (2014) reported QCM-D sensor coated fibronectin for the study of cytoskeleton changes [95]. Nowacki *et al* (2014) reported apoptosis-mediated cell death sense by QCM-D coated human breast cancer cells using staurosporine [96]. Furthermore, Kepp *et al* (2011) opened the way for the use of QCM-D for the study of cell cytotoxicity and drug efficacy of drugs [97]. Zhang *et al* (2015) reported QCM-D coated MCF-7 cells treated with resveratrol for the detection of cancer [98].

6.4.3 Detection of phenomena in cells

The QCM-D is a monitoring biological phenomena such as cell differentiation and cell migration. Zhang *et al* (2015) reported QCM-D to study adhesion of erythrocytes to endothelial cells. This study confirms that whether red blood cells (RBSs) are healthy or non-healthy in terms of cell adhesion in type 2 diabetic patients to check complications like vascular thrombosis [99]. Friedl and Gilmour reported cancer cell motility and collective cell migration morphogenesis, regeneration in cancer to give novel insights to quantify the metastatic potential of cancer cells [100]. Tarantola *et al* (2010) reported a QCM-based sensor to determine the cell motility of breast cancer lines [101].

6.4.4 Detection of VOCs and non-VOCs

The detection of alcohols, ethers, esters, NO_2, ammonia, halocarbons, chemical warfare agents, and toxic gases are very important, all of these are volatile organic compounds (VOCs) by QCM-based multianalyte detection systems. Lu *et al* (2009) reported a QCM chip sensor for the detection of volatile organic compounds, for example, butyric acid, acetic acid, ammonia, and benzene [102]. Alcohols are used in medicine, laboratories, and industry but prolonged exposure causes bad health. Ayad and Torad (2009) reported a QCM coated thin film polyaniline sensor for the detection of vaporous ethanol, methanol etc [103]. In addition to that Bello *et al* (2007) reported a QCM-based ethanol sensor using thin film of polyaniline as the sensing material for the detection of ethanol. Thus, it can be used as a quality control in bakery [104].

Kikuchi and Shiratori reported a QCM coated polyelectrolyte-coated sol–gel film for the detection of methyl mercaptan gas [105]. Ying *et al* reported a QCM coated polymer sensor array for the detection of chemical agents such as dimethyl methylphosphonate, *N,N*-dimethylacetamide, 1,5-dichloropentane, and dichloroethane [106].

Ying *et al* reported a poly (vinylidene fluoride) coated QCM sensor for dimethyl methylphosphonate vapor detection [107]. Koshets *et al* reported QCM coated calixarene films for the detection of volatile organic compounds such as ketones, and alcohols [108]. Matsuguchi and Uno reported a QCM MIP sensor for the detection of solvent molecules such as toluene and *p*-xylene [109]. Rabe *et al* reported a QCM array coated with polystyrene, β-cyclodextrin, and amyl-calixarene for the detection of toluene [110]. Dickert *et al* reported QCM sensor arrays for the detection of *m*-xylene and *p*-xylene [111]. Wyszynski *et al* reported QCM odor sensor coated PEGylated lipopolymers for the detection of a variety of alcohols, esters, acids, and aldehydes [112]. Park *et al* reported piezoelectric immunosensor for the detection of bisphenol A [113]. Tsuru *et al* reported a QCM sensor coated with MIP for the detection of Bisphenol A. They have suggested a stable MIP QCM sensor [114]. Kurosawa *et al* reported a QCM-based dioxin sensor [115]. Zeng *et al* reported a QCM sensor coated polymer for the detection of organophosphorous pesticide o,o-dimethyl-o-2,2-dichlorovinyl phosphate [116]. Yuan *et al* reported a QCM coated poly(3,4-ethylenedioxythiophene) (PEDOT)-conductive polymer film for the detection of urinary 1- and 2-naphthol using [117].

6.4.5 Detection of gaseous analytes

Matsuguchi *et al* (2007) reported a QCM coated morpholine-functional poly (styrene-co-chloromethylstyrene) copolymer sensor for the detection of HCl gas [118]. In another study, Matsuguchi *et al* (2008) reported a QCM coated poly (acrylamide) derivate sensor for the detection of HCl gas in air [119]. Sun *et al* (2009) reported a supramolecular cryptophane-A-based QCM sensor for the detection of methane [120]. Xie *et al* (2010) reported a QCM coated PANI/PdO composite for the detection of methane [121]. Palaniappan *et al* (2008) reported a QCM sensor coated cobalt phthalocyanine in a mesoporous silica matrix for the detection of nitric oxide [122].

Matsuguchi *et al* (2005) reported a QCM coated morpholine-functional cross-linked copolymer for the detection of nitrogen dioxide [123]. Ding *et al* (2004) reported a QCM sensor coated electrospun nanoporous membrane for the detection of ammonia [124]. Van Quy *et al* (2011) reported ZnO nanorods-coated QCM gold surface sensor for detecting NH_3 at room temperature [125]. Lee *et al* (2010) reported a QCM sensor coated TiO_2 and polyacrylic acid for the detection of amine odors [126]. Zhang *et al* (2011) reported electrospun nanoporous polystyrene fibers deposited on polyethyleneimine (PEI)-functionalized QCM for the detection of formaldehyde [127]. Guo *et al* (2009) reported a QCM sensor for the detection of mandelic acid [128]. Odor molecule approximation is a difficult task. However, Munoz-Aguirre *et al* reported QCM odor sensors coated lipids for the detection of the odor of orange and melon [129]. Ozmen *et al* (2006) reported QCM sensors coated phthalocyanine for the detection of gas mixtures such as ethanol–acetone, ethanol–trichloroethylene, and acetone–trichloroethylene [130]. Zhu *et al* (2010) reported QCM coated mesoporous silicate SBA-15 sensor for humidity detection [131]. Ayad *et al* (2010) reported QCM coated PANI film for the sensing of silver ions in aqueous media [132]. Escuderos *et al* (2011) reported eight QCM sensor arrays for olive oil sensory evaluation [133]. Reipa *et al* (2010) reported measurement of nanoparticle concentration in colloidal solution using quartz crystal microgravimetry [134].

6.4.6 Detection of bacteria/pathogen

Buchatip *et al* reported QCM immunosensor for the detection of shrimp pathogenic bacteria [135]. Yakovleva *et al* (2011) reported QCM coated lectins immobilized on the gold for the detection of several *Campylobacter jejuni* strains [136]. Wan *et al* (2010) reported QCM sensor coated vancomycin-functionalized magnetic nanoparticle for the detection of sulfate-reducing bacterium using external magnetic field [137]

6.4.7 Detection of biomolecules

Tang *et al* (2011) reported a QCM coated dextran-functionalized graphene for the detection of glucose molecules displace concanavalin A molecules [138]. Lin *et al* (2004) reported a QCM MIP sensor for the determination of albumin concentration in human serum [139]. Uludag and Tothill (2010) reported a QCM bound antibody with AuNPs for the detection of prostate-specific antigen and PSA–alpha 1-antichymotrypsin in human serum [45]. Kim *et al* (2010) reported a QCM immunosensor immobilized biotinylated antirat CRP antibody mixed with strepta-vidin-coated gold nanoparticle for the detection of C-reactive protein [140]. Chen *et al* (2011) reported a QCM immunosensor coated anti-EGFR for the detection of epidermal growth factor receptor [141]. Liu *et al* (2006) reported an enantioselective molecular imprinting polymer coated QCM for the detection of L tryptophan [142]. Yakovleva *et al* (2010) reported QCM-D bound thiol-modified Au electrodes to detect biospecific glycoprotein–lectin interactions [143]. Apodaca *et al* (2011) reported a QCM bis-terthiophene dendron sensing using a QCM probe coated with an electropolymerized MIP film [144].

6.5 Conclusions and future trends

The change in the resonant frequency of the microbalance (QCM) has increased the detection range and sensitivity when compared with label-free sensor technologies like surface plasmon resonance. The QCMs were initially used in applied physics to study metals in vacuum but later, they were used in chemistry, biology, materials science, medicine, and environmental monitoring. The QCM-based sensing method has demonstrated construction of simultaneous surface plasmon resonance (SPR) and QCM sensing platform reported by Kim *et al* (2010) [145].

The quartz crystal microbalance with dissipation (QCM-D) is real time, label-free measurements of molecular adsorption and/or interactions on various surfaces in a liquid environment. A device based on the simultaneous QCM and electrochemical measurements (EQCM) is useful for studying electroplated, evaporated, or sputtered materials. The QCM sensing concept using advanced analytical techniques such as SPR-based BIAcore instruments from GE Healthcare offer tremendous advantages in industries, academia, and healthcare. However, development of a combined system, such as QCM, QCM-D and SPR or QCM and EQCM measurement systems are useful analytical techniques. The changes in frequency, energy dis-sipation, and NPs will have a tremendous impact of QCM for the future applications. In this chapter the utility of nanoparticles in QCM biosensors has been discussed. A QCM measuring system is unique in offering an understanding of biological phenomena and biological performances. The QCM-D technology monitors cells in real time using a label-free method. Several phenomena can also be detected such as initial cell binding, focal adhesion formation, cell spreading, and complex changes in cytoskeleton.

Acknowledgement

The author would like to extend their gratitude of thanks to Vice-chancellor, Indira Gandhi National Tribal University, for providing facilities to prepare this chapter and is also thankful to all the faculty members of Department of Biotechnology, Indira Gandhi National Tribal University, Amarkantak, M.P., India for their support.

References

[1] Cady W G 1946 *Piezoelectricity* (New York: McGraw-Hill)

[2] Curie J and Curie P 1880 An oscillating quartz crystal mass detector *Rendu* **91** 294–7

[3] Lippman G 1881 Principe de conservation de lelectricite *Ann. Chim. Phys.* **24** 145–78

[4] Guilbault G G, Hock B and Schmid R A 1992 A piezoelectric immunobiosensor for atrazine in drinking water *Biosens. Bioelectron.* **7** 411–9

[5] O'Sullivan C K and Guilbault G G 1999 Commercial quartz crystal microbalances – theory and applications *Biosens. Bioelectron.* **14** 663–70

[6] Dirria F, Palombaa E, Longobardoa A, Zampettib E, Sagginc B and Scaccabarozzic D 2019 A review of quartz crystal microbalances for space applications *Sens. Actuators* A **287** 48–75

[7] Sauerbrey G Z 1959 Use of quartz vibration for weighing thin films on a microbalance *Phys. J.* **155** 206–12

[8] Rodahl M and Kasemo B 1996 A simple setup to simultaneously measure the resonant frequency and the absolute dissipation factor of a quartz crystal microbalance *Rev. Sci. Instrum.* **67** 3238–41

[9] Dixon M C 2008 Quartz crystal microbalance with dissipation monitoring: enabling real-time characterization of biological materials and their interactions *J. Biomol. Tech.* **19** 151

[10] Ward M D and Buttry D A 1990 In situ interfacial mass detection with piezoelectric transducers *Science* **249** 1000–7

[11] Lack F, Willard G and Fair I 1934 Some improvements in quartz crystal circuit elements *Bell Syst. Tech. J.* **13** 453–63

[12] Bradshaw L 2000 Understanding piezoelectric quartz crystals *RF Des.* **23** 50–9

[13] Warner A W and Stockbridge C D 1963 Quartz resonators; reduction of transient frequency excursion due to temperature change *J. Appl. Phys.* **34** 437–8

[14] Nomura T and Hattori O 1980 Determination of micromolar concentrations of cyanide in solution with a piezoelectric detector *Anal. Chim. Acta.* **115** 323–6

[15] Wegener J, Seebach J, Janshoff A and Galla H J 2000 Analysis of the composite response of shear wave resonators to the attachment of mammalian cells *Biophys. J.* **78** 2821–33

[16] Voinova M V, Rodahl M, Jonson M and Kasemo B 1999 Viscoelastic acoustic response of layered polymer films at fluid–solid interfaces: continuum mechanics approach *Phys. Scr.* **59** 391–6

[17] Cho N J, Frank C W, Kasemo B and Hook F 2010 Quartz crystal microbalance with dissipation monitoring of supported lipid bilayers on various substrates *Nat. Protoc.* **5** 1096–106

[18] Reviakine I, Johannsmann D and Richter R P 2011 Hearing what you cannot see and visualizing what you hear: interpreting quartz crystal microbalance data from solvated interfaces *Anal. Chem.* **83** 8838–48

[19] Kanazawa K K and Gordon J G II 1985 Frequency of a quartz microbalance in contact with liquid *Anal. Chem.* **57** 1770–1

[20] Syariena A, Salleh M M and Yahaya M 2008 The performance of quartz crystal microbalance coated TiO_2–porphyrin nanocomposite thin film gas sensors *Sens. Lett.* **6** 903–7

[21] Wang L 2020 Metal–organic frameworks for QCM-based gas sensors: a review *Sens. Actuators* A **307** 111984

[22] Chena Q, Xuab S, Liuc Q, Masliyahc J and Xuac Z 2016 QCM-D study of nanoparticle interactions *Adv. Colloid Interface Sci.* **233** 94–114
[23] Chen J Y, Penn L S and Xi J 2018 Quartz crystal microbalance: sensing cell–substrate adhesion and beyond *Biosens. Bioelectron.* **99** 593–602
[24] Liu Y, Jaiswal A, Poggi M A and Wilson W D 2011 Surface Plasmon Resonance and Quartz Crystal Microbalance Methods for Detection of Molecular Interactions. In *Chemosensors* (eds?B Wang, B Wang and E V Anslyn). http//doi.org/10.1002/9781118019580.ch16)
[25] Marx K A 2003 Quartz crystal microbalance: a useful tool for studying thin polymer films and complex biomolecular systems at the solution–surface interface *Biomacromolecules* **4** 1099–120
[26] Janshoff A, Galla H J and Steinem C 2000 Piezoelectric mass-sensing devices as biosensors. An alternative to optical biosensors *Angew. Chem. Int. Ed.* **39** 4004–32
[27] Braunhut S, McIntosh D, Vorotnikova E, Zhou T and Marx K A 2005 Detection of apoptosis and drug resistance of human breast cancer cells to taxane treatments using quartz crystal microbalance biosensor technology *Assay Drug Dev. Technol.* **3** 77–88
[28] Kim Y S, Niazi J H and Gu M B 2009 Specific detection of oxytetracycline using DNA aptamer-immobilized interdigitated array electrode chip *Anal. Chim. Acta.* **634** 250–4
[29] Fang L, Lu Z, Wei H and Wang E 2008 A electrochemiluminescence aptasensor for detection of thrombin incorporating the capture aptamer labeled with gold nanoparticles immobilized onto the thio-silanized ITO electrode *Anal. Chim. Acta.* **628** 80–6
[30] Yao C Y, Zhu T Y, Qi Y Z, Zhao Y H, Xia H and Fu W L 2010 Development of a quartz crystal microbalance biosensor with aptamers as bio-recognition element *Sens.* **10** 5859–71
[31] Wu V C H, Chen S H and Lin C S 2007 Real-time detection of *Escherichia coli* O157:H7 sequences using a circulating-flow system of quartz crystal microbalance *Biosens. Bioelectron.* **22** 2967–75
[32] Agasti S S, Rana S, Park M H, Kim C K, You C C and Rotello V M 2010 Nanoparticles for detection and diagnosis *Adv. Drug Deliv. Rev.* **62** 316–28
[33] Rounaghi G H, Mohamadzadehkakhki R and Azizi-Toupkanloo H 2012 Voltammetric determination of 4-nitrophenol using a modified carbon paste electrode based on a new synthetic crown ether/silver nanoparticles *Mater. Sci. Eng.* C **32** 172–7
[34] Ahirwal G K and Mitra C K 2010 Gold nanoparticles based sandwich electrochemical immunosensor *Biosens. Bioelectron.* **25** 2016–20
[35] Chu X, Zhao Z L, Shen G L and Yu R Q 2006 Quartz crystal microbalance immunoassay with dendritic amplification using colloidal gold immunocomplex *Sens. Actuators* B **114** 696–704
[36] Jin X, Jin X, Chen L, Jiang J, Shen G and Yu R 2009 Piezoelectric immunosensor with gold nanoparticles enhanced competitive immunoreaction technique for quantification of aflatoxin B1 *Biosens. Bioelectron.* **24** 2580–5
[37] Chu P T, Lin C S, Chen W J, Chen C F and Wen H W 2012 Detection of gliadin in foods using a quartz crystal microbalance biosensor that incorporates gold nanoparticles *J. Agric. Food Chem.* **60** 6483–92
[38] Kaewphinit T, Santiwatanakul S and Chansiri K 2012 Gold nanoparticle amplification combined with quartz crystal microbalance DNA based biosensor for detection of mycobacterium tuberculosis *Sens. Transducers J.* **146** 156–63

[39] Willner I, Patolsky F, Weimann Y and Willner B 2002 Amplified detection of single-base mismatches in DNA using microgravimetric quartz-crystal-microbalance transduction *Talanta.* **56** 847–56
[40] Hao R Z, Song H B, Zuo G M, Yang R F, Wei H P, Wang D B, Cui Z Q, Zhang Z, Cheng Z X and Zhang X E 2011 DNA probe functionalized QCM biosensor based on gold nanoparticle amplification for *Bacillus anthracis* detection *Biosens. Bioelectron.* **26** 3398–404
[41] Chen S H, Chuang Y C, Lu Y C, Lin H C, Yang Y L and Lin C S 2009 A method of layer-by-layer gold nanoparticle hybridization in a quartz crystal microbalance DNA sensing system used to detect dengue virus *Nanotechnology* **20** 215501
[42] Scodeller P, Flexer V, Szamocki R, Calvo E J, Tognalli N, Troiani H and Fainstein A 2008 Wired-enzyme core–shell au nanoparticle biosensor *J. Am. Chem. Soc.* **130** 12690–7
[43] Reimhult K, Yoshimatsu K, Risveden K, Chen S, Ye L and Krozer A 2008 Characterization of QCM sensor surfaces coated with molecularly imprinted nanoparticles *Biosens. Bioelectron.* **23** 1908–14
[44] Kong L J, Pan M F, Fang G Z, He X L, Yang Y K, Dai J and Wang S 2014 Molecularly imprinted quartz crystal microbalance sensor based on poly(o-aminothiophenol) membrane and Au nanoparticles for ractopamine determination *Biosens. Bioelectron.* **51** 286–92
[45] Uludag Y and Tothill I E 2010 Development of a sensitive detection method of cancer biomarkers in human serum (75%) using a quartz crystal microbalance sensor and nanoparticles amplification system *Talanta* **82** 277–82
[46] Ma Z F, Wu J L, Zhou T H, Chen Z H, Dong Y, Tang J T and Sui S F 2002 Detection of human lung carcinoma cell using quartz crystal microbalance amplified by enlarging Au nanoparticles *in vitro New J. Chem.* **26** 1795–8
[47] Chen Q, Tang W, Wang D, Wu X, Li N and Liu F 2010 Amplified QCM-D biosensor for protein based on aptamer-functionalized gold nanoparticles *Biosens. Bioelectron.* **26** 575–9
[48] Shan W Q, Pan Y L, Fang H T, Guo M L, Nie Z, Huang Y and Yao S Z 2014 An aptamer-based quartz crystal microbalance biosensor for sensitive and selective detection of leukemia cells using silver-enhanced gold nanoparticle label *Talanta* **126** 130–5
[49] Kaufman E D *et al* 2007 Probing protein adsorption onto mercaptoundecanoic acid stabilized gold nanoparticles and surfaces by quartz crystal microbalance and potential measurements *Langmuir* **23** 6053–62
[50] Su P G and Chang Y P 2008 Low-humidity sensor based on a quartz-crystal microbalance coated with polypyrrole/Ag/TiO_2 nanoparticles composite thin films *Sens. Actuators* B **129** 915–20
[51] Yang Y J, Jiang Y D, Xu J H and Yu J S 2007 Conducting polymeric nanoparticles synthesized in reverse micelles and their gas sensitivity based on quartz crystal microbalance *Polymer* **48** 4459–65
[52] Salam F, Uludag Y and Tothill I E 2013 Real-time and sensitive detection of *Salmonella typhimurium* using an automated quartz crystal microbalance (QCM) instrument with nanoparticles amplification *Talanta* **115** 761–7
[53] Guo X, Lin C S, Chen S H, Ye R and Wu V C H 2012 A piezoelectric immunosensor for specific capture and enrichment of viable pathogens by quartz crystal microbalance sensor, followed by detection with antibody-functionalized gold nanoparticles *Biosens. Bioelectron.* **38** 177–83
[54] Crooks R M and Ricco A J 1998 New organic materials suitable for use in chemical sensor arrays *Acc. Chem. Res.* **31** 219–27

[55] Chen S, Pei R, Zhao T and Dyer D J 2002 Gold nanoparticle assemblies by metal ion-pyridine complexation and their rectified quantized charging in aqueous solutions *J. Phys. Chem.* B **106** 1903–8

[56] Shen G, Wang H, Shen G and Yu R Q 2007 Au nanoparticle network-type thin films formed via mixed assembling and cross-linking route for biosensor application: quartz crystal microbalance study *Anal. Biochem.* **365** 1–6

[57] Liu H and Hu N F 2006 Interaction between myoglobin and hyaluronic acid in their layer-by-layer assembly: quartz crystal microbalance and cyclic voltammetry studies *J. Phys. Chem.* B **110** 14494–502

[58] Guleryuz H, Kaus I, Buron C C, Filiatre C, Hedin N, Bergstrom L and Einarsrud M A 2014 Deposition of silica nanoparticles onto alumina measured by optical reflectometry and quartz crystal microbalance with dissipation techniques *Colloids Surf.* A **443** 384–90

[59] Saitakis M and Gizeli E 2012 Acoustic sensors as a biophysical tool for probing cell attachment and cell/surface interactions *Cell. Mol. Life Sci.* **69** 357–71

[60] Tymchenko N, Nileba E, Voinova M V, Gold J, Kasemo B and Svedhem S 2012 Reversible changes in cell morphology due to cytoskeletal rearrangements measured in real-time by QCM-D *Biointerphases* **7** 43

[61] Westas E, Svanborg L M, Wallin P, Bauer B, Ericson M B and Wennerberg A 2015 Using QCM-D to study the adhesion of human gingival fibroblasts on implant surfaces *J. Biomed. Mater. Res.* A **103** 3139–47

[62] Kao W L, Chang H Y, Lin K Y, Lee Y W and Shyue J J 2017 Effect of surface potential on the adhesion behavior of NIH3T3 cells revealed by quartz crystal microbalance with dissipation monitoring (QCM-D) *J. Phys. Chem.* C **121** 533–41

[63] Kushiro K, Lee C H and Takai M 2016 Simultaneous characterization of protein–material and cell–protein interactions using dynamic QCM-D analysis on SAM surfaces *Biomater. Sci.* **4** 989–97

[64] Chronaki D, Stratiotis D I, Tsortos A, Anastasiadou E and Gizeli E 2016 Screening between normal and cancer human thyroid cells through comparative adhesion studies using the quartz crystal microbalance *Sens. Bio-Sens. Res* **11** 99–106

[65] Reipa V, Almeida J and Cole K D 2006 Long-term monitoring of biofilm growth and disinfection using a quartz crystal microbalance and reflectance measurements *J. Microbiol. Methods* **66** 449–59

[66] Olsson A L, van der Mei J H C, Busscher H J and Sharma P K 2010 Novel analysis of bacterium–substratum bond maturation measured using a quartz crystal microbalance *Langmuir* **26** 11113–7

[67] Olsson A L J, van der Mei H C, Busscher H J and Sharma P K 2011 Acoustic sensing of the bacterium–substratum interface using QCM-D and the influence of extracellular polymeric substances *J. Colloid Interface Sci.* **357** 135–8

[68] Joshi T, Voo Z X, Graham B, Spiccia L and Martin L L 2015 Real-time examination of aminoglycoside activity towards bacterial mimetic membranes using quartz crystal microbalance with dissipation monitoring (QCM-D) *Biochim. Biophys. Acta.* **1848** 385–91

[69] Tonda-Turo C, Carmagnola I and Ciardelli G 2018 Quartz crystal microbalance with dissipation monitoring: a powerful method to predict the *in vivo* behavior of bioengineered surfaces *Front. Bioeng. Biotechnol.* **6** 158

[70] Yao J, Feng B, Zhang Z, Li C, Zhang W, Guo Z, Zhao H and Zhou L 2018 Blood coagulation testing smartphone platform using quartz crystal microbalance dissipation method *Sens. (Basel)* **18** 3073

[71] Felgueiras H P, Murthy N S, Sommerfeld S D, Bras M M, Migonney V and Kohn J 2016 Competitive adsorption of plasma proteins using a quartz crystal microbalance *ACS Appl. Mater. Interfaces* **8** 13207–17

[72] Kompf D, Held J, Müller S F, Drechsel H R, Tschan S C, Northoff H, Mordmüller B and Gehring F K 2016 Real-time measurement of *Plasmodium falciparum*-infected erythrocyte cytoadhesion with a quartz crystal microbalance *Malar. J.* **15** 317

[73] Kojima T 2018 Surface modification enhanced reflection intensity of quartz crystal microbalance sensors upon molecular adsorption *Anal. Sci.* **34** 363–8

[74] Lin P H, Huang S C, Chen K P, Li B R and Li Y K 2018 Effective construction of a high-capacity boronic acid layer on a quartz crystal microbalance chip for high-density antibody immobilization *Sens. (Basel)* **19** 28

[75] Kobayashi J, Arisaka Y, Yui N, Akiyama Y, Yamato M and Okano T 2018 Effect of temperature changes on serum protein adsorption on thermoresponsive cell-culture surfaces monitored by a quartz crystal microbalance with dissipation *Int. J. Mol. Sci.* **19** 1516

[76] Tao W, Lin P, Liu S, Xie Q, Ke S and Zeng X 2017 1-Butyl-3-methylimidazolium tetrafluoroborate film as a highly selective sensing material for non-invasive detection of acetone using a quartz crystal microbalance *Sens. (Basel)* **17** 194

[77] Phan H T, Bartelt-Hunt S, Rodenhausen K B, Schubert M and Bartz J C 2015 Investigation of bovine serum albumin (BSA) attachment onto self-assembled monolayers (SAMs) using combinatorial quartz crystal microbalance with dissipation (QCM-D) and spectroscopic ellipsometry (SE) *PLoS One* **10** e0141282

[78] Rajaram K, Losada-Perez P, Vermeeren V, Hosseinkhani B, Wagner P, Somers V and Michiels L 2015 Real-time analysis of dual-display phage immobilization and autoantibody screening using quartz crystal microbalance with dissipation monitoring *Int. J. Nanomed.* **10** 5237–47

[79] Nielsen J E, Lind T K, Lone A, Gerelli Y, Hansen P R, Jenssen H, Cardenas M and Lund R 2019 A biophysical study of the interactions between the antimicrobial peptide indolicidin and lipid model systems *Biochim. Biophys. Acta Biomembr.* **1861** 1355–64

[80] Liu B, Yu T, Huang R, Su R, Qi W and He Z 2019 Interactions of transition metal dichalcogenide nanosheets with mucin: quartz crystal microbalance with dissipation, surface plasmon resonance, and spectroscopic probing *Front. Chem.* **7** 166

[81] Movilli J, Rozzi A, Ricciardi R, Corradini R and Huskens J 2018 Control of probe density at DNA biosensor surfaces using poly(L-lysine) with appended reactive groups *Bioconjug. Chem.* **29** 4110–8

[82] Miyake Y, Ishikawa S, Kimura Y, Son A, Imai H, Matsuda T, Yamada H, Toshimitsu A and Kondo T 2015 Pharmacokinetics of chiral dendrimer-triamine-coordinated Gd-MRI contrast agents evaluated by *in vivo* MRI and estimated by *in vitro* QCM *Sens. (Basel)* **15** 31973–86

[83] Alexander T E, Lozeau L D and Camesano T A 2019 QCM-D characterization of time-dependence of bacterial adhesion *Cell Surf* **5** 100024

[84] Silva J M, Caridade S G, Costa R R, Alves N M, Groth T, Picart C, Reis R L and Mano J F 2015 pH responsiveness of multilayered films and membranes made of polysaccharides *Langmuir* **31** 11318–28

[85] Browning K L, Lind T K, Maric S, Malekkhaiat-Häffner S, Fredrikson G N, Bengtsson E, Malmsten M and Cárdenas M 2017 Human lipoproteins at model cell membranes: effect of lipoprotein class on lipid exchange *Sci. Rep.* **7** 7478
[86] Bahmanzadeh S, Ruzgas T and Sotres J 2018 Proteolytic degradation of gelatin–tannic acid multilayers *J. Colloid Interface Sci.* **526** 244–52
[87] Heath G R, Li M, Polignano I L, Richens J L, Catucci G, O'Shea P, Sadeghi S J, Gilardi G, Butt J N and Jeuken L J 2016 Layer-by-layer assembly of supported lipid bilayer poly-L-lysine multilayers *Biomacromolecules* **17** 324–35
[88] Peiris D, Spector A F, Lomax-Browne H, Azimi T, Ramesh B, Loizidou M, Welch H and Dwek M V 2017 Cellular glycosylation affects Herceptin binding and sensitivity of breast cancer cells to doxorubicin and growth factors *Sci. Rep.* **7** 43006
[89] Lakshmanan R S, Efremov V, O'Donnell J S and Killard A J 2016 Measurement of the viscoelastic properties of blood plasma clot formation in response to tissue factor concentration-dependent activation *Anal. Bioanal. Chem.* **408** 6581–8
[90] Chouirfa H, Evans M D M, Castner D G, Bean P, Mercier D, Galtayries A, Falentin-Daudré C and Migonney V 2017 Grafting of architecture-controlled poly (styrene sodium sulfonate) onto titanium surfaces using bio-adhesive molecules: surface characterization and biological properties *Biointerphases* **12** 02C418
[91] Dubacheva G V, Araya-Callis C, Geert Volbeda A, Fairhead M, Codée J, Howarth M and Richter R P 2017 Controlling multivalent binding through surface chemistry: model study on streptavidin *J. Am. Chem. Soc.* **139** 4157–67
[92] Dalgarno P A *et al* 2019 Unveiling the multi-step solubilization mechanism of sub-micron size vesicles by detergents *Sci. Rep.* **9** 12897
[93] Geisler S, Barrantes A, Tengvall P, Messersmith P B and Tiainen H 2016 Deposition kinetics of bioinspired phenolic coatings on titanium surfaces. Polyphenols can form functional coatings on a variety of different materials *Langmuir* **32** 8050–60
[94] Fatisson J, Azari F and Tufenkji N 2011 Real-time QCM-D monitoring of cellular responses to different cytomorphic agents *Biosens. Bioelectron.* **26** 3207–12
[95] Kandel J, Lee H S, Sobolewski P, Tomczyk N, Composto R J and Eckmann D M 2014 Chemically grafted fibronectin for use in QCM-D cell studies *Biosens. Bioelectron.* **58** 249–57
[96] Nowacki L, Follet J, Vayssade M, Vigneron P, Rotellini L and Cambay F 2014 Real-time QCM-D monitoring of cancer cell death early events in a dynamic context *Biosens. Bioelectron.* **64** 469–76
[97] Kepp O, Galluzzi L, Lipinski M, Yuan J and Kroemer G 2011 Cell death assays for drug discovery *Nat. Rev. Drug Discov.* **10** 221–37
[98] Zhang S, Bai H, Pi J, Yang P and Cai J 2015 Label-free quartz crystal microbalance with dissipation monitoring of resveratrol effect on mechanical changes and folate receptor expression levels of living MCF-7 cells: a model for screening of drugs *Anal. Chem.* **87** 4797–805
[99] Zhang S, Bai H and Yang P 2015 Real-time monitoring of mechanical changes during dynamic adhesion of erythrocytes to endothelial cells by QCM-D *Chem. Commun.* **51** 11449–51
[100] Friedl P and Gilmour D 2009 Collective cell migration in morphogenesis, regeneration and cancer *Nat. Rev. Mol. Cell Biol.* **10** 445–57

[101] Tarantola M A, Marel K, Sunnick E, Adam H, Wegener J and Janshoff A 2010 Dynamics of human cancer cell lines monitored by electrical and acoustic fluctuation analysis *Integr. Biol.* **2** 139–50

[102] Lu H H, Rao Y K, Wu T Z and Tzeng Y M 2009 Direct characterization and quantification of volatile organic compounds by piezoelectric module chips sensor *Sens. Actuators* B **137** 741–6

[103] Ayad M M and Torad N L 2009 Alcohol vapours sensor based on thin polyaniline salt film and quartz crystal microbalance *Talanta* **78** 1280–5

[104] Bello A, Bianchi F and Careri M *et al* 2007 Potentialities of a modified QCM sensor for the detection of analytes interacting via H-bonding and application to the determination of ethanol in bread *Sens. Actuators* B **125** 321–5

[105] Kikuchi M and Shiratori S 2005 Quartz crystal microbalance (QCM) sensor for CH_3SH gas by using polyelectrolyte-coated sol–gel film *Sens. Actuators* B **108** 564–71

[106] Ying Z, Jiang Y, Du X, Xie G, Yu J and Tai H 2008 Polymer coated sensor array based on quartz crystal microbalance for chemical agent analysis *Eur. Polym. J.* **44** 1157–64

[107] Ying Z, Jiang Y, Du X, Xie G, Yu J and Wang H 2007 PVDF coated quartz crystal microbalance sensor for DMMP vapor detection *Sens. Actuators* B **125** 167–72

[108] Koshets I A, Kazantseva Z I, Shirshov Y M, Cherenok S A and Kalchenko V I 2005 Calixarene films as sensitive coatings for QCM-based gas sensors *Sens. Actuators* B **106** 177–81

[109] Matsuguchi M and Uno T 2006 Molecular imprinting strategy for solvent molecules and its application for QCM-based VOC vapor sensing *Sens. Actuators* B **113** 94–9

[110] Rabe J, Büttgenbach S, Schröder J and Hauptmann P 2003 Monolithic miniaturized quartz microbalance array and its application to chemical sensor systems for liquids *IEEE Sens. J.* **3** 361–8

[111] Dickert F L, Hayden O and Zenkel M E 1999 Detection of volatile compounds with mass-sensitive sensor arrays in the presence of variable ambient humidity *Anal. Chem.* **71** 1338–41

[112] Wyszynski B, Somboon P and Nakamoto T 2008 Chemisorbed PEGylated lipopolymers as sensing film supports for QCM odor sensors *Sens. Actuators* B **130** 857–63

[113] Park J W, Kurosawa S, Aizawa H, Goda Y, Takai M and Ishihara K 2006 Piezoelectric immunosensor for bisphenol A based on signal enhancing step with 2-methacrolyloxyethyl phosphorylcholine polymeric nanoparticle *Analyst* **131** 155–62

[114] Tsuru N, Kikuchi M, Kawaguchi H and Shiratori S 2006 A quartz crystal microbalance sensor coated with MIP for bisphenol A and its properties *Thin Solid Films* **499** 380–5

[115] Kurosawa S, Aizawa H and Park J W 2005 Quartz crystal microbalance immunosensor for highly sensitive 2,3,7,8-tetrachlorodibenzo-*p*-dioxin detection in fly ash from municipal solid waste incinerators *Analyst* **130** 1495–501

[116] Zeng H, Jiang Y, Xie G and Yu J 2007 'Polymer coated QCM sensor with modified electrode for the detection of DDVP *Sens. Actuators* B **122** 1–6

[117] Yuan Y K, Xiao X L and Wang Y S *et al* 2010 Quartz crystal microbalance with β-cyclodextrin/TiO_2 composite films coupled with chemometrics for the simultaneous determination of urinary 1- and 2-naphthol *Sens. Actuators* B **145** 348–54

[118] Matsuguchi M, Kadowaki Y, Noda K and Naganawa R 2007 HCl gas monitoring based on a QCM using morpholine-functional styrene-co-chloromethylstyrene copolymer coatings *Sens. Actuators* B **120** 462–6

[119] Matsuguchi M and Kadowaki Y 2008 Poly (acrylamide) derivatives for QCM-based HCl gas sensor applications *Sens. Actuators* B **130** 842–7

[120] Sun P, Jiang Y, Xie G, Du X and Hu J 2009 A room temperature supramolecular-based quartz crystal microbalance (QCM) methane gas sensor *Sens. Actuators* B **141** 104–8

[121] Xie G, Sun P, Yan X, Du X and Jiang Y 2010 Fabrication of methane gas sensor by layer-by-layer self-assembly of polyaniline/PdO ultra thin films on quartz crystal microbalance *Sens. Actuators* B **145** 373–7

[122] Palaniappan A, Moochhala S, Tay F E H, Su X and Phua N C L 2008 Phthalocyanine/silica hybrid films on QCM for enhanced nitric oxide sensing *Sens. Actuators* B **129** 184–7

[123] Matsuguchi M, Kadowaki Y and Tanaka M 2005 A QCM-based NO_2 gas detector using morpholine-functional cross-linked copolymer coatings *Sens. Actuators* B **108** 572–5

[124] Ding B, Kim J, Miyazaki Y and Shiratori S 2004 Electrospun nanofibrous membranes coated quartz crystal microbalance as gas sensor for NH_3 detection *Sens. Actuators* B **101** 373–80

[125] Van Quy N, Minh V A, Van Luan N, Hung V N and Van Hieu N 2011 Gas sensing properties at room temperature of a quartz crystal microbalance coated with ZnO nanorods *Sens. Actuators* B **153** 188–93

[126] Lee S W, Takahara N, Korposh S, Yang D H, Toko K and Kunltake T 2010 Nanoassembled thin film gas sensors. III. Sensitive detection of amine odors using TiO_2/poly(acrylic acid) ultrathin film quartz crystal microbalance sensors *Anal. Chem.* **82** 2228–36

[127] Zhang C, Wang X, Lin J, Ding B, Yu J and Pan N 2011 Nanoporous polystyrene fibers functionalized by polyethyleneimine for enhanced formaldehyde sensing *Sens. Actuators* B **152** 316–23

[128] Guo H S, Kim J M, Chang S M and Kim W S 2009 Chiral recognition of mandelic acid by L-phenylalanine-modified sensor using quartz crystal microbalance *Biosens. Bioelectron.* **24** 2931–4

[129] Munoz-Aguirre S, Yoshino A, Nakamoto T and Moriizumi T 2007 Odor approximation of fruit flavors using a QCM odor sensing system *Sens. Actuators* B **123** 1101–6

[130] Ozmen A, Fekce F, Ebeoglu M A, Tasaltin C and Ozturk Z Z 2006 Finding the composition of gas mixtures by a phthalocyanine-coated QCM sensor array and an artificial neural network *Sens. Actuators* B **115** 450–4

[131] Zhu Y, Yuan H, Xu J, Xu P and Pan Q 2010 Highly stable and sensitive humidity sensors based on quartz crystal microbalance coated with hexagonal lamelliform monodisperse mesoporous silica SBA-15 thin film *Sens. Actuators* B **144** 164–9

[132] Ayad M M, Prastomo N, Matsuda A and Stejskal J 2010 Sensing of silver ions by nanotubular polyaniline film deposited on quartz-crystal in a microbalance *Synth. Met.* **160** 42–6

[133] Escuderos M E, Sánchez S and Jiménez A 2011 Quartz crystal microbalance (QCM) sensor arrays selection for olive oil sensory evaluation *Food Chem.* **124** 857–62

[134] Reipa V, Purdum G and Choi J 2010 Measurement of nanoparticle concentration using quartz crystal microgravimetry *J. Phys. Chem.* B **114** 16112–7

[135] Buchatip S, Ananthanawat C, Sithigorngul P, Sangvanich P, Rengpipat S and Hoven V P 2010 Detection of the shrimp pathogenic bacteria, *Vibrio harveyi*, by a quartz crystal microbalance-specific antibody based sensor *Sens. Actuators* B **145** 259–64

[136] Yakovleva M E, Moran A P, Safina G R, Wadstrom T and Danielsson B 2011 Lectin typing of *Campylobacter jejuni* using a novel quartz crystal microbalance technique *Anal. Chim. Acta.* **694** 1–5

[137] Wan Y, Zhang D and Hou B 2010 Determination of sulphate-reducing bacteria based on vancomycin-functionalized magnetic nanoparticles using a modification-free quartz crystal microbalance *Biosens. Bioelectron.* **25** 1847–50

[138] Tang D, Li Q, Tang J, Su B and Chen G 2011 An enzyme-free quartz crystal microbalance biosensor for sensitive glucose detection in biological fluids based on glucose/dextran displacement approach *Anal. Chim. Acta.* **686** 144–9

[139] Lin T Y, Hu C H and Chou T C 2004 Determination of albumin concentration by MIP-QCM sensor *Biosens. Bioelectron.* **20** 75–81

[140] Kim N, Kim D K and Cho Y J 2010 Gold nanoparticle-based signal augmentation of quartz crystal microbalance immunosensor measuring C-reactive protein *Curr. Appl Phys.* **10** 1227–30

[141] Chen J C, Sadhasivam S and Lin F H 2011 Label free gravimetric detection of epidermal growth factor receptor by antibody immobilization on quartz crystal microbalance *Process Biochem.* **46** 543–50

[142] Liu F, Liu X, Ng S C and Chan H S O 2006 Enantioselective molecular imprinting polymer coated QCM for the recognition of L-tryptophan *Sens. Actuators* B **113** 234–40

[143] Yakovleva M E, Safina G R and Danielsson B 2010 A study of glycoprotein–lectin interactions using quartz crystal microbalance *Anal. Chim. Acta.* **668** 80–5

[144] Apodaca D C, Pernites R B, Ponnapati R R, Del Mundo F R and Advincula R C 2011 Electropolymerized molecularly imprinted polymer films of a bis-terthiophene dendron: folic acid quartz crystal microbalance sensing *ACS Appl. Mater. Interfaces* **3** 191–203

[145] Kim J, Kim S, Ohashi T, Muramatsu H, Chang S M and Kim W S 2010 Construction of simultaneous SPR and QCM sensing platform *Bioprocess. Biosyst. Eng.* **33** 39–45

IOP Publishing

Analytical Techniques for Biomedical Nanotechnology

Ajeet Kaushik, Sesha S Srinivasan and Yogendra Kumar Mishra

Chapter 7

Application of nuclear magnetic resonance spectroscopy in biomedical nanotechnology

Avtar Singh, Jaspreet Dhau, Rajeev Kumar, Kirandeep Singh and Amritpal Singh

Over the last few decades, the development of nanotechnology has attracted tremendous attention in the biomedical field. Biomedical nanotechnology promises a solution to the challenges associated with this field. In biomedical nanotechnology, various applications of nanotechnology-based materials proved their potential in reforming diagnostic techniques, drug delivery, nanodrugs, and prostheses and implants. Numerous FDA-approved nanomaterial-based products are widely used at commercial levels and clinical trials have staggeringly increased. In the biomedical nanotechnology field, analytical instrumentation techniques play a very important role in all steps from design to resulting products. This chapter provides an overview of the application of nuclear magnetic resonance in biomedical nanotechnology. The various applications of nuclear magnetic spectroscopy, such as in thiols-gold nanoparticles, in nanoclusters and in drug delivery systems, are discussed here. The objective of this chapter is to provide researchers with the knowledge of techniques of nuclear magnetic resonance that are required to apply in biomedical nanotechnology.

Abbreviations

AgNPs	Gold nanoparticles
AuNPs	Silver nanoparticles
AuNSs	Gold nanospheres
BTZ	Bortezomib
CD	Cyclodextrins
COSY	Correlation spectroscopy
DAU	Daunorubicin
DOSY	Diffusion ordered spectroscopy
DSC	Differential scanning calorimetry
FDA	Food and Drug Administration
FTIR	Fourier-transform infrared spectroscopy

doi:10.1088/978-0-7503-3379-5ch7

HPLC	High performance liquid chromatography
XRD	X-ray diffraction
CAP	Captopril
MALDI	Matrix-assisted laser desorption/ionization
NMR	Nuclear magnetic resonance
NOE	Nuclear Overhauser effect
NOESY	Nuclear overhauser effect spectroscopy
PEG	Poly(ethylene glycol)
REDOR	Rotational echo double resonance
ROESY	Rotating frame Overhauser enhancement spectroscopy
SAM	Self-assembled monolayers
SEM	Scanning electron microscopy
TEM	Transmission electron microscopy
TGA	Thermogravimetrical analysis
NPs	Nanoparticles
5FU	5-fluorouracil
PET	phenylethanethiol
ICPMS	Inductively coupled plasma mass spectrometry
ICPOES	Induvtively coupled plasma optical emission spectroscopy
MTAB	(16-mercaptohexadecyl)trimethylammonium bromide

7.1 Introduction

In biomedical research, researchers study human physiology and find ways to prevent and treat diseases for improvements in the lives of people and animals. Researchers continually devote efforts to explore new ways and techniques with the ultimate goal of developing effective treatment and cures [1–8]. In the last three decades, scientists have successfully used nanomaterial-based materials to design, develop, and apply these advanced materials in diverse fields of science [8–14]. Nanoparticles, which have one dimension less than 100 nm at least, have unique physical, chemical, and biological properties [15–18] and hold great promise for a variety of applications, including diagnostic techniques, drug delivery, nanodrugs, and prostheses and implants [19–23]. Currently, in diagnostic techniques, nanotechnology-based approaches for cancer diagnosis are in different phases of clinical trials [24]. Numerous nanoparticles which are approved by the FDA are widely used at a commercial level. Gold nanoparticles are used as label or probe molecules for detection in lateral flow immunoassay devices [25]. Nanotechnology-based drug delivery systems are another major application and have been gaining a lot of interest from researchers and industry [26, 27]. Carbon nanotubes, dendrimers, and liposomes are important tissue engineering scaffold materials and drug delivery systems and have the ability to control the release of a drug or therapeutic compound to impaired tissues [28].

In the biomedical nanotechnology field, analytical instrumentation techniques play a crucial role in synthesis, characterization, exploration of novel properties, application, and resulting devices. The major techniques include transmission electron microscopy, scanning electron microscopy, atomic force microscopy, dynamic light scattering, x-ray diffraction, mass spectroscopy, fluorescence spectroscopy, high performance liquid chromatography, and nuclear magnetic resonance spectroscopy [29–35]. In this chapter, we consider the application of nuclear magnetic resonance spectroscopy in the biomedical nanotechnology field.

Nuclear magnetic resonance spectroscopy has become a sophisticated and powerful analytical technique that has found a variety of applications in many disciplines of science. In the nanotechnology field, NMR spectroscopy is mainly helpful for investigation of step-by-step formation, shapes, composition, and size distribution of nanoparticles [36, 37]. The protecting ligands are also typically studied by NMR, and structural information pertaining to the interaction between a protecting ligand and a metallic surface is of potential significance for the understanding of the nanoparticle core for properties like electronic structure, atomic arrangement, or compositional framework [38, 39]. In the last decade, considerable research has been published using the application of NMR spectroscopy in the biomedical nanotechnology field. An overview of current research on the application of NMR spectroscopy in the biomedical nanotechnology is presented in this chapter.

7.2 Basics of NMR spectroscopy

The nuclear magnetic resonance spectroscopy technique was developed by Felix Bloch and Edward Mills Purcell in 1946, which won them a Nobel Prize in Physics in 1952 [40, 41]. Since then, it has grown to be one of the most powerful and valuable techniques for several scientific disciplines, i.e., chemistry, physics, biology, medicine, engineering, and materials research [42, 43]. NMR spectroscopy depends on the magnetic properties of the atomic nucleus [44]. The nuclear spin possesses a magnetic dipole moment, μ, that is proportional to its nuclear spin angular momentum, I

$$\mu \, \alpha \, I \Rightarrow \mu = \gamma \, I$$

where γ is constant, called the gyromagnetic constant, which is specific to each type of atomic nucleus. The higher the value of constant γ, the more sensitive will the active nucleus in NMR be. The magnitude of vector quantity, I is given by,

$$|\, I \,| = \hbar \sqrt{I} \, (I + 1)$$

In the above equation, I is the nuclear spin angular momentum quantum number, and $\hbar = h/2\pi i$, where h is Planck's constant. In the nucleus, both protons and neutrons have a spin quantum number of 1/2 and depending upon the orientation of particles (+1/2 or −1/2) in the nucleus, the resultant nucleus may have a zero or non-zero nuclear spin quantum number, I. Nuclei that have paired spin, means an even number of both neutrons and protons, there will be no net spin and the nuclear spin quantum number, I, will be zero. This type of nucleus has no magnetic dipole moment, μ, and is not NMR active. The distribution of positive charge in a nucleus of this type is spherical (figure 7.1). Typical examples include ^{4}He, ^{12}C, ^{16}O, and ^{32}S. If the spins of protons and neutrons are not paired, in that case nuclear spin quantum numbers have integer (1, 2, 3, etc) or half integer (1/2, 3/2, 5/2, 7/2, 9/2) values. When I is 1/2, there is one net unpaired spin and this unpaired spin imparts a nuclear magnetic moment, μ, to the nucleus. For nuclei with nuclear spin quantum

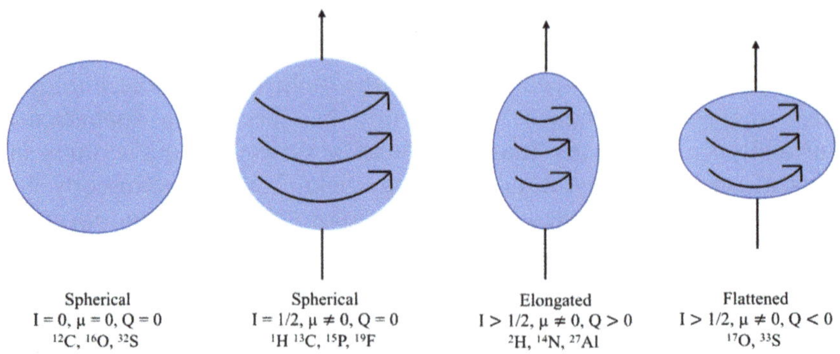

Figure 7.1. Types of nuclei.

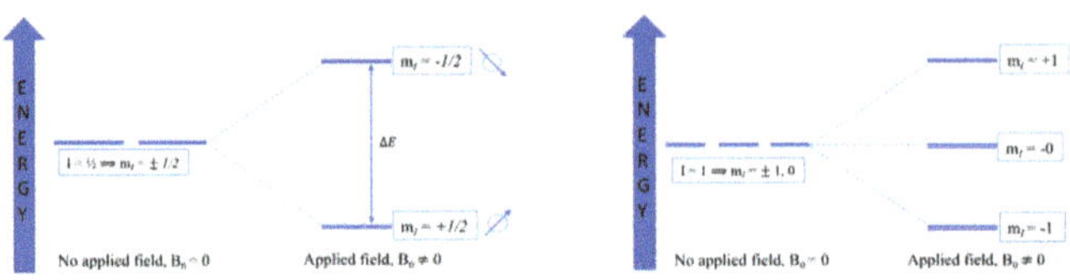

Figure 7.2. Splitting of m_I values in an external magnetic field.

number, *I*, greater than 1/2, the nuclear charge distribution of protons is non-spherical, which gives them an electric quadrupole moment in addition to their magnetic dipole moment (figure 7.1).

Nuclear magnetic resonance spectroscopy is often concerned with nuclei with $I = 1/2$, examples of which include ^{1}H, ^{13}C, ^{15}P, and ^{19}F. The allowed orientations of the nuclear magnetic moment vector in an external magnetic field are indicated by the nuclear spin angular momentum quantum number, m_I, which takes values, $+I$ to $-I$ with a difference of one.

For a ^{1}H nucleus with $I = ½$ ($m_I = \pm 1/2$), $+1/2$ state will be lower in energy and the $-1/2$ state higher, as indicated in figure 7.2. When $I = 1$, m_I has values of 1, 0, and -1, corresponding, respectively, to alignments with, perpendicular to, and opposed to the field (figure 7.2). In the absence of a magnetic field, all orientations of the nuclear moment are degenerate. In the presence of an external field, however, this degeneracy will be removed. NMR spectroscopy deals with bulk samples (more than 10^{14} molecules). The net magnetization, *M*, is a vector sum of individual moments ($\boldsymbol{\mu}$) in the sample.

$$\vec{\mathrm{M}} = \sum \vec{\mu}$$

When the static external magnetic field, B_0, is applied, the nucleus begins to precess about its own axis of spin with angular frequency, ω. This precession frequency is known as Larmor frequency, which is directly proportional to the strength of applied magnetic field. The precession of the nucleus generates an oscillating electric field. If radiofrequency waves of this frequency are supplied to the precessing nucleus, coupling of the oscillating electric field component of incoming radiation with the electric field generated by the precessing nucleus occurs (figure 7.3).

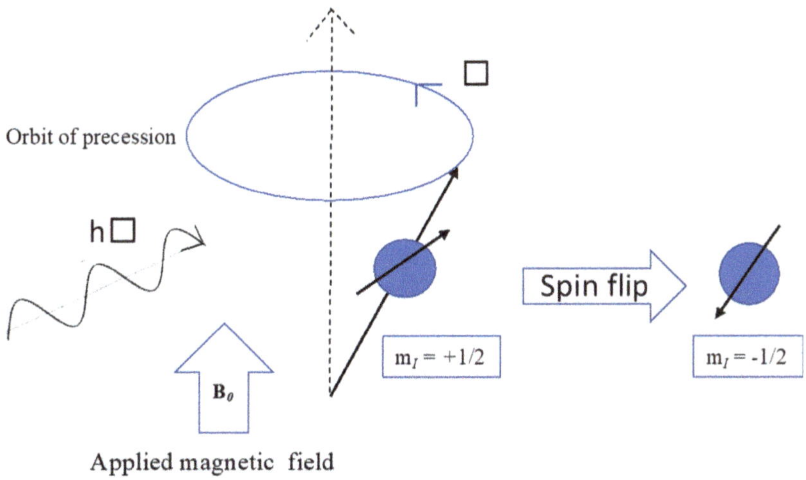

Figure 7.3. Mechanism for spin flipping in an external magnetic field.

The phase coherence among the spins returns to its equilibrium value of net magnetization (as given by the Boltzmann distribution) and is called relaxation. During relaxation electromagnetic energy is retransmitted, which produces an NMR signal. The relaxation process includes two mechanisms, one is longitudinal relaxation, corresponding to longitudinal magnetization recovery (spin–lattice relaxation, T_1) and the second is transverse relaxation corresponding to transverse magnetization decay (spin–spin relaxation, T_2).

7.3 Applications of NMR spectroscopy

NMR spectroscopy is a powerful tool for chemists, physicists, biologists, environmentalists interested in the characterization of particle structure, dynamics, hydrodynamic properties, and interactions from the atomic to supramolecular levels in solution [45]. There are various well-established mono- and multidimensional liquid and solid NMR techniques, which have proven to be very useful for the characterization of different aspects of nanoparticles and have helped to solve many complicated structural determinations. These techniques include cross-polarization, magic-angle spinning (MAS), DOSY, COSY, NOSEY, ROESY, REDOR. In this section, applications of nuclear magnetic resonance spectroscopy are divided into three parts (figure 7.4).

7.3.1 NMR application in gold-thiols nanoparticles

In the last two decades, NPs such as silver and gold have been studied extensively because of their wide applications in the biomedical field owing to their remarkable physicochemical properties [46–50]. These nanoparticles can be synthesized and functionalized with different ligands, including thiol, selenol, phosphine, and carbene-terminated ligands [51–55]. The surface chemistry of NPs depends upon metal–ligand chemical bonds or electrostatic interactions which play a major role

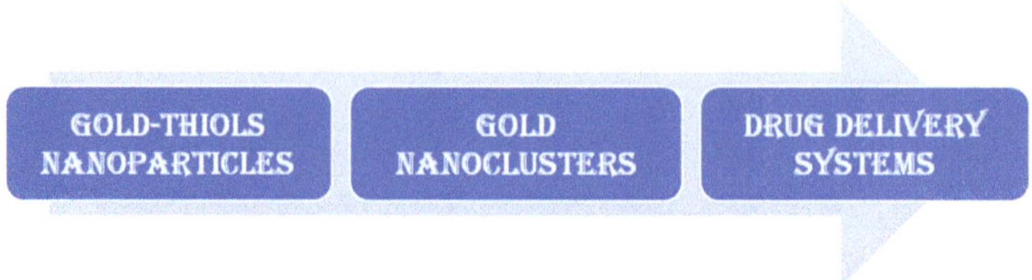

Figure 7.4. Applications of nuclear magnetic resonance spectroscopy.

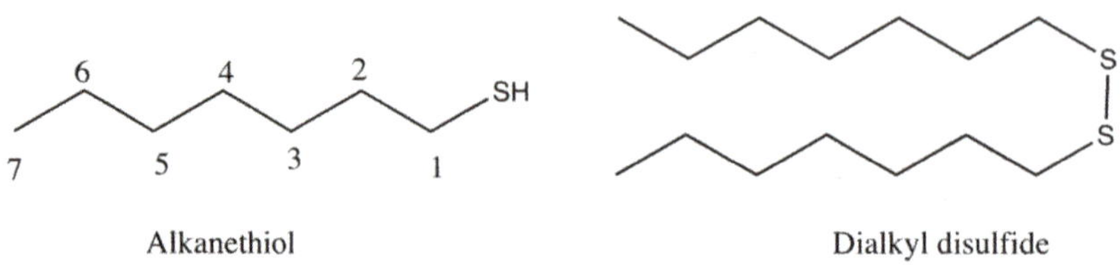

Figure 7.5. Structure of alkanethiol and dialkyl disulfide.

and impact almost every aspect like nucleation and growth of nanoparticles, optoelectronic properties, toxicity and chemical and colloidal stability. In the case of gold nanoparticles, the different ligands based upon thiol group-containing molecules like alkyl-/arylthiols or L-cysteine are well-studied compounds [56–59].

Several techniques have been developed in order to investigate the interaction between ligands and nanometal surfaces. For example, TEM and SEM are used to investigate morphology and size determination [60], optical spectroscopies are able to understand optical properties and quantitative descriptions of ligand shells [61], ICPMS and ICPOES have been used to monitor the ligand density of nano-structures, molecular formula for molecular-like nanoclusters [62], Single crystal x-ray crystallography is able to determine the size of the nanostructures [63] and the exact stacking patterns of atoms and TGA has also been applied to measure the number of ligands appended to nanoparticles [64]. NMR spectroscopy is the most powerful tool in chemical science. and provides great potential in elucidating the surface chemistry of ligand shells on nanoparticles [65–68]. The NMR technique has been increasingly used in recent years to elucidate the surface chemistry of ligand shells on nanoparticles.

SAMs are molecular assemblies, formed on some surfaces by adsorption and are organized into more or less large ordered domains. SAMs of thiols on gold have emerged as important elements to set up many systems that have various potential applications in the field of nanotechnology. Badia *et al* [69] studied alkylthiol SAMs formed on gold nanoparticles, and by using solid-state NMR, they provided evidence for the formation of sulfur–gold bonds. Before this study, metal–sulfur bonding in alkylthiol SAMs formed on gold surfaces was suggested through thiolates and dialkyl disulfides (figure 7.5). This ambiguous bonding mode was solved by Badia and co-workers by using solid-state NMR. The solid-state ^{13}C NMR spectra of unlabeled

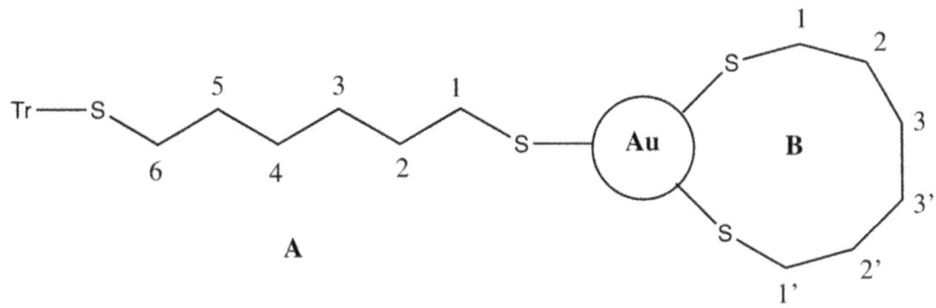

Figure 7.6. Mixed self-assembled monolayer stabilized gold nanoparticles with thiol functionalities.

short-chain (C_4) and isotopically-labeled long-chain (C_{14}) alkylthiols bound to gold nanoparticles were recorded. In $C_{14}S/Au$ nanoparticles, selective ^{13}C labeling of carbons 1 and 2 was used to enhance and resolve these signals which are weak as a result of extensive line broadening. In the [1-^{13}C]- and [2-^{13}C] labeled $C_{14}S/Au$ nanoparticles, ^{13}C resonances for the respective nuclei proximal to the sulfur showed noticeable downfield shift by 18 ppm for C1 and 12 ppm for C2 compared to the free thiol, which ruled out the possibility of other bonding modes. Many thiols-gold/silver studies have since been investigated using NMR spectroscopy, which confirms the validity of this technique in confirming thiol–NP interactions.

Wallner *et al* [70] used the one-pot single phase method for the preparation of stable mixed molecular-monolayer-coated gold nanoparticles, in which AuNPs were coated with R,ω-alkanedithiols whose outer ω-thiol is protected by a triphenylmethyl group (figure 7.6). The outer thiol groups at one terminus remain unbound, providing the opportunity for the covalent attachment of the nanoparticle to a surface or to a macromolecule. They exploited a combination of several one- and two-dimensional NMR spectroscopic techniques to identify and quantify mixed types of Au–S bonded alkanedithiols on gold nanoparticles. In NMR characterization, the ^1H NMR line widths for A-type molecules were compared with free molecules and slightly broader signals were found. Also, similar broadening was found for the ^{13}C NMR signals. The signals for B are much broader indicating the B molecule is attached to Au with both thiol groups which restricts their mobility in comparison to A. In the ^1H NMR spectrum, six different chemical shifts are observed in the aliphatic region because of six different methylene groups of A molecule (1,6-hexanedithiols with protected outer thiol). In contrast, for doubly Au–S linked, B molecules exhibited only three signals due to their symmetry. Diffusion NMR spectroscopic experiments were also performed to confirm bonding modes.

Cysteine is a non-essential amino acid containing a thiol group. This thiol group allows cysteine to bond with gold in a special way. Cysteine is an important molecule because it can be involved in hydrogen bonding with its neighbors. In order to avoid excessive broadening of solution state ^{13}C resonance caused by long rotational correlation times of gold nanoparticles, Abraham and co-workers [71] used the solid-state NMR technique characterization of the interaction between L-cysteine and 6.6 nm gold nanoparticles. The REDOR technique was used to detect ^{13}C–^{15}N dipolar couplings. Analysis of these couplings provides information about the

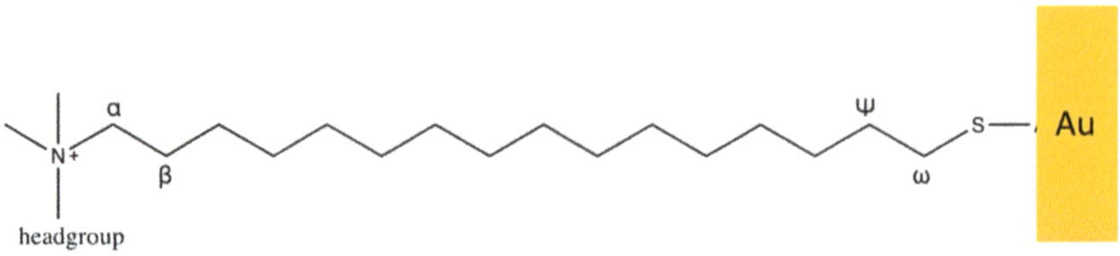

Figure 7.7. MTAB gold nanospheres.

evidence for two types of cysteine molecules in Au–cysteine, which is further supported by TGA. In their results they concluded that one type is attached to the gold surface by the sulfur and its charged amino and carboxyl groups are oriented away from the surface. The other type of cysteine molecules form an outer layer and the charged amino and carboxyl groups of the outer layer interact with their counterparts in the inner layer.

Meng Wu and co-workers [72] reported a solution NMR-based analysis to study ligand environments on larger nanoparticles. This study used (16-mercaptohexadecyl)trimethylammonium bromide (MTAB) self-assembled monolayers on colloidal AuNSs (figure 7.7). In order to investigate the role of surface curvature of nanoparticle on the ligand environment and to check the suitability of the presented method on the upper size limit of nanoparticles, MTAB AuNSs of sizes ranging from 1.4 to 25 nm were synthesized. ^{1}H NMR experiments performed for series of MTAB-AuNSs of given diameters in D_2O: (A) 1.2 ± 0.3 nm, (B) 4.8 ± 1.1 nm, (C) 6.4 ± 1.1 nm, (D) 8.2 ± 0.9 nm, (E) 10.8 ± 0.8 nm, (F) 13.4 ± 1.2 nm, (G) 19.3 ± 3.0 nm, (H) 25.0 ± 4.4 nm, and results were compared with ^{1}H NMR spectra of free MTAB ligand. In NMR spectra two broadened signals appeared, one at about 3 ppm for headgroup protons and another was centered at about 1.3 ppm for the main chain protons with more broadening because of a shorter distance from the core. In a series of different sizes of nanoparticles, the main chain proton signals gradually broaden into the baseline and the headgroup proton signals can still be detected for nanoparticles of sizes up to 25 nm. This study concluded that for MTAB-AuNSs, ~25 nm is the largest size that is suitable for solution NMR analysis.

7.3.2 NMR application in gold nanoclusters

Monolayer-protected metal clusters, also known as nanoclusters, are of a few tens to hundreds of metal atoms with dimensions in the nanometer range. They can be mono- or multi-elemental compounds. Nanoclusters (gold, silver, platinum, zinc, copper, etc) with sizes less than 2 nm possess special fluorescent properties making them suitable for biomedical applications [73–75]. Fluorescent gold nanoclusters have attracted much more attention than other metal nanomaterials because of biocompatibility, low cytotoxicity, high photostability, and are easily functionalized with other biomolecules. In the literature a number of studies reported using different techniques to investigate different nanoclusters. Few studies are available in which the NMR technique was employed to explore gold nanoclusters.

Salorinne and co-workers [76] presented DOSY to estimate the size of thiol stabilized gold nanoclusters in solution. The hydrodynamic radius and diffusion coefficient were determined for three well known monodisperse PET stabilized gold nanoclusters, and in their results they found the hydrodynamic diameters of 1.7, 2.2, and 3.1 nm for the $Au_{25}(PET)_{18}$, $Au_{38}(PET)_{24}$, and $Au_{144}(PET)_{60}$, respectively. These results agreed well with the theoretically predicted structures reported in the literature.

Pengo *et al* [77] investigated kinetic studies for exchange reactions between neutral $Au_{25}(SCH_2CH_2Ph)_{18}$ cluster and para substituted arylthiols. The Au_{25} cluster ($Au_{25}(SCH_2CH_2Ph)_{18}$) has six dimeric staples, which are symmetrically equivalent (figure 7.8). The ligands found at the inequivalent positions of the staple were labeled as inner (in) and outer (out). They explored the effect of the incoming thiol's structure on the reactivity of the inequivalent sites of the staple. The kinetic profiles were built by monitoring the time evolution of the integrals of the signals belonging to the protons on the outer site, the proton on the inner site and b-H of the 2-phenylethanethiol (6) formed during the reaction. In their results they found that site selectivity for exchange reaction depends on the structure of the incoming thiol employed. In the case of 4-fluorobenzylthiol as the incoming ligand, the outer position is more reactive than the inner position. The ligand exchange reaction with thiophenol has no site selectivity, both sites are equivalent. In a series of 4-substituted arylthiols, the outer reactivity increases with increasing electron donating properties of the substituent.

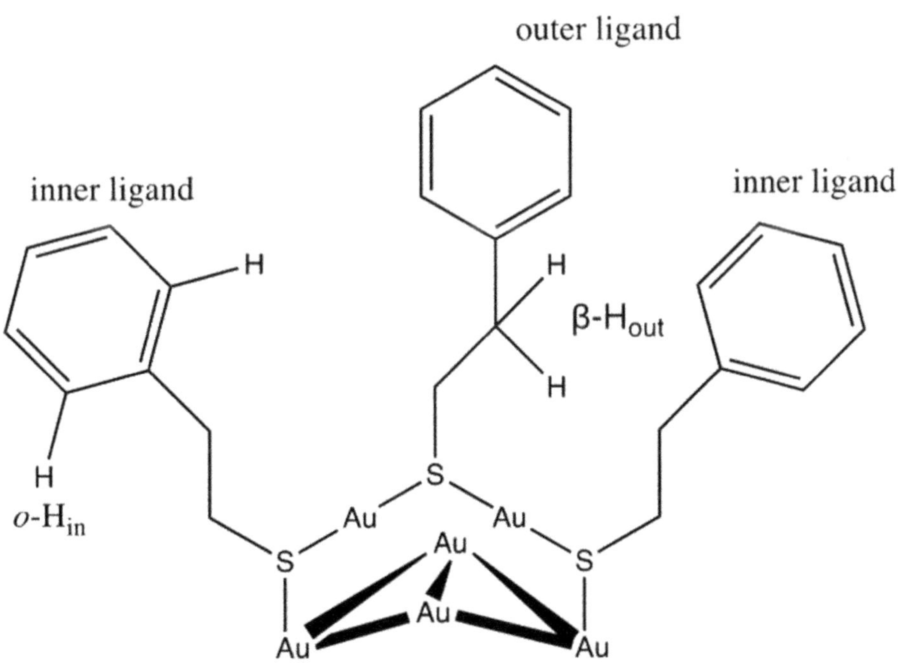

Figure 7.8. Structure of dimeric staple.

Salassa and co-workers [78] investigated the monolayer reactivity in $Au_{25}(SR)_{18}$ using NMR spectroscopy and MALDI mass spectrometry. They investigated the effects of several factors on the thiol exchange reaction, including stability of the thiols in solution, the affinity of the sulfur to the gold cluster, intermolecular interactions within the ligand layer.

A special feature of NMR is its possibility to study symmetric reactions like exchange reactions where starting materials and products are identical. Smith *et al* [79] used nuclear magnetic resonance spectroscopy methods to quantify the extent of ligand exchange between different types of thiolated molecules on the surface of gold nanoparticles and suggested that ligand addition mechanisms are strongly influenced by two factors, the first is the ligand functionalities directly interacting with the nanoparticle surface and second is intermolecular interactions within the ligand shell itself. In another study, Kluenker and co-workers [68] presented a proton NMR (^{1}H NMR) study on the ligand exchange of oleylamine by 1-octadecanethiol as a function of the particle size and repeated functionalization on AuNPs. In their results they showed efficient surface coverage depends on (i) repeated exchange reactions with large ligand excess, (ii) size of NPs, that is, the surface curvature and reactivity, and (iii) molecular size of the ligand.

7.3.3 Application of NMR in drug delivery systems

Bortezomib (BTZ) is a dipeptide boronic acid used as an anticancer drug. In the literature, AuNPs are confirmed as the drug delivery vehicle for BTZ in cancer therapy. Coelho *et al* [80] reported NMR spectroscopy in combination with FTIR, UV–Vis, DLS and TEM to study the structure and physicochemical properties of surface modified gold nanoparticles modified with poly(ethylene glycol) (PEG) which they designed for the drug delivery of the proteasome inhibitor BTZ in cancer therapy. They used NMR parameters such as spectral line shape, translation diffusion, the nuclear Overhauser effect (NOE), and spin–lattice relaxation (T_1) to explore intermolecular interactions and mechanisms of drug immobilization and location into surface modified gold nanoparticles. The results showed that two sets of BTZ protons (BTZ* and BTZ**) exist in the ^{1}H NMR spectrum of PEGAuNPs +BTZ, and no indication was found for chemical bonds between BTZ and PEGAuNPs. BTZ–PEGAuNPs interactions and the mechanism of drug incorporation were studied using diffusion ordered NMR spectroscopy and the NOE. The BTZ* molecules in PEGAuNPs+BTZ are distributed by weak H-bonds and/or dipole–charge interactions with polymer chains from the PEG layer coating of the AuNPs whereas BTZ** exist by adsorption on the surface of the gold nanoparticles.

Cyclodextrins can be used as drug delivery vehicles because of modifying physical, chemical, and biological properties. Cyclodextrin-containing drug formulations have been extensively studied and characterized with various techniques. Azevedo and co-workers reported the inclusion complex of CAP and three CDs and prepared different types of nanoparticles [81]. In addition to NMR, they used FTIR, DSC, XRD, and SEM to analyze the inclusion complexes. The complexation-induced chemical shifts of CAP were the first evidence of CAP inclusion in CDs.

Further they used ROESY and diffusion ordered spectroscopy experiments in order to find the inclusion mode of the complexes in aqueous solution.

Ivanova and colleagues used NMR spectroscopy for structural characterization and to determine particular intermolecular interactions and mechanisms of drug immobilization in the polymer matrix [82]. For this study, they used polymer-poly (butylcyanoacrylate) nanoparticles and drug-daunorubicin which is a chemotherapy medication. Diffusion ordered NMR spectroscopy and spin–lattice relaxation time (T_1) determinations allowed the exploration of intermolecular interactions between the drug and the polymer nanoparticles and the mechanism of drug immobilization. In their results they found the coexistence of three different types of interaction between daunorubicin and poly(butylcyanoacrylate) nanoparticles which are (i) association with the polymer chain by H-bonds and/or dipole–charge interactions, (ii) physical entrapment in the polymer matrix, and (iii) adsorption on the surface of the nanoparticles. In another study, Simeonova *et al* used two different drug loading approaches for loading two anticancer drugs 5FU and DAU on poly(butylcyanoacrylate) nanoparticles [83]. They reported results based upon NMR spectroscopy for structural determination and physicochemical characteristics of drug loaded polymer and concluded that a different composition and structure could be designed by different methods of preparation.

7.4 Conclusion

The use of nanotechnology has shown great potential in the biomedical field owing to their unique physicochemical properties. In the last two decades, there has been growing interest in the development of sensitive, selective, and powerful methods for characterizing nanomaterials and to discovering other aspects of nanomaterials. NMR spectroscopy has emerged as a sophisticated and powerful analytical technique that has found a variety of applications in biomedical nanotechnology. The objective of this chapter is to provide researchers with knowledge of the techniques of NMR required to apply it in biomedical nanotechnology. The applications presented in this chapter strongly emphasize the use of nuclear magnetic resonance spectroscopy in understanding the use of nanomaterials in the biomedical field and are divided into three parts: (1) application of NMR in gold–thiol nanoparticles, (2) application of NMR in gold nanoclusters, and (3) application of NMR in drug delivery systems.

References

[1] Tu Z, Zhong Y, Hu H, Shao D, Haag R, Schirner M, Lee J, Sullenger B and Leong K W 2022 Design of therapeutic biomaterials to control inflammation *Nat. Rev. Mater.* **7** 557–74

[2] Singh A, Kaushik A, Dhau J S and Kumar R 2022 Exploring coordination preferences and biological applications of pyridyl-based organochalcogen (Se, Te) ligands *Coord. Chem. Rev.* **450** 214254

[3] Perera A S and Coppens M-O 2019 Re-designing materials for biomedical applications: from biomimicry to nature-inspired chemical engineering *Phil. Trans. R. Soc.* A **377** 20180268

[4] Dhau J S, Singh A, Brandão P and Felix V 2021 Synthesis, characterization, X-ray crystal structure and antibacterial activity of bis[3-(4-chloro-*N*,*N*-diethylpyridine-2-carboxamide)] diselenide *Inorg. Chem. Commun.* **133** 108942

[5] Tibbitt M W, Rodell C B, Burdick J A and Anseth K S 2015 Progress in material design for biomedical applications *Proc. Natl Acad. Sci. USA.* **112** 14444–51

[6] Dhau J S, Singh A, Singh A, Sharma N, Brandão P, Félix V, Singh B and Sharma V 2015 A mechanistic study on synthesis, single crystal X-ray and anticarcinogenic potential of bis(2-pyridyl)selenides and-diselenides *RSC Adv.* **5** 78669–76

[7] Dhau J S, Singh A, Singh A and Sooch B S 2014 A study on the antioxidant property of pyridylselenium compounds and their slow release from poly(acrylamide) hydrogels *Phosphorus Sulfur, Silicon Relat. Elem* **189** 687–99

[8] Singh A, Singh P, Kumar R and Kaushik A 2022 Exploring nanoselenium to tackle mutated SARS-CoV-2 for efficient COVID-19 management *Front. Nanotechnol.* **4** 1004729

[9] Baig N, Kammakakam I and Falath W 2021 Nanomaterials: a review of synthesis methods, properties, recent progress, and challenges *Mater. Adv.* **2** 1821–71

[10] Salata O V 2004 Applications of nanoparticles in biology and medicine *J. Nanobiotechnol.* **2** 3

[11] Lastra L S, Sharma V, Farajpour N, Nguyen M and Freedman K J 2021 Nanodiagnostics: a review of the medical capabilities of nanopores *Nanomedicine: NBM* **37** 102425

[12] Singh T, Shukla S, Kumar P, Wahla V, Bajpai V K and Rather I A 2017 Application of nanotechnology in food science: perception and overview *Front. Microbiol* **8** 1501

[13] Singh A, Dhau J S and Kumar R 2021 Application of carbon-based nanomaterials for removal of hydrocarbons ed R Kumar, R Kumar and G Kaur *New Frontiers of Nanomaterials in Environmental Science* (Singapore: Springer)

[14] Mauter M S and Elimelech M 2008 Environmental applications of carbon-based nanomaterials *Environ. Sci. Technol.* **42** 5843–59

[15] Laurent S, Forge D, Port M, Roch A, Robic C, Elst L V and Muller R N 2010 Magnetic iron oxide nanoparticles: synthesis, stabilization, vectorization, physicochemical characterizations, and biological applications *Chem. Rev.* **110** 2574

[16] Jeevanandam J, Barhoum A, Chan Y S, Dufresne A and Danquah M K 2018 Review on nanoparticles and nanostructured materials: history, sources, toxicity and regulations *Beilstein J. Nanotechnol.* **9** 1050–74

[17] Yang L, Zhang L and Webster T J 2011 Nanobiomaterials: state of the art and future trends *Adv. Eng. Mater.* **6** B197–217

[18] Ren Q, Ga L, Lu Z, Ai J and Wang T 2020 Aptamer-functionalized nanomaterials for biological applications *Mater. Chem. Front.* **4** 1569–85

[19] Pelaz B, Alexiou C, Alvarez-Puebla R A, Alves F, Andrews A M and Ashraf S *et al* 2017 Applications of nanomedicine *ACS Nano* **11** 2313–81

[20] Laroui H, Rakhya P, Xiao B, Viennois E and Merlin D 2013 Nanotechnology in diagnostics and therapeutics for gastrointestinal disorders *Dig. Liver. Dis.* **45** 995–1002

[21] Onoue S, Yamada S and Chan H K 2014 Nanodrugs: pharmacokinetics and safety *Int. J. Nanomed.* **9** 1025–37

[22] Jahangirian H, Lemraski E G, Webster T J, Rafiee-Moghaddam R and Abdollahi Y 2017 A review of drug delivery systems based on nanotechnology and green chemistry: green nanomedicine *Int. J. Nanomed.* **12** 2957–78

[23] Gavaskar A, Rojas D and Videla F 2018 Nanotechnology: the scope and potential applications in orthopedic surgery *Eur. J. Orthop. Surg. Traumatol.* **28** 1257–60

[24] Engelberth S A, Hempel N and Bergkvist M 2014 Development of nanoscale approaches for ovarian cancer therapeutics and diagnostics *Crit. Rev. Oncog.* **19** 281–315

[25] Banerjee R and Jaiswal A 2018 Recent advances in nanoparticle-based lateral flow immunoassay as a point-of-care diagnostic tool for infectious agents and diseases *Analyst* **143** 1970–96

[26] Shi J, Votruba A R, Farokhzad O C and Langer R 2010 Nanotechnology in drug delivery and tissue engineering: from discovery to applications *Nano Lett.* **10** 3223–30

[27] Farokhzad O C and Langer R 2009 Impact of nanotechnology on drug delivery *ACS Nano* **3** 16–20

[28] Mody N, Tekade R K, Mehra N K, Chopdey P and Jain N K 2014 Dendrimer, liposomes, carbon nanotubes and PLGA nanoparticles: one platform assessment of drug delivery potential *AAPS Pharm. Sci. Tech* **15** 388–99

[29] Sandler S E, Fellows B and Mefford O T 2019 Best practices for characterization of magnetic nanoparticles for biomedical applications *Anal. Chem.* **91** 14159–69

[30] Hurley K R, Ring H L, Kang H, Klein N D and Haynes C L 2015 Characterization of magnetic nanoparticles in biological matrices *Anal. Chem.* **87** 11611–9

[31] Lopez-Cebral R, Martin-Pastor M, Seijo B and Sanchez A 2014 Progress in the characterization of bio-functionalized nanoparticles using NMR methods and their applications as MRI contrast agents *Prog. Nucl. Magn. Reson. Spectrosc* **79** 1–13

[32] Mourdikoudis S, Pallares R M and Thanh N T K 2018 Characterization techniques for nanoparticles: comparison and complementarity upon studying nanoparticle properties *Nanoscale* **10** 12871–934

[33] Anukiruthika T, Priyanka S, Moses J A and Anandharamakrishnan C 2020 Characterisation of green nanomaterials ed S Ahmed and W Ali *Green Nanomaterials. Advanced Structured Materials* vol 126 (Singapore: Springer)

[34] Dhau J S, Singh A, Singh A, Dhir R, Brandão P and Félix V 2014 Synthesis, characterization and antibacterial properties of pyridylseleniums: self-assembly of bis(3-bromo-2-pyridyl) diselenide via intermolecular secondary and π···π stacking interactions *J. Organomet. Chem.* **766** 57–66

[35] Singh A, Maximoff S N, Brandão P and Dhau J S 2021 Crystal structures of bis(2-methoxy-3-pyridyl) diselenide and bis(2-methoxy-3-pyridyl) ditelluride: an investigation by X-ray crystallography and DFT calculations *J. Mol. Struct.* **1240** 130568

[36] Marbella L E and Millstone J E 2015 NMR techniques for noble metal nanoparticles *Chem. Mater.* **27** 2721–39

[37] Sarker M, Fraser R E, Lumsden M D, Anderson D J and Rainey J K 2015 Characterization of variant soft nanoparticle structure and morphology in solution by NMR spectroscopy *J. Phys. Chem.* C **119** 7461–71

[38] Fei W, Antonello S, Dainese T, Dolmella A, Lahtinen M, Rissanen K, Venzo A and Maran F 2019 Metal doping of $Au_{25}(SR)_{18}$-clusters: insights and hindsights *J. Am. Chem. Soc.* **141** 16033–45

[39] Udayabhaskararao T, Bootharajua M S and Pradeep T 2013 Thiolate-protected Ag_{32} clusters: mass spectral studies of composition and insights into the Ag–thiolate structure from NMR *Nanoscale* **5** 9404–11

[40] Bloch F, Hansen W W and Packard M 1946 The nuclear induction experiment *Phys. Rev.* **70** 474–85

[41] Purcell E M, Torrey H C and Pound R V 1946 Resonance absorption by nuclear magnetic moments in a solid *Phys. Rev.* **69** 37–8

[42] Emsley J W and Feeney J 2007 Forty years of progress in nuclear magnetic resonance spectroscopy *Prog. Nucl. Magn. Reson. Spectrosc* **50** 179–98

[43] Blümich B 2016 Introduction to compact NMR: a review of methods *TrAC Trends Anal. Chem.* **83** 2–11

[44] Pavia D L, Lampman G M and Kriz G S 1979 *Introduction to Spectroscopy: A Guide for Students of Organic Chemistry* (Philadelphia, PA: W.B. Saunders)

[45] Rastrelli F, Jha S and Mancin F 2009 Seeing through macromolecules: T_2-filtered NMR for the purity assay of functionalized nanosystems and the screening of biofluids *J. Am. Chem. Soc.* **131** 14222–4

[46] Ivashchenko O, Gapiński J, Peplińska B, Przysiecka Ł, Zalewski T, Nowaczyk G, Jareka M, Marcinkowska-Gapińska A and Jurga S 2017 Self-organizing silver and ultrasmall iron oxide nanoparticles prepared with ginger rhizome extract: characterization, biomedical potential and microstructure analysis of hydrocolloids *Mater. Des.* **133** 307–24

[47] Dreaden E C, Alkilany A M, Huang X, Murphy C J and El-Sayed M A 2012 The golden age: gold nanoparticles for biomedicinew *Chem. Soc. Rev.* **41** 2740–79

[48] Song Y, Harper A S and Murray R W 2005 Ligand heterogeneity on monolayer-protected gold clusters *Langmuir* **21** 5492–500

[49] Udayabhaskararao T, Bootharaju M S and Pradeep T 2013 Thiolate-protected Ag_{32} clusters: mass spectral studies of composition and insights into the Ag–thiolate structure from NMR *Nanoscale* **5** 9404–11

[50] Mody V V, Siwale R, Singh A and Mody H R 2010 Introduction to metallic nanoparticles *J. Pharm. Bioallied Sci.* **2** 282–9

[51] Brust M, Walker M, Bethell D, Schiffrin D J and Whyman R 1994 Synthesis of thiol-derivatised gold nanoparticles in a two-phase liquid–liquid system *J. Chem. Soc.* **1994** 801–2

[52] Ulman A 1996 Formation and structure of self-assembled monolayers *Chem. Rev.* **96** 1533–54

[53] Thanneeru S, Ayers K M, Anuganti M, Zhang L, Kumar C V, Ung G and He J 2020 N-Heterocyclic carbene-ended polymers as surface ligands of plasmonic metal nanoparticles *J. Mater. Chem.* C **8** 2280–8

[54] Man R W Y, Li C H, Lean M W A M, Zenkina O V, Zamora M T, Saunders L N, Rousina-Webb A, Nambo M and Crudden C M 2018 Ultrastable gold nanoparticles modified by bidentate N-heterocyclic carbene ligands *J. Am. Chem. Soc.* **140** 1576–9

[55] Caragheorgheopol A and Chechik V 2008 Mechanistic aspects of ligand exchange in Au nanoparticles *Phys. Chem. Chem. Phys.* **10** 5029–41

[56] Pem B, Pongrac I M, Ulm L, Pavicic I, Vrcek V, Jurašin D D, Ljubojevic M, Krivohlavek A and Vrcek I V 2019 Toxicity and safety study of silver and gold nanoparticles functionalized with cysteine and glutathione *Beilstein J. Nanotechnol.* **10** 1802–17

[57] Schuetze B, Mayer C, Loza K, Gocyla M, Heggenc M and Epple M 2016 Conjugation of thiol-terminated molecules to ultrasmall 2 nm-gold nanoparticles leads to remarkably complex ^{1}H-NMR spectra *J. Mater. Chem.* B **4** 2179–89

[58] Yang Y, Serrano L A and Guldin S 2018 A versatile AuNP synthetic platform for decoupled control of size and surface composition *Langmuir* **34** 6820–6

[59] Meer S B, Loza K, Wey K, Heggen M, Beuck C, Bayer P and Epple M 2019 Click chemistry on the surface of ultrasmall gold nanoparticles (2 nm) for covalent ligand attachment followed by NMR spectroscopy *Langmuir* **35** 7191–204

[60] Rice S B *et al* 2013 Particle size distributions by transmission electron microscopy: an interlaboratory comparison case study *Metrologia* **50** 663–78

[61] Kumar S, Jagielski J, Marcato T, Solari S F and Shih C J 2019 Understanding the ligand effects on photophysical, optical, and electroluminescent characteristics of hybrid lead halide perovskite nanocrystal solids *J. Phys. Chem. Lett.* **10** 7560–7

[62] Wilschefski S C and Baxter M R 2019 Inductively coupled plasma mass spectrometry: introduction to analytical aspects *Clin. Biochem. Rev.* **40** 115–33

[63] Londoño-Restrepo S M, Jeronimo-Cruz R, Millán-Malo B M, Rivera-Muñoz E M and Rodriguez-García M E 2019 Effect of the nano crystal size on the x-ray diffraction patterns of biogenic hydroxyapatite from human, bovine, and porcine bones *Sci. Rep.* **9** 5915

[64] Mansfield E, Tyner K M, Poling C M and Blacklock J L 2014 Determination of nanoparticle surface coatings and nanoparticle purity using microscale thermogravimetric analysis *Anal. Chem.* **86** 1478–84

[65] Pagès G, Gilard V, Martino R and Malet-Martino M 2017 Pulsed-field gradient nuclear magnetic resonance measurements (PFG NMR) for diffusion ordered spectroscopy (DOSY) mapping *Analyst* **142** 3771–96

[66] Salassa G and Burgi T 2018 NMR spectroscopy: a potent tool for studying monolayer-protected metal nanoclusters *Nanoscale Horiz* **3** 457–63

[67] Sharma R, Holland G P, Solomon V C, Zimmermann H, Schiffenhaus S, Amin S A, Buttry D A and Yarger J L 2009 NMR characterization of ligand binding and exchange dynamics in triphenylphosphine-capped gold nanoparticles *J. Phys. Chem.* C **113** 16387–93

[68] Kluenker M, Mondeshki M, Tahir M N and Tremel W 2018 Monitoring thiol–ligand exchange on Au nanoparticle surfaces *Langmuir* **34** 1700–10

[69] Badia A, Demers L, Dickinson L, Morin F G, Lennox R B and Reven L 1997 Gold–sulfur interactions in alkylthiol self-assembled monolayers formed on gold nanoparticles studied by solid-state NMR *J. Am. Chem. Soc.* **119** 11104–5

[70] Wallner A, Jafri S H M, Blom T, Gogoll A, Leifer K, Baumgartner J and Ottosson H 2011 Formation and NMR spectroscopy of ω-thiol protected r,ω-alkanedithiol-coated gold nanoparticles and their usage in molecular charge transport junctions *Langmuir* **27** 9057–67

[71] Abraham A, Mihaliuk E, Kumar B, Legleiter J and Gullion T 2010 Solid-state NMR study of cysteine on gold nanoparticles *J. Phys. Chem.* C **114** 18109–14

[72] Wu M, Vartanian A M, Chong G, Pandiakumar A K, Hamers R J, Hernandez R and Murphy C J 2019 Solution NMR analysis of ligand environment in quaternary ammonium-terminated self-assembled monolayers on gold nanoparticles: the effect of surface curvature and ligand structure *J. Am. Chem. Soc.* **141** 4316–27

[73] Porret E, Guevel X L and Coll J L 2020 Gold nanoclusters for biomedical applications: toward *in vivo* studies *J. Mater. Chem.* B **8** 2216–32

[74] Lee S H and Jun B H 2019 Silver nanoparticles: synthesis and application for nanomedicine *Int. J. Mol. Sci.* **20** 865

[75] Lee K X, Shameli K, Yew Y P, Teow S Y, Jahangirian H, Rafiee-Moghaddam R and Webster T J 2020 Recent developments in the facile bio-synthesis of gold nanoparticles (AuNPs) and their biomedical applications *Int. J. Nanomed.* **15** 275–300

[76] Salorinne K, Lahtinen T, Koivisto J, Kalenius E, Nissinen M, Pettersson M and Häkkinen H 2013 Nondestructive size determination of thiol-stabilized gold nanoclusters in solution by diffusion ordered NMR spectroscopy *Anal. Chem.* **85** 3489–92

[77] Pengo P, Bazzo C, Boccalon M and Pasquato L 2015 Differential reactivity of the inner and outer positions of $Au_{25}(SCH_2CH_2Ph)_{18}$ dimeric staples under place exchange conditions *Chem. Commun.* **51** 3204–7

[78] Salassa G, Sels A, Mancin F and Bürgi T 2017 Dynamic nature of thiolate monolayer in Au_{25} $(SR)_{18}$ nanoclusters *ACS Nano* **11** 12609–14

[79] Smith A M, Marbella L E, Johnston K A, Hartmann M J, Crawford S E, Kozycz L M, Seferos D S and Millstone J E 2015 Quantitative analysis of thiolated ligand exchange on gold nanoparticles monitored by ^{1}H NMR spectroscopy *Anal. Chem.* **87** 2771–8

[80] Coelho S C, Rangel M, Pereira M C, Coelho M A N and Ivanova G 2015 Structural characterization of functionalized gold nanoparticles for drug delivery in cancer therapy: a NMR based approach *Phys. Chem. Chem. Phys.* **17** 18971–9

[81] Azevedo M B M, Tasic L, Fattori J, Rodrigues F H S, Cantos F C, Ribeiro L P, Paula V, Ianzer D and Santos R A S 2011 New formulation of an old drug in hypertension treatment: the sustained release of captopril from cyclodextrin nanoparticles *Int. J. Nanomed.* **6** 1005–16

[82] Ivanova G, Simeonova M, Cabrita E J and Range M 2011 NMR insight into the supramolecular structure of daunorubicin loaded polymer nanoparticles *J. Phys. Chem.* B **115** 902–9

[83] Simeonova M, Rangel M and Ivanova G 2013 NMR study of the supramolecular structure of dual drug-loaded poly(butylcyanoacrylate) nanoparticles *Phys. Chem. Chem. Phys.* **15** 16657–64

IOP Publishing

Analytical Techniques for Biomedical Nanotechnology

Ajeet Kaushik, Sesha S Srinivasan and Yogendra Kumar Mishra

Chapter 8

Mass spectroscopy in biomedical nanotechnology

Priyanka Mankotia, Kartikey Verma, Kashma Sharma, Vishal Sharma, Vijay Kumar and Rakesh Sehgal

In recent years, mass spectrometry (MS) has been extensively used in the characterization of various nanomaterials. MS is a very sensitive analytical technique with a number of applications in the various fields of science and technology. The high precision and resolution of the instrument have opened new opportunities in the examination of various biological compounds. In this chapter, first a brief introduction and historical background on MS is given, and then the fundamental and applied aspects of MS especially in the field of nanotechnology highlighting its versatile biomedical applications are covered. A specific consideration is given to the MS analysis of various nanoparticles such as silver, gold, metal oxides, engineered nanoparticles, tellurium biogenic nanoparticles, carbon-based nanoparticles, and their biomedical applications. The present status and the upcoming possibilities of the MS technique are examined in general along with appropriate examples drawn from the existing literature.

Abbreviations

MS	Mass spectroscopy
MALDI	Matrix-assisted laser desorption ionization
HDL	High-density lipoprotein
LDI	Laser desorption/ionization
LC–MS	Liquid chromatography–mass spectroscopy
MRI	Magnetic resonance imaging
SPR	Surface plasmon resonance
BBB	Blood–brain barrier
CNS	Central nervous system
MSI	Mass spectrometry imaging
HPCL	High-performance liquid chromatography

doi:10.1088/978-0-7503-3379-5ch8

GC/MS	Gas chromatography/mass spectrometry
SERS	Surface-enhanced Raman spectroscopy
CE	Capillary electrophoresis
LOD	Limit of detection
LOQ	Limit of quantification
RSD	Relative standard deviation
CHCA	α-cyano-4-hydroxycinnamic acid
MALDI-TOF MS	Matrix-assisted laser desorption/ionization-time of flight mass spectrometry
spICP-MS	Single-particle inductively coupled plasma mass spectrometry
ICPMS	Inductively coupled plasma mass spectrometry
FFF	Field-flow fractionation
HDC	Hydrodynamic chromatography

8.1 Introduction

Mass spectroscopy (MS) is a highly sensitive technique providing fast data acquisition speed and analysis of samples up to the picogram level [1–3]. It is one of the most significant conventional spectroscopic analytical tools and has been generally employed to investigate the chemical structures of organic materials and small biological molecules [3]. In addition, MS can give information on the molecular mass of a sample. MS has also been broadly used to dissect biological molecules and has developed into an irreplaceable tool for proteomics research [4]. The technique is being widely used in genomics and proteomics because of its high rate of reproducibility, reliability, broad application, and benefaction in modern biomedical sciences. The basic principle of MS lies in the effective ionization of chemical compounds followed by the separation of ions on the basis of mass to charge ratio [5]. Molecules are fragmented by the generation of ions by employing an energy and the formed ions are then isolated in the analyzers in the presence of electric and magnetic fields and subsequently recorded by the detector to give rise to a mass spectrum on the basis of their mass/charge ratio (figure 8.1) [2].

In this way, every molecule of the compound either purified or homogenate can easily be recognized and further its quantification can be done. To explain it in a simple way, a mass spectrum quantifies the mass in a sample via charging them during the measurement. To date MS has been utilized in numerous fields such as applied sciences and basic sciences including biomedical sciences. The identification of disordered proteins or metabolites for quantitative and qualitative analysis is possible using mass spectroscopy under experimental conditions [5].

The history of MS dates back to the 18th century by Eugen Goldstein. The mass spectrograph was developed by J J Thompson thereby providing a major contribution to the development of MS for various analytical applications [2, 3]. The word spectrograph derived through these devices was introduced internationally to the scientific community and was used in the scientific vocabulary from 1884 [6–8]. The modern MS techniques offer a more accurate analysis of atomic masses and structures of various compounds. Moreover, the discovery of new soft ionization techniques like electrospray mass ionization and matrix-assisted laser desorption

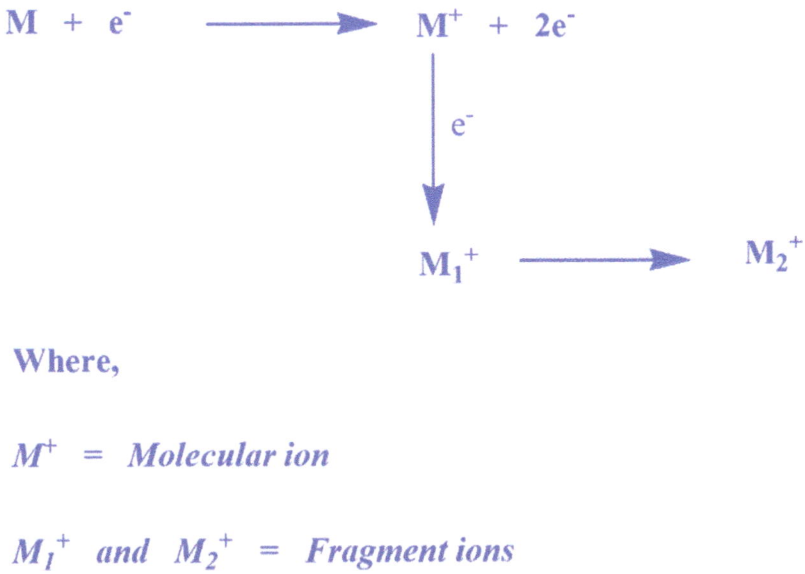

Figure 8.1. Ionization of molecules by energy application (here electron bombardment). Reproduced from [2]. CC BY 3.0.

ionization (MALDI), have made MS more precise in the analysis of the mass of high molecular weight compounds like polymers, nucleic acids (DNA and RNA), etc [3, 9–11]. MS has many advantages and has the potential to replace many techniques in the future. In the field of pharmacokinetics, MS is found to have a unique importance because of the complexity that the matrix provides for the analysis of samples like blood and urine [5]. Tandem MS is also utilized by researchers these days as it adds specificity to the drugs [12–14]. The pharmacokinetics of drugs present at various time intervals as well as their rate of clearance from the body can be analyzed and regulated via blood and urine [2]. However, the analyzers present in MS are highly sensitive which in turn efficiently helps the pharmacologists to study micro-dosing procedures. The wide implementation of MS will continue to benefit the advancement of a deep understanding of different biological processes followed by their molecular mechanisms. Additionally, MS-based proteomics and metabolomics have helped provide a deep understanding of various biologically occurring processes along with their mechanisms which will be helpful in clinical molecular diagnosis in the near future. Even in medical sciences, MS is useful for the examination of metabolites and the determination of the presence of abnormal proteins in patients [15, 16]. It requires a small sample for analysis and provides high sensitivity and precision to the analysis. All of the reasons stated above make MS the most reliable technique to be used in various laboratories worldwide [17–19]. MS has been used in the analysis of respiratory gas in patients and has shown accurate results [20]. It has been found that some of the MS instruments have been modified intentionally for reporting the composites of gases which are respired by a patient within a mass range of detection [21]. The highly accurate results obtained from MS have made it useful in the quantitative analysis, characterization, and sequencing of proteomic studies. With the help of electrospray ionization and MALDI, it is possible to fragment the proteins which can further be digested using trypsin enzyme followed by analysis for mass fingerprinting [8, 22]. Zhang *et al* [23] reviewed the studies on metabolomics for biomarker discovery demonstrating its role in the identification of biomarkers. Cheng *et al* [24] provided a detailed review of the developments of mass spectroscopy-based qualitative proteomics techniques, high-density lipoprotein (HDL) proteomics, and modification of lipoprotein for the discovery of a biomarker for the treatment of vascular disease—atherosclerotic. Godderis *et al* [25] demonstrated the mass spectroscopic application over the evaluation of DNA methylation and hydroxymethylation. They utilized the liquid chromatography–mass spectroscopy (LC–MS) method for quantification as well as for the simultaneous comparison of global methylation and hydroxymethylation in human DNA present in various tissues. In glycobiology, MS is found to be more reliable for the examination of the properties and structure of glycans [26]. The measurement of masses using laser desorption/ionization (LDI)/ MALDI MS and tandem MS is considered to be reliable for the identification of structures of peptides, carbohydrates, and lipids as they play an important role in biomedical applications having a molecular mass greater than 1000 Daltons. MS is now gaining a lot of attention for the characterization of nanoparticles (NPs). It provides information about the mass of ligands [27]. The combinations of LDI MS with MALDI has been successfully used for the determination of masses of small ligands present in gold (Au) NPs in biological samples [28]. The basic principle behind the working of the LDI/MALDI method is that the NPs tend to absorb energetic laser irradiation thereby causing ligands to ionize and be released to be detected by MS [28]. Nanotechnology has many applications in the research and development of matter at the macromolecular or atomic level having dimensions in the range of 1–100 nm. The materials at this scale show different quantum mechanical properties. The so-formed NPs need to be characterized for their functionality and toxicity. Therefore, the use of MS for the complete in-depth analysis of the structures with nanometer dimensions as well as the characterization of the surface composition of NPs is found to be highly beneficial in this area. This chapter deals with the detailed use of MS in the analysis of NPs for various biomedical applications. A detailed overview of all types of NPs and their characterization using MS has been discussed here.

8.2 Biomedical applications of nanoparticles

Nanoparticles can be defined as solid colloidal particles having a diameter range between 1 and 100 nm. Their wide employment for biomedical applications is due to the fact that they provide various advantages to the large-sized particles like large surface area and increased magnetic properties [29]. Recently, NPs have attracted a lot of interest in numerous biomedical applications like targeted drug delivery, photoablation therapy, hyperthermia, biosensors, and bio-imaging [30, 31]. NPs can be classified into four types of nano-systems, i.e., bimetallic nanoparticles, metallic nanoparticles, magnetic nanoparticles, and metal oxide nanoparticles as shown in figure 8.2, with each category contributing towards the applications in biomedical science.

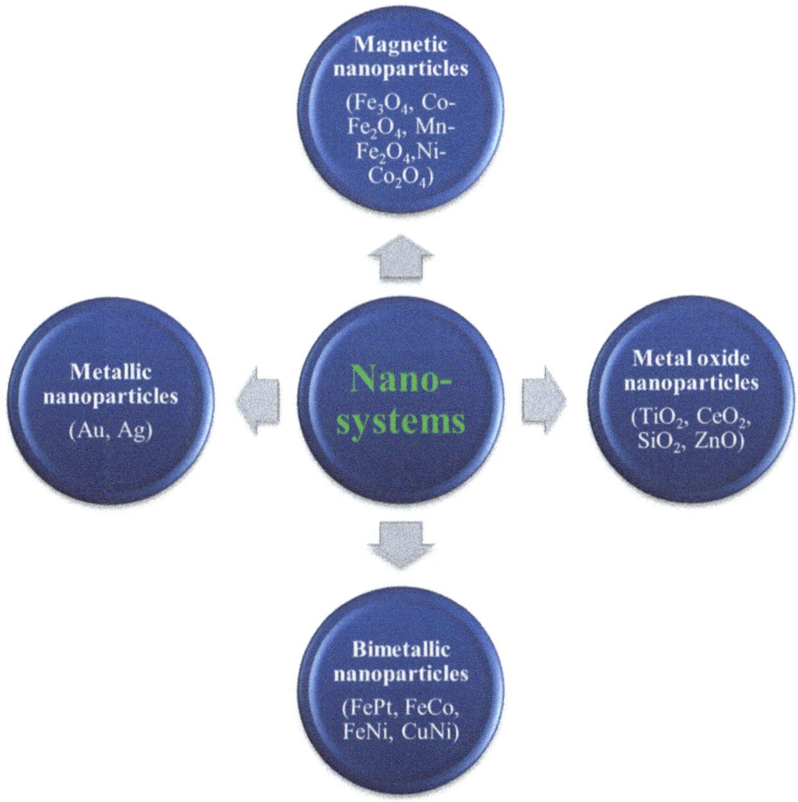

Figure 8.2. Schematic representation of classification of nano-systems.

8.2.1 Magnetic nanoparticles

These are considered to be the most common type of NPs employed for biomedical applications because of their distinctive chemical structure, biocompatibility, non-toxicity, chemical stability, high saturation magnetization, and high magnetic susceptibility [32]. Iron oxide comprises multiple states of oxidation like iron (II) oxide (FeO), iron (III) oxide (Fe_2O_3), and iron (II, III) oxide (Fe_3O_4). Fe_2O_3 consists of separate crystalline polymorphs of α-Fe_2O_3, β-Fe_2O_3, γ-Fe_2O_3 and ε-Fe_2O_3. Maghemite (γ-Fe_2O_3) and magnetite (Fe_3O_4) is found to be highly biocompatible, however, Fe_3O_4 has been used widely in biomedical applications [33]. It is easily oxidized; to prevent this coating on its surface with biocompatible shell-like metals, polymers, and ceramics are required [34–36]. Once the surface is shell coated, it provides many advantages like prevention of agglomeration, functionalization, and conjugation to enzymes, antibodies, anticancer drugs, and proteins. FeO NPs are effectively used for treating hyperthermia [37, 38], drug delivery [39–45], and magnetic resonance imaging (MRI) [46, 47]. Furthermore, the magnetic properties of FeO NPs can be enhanced through mixing with susceptible elements like cobalt, nickel, and manganese [48]. Of these, cobalt and manganese are widely used in the field of biomedical sciences. The $CoFe_2O_4$ nanoparticles consist of very large magneto-crystalline anisotropy, high Curie temperature, coercivity, considerable chemical stability, and moderate magnetization saturation [49–53]. The major applications of these NPs lie in the treatment of hyperthermia as well as important contrast agents for MRI [49–53]. Similarly, $MnFe_2O_4$ NPs show high magnetization, biocompatibility, and magnetic susceptibility. These have also been used for the possible treatment of magnetic hyperthermia [54–57].

8.2.2 Bimetallic nanoparticles

These include iron and cobalt-based NPs which show excellent magnetic properties like high Curie temperature, superparamagnetism, and high saturation magnetism. Despite these advantages, they have the major limitation of being easily oxidizable putting their biocompatibility into question. Coating the surface of NPs with some biocompatible material is the solution to the above problem. The iron–cobalt NPs have been utilized for many applications like contrast agents for MRI owing to their property of high saturation magnetism and hyperthermia [58–64]. Iron nickel-based NPs consist of a high Curie temperature along with some magnetization properties used majorly for MRI [65]. Copper–nickel NPs also come under bimetallic NPs having good magnetic properties being used for biomedical applications [65–68]. Bimetallic NPs like iron platinum (Fe–Pt) show a variety of chemical and magnetic properties like high Curie temperature, chemical stability, saturation magnetization, superparamagnetization, and high x-ray absorption [69–72]. It is due to these properties that the bimetallic NPs are ideally used for the treatment of hyperthermia [73, 74], MRI contrast agents [75–78], drug delivery [79–83] and biosensors [84].

8.2.3 Metallic nanoparticles

A new field of exploration has grown recently called 'plasmonics' that manages surface plasmon resonance (SPR) in the case of noble metals such as gold (Au) and silver (Ag) structures at the nanoscale dimensions. They show remarkable properties with a decrease in size and they have a large specific surface area, a high fraction of surface atoms, and large surface energy. These interesting properties of NPs have motivated researchers to use them in a variety of applications. Au and Ag NPs are being used for medical purposes. They have unique optical properties, electronic properties, chemical inertness, and an ability for surface functionalization because of the presence of negative charge over their surface [85–87]. They have been widely used for bio-imaging [88, 89], biosensors [90, 91], and photothermal therapy [92–94]. Au-NPs tend to conjugate easily with antibodies, drug molecules, and ligands for active or passive delivery [90–99]. The property of chemical inertness makes Au-NPs highly compatible with *in vitro* and *in vivo* applications. Similarly, Ag NPs have also been studied for various medicinal purposes because of their physicochemical properties like high electrical conductivity, chemical stability, thermal conductivity, chemical stability, antibacterial activity, catalytic activity, and optical properties [100]. The main applications of Ag NPs lie in electronic, antimicrobial, photonic, and disinfectant fields [101–108]. Ag NPs hold the excellent capability of antimicrobial activity which is why they are primarily used in wound dressings, textiles, and device coatings. Apart from this, they are also being used as biosensors [101–103], photothermal sensors, and targeted drug delivery applications [109–111].

8.2.4 Metal oxide nanoparticles

Titanium dioxide (TiO_2), cerium oxide (CeO_2), silicon dioxide (SiO_2), and zinc oxide (ZnO) are a few of the metal oxide-based nanoparticles used for a number of biomedical applications. Starting with TiO_2 NPs, they have important uses in various photovoltaic and photocatalytic devices, paint, food coloring, cosmetics, and toothpaste. They possess various properties like biocompatibility, optical properties, and chemical stability [112]. Due to these excellent properties, TiO_2 has been used for biomedical applications such as bio-imaging [113], drug delivery [112–117], biosensors [118], and photoablation therapy [119]. CeO_2 NPs are also known as nanoceria and have a characteristic switching properties in various oxidation states [120]. They report certain defects on their surface including oxygen vacancies resulting in a state of mixed valency of cerium (IV) and cerium (III) oxidation states coexisting on the surface. This leads to the nanoceria gaining catalytic activity. This has resulted in nanoceria being a prospective biological antioxidant. Nanoceria has been used as a biosensor and as an anticancer agent in various applications [121]. Another class of metal oxide NP includes SiO_2 NPs. These consist of large specific surface area, pore-volume, adjustable particle size, and great biocompatibility. Therefore, these properties of mesoporous silica make them an ideal material for drug delivery and bio-sensing applications [122, 123]. The use of ZnO NPs has become important recently but the surface of ZnO NPs is protected by a modification to prevent them from dissolving into acidic and neutral solutions. In order to use these NPs in fluorescence imaging, doping is required because they comprise of bandwidth in the UV region which makes it impossible for the UV light to penetrate the tissue [124].

8.3 Mass spectroscopy in biomedical applications

8.3.1 Mass spectroscopy for the detection of nanoparticles in neuroscience

The human brain is regarded as the controlling unit for the entire body, regulating the functioning of the organs and the entire system. With changes in lifestyle and an increase in life expectancy, the brain has been subjected to a prolonged aging process leading to a high risk of developing neurogenerative disorders like Alzheimer's, Parkinson's and dementia. Despite advancements in medical science, no effective therapy for the treatment of these neurogenerative disorders has been discovered because of the restriction imposed by the blood–brain barrier (BBB) [125–129]. The BBB is a semi-permeable membrane formed through tight junctions present on the endothelial membrane helping in the separation of blood vessels and the central nervous system (CNS) [125–129]. The major function of the BBB is in the protection of blood and blood vessels from the passage of harmful pathogens, toxins, or hormones. The BBB helps protect the brain by limiting the passage of toxins, hormones, and pathogens present in the blood. In a similar way, this filter inhibits the passage of therapeutic agents in reaching the brain, thereby prohibiting their treatment. The transmission of the drug across the BBB is crucial for the treatment of diseases like cancer, Parkinson's, Alzheimer's, and other neurological disorders. Recently, NPs have gained importance in the active release of drugs at targeted sites because of their ability to maintain drug levels in the therapeutic range and increasing their half-life, permeability, stability, and solubility [130]. NPs can be synthesized from various materials including polymers, lipids, proteins, plants, flowers, and semiconductors, thereby making their physicochemical properties suitable for targeted drug delivery as well as for imaging and therapeutic uses [131]. Therefore, monitoring of the working efficiency of NPs as drug carriers is an important step in the treatment of diseases and clinical translation. The need for an appropriate method which helps in imaging the nanocarriers in a certain interval of time will be helpful in keeping a check on the efficacy of the drug and treating the disorder.

Mass spectrometry imaging (MSI) has great importance in medical and clinical research with the detection and analysis of nanoparticles [132–134]. It has been investigated as an interdisciplinary technique consisting of physics, chemistry, and biology for analysing the molecular composition of various compounds [132–135]. MSI, a new technique that has been developed from MS, is useful for the visualization and study of the spatial distribution of various biological substances including proteins, peptides, metabolites, drugs, and lipids present in biological specimens. The molecular mass of a sample is taken as an intrinsic molecular parameter for label-free imaging using MS for the visualization of the distribution of biomolecules on the sample surfaces. The electric and magnetic fields are manipulated for this purpose and then the measurement of time of flight is done. The utilization of a mass spectrometer as an imaging instrument is done by equipping it with a desorption source and an ionization source which generates local information, an automated sample or beam manipulation system, automatic data acquisition, registration system, and visualization software. The signals so obtained are directly proportional to the compound concentration persistent in any sample. The mass spectra of each molecule represent its composition at x and y coordinates. An image dataset similar to pixels is obtained from the mass spectra of the tissue sample in the form of a digital photograph. Selective distribution of the compound inside the tissue section is visualized according to the mass to charge ratio at specific intensities noted from the obtained spectra. The amount of ion present in each pixel is visualized with the help of a color intensity scale in 2D maps. The data is extracted from the mass to charge ranges from the spatially obtained mass spectroscopy files to generate an image. Mass spectroscopy imaging is a suitable technique for studying the biodistribution in both large whole-body tissue samples as well as in small organs such as the liver, kidney, and eyes with a relatively high resolution [132].

Although the BBB restricts the entry of several molecules through them the employment of numerous methods has allowed the transit of drugs. Molecules smaller than 500 Dalton, being highly soluble in lipids, can efficiently penetrate the BBB barrier through passive diffusion. Using this strategy drugs can be easily delivered to the targeted site using liposome-based particles [136]. NPs can be easily fabricated up to nanoscale ranges and these are considered to be the most dominant ways to pass through the BBB and successfully reach the target site. All the physicochemical properties of NPs can be exploited for the facilitation of drug release at the target site with an optimal value. Till now the fluorescence imaging technique has been used for the detection of NPs inside the cellular organelles in cells. However, this technique has the disadvantage of not being able to carry out the imaging of the carrier and cargo molecules concurrently within the cell [137, 138]. To circumvent the disadvantages posed by the fluorescence imaging techniques, MSI is used. A three-dimensional molecular image of the cells and analytes of interest are easily obtained using MSI. The visualization of co-localized images of NPs along with the drugs of interest at a submicron level with a resolution at nanometer depth is possible using MSI. Figure 8.3 demonstrates an example of imaging of a composite Nano SIMS image of the HeLa cell lines incubated with 15 μM Cy15N-NP where 195Pt (red) and 15N enrichment (green) are overlaid on the image of secondary ion [138]. Yellow regions present specify the co-localization of

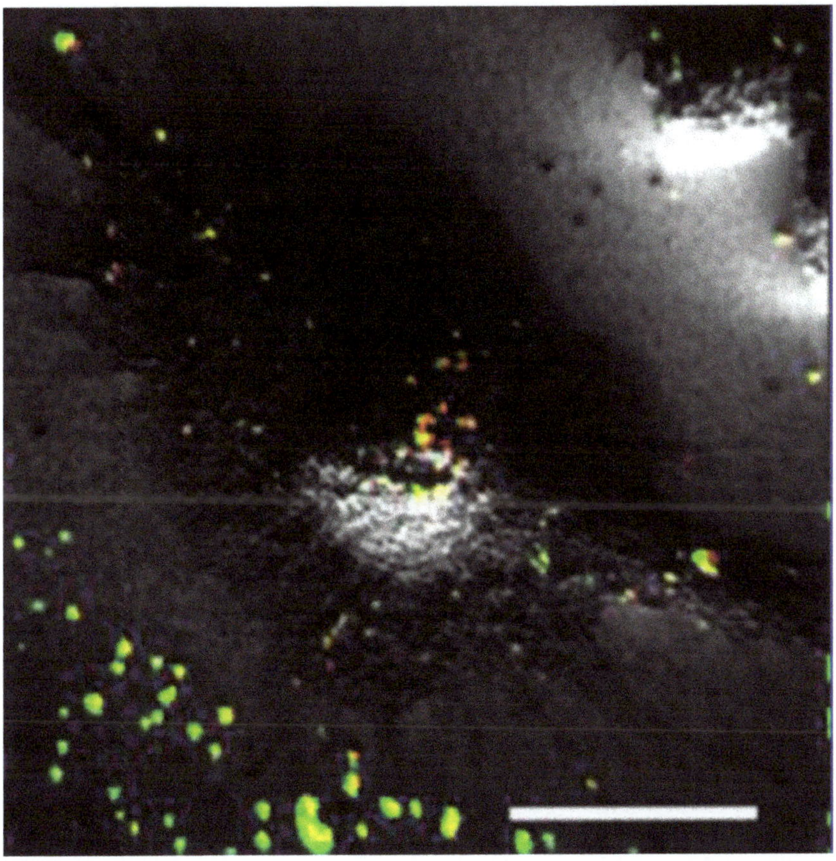

Figure 8.3. Composite nano image of a HeLa cell incubated with 15 μM $Cy^{15}N$-NP where ^{195}Pt (red) and ^{15}N enrichment (green) and overlaid on the secondary ion image. Yellow regions indicate co-localization of signals. The scale bar represents 10 μm. Reprinted with permission from [138]. Copyright (2016) American Chemical Society.

signals. The scale bar represents 10 μm. Therefore, the use of isotope labels is not required as the drug and its metabolites can be simultaneously detected using MSI. It can also be helpful in encountering problems with overlapping cell peaks. Apart from these qualitative characteristics, a quantitative estimation of the drug levels in tissue can also be done using MSI. Despite the wide variety of techniques used previously such as autoradiography, bioluminescent, and fluorescent receptors for the quantification of drugs in cells, they have many shortcomings which is why an alternative technique with high efficacy is required, so MSI offers various advantages in this regard. MSI has been reported to show the mechanism of optimization of designing therapeutic NPs along with the monitoring of pathogenesis of several neurodegenerative diseases thereby, making major contributions in neurosciences [138].

Xue *et al* [139] developed a novel label-free laser desorption/ionization MSI method for the imaging and measurement of the *in situ* drug release in tissues via examination of the intrinsic MS signal intensity ratio of the loaded drug over the nanocarriers. They loaded the anticancer drug doxorubicin (DOX) in MoS_2 nanosheets. They employed a label-free method for the simultaneous imaging of nanocarriers and release of drug as well as quantifying the amount of drug release in the targeted tissues. Furthermore, MoS_2-based nanocarriers additionally displayed extraordinary potential in gene therapy and other joined treatments [139–141]. Furthermore, large numbers of inorganic nanocarriers, such as Au-NPs, carbon nanotubes (CNTs), and phosphorus nanosheets, have been created and applied to biological frameworks, as a result of their high drug-loading ability and particular points of interest in combined therapy [142, 143]. Therefore, the trialing of these nanocarriers and loaded drugs in living systems is vital for biomedical investigations [139].

8.3.2 Mass spectroscopy for the analysis of sulfur drugs and biothiols using silver nanoparticles

It is a well-known fact that sulfur-containing peptides, amino acids, and drugs play an important role in human biological systems [144, 145]. For example, the homocysteine level present in blood serum is considered to be a risk factor for cardiovascular and Alzheimer's diseases. Furthermore, cysteine deficiency causes numerous health problems [146, 147]. A rise in the levels of thiol-containing amino acids and peptides in plasma are thought to cause HIV AIDS [148]. It is because of their crucial roles in the biological system a lot of emphasis is given to the detection of peptides and thiol-containing amino acids. Various analytical approaches have been employed for the detection of these compounds like high-performance liquid chromatography (HPLC), gas chromatography/mass spectrometry (GC/MS), surface-enhanced Raman spectroscopy (SERS), capillary electrophoresis (CE), and fluorescence measurements. However, these tools offer various disadvantages including extra derivatization steps before the analysis, lesser sensitivity and selectivity for the identification of biothiols from biological samples. MALDI MS is considered to be a highly reliable technique for the speedy analysis of nucleic acids, proteins, drugs, peptides, and environmental samples [149, 150]. The use of NPs as matrix and affinity probes for the analysis of peptides and proteins in

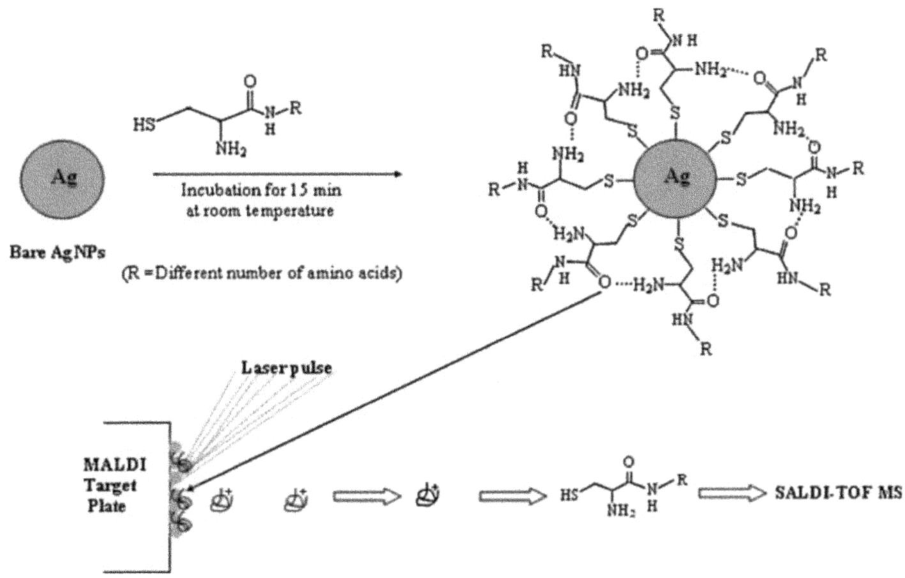

Figure 8.4. Diagrammatic representation of silver nanoparticles as preconcentrating probes and matrix for the SALDI-TOF mass spectroscopic analysis© of biothiols. Reprinted with permission from reference [151]. Copyright © 2008 John Wiley & Sons, Ltd.

MALDI MS is now becoming a popular technique. Kamlesh *et al* [151] worked on the synthesis of Ag NPS as matrix and affinity probes in MALDI MS for the determination of biothiols. The main reason behind using Ag NPs was that they have more affinity towards the sulfur atom and the –SH groups of cysteine-containing proteins and peptides can very well get attached to its surface via covalent bonding [152, 153]. They also proved the feasibility of the research by examining the urine samples collected from five volunteers. The interaction of Ag NPs with biothiols and their analysis using MS has been demonstrated in figure 8.4. The optical properties of Ag NPs along with the number of molecules adsorbed directly demonstrate the efficiency of ionization of biothiols. The values of the limit of detection (LOD) and limit of quantification (LOQ) for both the samples in urine, i.e., cysteine and homocysteine were calculated to be 7 and 22 nM, reporting a relative standard deviation (RSD) less than 10%. Upon the adsorption of biothiols over the surface of silver nanoparticles, an enhancement in the sensitivity of biothiols was reported to be around 4–15 fold. MS method offers various advantages over conventional methods such as simplicity, sensitivity, and rapidity for the examination of biological samples as it provides a high surface area and great photochemical properties for the Ag NPs which in turn effectively cause the release of drugs at the targeted sites.

8.3.3 Metal oxide nanoparticle-assisted laser desorption/ionization mass spectrometry for various medical applications

NPs having a core of metal oxides can successfully assist as analytes for ionizing molecules in LDI MS in the presence of glycerol [154]. For the examination of low molecular weight samples, ZnO NPs are found to be convenient using LDI MS [155]. The limitation of using ZnO NPs was that their shape was anisotropic (a combination of cubic and rectangular) and they have a large variation in size, i.e., from 20 to 200 nm. The utilization of uniform nanoparticles in MS analysis is yet to be explored. Shu *et al* [156] prepared MnO NPs which have a core of metal oxide coated with a functional silicate sheet. The purpose behind coating the NPs with a functional sheet is that it improves the transfer of energy between the metal oxide core and analyte meaning the analyte is only charged/ionized via nanoparticles. The synthesized NPs were dispersed instead of aggregated. The results obtained from UV absorption studies at 337 nm proved that the MnO NPs can be used as an ionization supporting reagent of analyte for the nanoparticle-assisted LDI MS. The value of zeta potential was calculated to be more than +30 mV which was regarded as the threshold value for electrostatic stabilization [157]. The efficiency of the NPs to be used as an ionization material was investigated via a reserpine drug, which is a substance P acetate hydrate peptide and insulin protein [158]. They found that the oxidation of reserpine happened because of air and light. Although it did not yield any strong signal. When α-cyano-4-hydroxycinnamic acid (CHCA) was added, a few signals at a low molecular range were observed. The results obtained proved that NPs can be used as ionization-assisting reagents for a variety of analytes. Therefore, it was proved that magnesium nanoparticles will be more satisfactory for analyzing the low molecular weight samples [156].

8.3.4 Mass spectrometry imaging of *Lepidium meyenii* using gold nanoparticles

Lepidium meyenii Walp also known as maca is a functional food having medicinal properties and has a high economic value. It has been consumed in Peru for 2000 years as a source of food and medicine. Maca contains various secondary metabolites in its hypocotyls region like glucosinolate, flavonoid, steroid, and alkaloid. Alkaloids have many effects on the health of humans and animals due to the presence of natural organic nitrogen bases. It also has aphrodisiac properties because of the presence of fatty acids and macamides [159–167]. Even the pentane extract of maca is comprised of macamides which in turn act on the endocannabinoid system via inhibitory activity on fatty acid amide hydrolase [168]. Many activities of the CNS are exerted by maca extract. Macapyrrolin present in maca having a benzyl substituent attached to the nucleus of pyrrole has been studied for its cytotoxicity against five human cancer cell lines [165]. The above-stated properties of maca make it an excellent material for the treatment of diabetes, female menopausal syndrome, benign prostatic hyperplasia, and osteoporosis in the elderly. Matrix-assisted laser desorption/ionization-time of flight mass spectrometry (MALDI-TOF MS) is used to analyze and locate the components of various molecules efficiently. Sihou *et al* [169] utilized Au-NPs as MALDI matrix for the analysis and location of components in maca root by MS. The size of the Au-NPs was calculated to be around 7–10 nm and because of the high absorption coefficient, they were utilized for MALDI mass spectroscopic examination of small molecules. The MALDI-TOF mass spectroscopy was used to distinguish between fresh maca

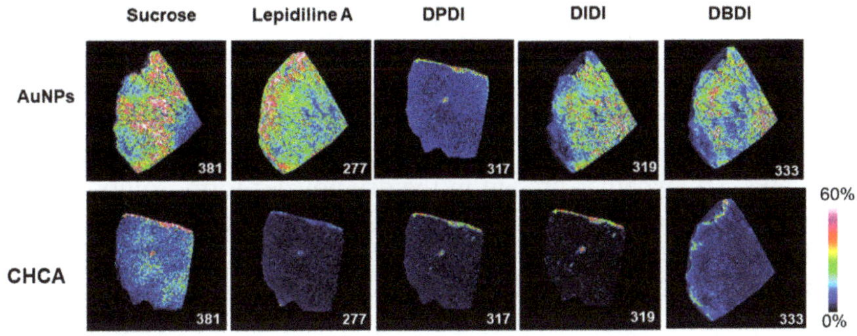

Figure 8.5. The ion distribution of compounds in maca root with gold nanoparticles and CHCA as matrices. Reprinted from [169], Copyright (2019), with permission from Elsevier.

and dry maca. The composition of maca having various constituents like sucrose, arginine, aspartic acid, etc using Fourier-transform ion cyclotron resonance mass spectroscopy. The use of Au-nanoparticles along with CHCA were used as matrices for the analysis of sucrose and alkaloids in dry maca root and the images proved that gold nanoparticles provided clearer images and spatial distribution in the efficient analysis of sucrose as demonstrated in figure 8.5. The position of various compounds in maca root tissue is vividly observable *in situ* by MALDI-MSI with gold nanoparticles as a matrix. Therefore, the use of MSI again provided a novel way of analyzing the medicinal properties of a compound for its use in the future for various applications [169].

8.3.5 Mass spectroscopy for the characterization of engineered nanoparticles

Engineered nanoparticles are being used in numerous consumer products which are currently on the market [170–173]. The most frequently employed inorganic nanomaterials include metallic NPs like Au and Ag, metal oxides such as TiO_2, and ZnO as discussed in section 8.2. The release of NPs from embedded matrices or as free entities is an area that needs to be analyzed using appropriate and sensitive instrumental techniques. The conventional techniques are not used for the characterization of NPs because of their unique physical and chemical properties. A well-established technique called single-particle inductively coupled plasma mass spectrometry (spICP-MS) is considered to be useful for the analysis of engineered NPs [174–177]. Its reliability, speed, and ability to size particles present at their lowest concentrations along with the side by side distinction between dissolved and particulate analytes make it an effective technique. If a separate separation step is required, the supplementary information about the nanoparticles can be obtained using spICP-MS. Therefore, obtaining information about size and quantifying the nanoparticles can be properly done if ICPMS is conjugated to some continuous separation techniques like field-flow fractionation (FFF) or hydrodynamic chromatography (HDC). When it comes to the synthesis of engineered NPs, size plays an important role [178, 179]. The shape of engineered NPs also plays a crucial role in a variety of applications like drug delivery, transport, targeting, and internalization

[180, 181]. Additionally, the chemical composition is also a crucial factor that is responsible for determining the toxicity of NPs [182]. Other properties like surface energy, wettability, surface charge, species absorbance, or adhesion are also considered to be some important parameters [183, 184]. The physicochemical characterization of the nanomaterials must be done by different physical states of engineered NPs, i.e., whether present in the dry powder form, solution form, or in suspension form and for this matter techniques for the determination of shelf life of engineered nanoparticles is essential [185–187]. The inorganic engineered NPs are characterized using the ICPMS technique as it provides very low detection limits up to nanograms per liter level. It usually involves the use of liquid phases which is why the solid samples need to be converted into a liquid through any process to be analyzed using the ICPMS technique. The practicability of direct study of suspension by ICPMS depends on the size and composition of the NPs [188]. It has the capability of carrying out rapid multi-element determination at the ultra-trace level making it beneficial for a variety of applications in various fields including environmental, chemical, medicinal, nuclear, metallurgical, biotechnology, and forensic science for toxicological and heavy metal poisoning studies. This technique is considered to be an innovative and emerging analytical approach for providing information about the elemental chemical composition of nanomaterials as well as their number concentration, size, and number size distribution. This is done on the basis of differences in signal to noise ratio produced for each particle. The spICP-MS technique has proven to be a highly reliable form of MS for the analysis of engineered NPs being further use for various applications. Mitrano *et al* [189] identified and quantified engineered Ag NPs in influent and effluent samples from wastewater treatment plants as the usage of consumer products can cause diseases in humans after their release into the environment. spICP-MS is capable of rapidly providing information about the size, distribution, and particle number concentration, elemental composition requiring minimal sample preparation providing high throughput and elemental specificity. It requires no instrumental modification and high detection ranges in terms of nanometer ranges [190].

8.3.6 Mass spectroscopy for the elucidation of tellurium biogenic nanoparticles

Tellurium usually designated as Te is a metalloid that belongs to group 16 in the periodic table and is used widely as an additive for manufacturing industrial materials like steel, optical disks, and solar panels [191, 192]. The metabolism of tellurium into organotellurium compounds is possible in various plants and one such widely studied plant for the metabolism of Te is garlic (Allium sativum) which is known for metabolizing various chalcogens like sulfur and selenium [193]. Tanaka *et al* [194] studied the elemental analysis of Te to determine its concentration in various parts of garlic using the ICPMS technique. The Te NPs were formed through the biological redox reactions in order to reduce its toxicity [193]. It is found that unambiguous observations of biogenic nanoparticles of tellurium were still lacking and there was a need for the investigation of the formation of insoluble NPs in garlic. The NPs were extracted from the clove and root samples by enzymatic digestion and were analyzed using ICPMS. Additionally, the tellurium oxyanions get converted into a zerovalent form in garlic whose reaction mechanism was still unexplained [194].

8.3.7 Mass spectrometry analysis of carbon nanomaterials for various applications

Carbon-based nanomaterials such as CNTs, carbon nanodots, and graphene have been widely used for a variety of applications in the field of tissue engineering, drug delivery, bio-sensing, and diagnostics [133, 195–208]. Currently used techniques for imaging of carbon nanoparticles include Raman spectroscopy, near-infrared fluorescence, and transient absorption, however, these techniques have certain limitations like weak signals, strong background interference, and slow imaging speed making them undesirable for the studies [201, 202]. LDI MS is currently being used for the analysis of a variety of biological components [133, 203]. Xu *et al* [209] worked on the employment of CNTs as an effective matrix in matrix-assisted laser desorption ionization mass spectroscopy to analyse small biomolecules. The CNTs acted as sample carrying matrices upon which the sample solution was dropped. This simplifies the sample preparation steps, helps in the reduction of background interference, and improves sensitivity [1]. Dong *et al* [210] prepared a graphene-based matrix for the characterization of small molecular compounds like steroids, polyamines, anticancer drugs, and nucleosides by MS. Hua *et al* [211] used graphene nanoflakes as a matrix for the determination of cancer cells using mass spectroscopic analysis. These produced a very good quality mass spectrum having no background noise thereby making the study successful. Chen *et al*, [212], employed carbon nanodots to evaluate low molecular weight molecules via MALDI-TOF mass spectroscopy using both positive and negative ion modes. They carried out successful quantification of glucose and uric acid present in a biological fluid. The matrix was found to be highly efficient in the analysis of a variety of molecules consisting of peptides, amino acids, β-agonists, and oligosaccharides. Polystyrene-based carbon nanotubes were utilized as a matrix material for LDI MS which studied the quantification of urine and water samples utilizing benzo[a]pyrene (BaP) and 1-hydroxypyrene (1-OHP) as probes and acted as a sorbent for thin-film microextraction [213]. Ma *et al* [214] prepared single-walled carbon nanomaterials for the analysis of urine samples via MS, utilizing adenosine triphosphate, fatty acids, and peptides as analytes. The limit of detection was found to be 1.0 μM for the urine samples. To summarize and include the remaining work done to date, table 8.1 represents the various NPs used in mass spectroscopy for highly selective analysis.

8.4 Conclusion

Mass spectroscopy is a highly reliable, effective, and accurate technique, and there are numerous approaches for mass spectrometry-based imaging. This chapter discusses the use of mass spectroscopy for the characterization, analysis, and use of nanoparticles as matrices for further applications in biomedical fields. The main four nanoparticles being utilized as effective components of biomedical applications have been discussed in detail, i.e., magnetic nanoparticles, bimetallic nanoparticles,

Table 8.1. Different nanomaterials and their characterization by mass spectroscopic techniques.

Nanomaterial	Analytes used	Instrumentation technique	Application	References
Silica NPs	Peptides, antiviral drugs	MALDI MS	On plate detection of various particles	[215]
Size selected Au-NPs	Peptides, small proteins	MALDI	Mixed with analyte solution as matrix	[216]
Au-film	Peptides, nucleotides, nucleosides	MALDI	On plate detection	[217]
Au-film coated on nanoporous aluminum oxide layers	Peptides	MALDI	On plate detection	[218]
Boronic acid-modified Au-NPs	HRP (horseradish peroxidase)	MALDI	On plate extraction and detection of particles	[219]
Au-based Ag NPs	Aminoglycosides	MALDI	Used as a mixture for analyte solution for extraction and detection	[220]
Ag NPs	Estrogens (3)	MALDI	Used as a mixture for analyte solution for extraction and detection	[221]
Platinum based nanoparticles	Peptides, phospholipids	MALDI	Mixed with the analyte solution as matrix	[222]
Titanium dioxide nanoparticles	Mouse brain tissue	MALDI MS	Deposition on tissue surface	[223]
Zinc oxide nanowires	Small molecule	MALDI MS	On plate detection	[224]
Silanized Fe_3O_4 NPs	Peptides	MALSI MS	Mixed with analyte solution as matrix	[225]
Pristine carbon nanotubes	Peptides, small proteins, organic compounds and β-cyclodextrin	MALDI MS	Mixed with analyte solution as matrix	[209, 226]
Acidic functionalized fullerene, $C60[(CH_2)_2COOH]_n$	Peptides	MALDI-TOF MS	Mixed with analyte solution as matrix	[227]
Graphene nanoparticles	Amino acids, peptides, acids, fatty acids, polyamines, estrogen, polycyclic aromatic hydrocarbons	MALDI-TOF MS	Mixed with analyte solution as matrix	[210, 228–230]
Magnetic graphene and CNT	Amino acids, sucrose	MALDI-TOF MS	Mixed with analyte solution as matrix	[231]
P-type h100i (boron) silicon with initiator BisF17	Clozapine, single cancer cell, biofluids, ketamine, tissues, *N*-desmethylclozapine, norketamine	MALDI	Laser-NIMS	[232, 233]

metallic nanoparticles, and metal oxide nanoparticles. It can be stated that the design and synthesis of nanoparticles with high selectivity, stability, and efficiency plays a major role in determining their efficacy for biomedical applications. The establishment of molecular imaging techniques was driven by uses for the analysis at the single-cell level for cells and tissues. Techniques including sp-MALDI MS, MALDI-TOF, ICPMS have been discussed briefly in the chapter. For certain applications, nanoparticles can act as a matrix in the mass spectrophotometer instrument thereby ionizing the drugs or its analytes of choice and distinguishing them on the basis of their mass to charge ratios. To date mass spectroscopy has been utilized in many applied and basic sciences and pure samples or complex mixtures in biomedical sciences. The identification of disordered proteins or metabolites for quantitative and qualitative analysis is possible using mass spectroscopy under experimental conditions. MALDI MS and tandem MS are more useful for various applications and are required for full structural identification of complex ligands which are of interest to biomedical applications. MS is currently gaining a lot of attention worldwide for the characterization of nanoparticles. It provides accurate information about the mass of the ligands. The nanomaterials need to be characterized for their functionality and toxicity, therefore the use of mass spectroscopy for the complete in-depth analysis of the film structures with nanometer dimensions as well as the characterization of the surface composition of nanoparticles is found to be highly beneficial. Hence, many potential benefits are possible by utilizing the mass spectroscopy techniques in the future for various biomedical applications and its related areas.

References

[1] Raftery D and Walker 2014 *Mass Spectrometry in Metabolomics-Methods and Protocols. Methods in Molecular Biology* (New York: Springer)

[2] Baghel U S, Singh A, Singh D and Sinha M 2017 *Application of Mass Spectroscopy in Pharmaceutical and Biomedical Analysis, Spectroscopic Analyses—Developments and Applications, Eram Sharmin and Fahmina Zafar* (Rijeka: Intech Open)

[3] Lu Y and Chen W 2015 *Anal. Chem.* **87** 10659–67

[4] Han X, Aslanian A and Yates Y R 2008 *Curr. Opin. Chem. Biol* **12** 483–90

[5] Vaiano F, Serpelloni G, Focardi M, Fioravanti A and Mari F 2015 *Forensic Sci. Int* **256** 1–6

[6] Webster M 2016 *Definition of Spectrograph* (Springfield, MA: Merriam Webster)

[7] Douglas H 2001 Spectrum *Online Etymology Dictionary*

[8] David S O 2000 *Mass Spectrometry Desk Reference* (Pittsburgh, PA: Global View Publishing)

[9] Konermann L, Ahadi E, Rodriguez A D and Vahidi S 2013 *Anal. Chem.* **85** 2–9

[10] Fenn J B 2003 *Angew. Chem. Int. Ed* **42** 3871–94

[11] Hsieh S, Dreisewerd K, van der Schors R C, Jimenez C R, Stahl-Zeng J R, Hillenkamp F, Jorgenson J W, Geraerts W P M and Li K W 1998 *Anal. Chem.* **70** 1847–52

[12] Mittal R D 2015 *Indian J. Clin. Biochem.* **30** 121–3

[13] Loos G, Schepdael A V and Cabooter D 2016 *Phil. Trans. R. Soc.* A **374** 20150366

[14] Beccaria M and Cabooter D 2020 *Analyst* **145** 1129-57

[15] Zhang X W, Li Q H, Xu Z D and Dou J J 2020 *RSC Adv* **10** 3092-104
[16] Nagana Gowda G A N, Zhang S, Gu H, Asiago V, Shanaiah N and Raftery D 2008 *Expert Rev. Mol. Diagn* **8** 617–33
[17] Covey T R, Lee E D and Henion J D 1986 *Anal. Chem.* **58** 2453-60
[18] Covey T R, Crowther J B, Dewey E A and Henion J D 1985 *Anal. Chem.* **57** 474-81
[19] Hsieh Y and Korfmacher W A 2006 *Curr. Drug Metab* **7** 479-89
[20] Riker J B and Haberman B 1976 *Crit. Care Med* **4** 223-29
[21] Gothard J W, Busst C M, Branthwaite M A, Davies N J and Denison D M 1980 *Anaesthesia* **35** 890-95
[22] Li Q Q, Tian K D, Tang G, Xiong Y M and Min S G 2016 [Multivariate calibration combined with mass spectrometry for rapid analysis] *Guang Pu Xue Yu Guang Pu Fen Xi* **36** 532–6 (in Chinese)
[23] Zhang A, Sun H, Yan G, Wang P and Wang X 2015 *BioMed Res. Int* **6** 354671
[24] Chang C T, Yang C Y, Tsai F J, Lin S Y and Chen C J 2015 *BioMed Res. Int* **13** 164846
[25] Godderis L, Schouteden C, Tabish A, Poels K, Hoet P, Baccarelli A A and Landuyt K V 2015 *BioMed Res. Int* **8** 854041
[26] Harvey D, Dwek R A and Rudd P M 2000 Determining the structure of glycan moieties by mass spectrometry *Curr. Protoc. Protein Sci.* **12** 12.7.1–18
[27] Unnikrishnan B, Chang C Y, Chu H W, Anand A and Huang C C 2016 *Anal. Methods* **8** 8123–33
[28] Marsico A L M, Elci G S, Moyano D F, Yesilbag Tonga G, Duncan B, Landis R F, Rotello V M and Vachet R W 2015 *Anal. Chem.* **87** 12145–50
[29] Sun C, Lee J S and Zhang M 2008 *Adv. Drug Delivery Rev.* **60** 1252
[30] Karimi Z, Karimi L and Shokrollahi H 2013 *Mater. Sci. Eng.* C **33** 2465
[31] Tural B, Ozkan N and Volkan M 2009 *J. Phys. Chem. Solids* **70** 860
[32] Chen Z P, Zhang Y, Zhang, Xia J G, Liu J W, Xu K and Gu N 2008 *Colloids Surf.* A **316** 210
[33] Namara K M and Tofail S A M 2013 Biomedical applications of nanoalloys , *Nanoalloys: From Fundamentals to Emergent Applications* ed C Florent (Oxford: Elsevier) pp 345
[34] Ahmad T, Bae H, Rhee I, Chang Y and Jin S U 2012 *J. Nanosci. Nanotechnol* **12** 5132
[35] Iqbal M Z, Ma X and Chen T 2015 *J. Mater. Chem.* B **3** 5172
[36] Qu J, Liu G, Wang Y and Hong R 2010 *Adv. Powder Technol* **21** 461
[37] Barick K C, Singh S, Bahadur D, Lawande M A, Patkar D and Hassan P A 2014 *J. Colloid Interface Sci.* **418** 120
[38] Jiang Q L *et al* 2014 *Appl. Surf. Sci.* **307** 224
[39] Jia Y *et al* 2012 *Int. J. Nanomedicine* **7** 1697
[40] Akbarzadeh A, Samiei M, Joo S W, Anzaby M, Hanifehpour Y, Nasrabadi H T and Davaran S 2012 *J. Nanobiotechnol* **10** 1
[41] Mohammadi-Samani S, Miri R, Salmanpour M, Khalighian N, Sotoudeh S and Erfani N 2013 *Res. Pharm. Sci.* **8** 25
[42] Li G, Cao L, Zhou Z, Chen Z, Huang Y and Zhao Y 2015 *Colloids Surf.* B **128** 379
[43] Karamipour S, Sadjadi M S and Farhadyar N 2015 *Spectrochim. Acta Mol. Biomol. Spectrosc* **148** 146
[44] Mancarella S, Greco V, Baldassarre F, Vergara D, Maffia M and Leporatti S 2015 *Macromol. Biosci.* **15** 1365
[45] Zou Y, Liu P, Liu C H and Zhi X T 2015 *Biomed. Pharmacother* **69** 355

[46] Zhao G, Wang J, Peng X, Li Y, Yuan X and Ma Y 2014 *Chem. Asian* J **9** 546
[47] Chen W, Wen X, Zhen G and Zheng X 2015 *RSC Adv* **5** 69307
[48] Sabale S, Jadhav V, Khot V, Zhu X, Xi M and Chen H 2015 *J. Mater. Sci. Mater. Med* **26** 1
[49] Lee J H *et al* 2006 *Nat. Med* **13** 95
[50] Joshi H M, Lin Y P, Aslam M, Prasad P V, Schultz-Sikma E A, Edelman R, Meade T and Dravid V P 2009 *J. Phys. Chem.* C **113** 17761
[51] Wu H, Liu G, Wang X, Zhang J, Chen Y, Shi J, Yang H, Hu H and Yang S 2011 *Acta Biomater* **7** 3496
[52] Kim D H, Nikles D E, Johnson D T and Brazel C S 2008 *J. Magn. Magn. Mater* **320** 2390
[53] Surendra M K, Annapoorani S, Ansar E B, Varma P H and Rao M R 2014 *J. Nanoparticle Res* **16** 1
[54] Shah S A, Asdi M H, Hashmi M U, Umar M F and Awan S U 2012 *Mater. Chem. Phys.* **137** 365
[55] Doaga A, Cojocariu A M, Amin W, Heib F, Bender P, Hempelmann R and Caltun O F 2013 *Mater. Chem. Phys.* **143** 305
[56] Lu J *et al* 2009 *Biomaterials* **30** 2919
[57] Yang H, Zhang C, Shi X, Hu H, Du X, Fang Y, Ma Y, Wu H and Yang S 2010 *Biomaterials* **31** 3667
[58] Jing Y, Sohn H, Kline T, Victora J P and Wang J P 2009 *J. Appl. Phys.* **105** 305
[59] Lacroix L M, Malaki R B, Carrey J, Lachaize S, Respaud M, Goya G F and Chaudret B 2009 *J. Appl. Phys.* **105** 023911
[60] Kline T L, Xu Y H, Jing Y and Wang J P 2009 *J. Magn. Magn. Mater* **321** 1525
[61] Mehdaoui B, Carrey J, Stadler M, Cornejo A, Nayral C, Delpech F, Chaudret B and Respaud M 2012 *Appl. Phys. Lett.* **100** 052403
[62] Shokuhfar A and Afghahi S S S 2014 *Adv. Mater. Sci. Eng* **2014** 1
[63] Alonso J, Khurshid H, Sankar V, Nemati Z, Phan M H, Garayo E H and Srikanth H 2015 *J. Appl. Phys.* **117** 17113
[64] An L, Yu Y, Li X, Liu W, Yang H, Wu D and Yang S 2014 *Mater. Res. Bull* **49** 285
[65] Yang H, Li X, Zhou H, Zhuang Y, Hu H, Wu H and Yang S 2011 *J. Alloys Compd* **509** 1217
[66] Ban I, Stergar J, Drofenik M, Ferk G and Makovec D 2011 *J. Magn. Magn. Mater* **323** 2254
[67] Stergar J, Ferk G, Ban I, Drofenik M, Hamler A, Jagodič M and Makovec D 2013 *J Alloys Compd.* **576** 220
[68] Amrollahi P, Ataie A, Nozari A, Seyedjafari E and Shafiee A 2015 *J. Mater. Eng. Perform* **4** 1220
[69] Kim D K, Kan D, Veres T, Normadin F, Liao J K, Kim H H, Lee S H, Zahn M and Muhammed M 2205 *J. Appl. Phys.* **97** 918
[70] Sun S 2006 *Adv. Mater* **18** 393
[71] Chiang P C, Hung D S, Wang J W, Ho C S and Yao Y D 2007 *IEEE Trans. Magn* **43** 2445
[72] Shi Y, Lin M, Jiang X and Liang S 2015 *Biomedicine* **21** 22
[73] Maenosono S and Saita S 2006 *IEEE Trans. Magn* **42** 1638
[74] Seehra M S, Singh V, Dutta P, Neeleshwar S, Chen Y Y, Chen C L, Chou S W and Chen C C 2010 *J. Phys. D: Appl. Phys.* **43** 145002
[75] Maenosono S, Suzuki Tand S and Saita J 2008 *Magn. Magn. Mater* **320** 79

[76] Taylor R M, Huber D L, Monson T C, Esch V and Sillerud L O 2012 *J. Vac. Sci. Technol.* B **30** 02C101

[77] Yang H, Zhang J, Tian Q, Hu H, Fang Y, Wu H and Yang S 2010 *J. Magn. Magn. Mater* **322** 973

[78] Chou S W, Shau Y H, Wu P C, Yang Y S, Shieh D B and Chen C C 2010 *J. Am. Chem. Soc* **132** 13270

[79] Fuchigami T, Kawamura R, Kitamoto Y, Nakagawa M and Namiki Y 2012 *Biomaterials* **33** 1682

[80] Chen C L, Kuo L R, Lee S Y, Hwu Y K, Chou S W, Chen C C, Chang F H, Lin K H, Tsai D H and Chen Y Y 2013 *Biomaterials* **34** 1128

[81] Sun H *et al* 2012 *Int. J. Nanomed.* **7** 3295

[82] Seemann K M, Luysberg M, Revay Z, Kudejova P, Sanz B, Cassinelli N, Loidl A, Ilcic K, Multhoff G and Schmid T E 2015 *J. Control. Release* **197** 131

[83] Zheng Y, Tang Y, Bao Z, Wang H, Ren F, Guo M, Quan H and Jiang C 2015 *Int. J. Nanomed.* **10** 6435

[84] Moghimi N and Leung K T 2013 *Anal. Chem.* **85** 5974

[85] Bhattacharya R *et al* 2007 *Nanomed. Nanotechnol. Biol. Med* **3** 224

[86] Patra C R, Bhattacharya R, Mukhopadhyay D and Mukherjee P 2010 *Adv. Drug Delivery Rev.* **62** 346

[87] Muddineti O S, Ghosh B and Biswas S 2015 *Int. J. Pharm* **484** 252

[88] Bertok T, Sediva A, Katrlik J, Gemeiner P, Mikula M, Nosko M and Tkac J 2013 *Talanta* **108** 11

[89] Lepinay S, Staff A, Ianoul A and Albert J 2014 *Biosen. Bioelectron* **52** 337

[90] Sun I C, Na J H, Jeong S Y, Kim D E, Kwon I C, Choi K, Ahn C H and Kim K 2014 *Pharmaceut. Res* **31** 1418

[91] Meir R, Shamalov K, Betzer O, Motiei M, Horovitz-Fried M, Yehuda R, Popovtzer A, Popovtzer R and Cohen C J 2015 *ACS Nano* **9** 6363

[92] Choi W I, Sahu A, Kim Y H and Tae G 2012 *Ann. Biomed. Eng* **40** 534

[93] Jung S, Nam J, Hwang S, Park J, Hur J, Im K, Park N and Kim S 2013 *Anal. Chem.* **85** 7674

[94] Curry T, Kopelman R, Shilo M and Popovtzer R 2014 *Contrast Media Mol. Imaging* **9** 53

[95] Wang F, Wang YC S, Dou S, Xiong M H, Sun T M and Wang J 2011 *ACS Nano* **5** 3679

[96] Lee J, Chatterjee D K, Lee M H and Krishnan S 2014 *Cancer Lett.* **347** 46

[97] Khan A K, Rashid R, Murtaza G and Zahra A 2014 *Trop. J. Pharm. Res* **13** 1169

[98] Ajnai G, Chiu A, Kan T, Cheng C C, Tsai T H and Chang J 2014 *J. Exp. Clin. Med* **6** 172

[99] Elbialy N, Fathy N M and Khalil W M 2015 *Int. J. Pharm* **490** 190

[100] Ge L, Li Q, Wang M, Ouyang J, Li X and Xing M M 2014 *Int. J. Nanomed.* **9** 2399

[101] Jun B H *et al* 2010 *Small* **6** 119

[102] Numnuam A 2014 *Anal. Bioanal. Chem.* **406** 3763

[103] Huang K J, Liu Y J, Wang H B and Wang Y Y 2014 *Electrochim. Acta* **118** 130

[104] Tian J, Wong K K, Ho C M, Lok C N, Yu W Y, Che C M, Chiu J F and Tam P K 2007 *Chem. Med. Chem.* **2** 129

[105] Kalishwaralal K, BarathManiKanth S, Pandian S R K, Deepak V and Gurunathan S 2010 *Colloids Surf.* B **79** 340

[106] Ragaseema V M, Unnikrishnan S, Krishnan V K and Krishnan L K 2012 *Biomaterials* **33** 3083

[107] Park S, Park H H, Kim S Y, Kim S J, Woo K and Ko G 2014 *Appl. Environ. Microbiol* **80** 2343
[108] Podbielska H, Wysocka K, Kowal K and Bauer J 2009 *World J. Eng* **6** 1
[109] Sahu S C, Zheng J, Graham L, Chen L, Ihrie J, Yourick J J and Sprando R L 2014 *J. Appl. Toxicol* **34** 1155
[110] Patra S, Mukherjee S, Barui A K, Ganguly A, Sreedhar B and Patra C R 2015 *Mater. Sci. Eng.* C **53** 298
[111] Benyettou F *et al* 2015 *J. Mater. Chem.* B **3** 7237
[112] Yin Z F, Wu L, Yang H G and Su Y H 2013 *Phys. Chem. Chem. Phys.* **15** 4844
[113] Wu K C W, Yamauchi Y, Hong C Y, Yang Y H, Liang Y H, Funatsu T and Tsunoda M 2011 *Chem. Commun* **47** 5232
[114] Qin Y, Sun L, Li X, Cao Q, Wang H, Tang X and Ye L J 2011 *Mater. Chem.* **21** 18003
[115] Wang T, Jiang H, Wan L, Zhao Q, Jiang T, Wang B and Wang S 2015 *Acta Biomater* **13** 354-63
[116] Zhang H, Wang C, Chen B and Wang X 2012 *Int. J. Nanomed.* **7** 235
[117] Ren W *et al* 2013 *RSC Adv* **3** 20855
[118] Shen Q, You S K, Park S G, Jiang H, Guo D, Chen B and Wang X 2008 *Electroanalysis* **20** 2526
[119] Meinhardt M, Krebs R, Anders A, Heinrich U and Tronnier H 2008 *J. Biomed. Opt* **13** 044030
[120] Karakoti A S, Monteiro-Riviere N A, Aggarwal R, Davis J P, Narayan R J, Self W T, McGinnis J and Seal S 2008 *JOM* **60** 33
[121] Renu G, Rani V V, Nair S V, Subramanian K R V and Lakshmanan V K 2012 *Adv. Sci. Lett.* **6** 17
[122] Chen J F, Ding H M, Wang J X and Shao L 2004 *Biomaterials* **25** 723
[123] Slowing I I, Trewyn B G, Giri S and Lin V Y 2007 *Adv. Funct. Mater* **17** 1225
[124] Rasmussen J W, Martinez E, Louka P and Wingett D G 2010 *Expert Opin. Drug Deliv* **7** 1063
[125] Bourganis V, Kammona O, Alexopoulos A and Kiparissides C 2018 *Eur. J. Pharm. Biopharm* **128** 337-62
[126] Daneman R and Prat A 2015 The blood–brain barrier , *Cold Spring Harb. Perspect. Biol* **7** 020412
[127] Upadhyay R K 2014 *BioMed Res. Int* **2014** 869269
[128] Bhowmik A, Khan R and Ghosh M K 2015 *BioMed Res. Int* **2015** 20
[129] Jena L, McErlean E and McCarthy H 2020 *Drug Deliv. Transl. Res* **10** 304–18
[130] Pardridge W M 2007 Drug targeting to the brain . *Pharm. Res* **24** 1733-44
[131] Cheng Y, Morshed R A, Auffinger B, Tobias A L and Lesniak M S 2014 *Adv. Drug Deliv. Rev.* **66** 42–57
[132] Florian P Y, Ron M A and Potočnik N O 2017 *Curr. Pharm. Des.* **23** 1–11
[133] Chughtai K and Heeren R M A 2010 *Chem. Rev.* **110** 3237–77
[134] Gemperline E, Chen B and Li L 2014 *Bioanalysis* **6** 525–40
[135] Boughton B A, Thinagaran D, Sarabia D, Bacic A and Roessner U 2016 *Phytochem. Rev.* **15** 445–88
[136] Masserini M and Masserini M 2013 *ISRN Biochem.* **2013** 238428
[137] Kaur I P, Bhandari R, Bhandari S and Kakkar V 2008 *J. Control. Release* **127** 97–109
[138] Proetto M T *et al* 2016 *ACS Nano* **10** 4046–54

[139] Xue J, Liu H, Chen S, Xiong C, Zhan L, Sun J and Nie Z 2017 *Sci. Adv* **2018** 9039
[140] Li X, Shan J, Zhang W, Su S, Yuwen L and Wang L 2017 *Small* **13** 1602660
[141] Chen H, Liu T, Su Z, Shang L and Wei G 2018 *Nanoscale Horiz* **3** 74–89
[142] Pelaz B *et al* 2017 Diverse applications of nanomedicine *ACS Nano* **11** 2313–81
[143] Chen S, Xiong C, Liu H, Wan Q, Hou J, He Q, Badu-Tawiah A and Nie Z 2015 *Nat. Nanotechnol* **10** 176–82
[144] Wu G, Fang Y Z, Yang S, Lupton J R and Turner N D 2004 *J. Nutr* **134** 489
[145] Carmel R and Jacobsen D W 2001 *Homocysteine in Health and Disease* (Cambridge: Cambridge University Press)
[146] Refsum H, Ueland P M, Nygard O and Vollset S E 1998 *Annu. Rev. Med* **49** 31
[147] Seshadri S, Beiser A, Selhub J, Jacques P F, Rosenberg I H, D'Agostino R B and Wilson P W F 2002 *N. Engl. J. Med* **346** 476
[148] Staal F J T, Ela S, Roedere M, Anderson M T and Herzenberg L A 1992 *Lancet* **339** 909
[149] Berkenkamp S, Kirpekav F and Hillenkamp F 1998 *Science* **281** 260
[150] Shrivas K and Wu H F 2007 *Rapid Commun. Mass Spectrom* **21** 3108
[151] Shrivas K and Wu H F 2008 *Rapid Commun. Mass Spectrom* **22** 2863–72
[152] Tokareva I and Hutter E 2004 *J. Am. Chem. Soc* **126** 15784
[153] Vidal B C, Deivaraj T C, Yang J, Too H P, Chow G M, Gan L M and Lee J Y 2005 *New J. Chem.* **29** 812
[154] Tanaka K, Ido Y, Akita S, Yoshida Y and Yoshida T 1987 *Proc. 2nd Japan–China Joint Symp. on Mass Spectrometry* pp 185
[155] Watanabe T, Kawasaki H, Yonezawa T and Arawaka R 2008 *J. Mass Spectrom* **43** 1063
[156] Taira S, Kitajima K, Katayanagi H, Ichiishi E and Ichiyanagi Y 2009 *Sci. Technol. Adv. Mater* **10** 034602
[157] Cunningham D, Littleford R E, Smith W E, Lundahl P J, Khan I, McComb D W, Graham D and Laforest N 2006 *Faraday Discuss* 132–35
[158] Pasilis S P, Kertesz V and Berkel G J V 2008 *Anal. Chem.* **80** 1208
[159] Zheng B L, He K, Kim C H, Rogers L, Shao Y, Huang Z Y, Lu Y, Yan S J, Qien L C and Zheng Q Y 2000 *Urology* **55** 598–602
[160] Zhao M J, Dunbar D C and Khan I A 2002 *Phytochemistry* **59** 105–10
[161] Zhao J P, Muhammad I, Dunbar D C, Mustafa J and Khan I A 2005 *J. Agric. Food Chem.* **53** 690–3
[162] Piacente S, Carbone V, Plaza A, Zampelli A and Pizza C 2002 *J. Agric. Food Chem.* **50** 5621–5
[163] Cui B, Zheng B L, He K and Zheng Q Y 2003 *J. Nat. Prod* **66** 1101–3
[164] Yu M, Qin X J, Shao L D, Peng X R, Li L, Yang H and Qiu M H 2017 *Tetrahedron Lett.* **58** 1684–6
[165] Zhou M, Zhang R Q, Chen Y J, Liao L M, Sun Y Q, Ma Z H, Yang Q F, Li P, Ye Y Q and Hu Q F 2018 *Phytochem. Lett.* **25** 137–40
[166] McCollom M M, Villinski J R, McPhail K L, Craker L E and Gafner S 2005 *Phytochem. Anal* **16** 463–9
[167] Alasmari M, Böhlke M, Kelley C, Maher T and Figueroa A P 2019 *Mol. Neurobiol* **56** 1770–81
[168] Li J, Liu J, Liu Z, Tan Y, Liu X and Wang F 2017 *Chem. Commun* **53** 12688–91
[169] Yang S, Zhan L, Liu C, Fu L, Chen R and Nie Z 2019 *Microchem.* J **150** 104190
[170] Nile S H, Baskar V and Selvaraj D 2020 *Nano-Micro Lett.* **12** 45

[171] Kessler R 2011 *Environ. Health Perspect* **119** A120–5
[172] Domercq P, Praetorius A and Boxall A B A 2018 *Environ. Sci.: Nano* **5** 533-43
[173] Pourzahedi L, Vance M and Eckelman M J 2017 *Environ. Sci. Technol* **51** 7148–58
[174] Laborda F, Bolea E and Lamana J J 2014 *Anal. Chem.* **86** 2270–8
[175] Mozhayeva D and Engelhard C 2020 *J. Anal. At. Spectrom* **35** 1740-83
[176] Montaño M D, Olesik J W and Barber A G 2016 *Anal. Bioanal. Chem.* **408** 5053–74
[177] Bustos A R M and Winchester M R 2016 *Anal. Bioanal. Chem.* **408** 5051–2
[178] Powers K W, Brown S C, Krishna V B, Wasdo S C, Moudgil B M and Roberts S M 2006 *Toxicol. Sci.* **90** 296–303
[179] Shekunov B Y, Chattopadhyay P, Tong H H and Chow A H 2007 *Pharm. Res* **24** 203–27
[180] Champion J A, Katare Y K and Mitragotri S 2007 *J. Control. Release* **121** 3–9
[181] Decuzzi P, Pasqualini R, Rap W and Ferrari M 2009 *Pharm. Res* **26** 235–43
[182] Buzea C, Pacheco I and Robbie K 2007 *Biointerphases* **2** 17–71
[183] Brodbeck W G, Shive M S, Calton E, Nakayama Y, Matsuda T and Anderson J M 2001 *J. Biomed. Mater. Res* **55** 661–8
[184] Patri A, Dobrovolskais M, Stem S, McNeil S and Amiji M 2006 Preclinical characterization of engineered nanoparticles intended for cancer therapeutics *Nanotechnology for Cancertherapy* (Boca Raton, FL: CRC Press) pp 105–38
[185] Lin P, Lin S, Wang P C and Sridhar R 2014 *Biotechnol. Adv* **32** 711–26
[186] Laborda F, Bolea E and Jimenez J 2014 *Anal. Chem.* **86** 2270–8
[187] Laborda F, Bolea E, Cepria G, Gomoz M T, Jimenez M S, Perez J and Castillo J R 2016 *Anal. Chim. Acta* **904** 10–32
[188] Lee W W and Chan W T 2015 *J. Anal. At. Spectrom* **30** 1245–54
[189] Mitrano D M, Barber A, Bednar A, Westerhoff P, Higgins C P and Ranville J F 2012 *J. Anal. At. Spectrom* **27** 1131–42
[190] Kaushik S, Djiwanti S R and Skotti E 2019 *Nanotechnology in the Life Sciences* (Cham: Springer)
[191] Ruan J, Song H, Qian Q, Li C, Wang K, Bao C and Cui D 2012 *Biomaterials* **33** 7093–102
[192] Ogra Y, Awaya Y and Anan Y 2015 *Environ. Contam. Toxicol* **94** 604–8
[193] Najimi S, Shakibaie M, Jafari E, Ameri A, Rahimi N, Forootanfar H, Yazdanpanah M and Rahimi H R 2017 *Regul. Toxicol. Pharmacol* **90** 222–30
[194] Tanakaa Y K, Takadaa S, Kumagaib K, Kobayashib K, Hokurac A and Ogra Y 2020 **62** 126628
[195] Jariwala D, Sangwan V K, Lauhon L J, Marks T J and Hersam M C 2013 *Chem. Soc. Rev.* **42** 2824–60
[196] Allen M J, Tung V C and Kaner R B 2010 *Chem. Rev.* **110** 132–45
[197] Abarrategi A 2008 *Biomaterials* **29** 94–102
[198] Miyako E 2012 *Nat. Commun* **3** 1226
[199] Baker S N and Baker G A 2010 *Angew. Chem. Int. Ed* **49** 6726–44
[200] Bianco KK A and Prato M 2009 *Nat. Nanotechnol.* **4** 626–33
[201] Georgin D 2009 *J. Am. Chem. Soc* **131** 14658–9
[202] Avti P K 2012 *PLoS One* **7** e35064
[203] Berry K A 2011 *Chem. Rev.* **111** 6491–512
[204] Chen S 2013 *Anal. Chem.* **85** 6646–52
[205] Belau L 2007 *J. Am. Chem. Soc* **129** 10229–43
[206] Lagarrigue M 2014 *Anal. Chem.* **86** 5775–83

[207] Yang X, Ren J, Qu K and Qu X 2012 *Adv. Mater* **24** 1722–8
[208] Chen S, Xion C, Liu H, Wan Q, Hou J, He Q, Tawiah A B and Nie Z 2005 *Nat. Nanotechnol* **5** 176–82
[209] Xu S Y, Li Y F, Zou H F, Qiu J S, Guo Z and Guo B C 2003 *Anal. Chem.* **75** 6191–5
[210] Dong X L, Cheng J S, Li J H and Wang Y S 2010 *Anal. Chem.* **82** 6208–14
[211] Hua P-Y, Manikandan M, Abdelhamid H N and Wu H-F 2014 *J. Mater. Chem.* B **2** 7334–43
[212] Chen S, Zheng H, Wang J, Hou J, He Q and Liu H 2013 *Anal. Chem.* **85** 6646–52
[213] He X-M, Zhu G-T, Yin J, Zhao Q, Yuan B-F and Feng Y-Q 2014 *J. Chromatogr.* A **1351** 29–36
[214] Ma R N, Lu M H, Ding L, Ju H X and Cai Z W 2013 *Chem. Eur.* J **19** 102–8
[215] Wei J, Buriak J M and Siuzdak G 1999 *Nature* **399** 243–6
[216] McLean J A, Stumpo K A and Russell D H 2005 *J. Am. Chem. Soc* **127** 5304–5
[217] Wah M C, Kim H S, Wood T D, Guan S H and Marshall A G 1993 *Anal. Chem.* **65** 3669–76
[218] Nayak R and Knapp D R 2007 *Anal. Chem.* **79** 4950–6
[219] Tang J, Liu Y C, Qi D W, Yao G P, Deng C H and Zhang X M 2009 *Proteomics* **9** 5046–55
[220] Teng C H, Ho K C, Lin Y S and Chen Y C 2004 *Anal. Chem.* **76** 4337–42
[221] Chiu T C, Chang L C, Chiang C K and Chang H T 2008 *J. Am. Soc. Mass Spectrom* **19** 1343–6
[222] Kawasaki H, Yonezawa T, Watanabe T and Arakawa R 2007 *J. Phys. Chem.* C **111** 16278–83
[223] Shrivas K, Hayasaka T, Sugiura Y and Setou M 2011 *Anal. Chem.* **83** 7283–9
[224] Shin W J, Shin J H, Song J Y and Han S Y 2010 *J. Am. Soc. Mass Spectrom* **21** 989–92
[225] Chen W Y and Chen Y C 2006 *Anal. Bioanal. Chem.* **386** 699–704
[226] Chen W Y, Wang L S, Chiu H T, Chen Y C and Lee C Y 2004 *J. Am. Soc. Mass Spectrom* **15** 1629–35
[227] Ugarov M V *et al* 2004 *Anal. Chem.* **76** 6734–42
[228] Lu M, Lai Y, Chen G and Cai Z 2011 *Anal. Chem.* **83** 3161–9
[229] Tang L A L, Wang J and Loh K P 2010 *J. Am. Chem. Soc* **132** 10976–7
[230] Zhang J, Dong X, Cheng J, Li J and Wang Y 2011 *J. Am. Soc. Mass Spectrom* **22** 1294–8
[231] Shi C, Meng J and Deng C 2012 *J. Mater. Chem.* **22** 20778–85
[232] Northen T R, Yanes O, Northen M T, Marrinucci D, Uritboonthai W, Apon J, Golledge S L, Nordstrom and Siuzdak A G 2007 *Nature* **449** 1033–6
[233] Yanes O *et al* 2009 *Anal. Chem.* **81** 2969–75

IOP Publishing

Analytical Techniques for Biomedical Nanotechnology

Ajeet Kaushik, Sesha S Srinivasan and Yogendra Kumar Mishra

Chapter 9

Magnetic measurement systems for biomedical nanotechnology

Md Mottahir Alam, Mohd Imran, Akhilesh Kumar Gupta, Afzal Khan, Tansir Ahamad and Ajeet Kaushik

Over the last few decades, magnetic nanostructures have been providing the platform to develop magnetically guided systems for biomedical nanotechnology and applications such as biosensors, nanomedicine, targeted drug delivery, etc. Magnetic nanoparticles especially super-paramagnetic iron oxide nanoparticles (SPIONs) have gained more importance in biomedical applications. This chapter discusses the biomedical uses of magnetic nanoparticles. The use of magnetic nanoparticles in hyperthermia, drug delivery, imaging tools, MRI, electrochemical sensors, cell and gene therapy for cancer treatment are discussed after reviewing some of the basic principles of magnetism. Finally, a summary of the magnetic nanostructure based biomedical nanotechnology is presented by examining current possibilities in this area, especially the huge hurdles faced when implementing laboratory-tested technologies.

9.1 Introduction

Magnetic nanoparticles (MNPs) due to their outstanding magnetic properties, sizes comparable to that of biological entities like cells, proteins, genes, viruses, and their excellent biocompatibility offer several exciting biomedical applications. Magnetic nanoparticles, owing to their magnetic nature, obey Coulomb's law, and hence may be monitored through an external magnetic field [1]. Functional groups may be coated on magnetic nanoparticles to modify their physical and chemical properties and achieve versatility. These functionalized MNPs offer new potential methods for bio-separation, bio-detection, and drug administration by enabling biomolecules to be tagged, detected, and controlled magnetically. Magnetic nanoparticles can be used for the transport of magnetically tagged biological entities to a specific part of the body, such as a tumorous cell. Magnetic nanoparticles may be engineered to

doi:10.1088/978-0-7503-3379-5ch9

resonantly respond to a high-frequency variable magnetic field, resulting in beneficial energy transfer from the stimulating magnetic field to the magnetic nanoparticles. Thus, magnetic nanoparticles can be used in magnetic-induced hyperthermia by providing very high thermal energy at the nanoscale to targeted areas like tumors, or as enhancement agents in magnetic nanoparticle enhanced chemotherapy and radiotherapy, where a reasonable extent of tissue warming results in cancer cell destruction and can debar the uncontrolled growth of tumor cells to different parts of the body. Magnetic nanoparticles are also employed as contrast-enhancing agents for enhancing the sensitivity of magnetic resonance imaging (MRI). In addition, magnetic nanoparticles are widely used for drug delivery, imaging tools, electrochemical sensors, cell and gene therapy, oncology, cardiovascular, magnetic separation of cell, etc [2–5]. Hence, because of the unique tunable physicochemical, thermal, and mechanical characteristics of magnetic nanoparticles, these and many more potential biomedical uses are now conceivable. This chapter discusses the core concepts involved in the biomedical applications of magnetic nanoparticles. After reviewing some of the fundamental concepts of magnetism, we will discuss various biomedical applications such as hyperthermia, drug delivery, imaging tools, MRI, electrochemical sensors, cell and gene therapy, and oncology. We will wrap up with an assessment of prospects in this field, particularly in light of the obstacles involved in putting existing laboratory-tested technology into widespread usage.

9.1.1 Basic characteristics of magnetic materials

The fundamental physics of magnetic nanoparticle biomedical applications will be discussed in this section.

9.1.1.1 Magnetization curve of magnetic materials

When a magnetic material is exposed to a magnetic field, its magnetic dipoles align to produce a response magnetization, which combines with the applied field to produce magnetic induction. There are two types of magnetization curve generated in response to an applied field. *M–H* curves focus on the internal response of the magnetic material, while *B–H* curves focus on the magnetic induction. In the *B–H* curve, the flux density of the magnetic sample *B* (in tesla) is plotted against the externally applied magnetic field (in A m^{-1}). By studying the hysteresis loop in depth, we may understand a variety of other magnetic ideas and principles. If a magnetic substance is placed in a magnetic field strength *H*, the overall magnetic induction is the sum of individual atomic moment in the substance [6], that is,

$$B = \mu_0(H + M)$$

where μ_0 is the magnetic permeability of free space, having SI unit as henries per meter (H m^{-1}) and *M* is called magnetization (magnetic moment per unit volume), written as:

$$M = m/V$$

where m is the magnetic moment on a volume V of the material, and M is the magnetization induced in a material by an external magnetic field H. All materials, based on their atomic structure and temperature, are magnetic to a certain degree. They may be suitably categorized on the basis of their volumetric magnetic susceptibility, χ, defined by the relation:

$$M = \chi H$$

In SI units, χ is dimensionless and both M and H are expressed in A m^{-1}.

The *B–H* curve is often used to explain the nonlinear magnetization behavior of a ferromagnetic material in response to an applied magnetic field. It is usually used to describe the magnetization properties at a specific temperature of magnetic materials by characterizing the magnetic permeability (μ). Magnetic permeability is the measure of a material to allow its magnetization against an applied magnetic field. It can be defined as a relative increase or decrease in the resultant magnetic field (B) of a magnetic material due to an applied magnetizing field (H) in which the given material is located. *B–H* curve can be linear or nonlinear. When the applied magnetic field is cycled, however, the response is nonlinear, and hysteresis curves occur.

Figure 9.1(a) shows schematically what happens when a magnetic field (H) is applied to a magnetic material. As the field increases in strength, the magnetic moment of the material (B) increases as well, as the magnetic dipoles begin to align with the applied magnetic field. That is, the material is becoming magnetically polarized. Since M is increasing, the corresponding magnetic induction (B) increases

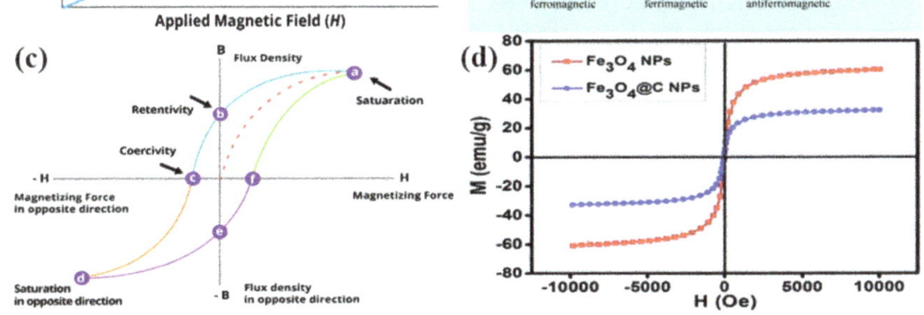

Figure 9.1. (a) Initial magnetization curve. (b) Schematic depiction of magnetic dipole configurations in diamagnetic, paramagnetic, ferromagnetic, ferrimagnetic, and antiferromagnetic materials in the presence and absence of an external magnetic field (H). (c) Typical magnetization curve for ferromagnetic nanoparticles and (d) magnetization curve and magnetic response of the magnetite nanoparticles against an external magnetic field (magnet). Reproduced from [20]. CC BY 3.0.

as well. Eventually, when the magnetic dipoles are fully aligned with the field, B can increase no more. This is known as the saturation magnetization (M_s). Based on the magnetic permeabilities, materials can be classified as: diamagnetic, paramagnetic, or ferromagnetic. Diamagnetic materials have a constant relative magnetic permeability slightly lesser than one. For example, when bismuth is placed in a magnetic field, a magnetic field in opposition of an externally applied magnetic field is created, producing a repulsive effect. Paramagnetic materials have a constant relative permeability which is slightly more than one. When a paramagnetic material such as platinum is placed in a magnetic field, it becomes magnetized in the direction of the external magnetic field. Ferromagnetic materials do not have a constant relative permeability. When a ferromagnetic material such as iron is placed in an external magnetic field, the magnetizing field increases, and the relative permeability also increases reaching a maximum and then decreases. Many magnetic alloys including purified iron have a maximum relative permeability of over 100 000. The magnetic permeability of a material is affected by several factors such as the nature of the material, humidity, temperature, frequency of the applied force, and the magnetic field etc. Magnetic susceptibility is the degree to which a material can be magnetized in an external magnetic field. If the ratio between the induced magnetization and the inducing field is expressed per unit volume. It can be expressed as: $k = M/H$, where M is the volume magnetization induced in a material of susceptibility k by the applied external field H. It is crucial to comprehend the basic characteristics of magnetic nanoparticles, as well as the impact of physical and chemical characteristics on their magnetic properties for its use in different applications. Based on the arrangement of magnetic dipoles in the presence or absence of an external magnetic field, magnetic nanomaterials are categorized as: diamagnetic, paramagnetic, ferromagnetic, ferrimagnetic, and antiferromagnetic, as shown in figure 9.1(b) [7]. Diamagnetic nanoparticles produce magnetic dipoles in the opposite direction of the external magnetic field, whereas the magnetic dipoles of paramagnetic nanoparticles align in the same direction as the external field. In the case of ferromagnetic nanoparticles, permanent magnetic dipoles exist either with or without an external magnetic field, ferromagnetic materials have permanent magnetic dipoles. In the absence of a magnetic field, certain weak magnetic dipoles may be found antiparallel to adjacent stronger dipoles in ferrimagnetic materials. In the absence of a magnetic field, adjacent dipoles in the antiferromagnetic material are antiparallel and neutralize each other. The saturation magnetization (M_s), the remanent magnetization (M_r), and the coercivity (H_c), are all shown on the magnetization curve of ferromagnetic particles [7]. Above the blocking temperature, ferromagnetic and ferrimagnetic materials show super-paramagnetic behavior (T_B). The merging points of the zero-field-cooled (ZFC) and field-cooled (FC) magnetization curves [7] are used to calculate the value of this temperature. The following formula may be used to determine the blocking temperature: $T_B = KV/25k_B$, where K denotes the anisotropy constant, V the magnetic particle's volume, and k_B the Boltzmann constant. Researchers have employed super-paramagnetic, ferromagnetic, and ferromagnetic nanomaterials for a variety of biomedical applications.

The uses of nanomaterials for different applications are based on different parameters like the size, shape, and composition of the magnetic nanoparticles, the magnetic anisotropy constant (K_T), the volume of the nanoparticles (V), and the magnetization saturations of the nanoparticles ($M_S(T)$) [5, 8, 9]. The magnetization of saturation increases according to the size of the nanoparticle to some degree. As a consequence, monodispersed, large-size nanoparticles are magnetically saturated, which increases the heating capacity of the nanoparticles. As a result, a small species absorption rate (SAR) of magnetic nanoparticles with a size below 7 nm (e.g., iron oxide) means that, whereas a significantly greater value for SAR in 14–16 nm magnetic nanoparticles is found they are much better at producing sufficient heat for effective hyperthermia therapy without major side effects [10, 11]. This form of nanoparticles is being considered for applications requiring heat production. Low magnetic anisotropy (K_T) and high M_S (T) results in reduced energy surface facets in magnetic nanoparticles which increases the heating efficiency of these nanoparticles. That is why, nanoparticles of spherical iron oxide have lower SAR values than those of cubic nanoparticles of the same volume [12, 13]. Nanoparticles may also be modified for magnetic effect to alter the chemical makeup. Nanoparticles with metal ions doping ferrite (Fe_2O_3) is a popular method used to increase saturation magnetization and, therefore, to improve SAR measurements. The SAR value of Zn and/or Mn-doped iron oxide nanoparticles is four times greater than the traditional iron oxide nanoparticles [14]. The magnetic response of magnetic nanoparticles to an external field is determined by the degree of magnetic ordering and its temperature [15]. The magnetization, or magnetic moment per unit volume of particle, can be described on the basis of spin or orbital energy possessed by the magnetic dipole. To maintain the lowest energy state, particles with large crystallite sizes have dipoles organized in numerous domains separated by a domain wall. The formation of domain barriers is energetically unfavorable below a certain size (usually less than 100 nm), resulting in single domain nanoparticles [16]. Under an external magnetic field, a hysteresis curve is not exhibited by nanoparticles in the single domain range. Magnetic spins of magnetic nanoparticles try to align in the direction of the externally applied magnetic field leading to induced magnetization [17]. The highest induced magnetization of a sample is called the saturation magnetization. The induced magnetization may persist after the magnetic field is withdrawn, which is known as remanent magnetization. Remanence is the magnetic field that still remains in the magnetic material after the applied magnetic field is decreased to zero. The raw value of remanence and the shape of hysteresis curve help to determine whether a given material displays hard or soft magnetic behavior. The value of external magnetic field (H) required returning the magnetization (B) to zero is called coercivity. It can be also called the resistance of a material to changes in magnetization. Soft magnetic materials have a low coercivity, whereas hard magnetic materials have a high coercivity. This implies that the hysteresis curve of soft magnetic materials is extremely narrow, while the hysteresis curve of hard magnetic materials is quite wide. Hysteresis is common in nanoparticles with ferro- and ferrimagnetic properties. Remanence and coercive field are minimal in nanoparticles that show superparamagnetism.

Figure 9.1(c) shows a schematic diagram of characteristic magnetization curve for ferromagnetic nanoparticles. It shows a magnetic material's capacity to act in response to an applied magnetic field H. The magnetization curve, as shown in figure 9.1(c) gives the major magnetic characteristics parameters such as saturation magnetization ($M_s(T)$), the exchange constant ($A(T)$), the anisotropy ($K(T)$), coercivity, the Curie temperature (T_c), and remanence. The magnitude of magnetic susceptibility is determined by the slope of the magnetization curve at H tends to zero. Figure 9.1(d) illustrates the magnetic response of magnetite nanoparticles due to a magnet and the magnetization curve of the sample using a vibrating sample magnetometry (VSM) [20]. The saturation magnetization of magnetite nanoparticles (76 emu g^{-1}) was found to be lower than that of bulk magnetite (92 emu g^{-1}). The saturation magnetization of ferrite nanoparticles is also reported to drop dramatically with decreasing particle size, although the cause of this phenomenon is unknown and under research. Magnetite nanoparticles lose their bulk ferromagnetism and become super-paramagnetic when their diameter is reduced to less than a threshold value (usually less than 35 nm). The average diameter of the produced magnetite nanoparticles is around 25 nm, which is smaller than the top limit for super-paramagnetic property. As a result, most of these nanoparticles are super-paramagnetic [19, 20].

9.1.1.2 Vibrating sample magnetometer/magnetometry

The vibrating sample magnetometer is employed as the most common instrument for measuring magnetization, hysteresis loop, magnetization curve, demagnetization curve, temperature rise and fall curve, etc in a magnetic material. The values of various magnetic measurement parameters such as saturation magnetization, residual magnetization, Curie temperature, coercivity, magnetic energy product and permeability, etc can be measured when a magnetic material is vibrated perpendicularly to a uniform magnetizing field. It was invented by Simon Foner at MIT Lincoln Laboratory in 1955, and is, therefore, also called the Foner magnetometer [21]. Several improvements and additions have been made for this instrument since its invention, but the underlying concept has remained the same. The magnetic properties of materials of diverse sample sizes and shapes, such as powder, particles, films, liquids, and single crystals, can be measured with this device. The VSM can monitor the variations in magnetic strength with changes in temperature from −196 °C to 900 °C. The magnetometer is based on Faraday's law of electromagnetic induction. The inductive detection process of this magnetic moment mechanism is closely linked with the pick-up coil design, physical sizes, and cross-section of the spools. This is known as inductive detection. The different types of materials measured by a typical vibrating sample magnetometer are as follows:

a. Magnetic materials, such as paramagnetic, diamagnetic, ferromagnetic, ferrimagnetic, and antiferromagnetic, or anisotropic materials.
b. Particle based or continuous thin film based magnetic recording materials, CMR, giant magnetoresistance (GMR), spin valve and exchange-based materials.
c. Magnetic–optical materials.
d. Single crystals, thin films, powders, bulk materials, and liquids.

9.1.2 Biomedical nanotechnology

MNPs have recently been the focus of intense research for biomedical applications [22, 23]. The development of the magnetic domain theory in the early 20th century and the magnetism of particles have been the subject of considerable study. The hypothesis demonstrates that the size of magnetic particles substantially affects how they behave in a magnetic field. When their size is less than the actual size for exchange interactions (usually 10–15 nm), they exhibit super-paramagnetic behavior throughout a small temperature range [24]. Magnetic nanostructures and nanoparticles are critical components of biology and technology. Moreover, the appropriate surface functionalization of nanoparticles (NPs) enables the selective bonding of magnetic forces to a wide variety of cellular structures and biomolecules.

Generally, MNPs are classified into three types: metal oxides, pure metals, and magnetic nanocomposite. The most often utilized MNPs in the biomedical sector include metal alloys of Fe, Co, Ti, Ni, iron oxide, and ferrite ($BaFe_{12}O_{19}$, $CoFe_2O_4$). Among them, iron oxide nanoparticles (often Fe_3O_4 or Fe_2O_3) have received the greatest attention due to their low toxicity [25]. Additionally, MNPs are a type of nanoparticle that have a high surface-to-volume ratio, enabling them to adsorb proteins or load medicines. They also possess a unique super-paramagnetic feature that allows them to respond to an external magnetic field. MNPs can be easily separated from other components of the mixture using magnets. This chapter describes different types of MNPs, most notably iron oxide nanoparticles and magnetic nanocomposites. Further, MNPs have been used in several biomedical applications such as MRI, drug delivery, tissue engineering, and biosensors, as shown in figure 9.2.

Internal organ imaging with a high spatial resolution is critical for accurate medical diagnosis and therapy. MRI is a vital imaging technology because it provides unprecedented temporal and spatial resolution without invasive procedures [27]. Computer-assisted imaging is accomplished in MRI by excitation of proton spins within the human body by radiofrequency waves in a high magnetic field. While MRI produces precise images, it is not always reliable, as normal tissues and tumors frequently exhibit only minor changes in relaxation time. To address this, MRI contrast agents can be employed to enhance image clarity and facilitate interpretation. In addition, the increased recognition of magnetic nanoparticles as MRI contrast agents enables detection of disease of specific biomarkers at the molecular and cellular level [25]. The nanoparticle's core can be entirely encased using a surface-capsulation technique to overcome the end-grafting strategy's constraints. Although imaging of sentinel lymph nodes (SLNs) is challenging, mainly when they are located deep within tissue, it is critical for understanding how cancer cells flow through them [28, 29]. While positron emission tomography (PET) is a susceptible imaging technology, it provides little anatomical information. The precise location of a brachial lymph node (LN) within the context of the rat's anatomical form is only apparent when PET and MR images are superimposed. We dissected and reexamined the brachial LNs on both the right and left sides using PET and MRI to corroborate the above imaging findings as shown in figures 9.3(A) and (B).

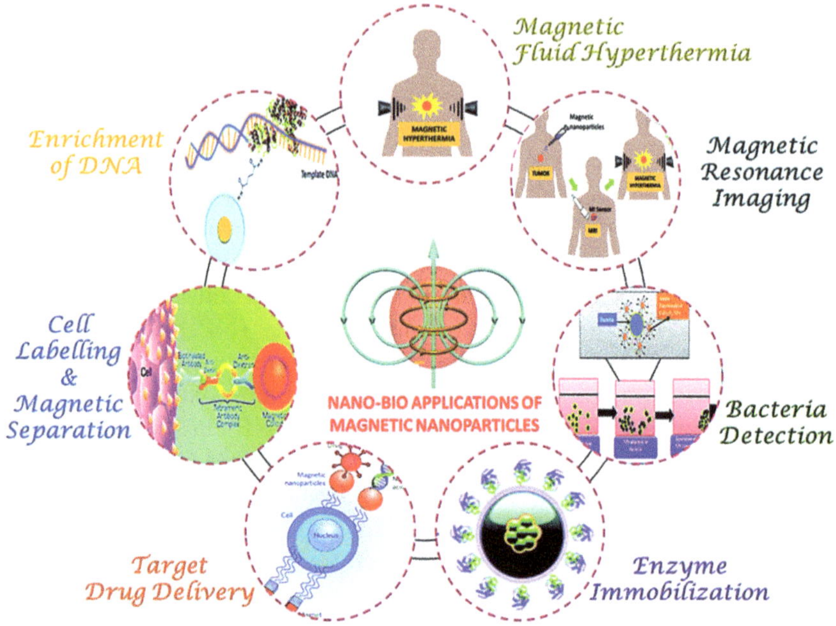

Figure 9.2. Magnetic nanoparticles and their different biomedical applications. Reproduced from [26] with permission of The Royal Society of Chemistry.

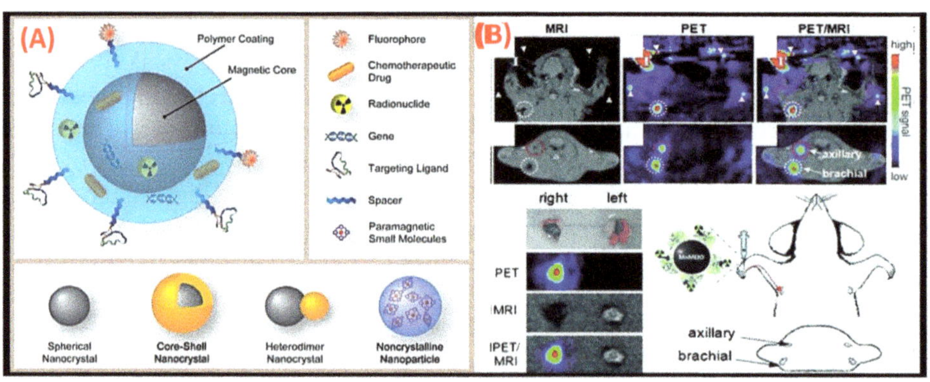

Figure 9.3. (A) Graphic illustration of the structure of a multifunctional MNP and different types of magnetic cores. Reproduced from [30] with permission of The Royal Society of Chemistry. (B) PET/MR images of rat [28]. Copyright © 2008 WILEY-VCH Verlag GmbH & Co. KGaA, Weinheim.

Cancer is a leading cause of death worldwide, accounting for ten million fatalities. Over the last several decades, remarkable advances in understanding how cancer begins and progresses have improved diagnosis and therapy methods. The physicochemical properties of nanoparticles can also be tuned by altering their chemical compositions, sizes, morphologies, and surface properties. Numerous similar delivery methods have been approved for use in clinical trials or preclinical evaluations for cancer therapy. Nanoparticle-based medicines can drastically

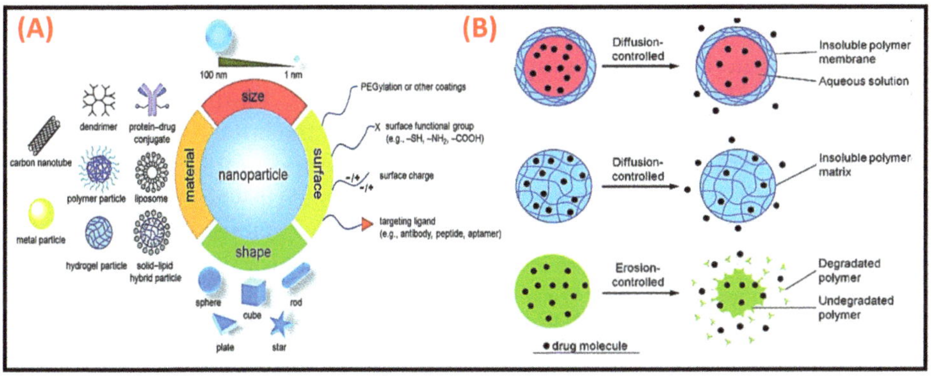

Figure 9.4. (A) A summary of nanoparticles carriers for drug delivery in cancer therapy and (B) three major mechanisms for achieving sustained drug release [24]. © 2014 WILEY-VCH Verlag GmbH & Co. KGaA, Weinheim.

improve the treatment outcomes for oncological disorders, reshaping the pharmaceutical industry's environment, as shown in figure 9.4(A).

Diffusion-controlled release prevents the drug molecules packed inside a nanoparticle from exiting the aqueous environment due to an insoluble substance acting as a barrier, as shown in figure 9.4(B). By switching to colloidal hollow particles, the concept of this release system can readily be extended to nanosized carriers. Typically, the initially loaded drug molecules in the reservoir can only diffuse out through the membrane. The rate of drug release is determined by the membrane's physicochemical qualities and the loaded drug, as well as the membrane's thickness. Despite their simplicity in terms of the release mechanism and ability to ensure steady-state release, polymer-membrane-based devices are significantly disadvantaged due to the dose generated by pinholes and cracks in the membrane.

9.2 Magnetic materials

Magnetic particles have been used in medicine since early times. Thales of Miletus, an ancient Greek philosopher, believed that man and the magnet were linked in some way and that each had a soul. Hippocrates of Kos, the father of medicine, utilized the styptic iron oxides magnetite and hematite to halt bleeding and reduce hemorrhage [31]. William Gilbert, who compiled all the information about magnetism and electricity known at his time in a six-volume treatise, was a physician—in fact, Queen Elizabeth's personal physician. At present, owing to the excellent physical and chemical properties of magnets and magnetic particles, they are used extensively in the areas of dentistry, cardiology, neurology, cancer, and radiology, to name just a few. The most commonly used magnetic nanoparticles for biomedical applications include iron oxide based nano-crystalline structures of magnetite (Fe_3O_4) and/or maghemite (γ-Fe_2O_3) coated with polysaccharide, organic or polymeric stabilizers, or inorganic coatings. Apart from these, metallic nanoparticles (such as Fe, Cu, Ag, Au, or Cr), metallic oxide nanoparticles (such as α-Fe_2O_3, CuO, ZnO, TiO_2, CeO_2 SiO_2) are also used.

9.2.1 Synthesis of magnetic nanomaterials

Two primary methods exist for creating nanoparticles in the size range of 1–100 nm: 'top-down' technology and 'bottom-up' synthesis [32]. In the former, the bulk materials are chopped down to the nanoscale, while in the latter, nanoscale particles are created from smaller particles. One of the most important differences between the two methods is that only the same basic attributes exist when trying to regulate the size of nanoparticles and when using energies to manufacture the nanoparticles. Top-down technologies originate from the semiconductor industry, particularly lithography, employed in the fabrication of chips. To create different nanostructures, light with an electron beam is utilized to eliminate unwanted microstructures from the precursor materials. Also, the use of the ball milling and sputtering processes are top-down technologies. The second technique is bottom-up, beginning with molecules or atoms. Major techniques in the bottom-up approach are: plasma arcing, chemical vapor deposition (CVD), and microwave-assisted plasma chemical vapor deposition (MWPCVD). Additionally, sol–gel synthesis, the co-precipitation method, the microemulsion method, the hydrothermal method, and the reduction method can be used to make nanoparticles in the bottom-up approach. Some of the synthesis methods are described below.

9.2.1.1 Ball mill method

Ball milling is the method of reducing particle size by impact from falling balls. Using this conventional method, micro and nano size particle production is ecologically benign at a relatively low cost. This method is both cost-effective and simple and may generate a variety of nanostructures. Ball milling involves many variables, such as the milling rate, quantity and size of milling balls, milling duration, and the milling material [33, 34].

9.2.1.2 Chemical vapor deposition

This method consists of depositing thin films of various mixed components. It is used to create crystalline, polycrystalline, and amorphous films. The compound is heated up, vapor of its component is placed on a substrate, and the compound is evaporated. When heating is used, it may result in plasma arc discharge, resulting from laser or other heating methods. MWPCVD is an essential technology. One established fact about the power of the microwave is that it can establish a certain temperature, at which the component has to be deposited into its vapor states. Once the components have been deposited into their vapor states, the metal or metal oxides are then formed into the thin film. The thin film of metal oxides is formed using MWPCVD from a metallic thin film that was initially synthesized by sputtering methods (RF sputtering, DC magnetron sputtering) [35–37].

9.2.1.3 Co-precipitation method

When metal salt is added to an alkali solution, it results in a precipitate, according to the process known as chemical co-precipitation. To regulate the form and size of nanoparticles, this precipitate is maintained at various pH and other conditions.

The production of metal oxide nanoparticles is a relatively easy and fast process using this method. Most often, the above methods yield metal oxide compounds, such as iron oxide, copper oxide, and the like. In the production of nanoparticles, the pH is very critical since it affects the form and size of the particles [38–43].

9.2.1.4 Sol–gel method

Inorganic and organic nanoparticles that have highly controlled nanostructures and customized surface chemistry are synthesized using the sol–gel method. The percursor used in this technique is either a metal alkoxide or metal chloride. In addition, tetraethyl orthosilicate (TEOS) which is an organic liquid is used for hydrolysis in the case of silica nanoparticles. After hydrolysis, oligomerization occurs, leading to the formation of a sol. When a solution of sol is cross-linked, a gel is produced [44–46].

9.2.1.5 Hydrothermal synthesis

This method was implemented through the use of an autoclave. This process is done in a closed, water-filled chamber to make use of an eco-friendly reaction media. The majority of hydrothermal techniques are often used to regulate the size, shape, phase, and crystallinity of particles. The surface modification or surface coating of inorganic particles such as carbon easily takes place by this technique. In comparison to other methods, it produces smaller sizes, better stability, and a larger specific area [47–49].

9.2.1.6 Microemulsion method

In this procedure, oil is mixed with an aqueous solution of metal salts to create an oil-in-water or water-in-oil microemulsion. Surfactants in both phases help to prevent phase separation (organic or inorganic). Upon the addition of an aqueous solution of alkali, precipitates are formed in the stabilized solution. Once these precipitates have been cleaned and calcined in an oven, they are dried in a stream of air. Using this ecologically friendly method, uniformity and shape and regulated crystallinity may be accomplished [50–52].

9.2.1.7 Reduction method

Typically, chemical reduction involves the reduction of metal ions in a solvent using a reducing agent. It is commonly used to prepare magnetic metal nanoparticles, such as iron, cobalt, and nickel nanoparticles. By reducing silver nitrate with ethylene glycol in the presence of poly(vinyl pyrrolidone) (PVP), large quantities of monodisperse samples of silver nanocubes have been synthesized [53]. PVP acts as a surface stabilizer, a growth modifier, a nanoparticle dispersant, and a reducing agent. This technique allows nanoparticle size, morphology, and crystallinity to be altered. A strong correlation exists between metal nanoparticles' size, shape, and structure and their electrical, optical, and catalytic properties, making regulating these parameters technologically essential [53, 54].

9.2.2 Characterization techniques

These methods are critical for characterizing nanoparticles for many purposes, including, shape surface, crystallinity, size, and materials characteristics, and so on.

The characterization methods utilized for the nanoparticles includex-ray diffraction (XRD), UV–visible spectroscopy, Fourier-transform infrared spectroscopy (FT-IR), scanning electron microscope (SEM), Raman scattering Spectroscopy, atomic force microscopy (AFM), and Brunauer–Emmett–Teller (BET) surface area analysis. Here are a few key characterization methods for materials and nanomaterials. XRD is the characterization method which gives information on crystal size, crystalline characteristics, and phase of nanoparticles [39, 54]. Scherrer's formula allows us to determine the crystal size of the nanoparticles since the necessary value may be input. The most significant method for liquids is UV–visible spectroscopy, which is also known as absorption/reflectance spectroscopy if UV and visible light are used. During this process, light is absorbed or reflected, and this excites or restabilizes atoms or molecules. Most diluted samples have these characteristics. FT-IR may be utilized for solid, liquid, and gas samples. This is an absorption/emission method where spectrum is acquired. FT-IR spectroscopy may be used to examine various organic substances. The FT-IR spectroscopy has more importance, since it assesses the intensity across a much wider range of wavelengths all at once [39–42]. Scanning electron microscopy can examine the shape and surface properties of the nanoparticles. Also, SEM studies nanoparticle structure and shape. Structural topography and composition analysis is done using SEM. Figures 9.5(a)–(e) illustrate the different characterizations of Fe_3O_4 nanoparticles. One of the most vital characterization methods used to get information on nanoparticle size and shape is TEM [20]. To investigate the local structures, dispersion of multicomponent polymers, morphology, and cross sections and crystallizations of metallic alloys, semiconductors, microstructure of composites, TEM is a useful characterization technique (figure 9.6).

AFM is a kind of scanning probe microscopy (SPM) with nanometer-scale resolution. It is a highly resolved method for classifying nanoparticles. Probing the substrate with a mechanical probe provides access to the data. Measurements like stiffness, Young modulus, and so on may be made using atomic force microscopy. AFM also gives information about atoms on the surface, about adjacent atoms, about interactions, and about physical characteristics. Molecular biology and cellular biology utilize AFM to examine the surface and mechanical characteristics

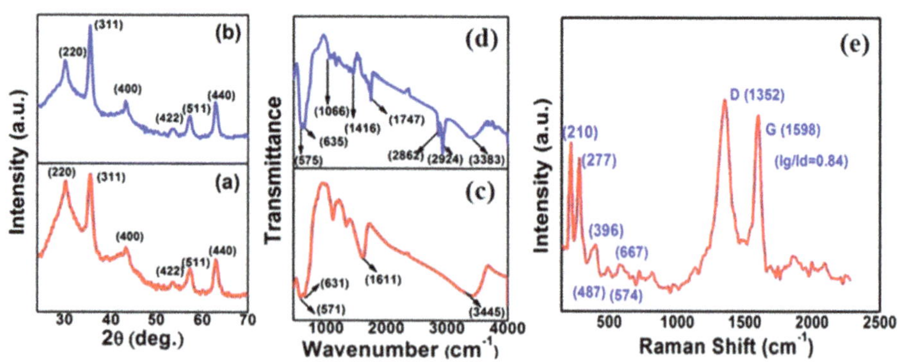

Figure 9.5. XRD patterns of (a) Fe_3O_4 and (b) Fe_3O_4@C core–shell NPs. FT-IR spectra of (c) Fe_3O_4 and (d) Fe_3O_4@C core–shell NPs and (e) Raman spectrum of Fe_3O_4@C core–shell NPs. Reproduced from [20]. CC BY 3.0.

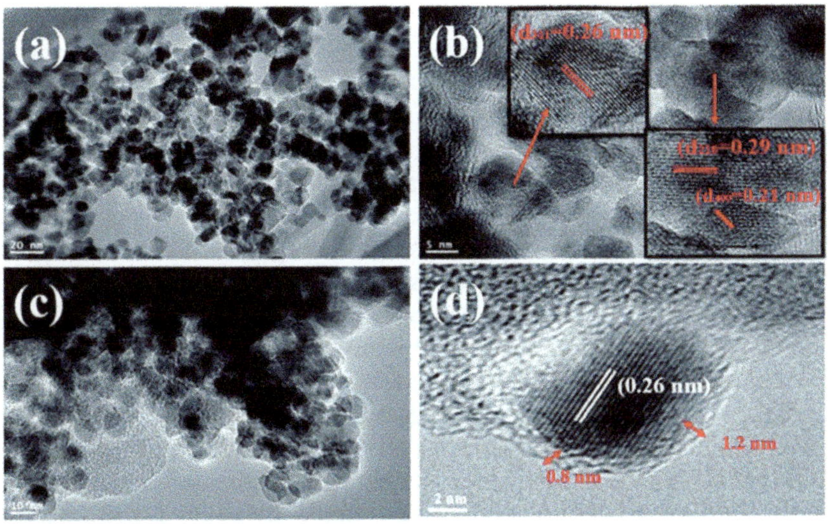

Figure 9.6. High-magnification TEM images of (a) Fe_3O_4 NPs and (c) Fe_3O_4@C core–shell NPs. (b) and (d) HRTEM images of Fe_3O_4 NPs and a random Fe_3O_4@C core–shell NP. Reproduced from [20]. CC BY 3.0.

of protein complexes and assemblies. When analyzing nanoparticles, particularly inorganic nanoparticles, Raman spectroscopy provides additional information that allows identifying atoms or molecules. The primary use of Raman spectroscopy is to detect molecules and chemical bonds. Raman spectroscopy is used to explore low-frequency modes in systems. Raman spectroscopy revealed the identification of the compounds [36]. Lastly, surface area analysis uses the BET model, which describes the computation of specific surface area and pore size. To quantify the specific surface area of a sample, utilizing a gaseous adsorbate such as N_2, argon, and other inert gases is required.

9.3 Applications of MNPs in medical biotechnology

Over the last two decades, MNPs have garnered increasing interest in biomedical applications. MNPs must consider various chemical, physical, physiological, and biological aspects and situations to be employed in the biomedical area.

9.3.1 Magnetic fluid hyperthermia

Magnetic fluid hyperthermia (MFH) or hyperthermia is a heat treatment technique to the cell or tissue which is affected by a tumor or cancer. A class of magnetic nanoparticles is intended to generate the heat under the applied magnetic field. The generated heat is utilized to treat the cancer cell within the body in such a way that healthy tissues are not damaged. Therefore, this therapy has widened the area of treating cancer cells by injecting magnetic nanoparticles into the area which is affected by cancer and the applied magnetic field causes heating enhancement up to 42 °C–45 °C which is enough to destroy a cancer cell [55–67]. The magnetic nanoparticles which are dispersed in different media are utilized in treating cancer cells *in vivo* and *in vitro* applications. For hyperthermia, magnetic nanoparticles are dispersed in a liquid medium and then injected within tissue under the applied magnetic field. Gilchrist *et al* [68] have for the first time used MFH based therapy for cancer treatment in 1957. The dispersed magnetic nanoparticles especially iron oxide based nanoparticles are termed ferrofluids. Therefore, ferrofluids are more susceptible to generate heat under an applied magnetic field and enhance the temperature enough to damage the affected tissue or cell in the region of cancer or tumor. The γ-Fe_2O_3 (maghemite) NPs of varying sizes in the range 20–100 nm, were exposed to the 1.2 MHz magnetic field which increased the temperature to 43 °C–46 °C. This technique was used to treat lymphatic nodes by destroying metastases. The MFH technique, which was established approximately 70 years ago to treat cancer, today is used in clinical phase trials for neck and brain tumors as well as esophagus and prostate cancer [69]. Other types of cancer are under clinical prophase and animal based experimental stages [70]. Due to the advantage of accurate targeting of cancer cell, the MFH technique is considered to be a novel therapy which has minimal damage on healthy tissue compared with the conventional therapies such as chemotherapy, radiotherapy and surgery [71]. The specific power absorption rate (SAR) or intrinsic power loss (ILP) determine the energy absorption efficiency of magnetic nanoparticles. The factors which may have an effect on the hyperthermia efficiency are the size of magnetic nanoparticles, magnetic field intensity, nature of magnetic materials and viscosity of dispersed nanoparticles fluids [72–76]. The SAR is measured in W g^{-1} and ILP is measured in nHm^2 kg^{-1} of magnetic materials. The SAR can be calculated according to the following equation:

$$\mathrm{SAR} = \frac{dT}{dt} \times \frac{C}{m}$$

where dT/dt is the initial slope, from the heating curve, C is the specific heat capacity in J kg^{-1} K^{-1} and m is the normalized mass of Fe per unit mass of the sample.

The intrinsic loss power ILP can be determined by the relation between SAR value and the applied magnetic field. The ILP can be calculated using the following equation:

$$\mathrm{ILP} = \frac{\mathrm{SAR}}{H^2 f}$$

where H^2 is alternating magnetic field and f is the frequency.

The MFH studies are mostly based on iron oxide nanoparticles, ferrites and other magnetic nanoparticles and ferrofluids as well. These magnetic nanoparticles are non-toxic and biocompatible materials which are simply processed at low-cost; examples are Fe_3O_4 NPs and cobalt ferrite based ferrofluids [64–67]. A few studies based on recent data are describe here. Kandasamy *et al* [55] have synthesized superparamagnetic iron oxide nanoparticles (SPIONs) of 10–12 nm coated with terephthalic acid (TA). The synthesized NPs were dispersed in water and triethylene glycol individually for magnetic fluid hyperthermia studies. The SAR and ILP value for water based ferrofluids were obtained as 23.4–160.7 W $g_{Fe}{}^{-1}$ and 2.5 nHm^2 kg^{-1}

respectively. Similarly, Lahiri *et al* [56] syntheisized Fe_3O_4 NPs of 10 nm and coated with them by tetramethyl ammonium hydroxide (TMAH). They were then ispersed in water and MFH studies were performed using infrared thermography (IRT). The SAR value was obtained as 135.98 (±4.6) W g_{Fe}^{-1}. The results validate the universal applicability and efficacy of IRT as an alternate and non-contaminated hyperthermia technique. In another study, Guibert *et al* [66] synthesized γ-Fe_2O_3 nanoparticles of two different sizes: 10 nm and 20 nm. The maghemite nanoparticles were dispersed in a water and glycerol medium to obtain well dispersed ferrofluids. These ferrofluids were explored for the MFH studies and found that SAR does not depend on the viscosity of the ferrofluids. The MFH studies were performed using two different techniques called calorimetric and dynamic hysteresis measurement techniques. The results obtained by the two different techniques were in good agreement. Kandasamy *et al* [77] have produced iron oxide nanoclusters (IONCs) based ferrofluids via one pot pyrolysis of iron acetylacetonate using triethanolamine (TEA) and diethylene glycol (DEG)/tetraethylene glycol (TTEG) mixtures. The prepared ferrofluids are assigned as NCAFF-1 (TEA:DEG, 8:2), NCAFF-2 (TEA: TTEG, 8:2) and NCAFF-3 (TEA:TTEG, 7:3). These ferrofluids are exposed to an applied magnetic field of ~2.4–9.9 GA m^{-1} s^{-1} intensity and results were obtained through calorimetry. In figures 9.7(A)–(C) the heating curve for the above mentioned ferrofluids are demonstrated and the SAR/ILP value was determined. Further, figure 9.7(D(i)) shows the concentration of ferrofluids versus time taken by ferrofluids to reach 42 °C and figure 9.7(D(ii)) shows the concentration versus SAR (heating efficiency) of the ferrofluids. The values of SAR and ILP are in the ranges 142.4–909.4 W g_{Fe}^{-1} and 4.2–14.7 nHm^2 kg^{-1}, respectively with NCAFF-3 (0.5 mg ml^{-1} concentration) on exposure to the AMFs with H^*f values ranging from 2.4 to 9.9 GA m^{-1} s^{-1}. From the graph it is clear that as the concentration of ferrofluid ($\phi 1$ to $\phi 5$) increases, the time taken to attain 42 °C decreases. Moreover, figure 9.7(E) represents the heating curves for NCAFF-3 at $\phi 1$ = 0.5 mg ml^{-1} concentration on varying the alternating magnetic field. It is concluded from the study that NCAFF-3 has found to be excellent heating efficiency which is reached 42 °C within 0.7–9.7 min as compared to NCAFF-1 and NCAFF-2. *In vitro* MFH study has also done by using NCAFF-3 for HepG2 cancer cells. Therefore, it is found that NCAFF-3 is the most promising candidate for hyperthermia treatment for cancer treatment.

The effect of texturing and orientational ordering of MNPs also plays an important role in hyperthermia efficiency. Lahiri *et al* [78] studied the 200 nm size nanoemulsion which was loaded with super-paramagnetic NPs in an agar matrix. The SAR value was found to be ~73 ±2 W g_{Fe}^{-1} when the droplet and applied magnetic field were paralleled to each other. It was also observed that 20%–30% SAR efficiency was performed when the field was parallel to the nanoemulsion droplet orientation as compared to when the applied field was perpendicular to the droplet. Moreover, Conde-Leborn *et al* [79] investigated the effect of magnetization orientation in easy axes anisotropy with MNP interactions. The effect of particle chain formation on the normalized heating properties, or specific loss power (SLP), was studied by Branquinho *et al* [80] for manganese ferrite-based ferrofluids. They found that specific loss power (SLP) was decreased as the concentration of NPs

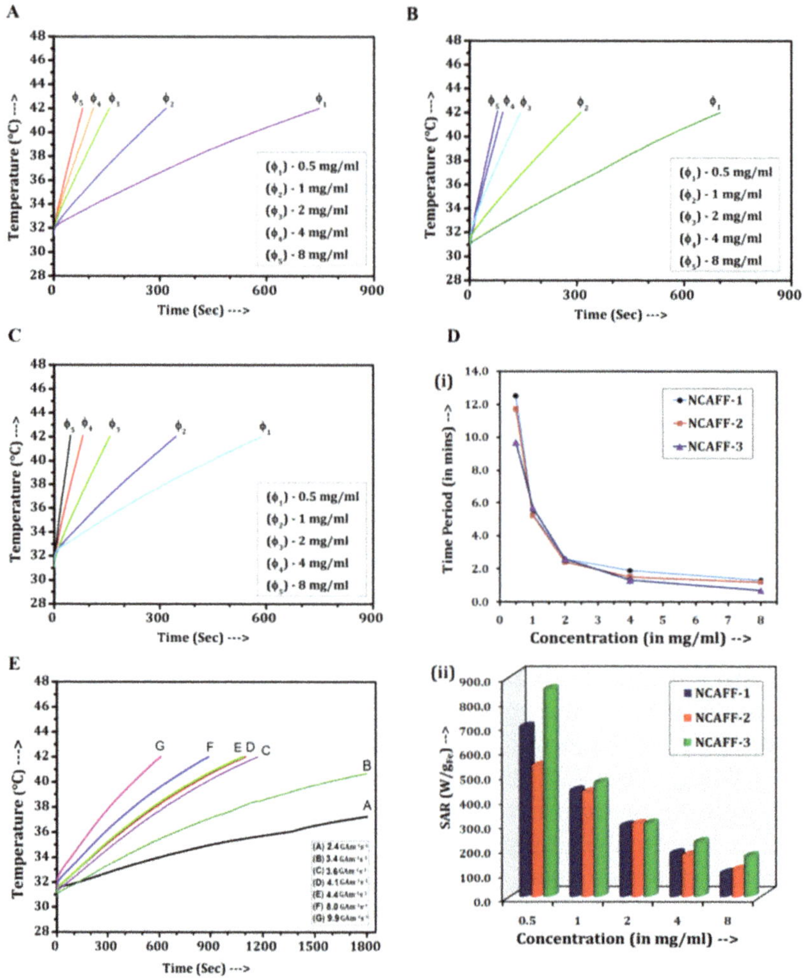

Figure 9.7. (A–C) Heating curves for NCAFF-1, NCAFF-2 and NCAFF-3, (D(i)) ferrofluids concentration vs time reached to 42 C, (D(ii)) concentration vs SAR (heating efficacy) and (E) the heating curves for NCAFF-3 at varying alternating magnetic fields. Reprinted from [77], Copyright (2019), with permission from Elsevier.

increased. This is due to the fact that as the NP concentration increases, the chain length increases which was investigated by ferromagnetic resonance (FMR). The heating effect of ferrofluids against applied magnetic field was studied by Rosensweig [81] who found that orientational relaxation of NPs caused power dissipation. The power dissipation was estimated by establishing analytical equations. Heating efficiency of Neel relaxation, Brownian relaxation and hysteresis loss in magnetic NPs hyperthermia was investigated by Deatsch *et al* [82]. The shape, size, crystallographic anisotropy and level of aggregation of MNPs have a significant effect on these processes in hyperthermia. It is noted that as the MNP concentration decrease, the magnetic relaxation period was reduced in both Neel and Brownian dominated regimes.

9.3.2 Drug delivery

The functionalization of magnetic NPs especially iron oxide NPs enables them to be used for drug delivery applications. Drugs or drug-attracted molecules can be easily attached to the surface of magnetic iron oxide NPs. The dispersed drug-loaded NPs into a biocompatible fluid-like serum enters through the intravenous system and is guided through an external magnetic field. Among a variety of anticancer and antitumor drugs, doxorubicin (DOX) is found to be actively involved in chemotherapy/targeted drug delivery as an antitumor/anticancer agent for a variety of cancer cells [83–86]. Several studies have been performed for targeted delivery of DOX with the help of SPION based ferrofluid [83] and iron oxide NPs [84–86]. For example, a SPION based ferrofluid loaded with DOX was studied by Munnier *et al* for magnetically targeted drug delivery for breast cancer cells [83]. The SPION had an average diameter of 8±2 nm and consisted of ~60% magnetite (Fe_3O_4) and ~40% maghemite (γ-Fe_2O_3) which constituted the inner nucleus and the outer layer of each NP, respectively. Since the maghemite crystal is composed of Fe^{3+} and O^{2-} ions, the use of Fe^{2+} was preferred over Fe^{3+} to avoid the undesirable oxidation of DOX. The interaction of DOX with iron on the NP surface was hindered by a layer of water and hydroxyl species, therefore DOX was attached to the NP surface using a preformed DOX–Fe^{2+} complex. Hence, the Fe^{2+} ion played the role of an intermediate between DOX and NP as shown in figure 9.8. Figure 9.9(a) shows the DOX loading as a function of the amount of DOX initially used during incubation. The DOX loading exceeded 14% for DOX/SPION (w/w) ratio of 0.95. Figure 9.9(b) shows the *in vitro* release of DOX from loaded SPION ferrofluids in Tris buffer pH 7.4 (pH of blood plasma) at 37 ¼C. The DOX–Fe^{2+} complex was favored by pH and the drug was gradually released from the SPION surface via hydrolysis. The DOX–SPION binding could be easily reversed at physiological pH and the DOX–SPION aqueous ferrofluids released 85%±9.1% of loaded DOX in 1 h. Figure 9.10 shows the biological activity of DOX solutions and DOX–SPION ferrofluids carrying the same amount of the drug by measuring their cytotoxicity on MCF-7 cancer cells. DOX and DOX–SPION exhibited similar activity at higher drug concentrations; however, DOX–SPION killed more cancer cells at lower drug concentrations. The enhanced cytotoxic activity of DOX–SPION may be attributed to the drug release on the cellular membrane and even its delivery inside the cells by internalized NPs.

Recently (2020), Norouzi *et al* [84] loaded DOX with trimethoxysilylpropylethylenediaminetriacetic acid (EDTA) stabilized iron oxide NPs to release the drug for glioblastoma (GBM) chemotherapy in the brains of mice. The DOX–EDTA–IONPs were found to be effective for more than 90% apoptotic induced-cell death in GBM within 48 h of the release of the drugs. Similarly, Lungu *et al* [85] used carboxymethylcellulose sodium (CMCNa) stabilized γ-Fe_2O_3 NPs and loaded with DOX as an anticancer potential agent in the treatment of breast cancer. The DOX conjugated CMCNa coated γ-Fe_2O_3 is an effective anticancer agent which inhibits the tumoral cell proliferation, reduces the effect on normal breast cells, disrupts the cellular membrane and induces cell death. A 50% reduction of cancer cell viability and increased cytotoxicity were observed. Moreover, a multifunctional nano vector

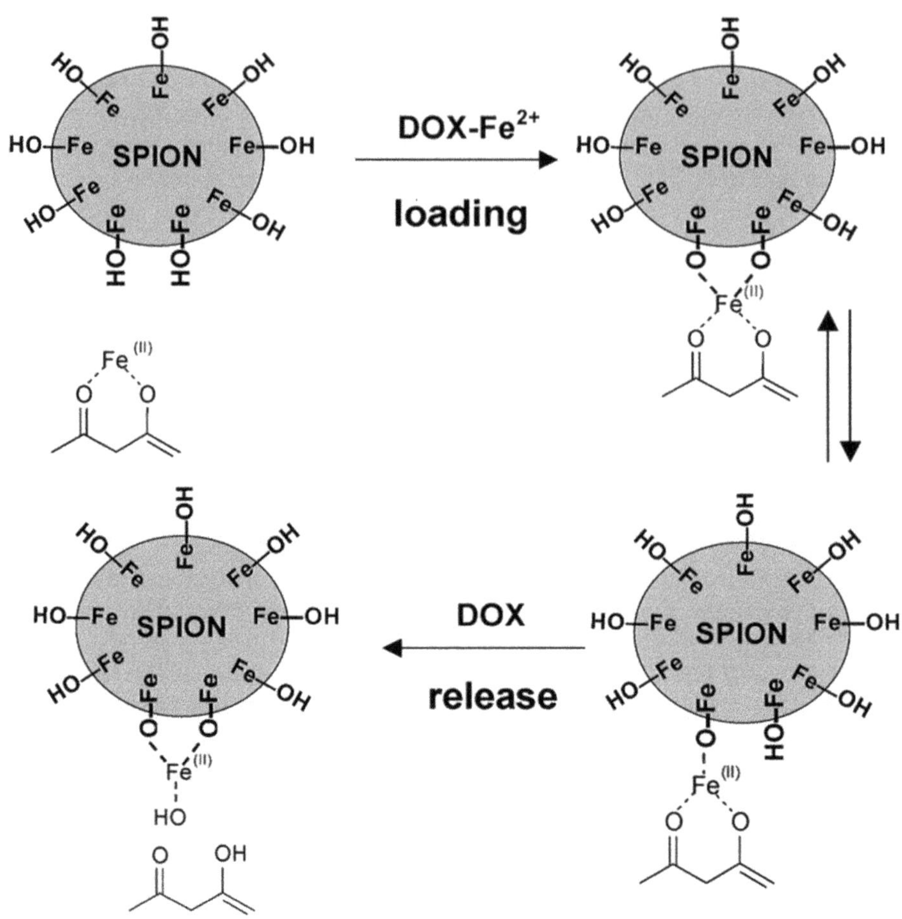

Figure 9.8. Schematic diagram of DOX–Fe^{2+} binding to the SPION surface (pH 6–8) and of subsequent drug release. Reprinted from [83], Copyright (2008), with permission from Elsevier.

can be used as a specific targeted delivery of functionalized DOX drugs as reported by Wu *et al* [86]. Fe_3O_4 NPs were functionalized with *N*-isopropylacrylamide (NIPAM) and polymethylmethacrylate (PMMA) and loaded with DOX. The functional materials (DOX–PNIPAM–PMMA@Fe_3O_4) were analyzed *in vitro* and exhibited enhanced drug release efficiency in acidic and warm conditions. The cell viability and cellular uptake studies were performed through different treatments in an MDA-MB 231 cell line.

9.3.3 Magnetic resonance imaging

Super-paramagnetic NPs can enhance the proton nuclear relaxation rates, which in turn increases the contrast of the image. The efficiency of the contrasted image is determined by their NMR-Dispersion (NMRD) profile, which is based on the measurement of longitudinal (r_1) and transverse (r_2) relaxivities in terms of frequency [88]. The efficiency of the contrasted image is also based on the

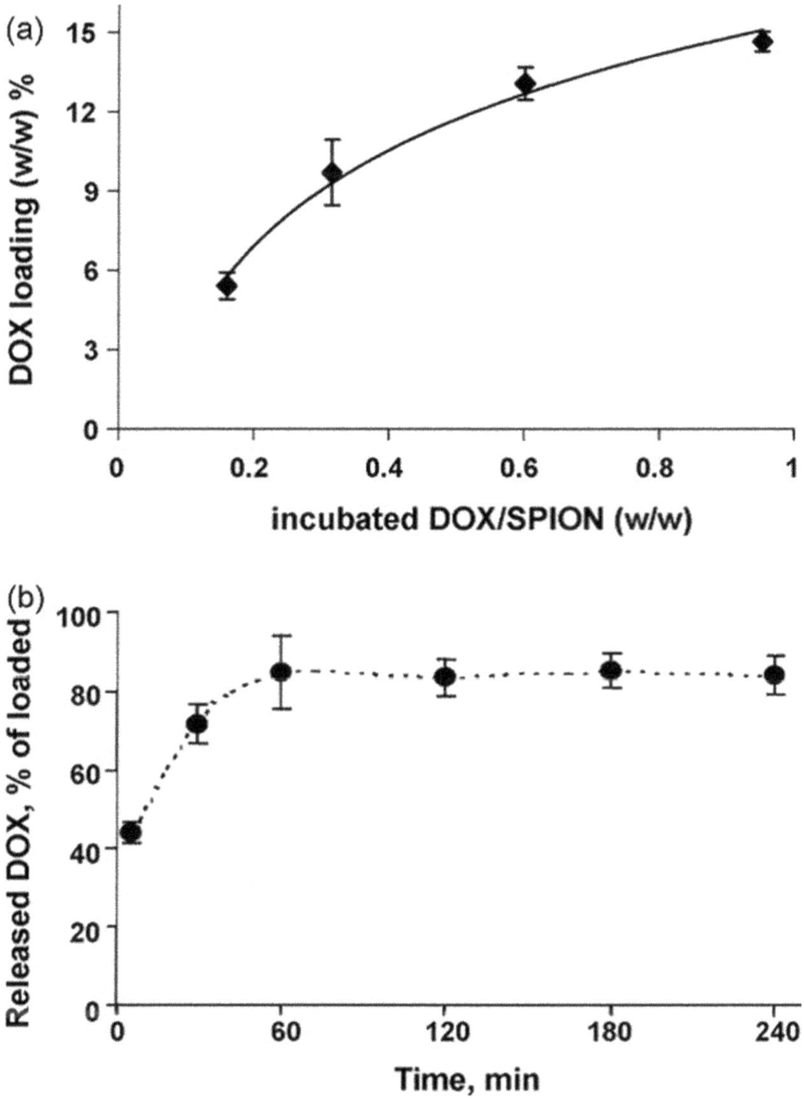

Figure 9.9. Binding of DOX–Fe^{2+} complex to citrate-stabilized SPION: (a) DOX loading vs initial drug/SPION weight ratio; (b) release of doxorubicin *in vitro* (Tris buffer pH 7.4) from drug-loaded SPION ferrofluids. Reprinted from [83], Copyright (2008), with permission from Elsevier.

measurement of longitudinal (T_1) and transverse (T_2) nuclear relaxation times. SPION based ferrofluids possess great potential to be utilized in MRI for the diagnosis of various diseases as they are good contrast-enhancing agents [87, 88]. Such studies involve both *in vitro* and *in vivo* tests, where high-resolution MR images with improved transverse relaxation T_2 can be observed. For *in vitro* MRI studies, a novel ferrofluid called magnetic nanobubbles (MNBs) embedded with SPIONs has been used [89–92]. Recently, Li *et al* (2021) prepared assembled MNBs embedded

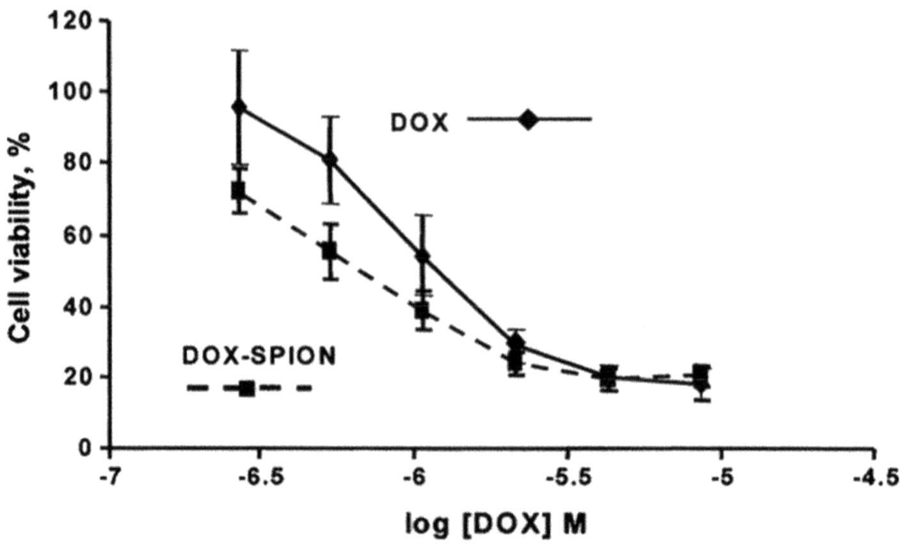

Figure 9.10. *In vitro* cytotoxic activity profiles of DOX-loaded SPION ferrofluids (DOX–SPION) compared to drug in solution (DOX), when applied for 24 h on the MCF-7 cancer cells in culture. The differences are statistically significant for concentrations $\leqslant 10^{-6}$ M. Reprinted from [83], Copyright (2008), with permission from Elsevier.

with SPIONs by a repeated compression method [89]. A 2 ml of DI water with different concentrations of SPIONs were taken into a 4 ml glass vials. In the upper part of the vial, the air layer was replaced with SF_6 gas and the vial was sealed. Next, 3 ml of SF_6 gas contained in a syringe with a needle was inserted into the vial. The tip of the needle remained below the surface of water during the whole process. To acquire the optimal conditions for assembly, the moving speed of the piston, the number of compression cycles, and the concentration of SPIONs were measured. Under the condition of 150 compression cycles, the NBs concentration could reach about 6.12×10^9 ml^{-1}. The mechanism during the process of self-assembly of SPIONs with NBs is shown in figure 9.11. SPIONs were treated with ultra-pure water so that their surfaces have the same electric charge. Figure 9.11(a) shows that the SPIONs are repelled due to the electrostatic force and uniformly dispersed in the water. Therefore, they could easily pass through the 1000 KD ultrafiltration tube, and the concentration of iron was measured as 11.25 mg l^{-1}. Since the sample was prepared by the cyclic compression method, a gas layer was deposited on the surface of the NP as shown in figure 9.11(b). Hence, there was a strong attraction between the NPs with gas layer and NBs as shown in figure 9.11(c), and finally NPs adsorbed on the NB as shown in figure 9.11(d). The assembled MNBs exhibited good MR contrast capability. The assembled MNBs with different concentrations of SPIONs (0.002, 0.02, and 0.20 mM) caused the T_2 signal to decrease by different amounts as compared to the blank control of water as shown in figure 9.12(a). Figure 9.12(b) shows the gray values of iron concentration at 0.20 mM and 0.02 mM, which exhibits a significant difference as compared to the blank control water. The SPIONs

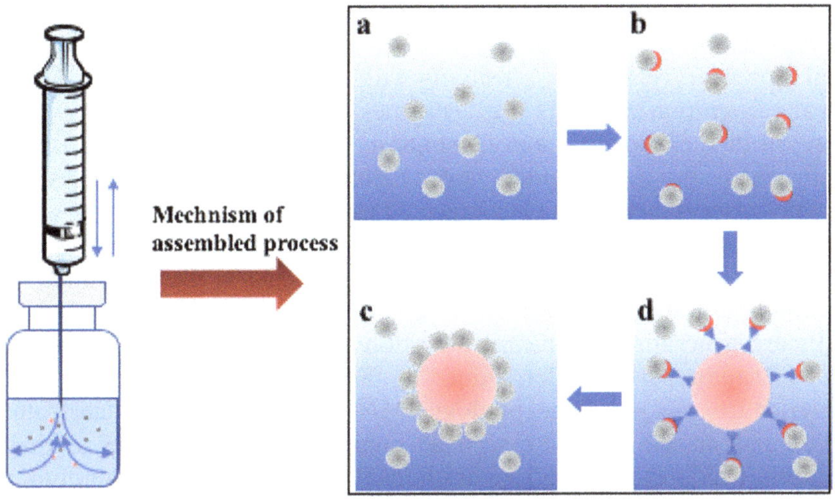

Figure 9.11. Mechanism of assembled process for assembled nanobubbles. (a) SPIONs in water solution before compression; (b) a gas layer deposited on the surface of the nanoparticles during repeat compressions; (c) attractions between nanoparticles and nanobubbles; and (d) the assembled nanobubbles structures. Reprinted from [89], Copyright (2021), with permission from Elsevier.

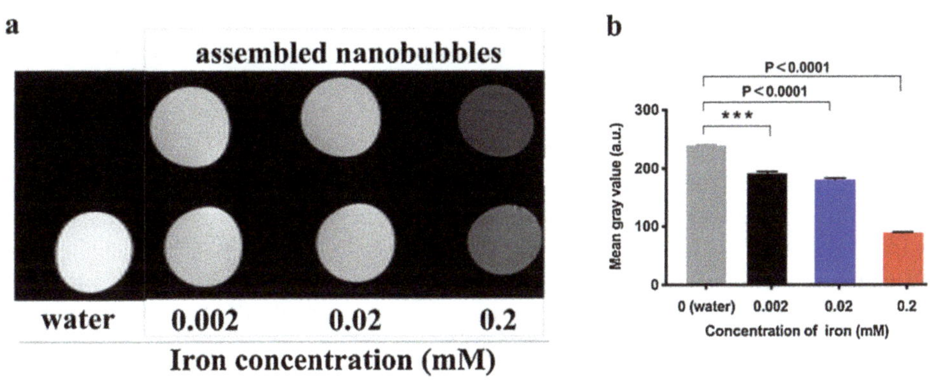

Figure 9.12. MR and ultrasound imaging of assembled nanobubbles. (a) Fe concentration-dependent T_2-weighted magnetic resonance images in a 7.0 T MR scanner, and the average mean gray value of T_2 signal (b). All bars represent mean ± SD, and three independent experiments ($n = 3$) were performed; and the statistical significance is indicated by $***p < 0.001$ and $****p < 0.0001$. Reprinted from [89], Copyright (2021), permission from Elsevier.

based assembled MNBs at the higher concentration indicated better MRI capabilities and could be used as a good MRI contrast agent.

9.3.4 Electrochemical sensors

Electrochemical biosensors have been shown to be promising as *in situ* and real-time detection tools in biomedical applications [93–95]. Moreover, technological advancements and high-quality research continue to transform healthcare standards. These devices are easily miniaturized and have a rapid response time, critical characteristics for point-of-care (POC) technology. Additionally, electrochemical biosensors relate their sensitivity with the high specificity and selectivity of biological recognition elements (i.e., enzymes, nucleic acids, antibodies, etc) [95]. They use all of these magnificent elements to provide analytical measurements in straightforward and user-friendly ways. Electrochemical-based devices currently lead the biosensors market, which is expected to expand at a 7.4% yearly growth rate between 2021 and 2027. The market for electrochemical biosensors is driven by diagnostic and health monitoring applications, particularly the burgeoning demand for point-of-care testing.

MNPs are generating significant attention and demand in this area [96]. The behavior of nanomaterials is determined by their chemical composition and shape, crystal structure, size, and morphology. MNPs exhibit superior electromagnetic properties and unique behavior such as quantum-size effects due to their large surface area, which exhibits super-paramagnetic and magnetized quantum tunneling. Apart from collecting and separating the analyte, MNPs have garnered considerable attention from researchers for their ability to generate the signal. This behavior translates into superior sensor performance for ultralow detection of a wide variety of analytes, including nucleic acids, proteins, and small analytes with a variety of transduction principles. In terms of signal generation, one of the most extensively utilized methods is to monitor the magnetic field of MNPs, which is often accomplished using magnetosensors and *in vivo* imaging technology. Additionally, MNPs can enhance electrochemical signals by obstructing an underlying electrode or providing conductivity after coating [97].

In general, electrochemical sensors work by causing a redox reaction between the species on the electrode surface, which results in the production of an electrical signal that is proportional to the concentration of the analyte species on the electrode surface.

We concentrated on applying magnetic nanoparticles to the analysis of inorganic and organic species and biomolecules in a variety of biological samples, including blood, serum, plasma, tissue extracts, urine, and milk, as shown in figure 9.13(a). Numerous papers have been published over the last several decades describing how to produce magnetic iron oxide nanoparticles using either pure iron oxide or a hybrid material. Magnetic nanoparticles are synthesized using the method(s) depicted in figure 9.13(b), depending on the shape and stability of the final product, the application, and the available infrastructure. Further, magnetic nickel-based nanoparticles have been employed to synthesize magnetic molecularly imprinted polymers (MMIPs) and create electrochemical sensors. Special consideration should be made of graphene oxide (GO), a fascinating nanomaterial with excellent water solubility, high electrical conductivity, high mechanical strength, chemical stability, and a large surface area with numerous active sites. These characteristics make GO an excellent choice for use as supporting material in preparing imprinted materials. MIPs have a large surface area, which is advantageous if the polymerization occurs at the GO surface. The binding sites on the outer layer of the MIPs composite enable the complete removal of templates, improve target species accessibility, and reduce

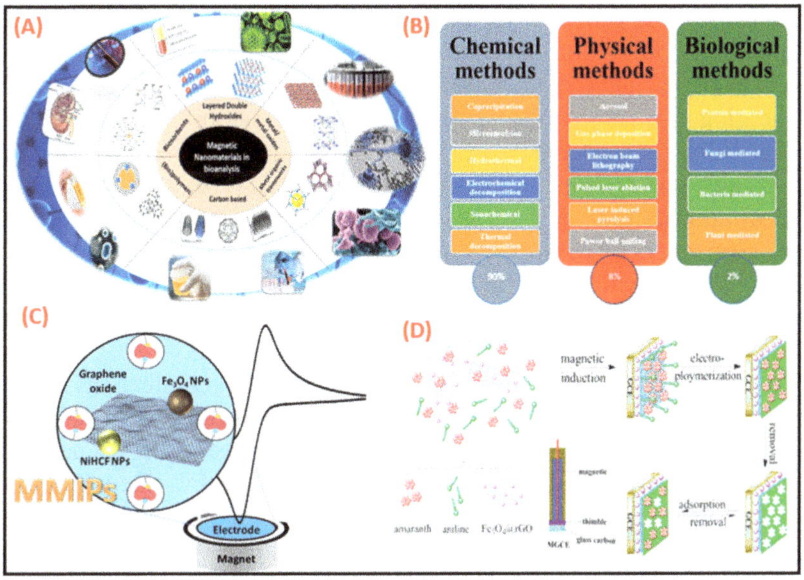

Figure 9.13. (A) Schematic illustration of the usability of Mag-NMs for magnetic solid-phase extraction (MSPE) and sensor applications. (B) Schematic representation of the different synthesis methods used in the literature for magnetic nanoparticles. Reprinted from [98], with permission from Elsevier. (C) MMIP based electrochemical sensor. Reprinted from [97], with permission from Elsevier. (D) Schema of MIES preparation to detect amaranth in the fruit drinks. Reprinted from [96], with permission from Elsevier.

binding time, as shown in figure 9.13(c). A complex containing aniline function monomer, amaranth, and Fe_3O_4@rGO template was preassembled by π–π stacking and hydrogen bonding interactions in the molecular imprinting electrochemical sensor (MIES) has been self-assembled over the magnetic field induction. The fabricated route of MIES showed acceptable selectivity, sensitivity, efficiency, and reproducibility to detect amaranth, as shown in figure 9.13(d).

Apart from facilitating simple, reproducible, and rapid fabrication, electrochemical sensors based on MSPE and MMIPs sensors have proven tol have significant potential for the highly selective and sensitive detection of analytes of interest in the environment of food therapeutic areas. Additionally, considering the rapid advancement of novel nanomaterials and the promising possibilities for sensitivity, selectivity, and simplicity given by MMIPs based electrochemical sensors. According to current predictions, the development and implementation of new electrochemical sensing scaffolds based on unique multifunctional-MMIPs will become increasingly popular in the near future.

9.3.5 Gene therapy

Gene therapy refers to a therapeutic technique in which genetic material is directly transferred into tissues or cells to treat various hereditary illnesses and acquired diseases. Using genetic information, gene therapy attempts to alter the phenotypic of cells by replacing a malfunctioning or abnormal gene with a functional and healthy one. To achieve this, genetically engineered cells (*in vitro* or *ex vivo*) are used to deliver therapeutic DNA into the nucleus where it is transcribed alongside genomic DNA [99].

The emerging area of gene therapy is used to treat uncommon and sometimes life-threatening genetic disorders such as hemophilia, cystic fibrosis, cancer, sickle cell anemia, Huntington's disease, Parkinson's disease, Alzheimer's disease, severe combined immunodeficiency (SCID), chronic granulomatous disorder, etc, where traditional treatments have shown very modest improvements [100–102].

Wei *et al* [103] evaluated the feasibility and efficacy of using TNF-related apoptosis-inducing ligand (TRAIL) gene to treat breast cancer mediated with PEI-coated magnetic iron oxide nanoparticles (polyMAG-1000). The magnetic iron oxide nanoparticles were used as a gene carrier to transfect the TRAIL gene into MCF-7 cells. Fouriki *et al* [101] evaluated the viability of oscillating nano-magnetic gene transfection systems for enhancing transfection efficiency in NIH_3T_3 mouse embryonic fibroblastic cells (MEFs). The NIH_3T_3 cells line was derived from NIH Swiss mouse embryo cultures, which are known for their relatively strong contact inhibition. The mechanism of oscillating nanomagnetic transfection is illustrated in figure 9.14. Attached to magnetic nanoparticles are plasmid DNA or small interfering RNA (siRNA), and then the samples are incubated with cells in culture (left) promoting endocytosis (iii). When the particle/DNA combination is endocytosed, a proton sponge effect causes the endosome to rupture, releasing the DNA. This process causes the DNA to synthesize the protein that the DNA is targeting (vi). The 30 min technique retained transfection efficiency similar to untreated samples and greater transfection efficiency than Lipofectamine 2000 in comparison to Lipofectamine 2000 at 6 h. It was deduced that non-viral transfection

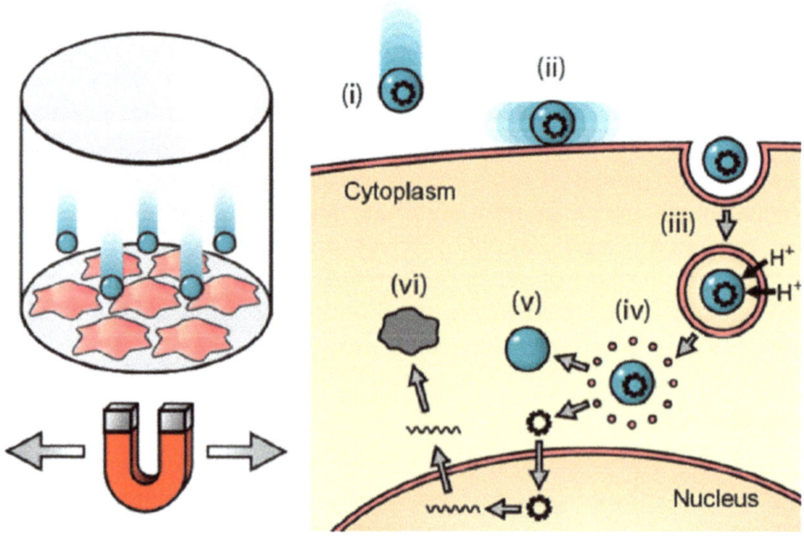

Figure 9.14. The mechanism of oscillating nanomagnetic transfection. Reprinted from [101]. CC BY 3.0.

of mouse embryonic fibroblasts may be accomplished via nanomagnetic transfection (NIH_3T_3).

In order to see whether spherical and rod-like magnetic mesoporous silica nanoparticles (M-MSNs) are useful in suicide gene therapy, Wang *et al* [104] produced these particles and then investigated their ability to treat hepatocellular cancer (HCC). For combining several suicide gene therapies, magnetic hyperthermia treatment, and MRI therapies into a single system, nanoplatforms with various geometries were developed as shown in figure 9.15. The rod-like MSNs had greater drug-loading efficiency, a quicker drug-release pattern, and improved gene delivery in the presence of an external magnetic field. Importantly, the rod-like MSNs showed better magnetic targeting and more magnetic hyperthermia-enhanced suicide gene therapy effectiveness *in vitro* and *in vivo*. MSNs may both turn into sphere-like and rod-like HCC theranostics. The study concluded that the sphere-like and rod-like MSNs possess the capability to grow to be viable, effective, and safe HCC theranostics.

Zhang *et al* [105] built thermally induced manganese-doped magnetic nano-carriers utilizing a microemulsion approach and electrostatic interaction, as illustrated in figure 9.16. HMM-siRNA NCs were created by co-loading $Mn_{0.8}Fe_{2.2}O_4$ NPs and photosensitizer ICG into the matrix of poly (lactic-co-glycolic acid)-polyetherimide and exposed positively surfaces where positively charged siRNA is captured by electrostatic contact. To track the metabolism, tumor enrichment, and drug release of HMM-siRNA NCs in HCC tumor tissue, real-time NIR and MR imaging from the implanted ICG and $Mn_{0.8}Fe_{2.2}O_4$ NPs will be used. Under 808 nm laser irradiation, constant heat produced by ICG may cause HMM-siRNA NCs to

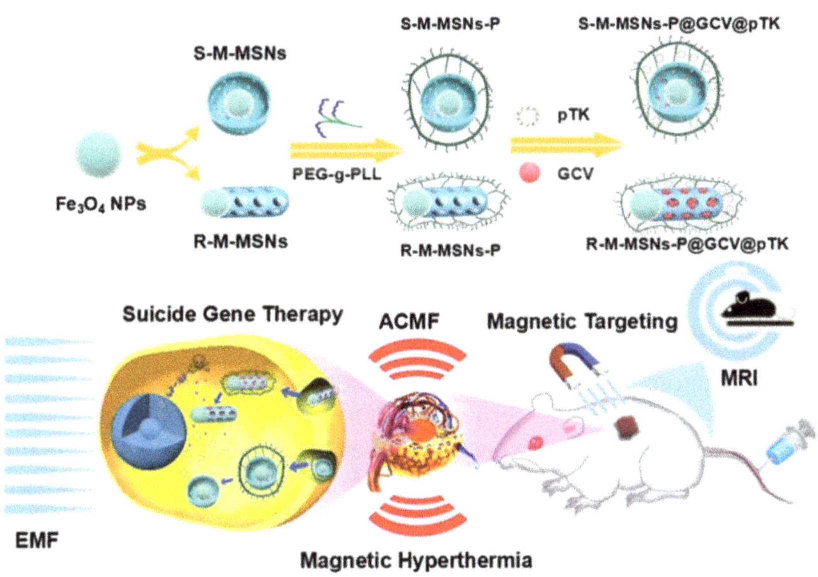

Figure 9.15. Graphical depiction of M-MSNs for M-MSN of various shapes for suicide gene therapy approach for hepatocellular cancer. Reprinted from [104], Copyright (2018), with permission from Elsevier.

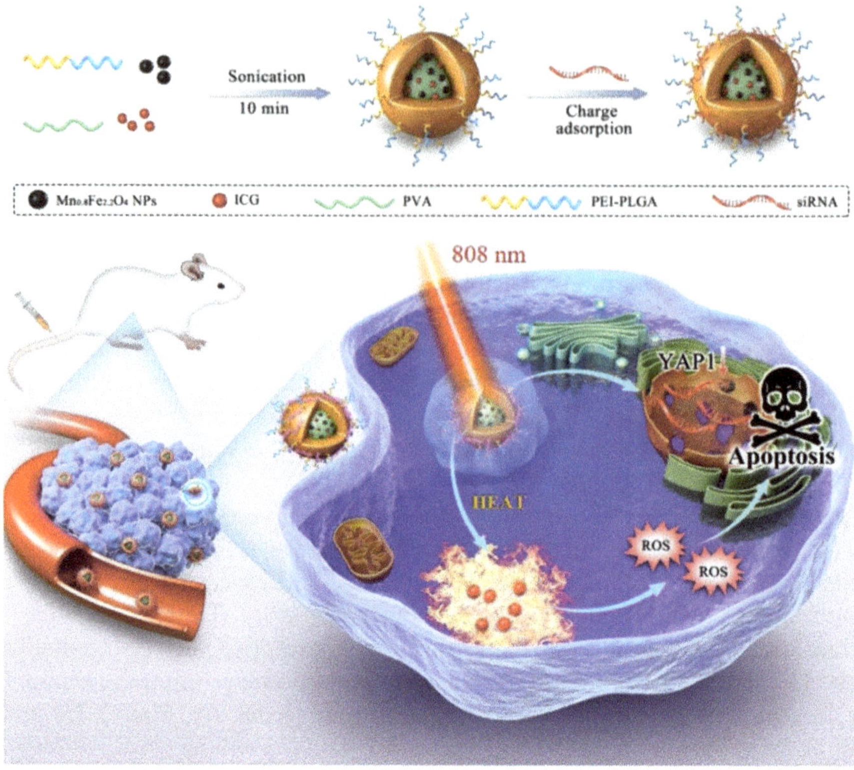

Figure 9.16. Graphical depiction of the MRI/NIR guided therapy for hepatocellular carcinoma (HCC) combined with YAP1 siRNA and the YAP1 regulation. Reprinted from [105], Copyright (2021), with permission from Elsevier.

release their cargo. ICG produced heat may lead to the cell death via a PTT action whereas siRNA may help reduce YAP1 expression in HCC cells, ultimately resulting in cell proliferation and migration. Thus, our proposed thermally induced HMM-siRNA NCs may allow for MRI/NIR guided, low-temperature PTT effectiveness in HCC cells, which may lead to a multimodal diagnosis-guided therapy to treat cancer.

9.4 Conclusion

The synthesis, characterization, and biomedical uses of magnetic nanoparticles are described in this study. The fast growth of nanotechnology has a lot to do with the idea of using magnetic nanoparticles in biomedical applications. On the one hand, highly desired properties may be obtained by selecting certain experimental conditions, while on the other hand, surface functionalization of magnetic nanoparticles has been discovered and developed via the combination of both composition and molecular structure. Using the unique magnetic properties, these functionalized magnetic nanoparticles with high selectivity, high sensitivity, and special applications enhance the efficiency and accuracy, as well as the specificity and damage reduction in drug delivery and hyperthermia *in vivo* treatment.

Although there are many exciting and promising advancements in the field of magnetic nanoparticles, as detailed in this study, this is only the beginning of the journey with many hurdles still to be cleared. Moreover, clinical trials are very restrictive since toxicity and biocompatibility are key when it comes to the use of medical devices. Although many magnetic nanoparticles are found in the scientific literature, very few *in vitro* or *in vivo* investigations have been conducted to date. Another concern is that functional molecules such as DNA, RNA, or antibodies bound to the surfaces of the magnetic nanoparticles are highly prone to becoming unstable and denatured by the surrounding conditions. To achieve long-term environmental stability, a new approach is required. Another key component in biomedical drug development is 'druggability', which is the potential to alter the target with a small molecule medication. Current drug discovery methods rely on just 10% of the human genome, which is druggable, and only half of those regions are linked to diseases. As a result, it is critical to be able to anticipate whether a novel target is a druggable target in the early stages of drug research. With the addressing of these concerns, the design and development of multifunctional magnetic nanoparticles with unique characteristics of wide flexibility, biocompatibility, and multifunctional features will play a key role in future biomedicine endeavors.

Acknowledgement

All authors acknowledge their respective institution for support.

References

[1] Pankhurst Q A, Connolly J, Jones S K and Dobson J 2003 Applications of magnetic nanoparticles in biomedicine *J. Phys.* D **36** R167–81

[2] Guo T *et al* 2018 The recent advances of magnetic nanoparticles in medicine *J. Nanomater.* **2018** 1–8

[3] Wu K, Su D, Liu J, Saha R and Wang J-P 2019 Magnetic nanoparticles in nanomedicine: a review of recent advances *Nanotechnology* **30** 1–47

[4] Torres-Lugo M and Rinaldi C 2013 Thermal potentiation of chemotherapy by magnetic nanoparticles *Nanomedicine* **8** 1689–707

[5] Das P, Colombo M and Prosperi D 2019 Recent advances in magnetic fluid hyperthermia for cancer therapy *Colloids Surf.* B **174** 42–55

[6] Pankhurst Q A, Connolly J, Jones S K and Dobson J 2003 Applications of magnetic nanoparticles in biomedicine *J. Phys.* D **36** R167

[7] Jeong U, Teng X, Wang Y, Yang H and Xia Y 2007 Superparamagnetic colloids: controlled synthesis and niche applications *Adv. Mater.* **19** 33–60

[8] Laurent S, Dutz S, Häfeli U O and Mahmoudi M 2011 Magnetic fluid hyperthermia: focus on superparamagnetic iron oxide nanoparticles *Adv. Colloid Interface Sci.* **166** 8–23

[9] Kumar C S and Mohammad F 2011 Magnetic nanomaterials for hyperthermia-based therapy and controlled drug delivery *Adv. Drug Delivery Rev.* **63** 789–808

[10] Fortin J P, Wilhelm C, Servais J, Ménager C, Bacri J C and Gazeau F 2007 Size-sorted anionic iron oxide nanomagnets as colloidal mediators for magnetic hyperthermia *J. Am. Chem. Soc.* **129** 2628–35

[11] Lartigue L, Innocenti C, Kalaivani T, Awwad A, Sanchez Duque M D M, Guari Y and Sangregorio C 2011 Water-dispersible sugar-coated iron oxide nanoparticles. An evaluation of their relaxometric and magnetic hyperthermia properties *J. Am. Chem. Soc.* **133** 10459–72

[12] Martinez-Boubeta C, Simeonidis K, Makridis A, Angelakeris M, Iglesias O, Guardia P and Baldomir D 2013 Learning from nature to improve the heat generation of iron-oxide nanoparticles for magnetic hyperthermia applications *Sci. Rep.* **3** 1–8

[13] Guardia P, Di Corato R, Lartigue L, Wilhelm C, Espinosa A, Garcia-Hernandez M and Pellegrino T 2012 Water-soluble iron oxide nanocubes with high values of specific absorption rate for cancer cell hyperthermia treatment *ACS Nano* **6** 3080–91

[14] Jang J T, Nah H, Lee J H, Moon S H, Kim M G and Cheon J 2009 Critical enhancements of MRI contrast and hyperthermic effects by dopant-controlled magnetic nanoparticles *Angew. Chem. Int. Ed.* **48** 1234–8

[15] Maldonado-Camargo L *et al* 2017 Magnetic characterization of iron oxide nanoparticles for biomedical applications. *Methods Mol. Biol.* **1570** 47–71

[16] Krishnan K M 2010 Biomedical nanomagnetics: a spin through possibilities in imaging, diagnostics, and therapy *IEEE Trans. Magn.* **46** 2523–58

[17] Jiles D 2015 *Introduction to Magnetism and Magnetic Materials* (Boca Raton, FL: CRC Press)

[18] Philippova O, Barabanova A, Molchanov V and Khokhlov A 2011 Magnetic polymer beads: recent trends and developments in synthetic design and applications *Eur. Polym. J.* **47** 542–59

[19] Khatiri R, Reyhani A, Mortazavi S Z and Hossainalipour M 2013 Immobilization of serum albumin on the synthesized three layers core–shell structures of super-paramagnetic iron oxide nanoparticles *J. Ind. Eng. Chem.* **19** 1642–7

[20] Imran M, Zouli N, Ahamad T, Alshehri S M, Chandan M R, Hussain S and Khan A 2021 Carbon-coated Fe_3O_4 core–shell super-paramagnetic nanoparticle-based ferrofluid for heat transfer applications *Nanoscale Adv.* **3** 1962–75

[21] Foner S 1959 Versatile and sensitive vibrating-sample magnetometer *Rev. Sci. Instrum.* **30** 548–57

[22] Mukhtar A, Wu K, Cao X and Gu L 2020 Magnetic nanowires in biomedical applications *Nanotechnology* **31** 433001

[23] Wu K, Su D, Liu J, Rand S and Wang J P 2019 Magnetic nanoparticles in nanomedicine: a review of recent advances *Nanotechnology* **30** 502003

[24] Sun T, Zhang Y S, Pang B, Hyun D C, Yang M and Xia Y 2014 Engineered nanoparticles for drug delivery in cancer therapy *Angew. Chem. Int. Ed* **53** 12320–64

[25] Li X, Wei J, Aifantis K E, Fan Y, Feng Q, Cui F Z and Watari F 2016 Current investigations into magnetic nanoparticles for biomedical applications *J. Biomed. Mater. Res.* A **104** 1285–96

[26] Bohara R A, Thorat N D and Pawar S H 2016 Role of functionalization: Strategies to explore potential nano-bio applications of magnetic nanoparticles *RSC Adv.* **6** 43989–4012

[27] Chatterjee K, Sarkar S, Jagajjanani Rao K and Paria S 2014 Core/shell nanoparticles in biomedical applications *Adv. Colloid Interface Sci.* **209** 8–39

[28] Choi J S, Park J C, Nah H, Woo S, Oh J, Kim K M, Cheon G J, Chang Y, Yoo J and Cheon J 2008 A hybrid nanoparticle probe for dual-modality positron emission tomography and magnetic resonance imaging *Angew. Chem. Int. Ed* **47** 6259–62

[29] Corr S A, Rakovich Y P and Gun'Ko Y K 2008 Multifunctional magnetic-fluorescent nanocomposites for biomedical applications *Nanoscale Res. Lett.* **3** 87–104

[30] Fang C and Zhang M 2009 Multifunctional magnetic nanoparticles for medical imaging applications *J. Mater. Chem.* **19** 6258–66

[31] Hafeli U 2007 The history of magnetism in medicine ed W Andrä, and H Nowak *Magnetism in Medicine: A Handbook* 2nd edn (Weinheim: Wiley-VCH) pp 1–25

[32] Arole V M and Munde S V 2014 Fabrication of nanomaterials by top-down and bottom-up approaches—an overview *J. Mater. Sci.* **1** 89–93

[33] Amirkhanlou S, Ketabchi M and Parvin N 2012 Nanocrystalline/nanoparticle ZnO synthesized by high energy ball milling process *Mater. Lett.* **86** 122

[34] Sina B, Arsalani N, Khataee A and Tabrizi A G 2018 Comparison of ball milling hydrothermal and hydrothermal methods for synthesis of ZnO nanostructures and evaluation of their photocatalytic performance *J. Ind. Eng. Chem.* **62** 265–72

[35] Ansari A R, Imran M, Yahia I S, Abdel-Wahab M S, Alshahrie A, Khan A H and Sharma C 2018 Effect of microwave power on morphology of AgO thin film grown using microwave plasma CVD *Int. J. Surf. Sci. Eng.* **12** 1–2

[36] Ansari A R, Hussain S, Imran M, Abdel-wahab M S and Alshahrie A 2018 Synthesis, characterization and oxidation of metallic cobalt (Co) thin film into semiconducting cobalt oxide (Co_3O_4) thin film using microwave plasma CVD *Mater. Res. Exp.* **5** 065003

[37] Matsumura H 2019 Current status of catalytic chemical vapor deposition technology—history of research and current status of industrial implementation *Thin Solid Films* **679** 42–8

[38] Kaushik A, Khan R, Solanki P R, Pandey P, Alam J, Ahmad S and Malhotra B D 2008 Iron oxide nanoparticles–chitosan composite-based glucose biosensor *Biosens. Bioelectron.* **24** 676–83

[39] Sharma R, Agrawal V V, Srivastava A K, Govind, Nain L, Imran M, Kabi S R, Sinha R K and Malhotra B D 2013 Phase control of nanostructured iron oxide for application to biosensor *J. Mater. Chem.* B **1** 464

[40] Javed M, Shaik A H, Khan T A, Imran M, Aziz A, Ansari A R and Chandan M R 2018 Synthesis of stable waste palm oil based CuO nanofluid for heat transfer applications *Heat Mass Transfer* **54** 1–7

[41] Imran M, Ansari A R, Shaik A H, Hussain S, Khan A and Chandan M R 2018 Ferrofluid synthesis using oleic acid coated Fe_3O_4 nanoparticles dispersed in mineral oil for heat transfer applications *Mater. Res. Exp.* **5** 036108

[42] Imran M, Shaik A H, Ansari A R, Aziz A, Hussain S, Abouatiaa A F, Khan A and Chandan M R 2018 Synthesis of highly stable γ-Fe_2O_3 ferrofluid dispersed in liquid paraffin, motor oil and sunflower oil for heat transfer applications *RSC Adv.* **8** 13970–5

[43] Hussain S, Alam M M, Imran M, Zouli N, Aziz A, Irshad K and Khan A 2020 Fe_3O_4 nanoparticles decorated multi-walled carbon nanotubes based magnetic nanofluid for heat transfer application *Mater. Lett.* **274** 128043

[44] Solanki P R, Dhand C, Kaushik A, Ansari A A, Sood K N and Malhotra B D 2009 Nanostructured cerium oxide film for triglyceride sensor *Sensors Actuators* B **141** 551–6

[45] Ansari A A, Kaushik A, Solanki P R and Malhotra B D 2010 Nanostructured zinc oxide platform for mycotoxin detection *Bioelectrochemistry* **77** 75–81
[46] Sayilkan F, Erdemoglu S, Asilturk M, Akarsu M, Sener S, Sayilkan H, Erdemogl M and Mater E A 2006 Photocatalytic performance of pure anatasenanocrystallite TiO_2 sythesized under low temperature hydrothermal conditions *Res. Bull.* **41** 2276–85
[47] Yu J G, Wang G H, Cheng B and Zhou M H 2007 Effects of hydrothermal temperature and time on the photocatalytic and microstructures of bimodal mesoporous TiO_2 powders *Appl. Catal.* B **69** 171–80
[48] Rooymans J M 1972 ed P Hagenmuller *Preparative Methods in Solid State Chemistry* (New York: Academic)
[49] Asilturk M, Sayilkan F, Erdemoglu S, Akarsu M, Sayilkan H, Erdemoglu M and Arpac E 2006 *J. Hazard. Mater.* **129** 164–70
[50] Yalc¸ınoz S and Erc¸elebi E 2018 Potential applications of nano-emulsions in the food systems: an update *Mater. Res. Exp.* **5** 062001
[51] Asgari S, Saberi A H, McClements D J and Lin M 2019 Microemulsions as nanoreactors for synthesis of biopolymer nanoparticles *Trends Food Sci. Technol.* **86** 118–30
[52] Ahmad T, Wani I A, Al-Hartomy O A, Al-Shihri A S and Kalam A 2015 Low temperature chemical synthesis and comparative studies of silver oxide nanoparticles *J. Mol. Struct.* **1084** 9–15
[53] Suriati G, Mariatti M and Azizan A 2014 Synthesis of silver nanoparticles by chemical reduction method: effect of reducing agent and surfactant concentration *Int. J. Automot. Mech. Eng.* **10** 1920
[54] Sun Y and Xia Y 2002 Shape-controlled synthesis of gold and silver nanoparticles *Science* **298** 2176–9
[55] Kandasamy G, Sudame A, Bhati P, Chakrabarty A, Kale S N and Maity D 2018 Systematic magnetic fluid hyperthermia studies of carboxyl functionalized hydrophilic superparamagnetic iron oxide nanoparticles based ferrofluids. *J. Colloid Interface Sci.* **514** 534–43
[56] Lahiri B B, SurojitRanoo and Philip J 2017 Magnetic hyperthermia study in water based magnetic fluids containing TMAOH coated Fe_3O_4 using infrared thermography. *Infrared Phys. Technol.* **80** 71–82
[57] Diamantopoulos G, Basina G, Tzitzios V, Karakosta E, Fardis M, Jaglicic Z, Lazaridis N and Papavassiliou G 2013 Magnetic hyperthermia of laponite based ferrofluid. *J. Magn. Magn. Mater.* **336** 71–4
[58] Kandasamy G and Maity D 2015 Recent advances in superparamagnetic iron oxide nanoparticles (SPIONs) for *in vitro* and *in vivo* cancer nanotheranostics. *Int. J. Pharm.* **496** 191–218
[59] Barick K C, Singh S, Bahadur D, Lawande M A, Patkar D P and Hassan. P A 2014 Carboxyl decorated Fe_3O_4 nanoparticles for MRI diagnosis and localized hyperthermia. *J. Colloid Interface Sci.* **418** 120–25
[60] Stone R, Willi T, Rosen Y, Mefford O T and Alexis F 2011 Targeted magnetic hyperthermia. *Ther. Deliv.* **2** 815–38
[61] Kaur P, Aliru M L, Chadha A S, Asea A and Krishnan S 2016 Hyperthermia using nanoparticles–promises and pitfalls. *Int. J. Hyperth.* **32** 76–88
[62] Kozissnik B, Bohorquez A C, Dobson J and Rinaldi C 2013 Magnetic fluid hyperthermia: advances, challenges, and opportunity. *Int. J. Hyperth.* **29** 706–14

[63] Mosayebi J, Kiyasatfar M and Laurent S 2017 Synthesis, functionalization, and design of magnetic nanoparticles for theranostic applications. *Adv. Healthcare Mater.* **6** 1700306

[64] Zayed M A, Ahmed M A, Imam N G and El Sherbiny D H 2016 Preparation and structure characterization of hematite/magnetite ferro-fluid nanocomposites for hyperthermia purposes. *J. Mol. Liq.* **222** 895–905

[65] Lahiri B B, Muthukumaran T and Philip J 2016 Magnetic hyperthermia in phosphate coated iron oxide nanofluids. *J. Magn. Magn. Mater.* **407** 101–13

[66] Guibert C, Fresnais J, Peyre V and Dupuis V 2017 Magnetic fluid hyperthermia probed by both calorimetric and dynamic hysteresis measurements. *J. Magn. Magn. Mater.* **421** 384–92

[67] Lahiri B B, SurojitRanoo and Philip J 2016 Infrared thermography based magnetic hyperthermia study in Fe_3O_4 based magnetic fluids. *Infrared Phys. Technol.* **78** 173–84

[68] Gilchrist R K, Medal R, Shorey W D, Hanselman R C, Parrott J C and Bruce Taylor C 1957 Selective inductive heating of lymph nodes. *Ann. Surg.* **146** 596

[69] Hedayatnasab Z, Abnisa F and Daud W M A W 2017 Review on magnetic nanoparticles for magnetic nanofluid hyperthermia application. *Mater. Des.* **123** 174–96

[70] Pang C L K 2015 *Hyperthermia in Oncology* (Boca Raton, FL: CRC Press)

[71] Hergt R, Dutz S and Röder M 2008 Effects of size distribution on hysteresis losses of magnetic nanoparticles for hyperthermia. *J. Phys. Condens. Matter* **20** 385214

[72] Pollert E, Veverka P, Veverka M, Kaman O, Závěta K, Vasseur S, Epherre R, Goglio G and Duguet E 2009 Search of new core materials for magnetic fluid hyperthermia: preliminary chemical and physical issues. *Prog. Solid State Chem.* **37** 1–14

[73] Giri J, Pradhan P, Sriharsha T and Bahadur D 2005 Preparation and investigation of potentiality of different soft ferrites for hyperthermia applications. *J. Appl. Phys.* **97** 10Q916

[74] Purushotham S and Ramanujan R V 2010 Thermoresponsive magnetic composite nanomaterials for multimodal cancer therapy. *Acta Biomater.* **6** 502–10

[75] Amiri S and Shokrollahi H 2013 The role of cobalt ferrite magnetic nanoparticles in medical science. *Mater. Sci. Eng.* C **33** 1–8

[76] Fardis M, Rabias I, Diamantopoulos G, Boukos N, Tsitourli D, Papavassiliou G and Niarchos D 2007 Magnetic nanoparticles for biomedical applications. *J. Optoelectron. Adv. Mater.* **9** 527

[77] Kandasamy G, Khan S, Giri J, Bose S, Veerapu N S and Maity D 2019 One-pot synthesis of hydrophilic flower-shaped iron oxide nanoclusters (IONCs) based ferrofluids for magnetic fluid hyperthermia applications. *J. Mol. Liq.* **275** 699–712

[78] Lahiri B B, Ranoo S and Philip J 2018 Effect of orientational ordering of magnetic nanoemulsions immobilized in agar gel on magnetic hyperthermia. *J. Magn. Magn. Mater.* **451** 254–68

[79] Conde-Leborán I, Serantes D and Baldomir D 2015 Orientation of the magnetization easy axes of interacting nanoparticles: influence on the hyperthermia properties. *J. Magn. Magn. Mater.* **380** 321–24

[80] Branquinho L C, Carrião M S, Costa A S, Zufelato N, Sousa M H, Miotto R, Ivkov R and Bakuzis A F 2013 Effect of magnetic dipolar interactions on nanoparticle heating efficiency: Implications for cancer hyperthermia. *Sci. Rep.* **3** 1–11

[81] Rosensweig R E 2002 Heating magnetic fluid with alternating magnetic field. *J. Magn. Magn. Mater.* **252** 370–74

[82] Deatsch A E and Benjamin A E 2014 Heating efficiency in magnetic nanoparticle hyperthermia. *J. Magn. Magn. Mater.* **354** 163–72

[83] Munnier E, Cohen-Jonathan S, Linassier C, Douziech-Eyrolles L, Marchais H, Soucé M, Hervé K, Dubois P and Chourpa I 2008 Novel method of doxorubicin–SPION reversible association for magnetic drug targeting. *Int. J. Pharm.* **363** 170–76

[84] Norouzi M, VinithYathindranath J A, Thliveris B M, Kopec T J, Siahaan and Miller D W 2020 Doxorubicin-loaded iron oxide nanoparticles for glioblastoma therapy: a combinational approach for enhanced delivery of nanoparticles. *Sci. Rep.* **10** 1–18

[85] Lungu I I, Nistorescu S, Badea M A, Petre A-M, Udrea A-M, Banici A-M and Fleacă C *et al* 2020 Doxorubicin-conjugated iron oxide nanoparticles synthesized by laser pyrolysis: *in vitro* study on human breast cancer cells. *Polymers* **12** 2799

[86] Wu T-C, Lee P-Y, Lai C-L and Lai C-H 2021 Synthesis of multi-functional nano-vectors for target-specific drug delivery. *Polymers* **13** 451

[87] Casula M F, Corrias A, Arosio P, Lascialfari A and Sen T *et al* 2011 Design of water-based ferrofluids as contrast agents for magnetic resonance imaging *J. Colloid Interface Sci.* **357** 50–5

[88] Vuong T K O, Le T T, Do H D, Nguyen X T and Nguyen X C *et al* 2020 PMAO-assisted thermal decomposition synthesis of high-stability ferrofluid based on magnetite nanoparticles for hyperthermia and MRI applications *Mater. Chem. Phys.* **245** 122762

[89] Li J, Feng Z, Gu N and Yang F 2021 Superparamagnetic iron oxide nanoparticles assembled magnetic nanobubbles and their application for neural stem cells labeling *J. Mater. Sci. Technol.* **63** 124–32

[90] Yi X, Abenojar E C, Zhu J, Zheng Y and Exner A A 2019 In vitro preparation and characterization of magnetic nanobubbles *2019 IEEE Int. Ultrasonics Symp. (IUS).* (Piscataway, NJ: IEEE) pp 392–95

[91] Ficiarà E, Ansari S A, Argenziano M, Cangemi L, Monge C, Cavalli R and D'Agata F 2020 Beyond oncological hyperthermia: physically drivable magnetic nanobubbles as novel multipurpose theranostic carriers in the central nervous system. *Molecules* **25** 2104

[92] Guo X-M, Chen J-L, Zeng B-H, Lai J-C, Lin C-Y and Lai M-Y 2020 Ultrasound-mediated delivery of RGD-conjugated nanobubbles loaded with fingolimod and superparamagnetic iron oxide nanoparticles: targeting hepatocellular carcinoma and enhancing magnetic resonance imaging. *RSC Adv.* **10** 39348–58

[93] Li Y, Huang L, Wang X and Chen Y 2017 A study of electrochemical sensor based on BHb-imprinted magnetic nanoparticles *Anal. Sci.* **33** 1105–10

[94] Mollarasouli F, Zor E, Ozcelikay G and Ozkan S A 2021 Magnetic nanoparticles in developing electrochemical sensors for pharmaceutical and biomedical applications *Talanta* **226** 122108

[95] Romanholo P V V, Razzino C A, Raymundo-Pereira P A, Prado T M, Machado S A S and Sgobbi L F 2021 Biomimetic electrochemical sensors: New horizons and challenges in biosensing applications *Biosens. Bioelectron.* **185** 113242

[96] Garkani Nejad F, Tajik S, Beitollahi H and Sheikhshoaie I 2021 Magnetic nanomaterials based electrochemical (bio)sensors for food analysis *Talanta* **228** 122075

[97] Yáñez-Sedeño P, Campuzano S and Pingarrón J M 2017 Electrochemical sensors based on magnetic molecularly imprinted polymers: a review *Anal. Chim. Acta* **960** 1–17

[98] Yilmaz E, Sarp G, Uzcan F, Ozalp O and Soylak M 2021 Application of magnetic nanomaterials in bioanalysis *Talanta* **229** 122285

[99] Worgall S and Crystal R G 2014 Gene therapy ed R Lanza, R Langer and J P Vacanti *Principle of Tissue Engineering* 4th edn (New York: Academic) pp 657–86

[100] Dobson J 2006 Gene therapy progress and prospects: magnetic nanoparticle-based gene delivery *Gene Ther.* **13** 283–7

[101] Fouriki A and Dobson J 2013 Nanomagnetic gene transfection for non-viral gene delivery in NIH 3T3 mouse embryonic fibroblasts *Materials* **6** 255–64

[102] Ginn S L, Amaya A K, Alexander I E, Edelstein M and Abedi M R 2018 Gene therapy clinical trials worldwide to 2017: an update *J. Gene Med.* **20** e3015

[103] Wei W, Xu C and Wu H 2006 Magnetic iron oxide nanoparticles mediated gene therapy for breast cancer—an *in vitro* study *J. Huazhong Univ. Sci. Technol* **26** 728–30

[104] Wang Z *et al* 2018 Shape-controlled magnetic mesoporous silica nanoparticles for magnetically-mediated suicide gene therapy of hepatocellular carcinoma *Biomaterials* **154** 147–57

[105] Zhang Q, Zhao W, Cheng J, Deng Z, Zhang P, Zhang A, Xu Z, Pan S, Liao X and Cui D 2021 Heat-induced manganese-doped magnetic nanocarriers combined with Yap-siRNA for MRI/NIR-guided mild photothermal and gene therapy of hepatocellular carcinoma *Chem. Eng. J.* **426** 130746

Chapter 10

Application of x-ray diffraction for biomedical nanotechnologies: current insights and perspectives

Rahul Bhattacharjee, Priya Mitra, Srija Chakrabarty, Radheka Bhaduri, Sulagna Kar and Abhijit Dey

The nanoparticle has been a matter of interest in recent times owing to its vast application in varied biomedical sectors and their characteristics which include size, crystal shape, and physical attributes. X-ray diffraction (XRD) is one such technique used for the characterization of nanoparticles providing valuable insights on phase, structure, orientation, and aberration on the crystal. It is a powerful non-destructive interference technique produced by the interference of scattering x-ray beam upon crystal lattice and determined by the distribution of atoms in the lattice. Here in this book chapter, we have elucidated the instrumentation and sampling of XRD and its application in biomedical nanotechnologies.

10.1 Introduction

X-ray diffraction (XRD) is the most remarkable non-destructive process for determining atomic spacing by crystal structure analysis along with their preferred texture orientations, dimensions, crystal defects, and crystallinity strain [1]. X-ray imaging involves energy-resolved x-ray imaging owing to its major benefits to fluency in detection as well as its application in including security, health, and resolution of protein structure [2, 3]. The cross-sections of attenuated bone, metals, liquids in x-ray imaging are dependent on the wavelength of the x-ray beam, contributing composition-specific contrast which is generally inaccessible from the measured intensity [4]. XRD is based on the constructive interference of monochromatic x-ray beams scattering at a specified angle from lattice planes of crystalline samples for the formation of diffraction peaks [5]. The maximum intensity, known as peak intensity, is illustrated by the atomic spacing in the lattice, making XRD pattern the fingerprint of atomic configurations in a particular

doi:10.1088/978-0-7503-3379-5ch10

constituent. The cathode ray tube produces x-rays, filtered to provide monochromatic radiation, and collimated to intensify by aiming at the sample [5].

Max von Laue witnessed crystallographic XRD for the first time in 1912 exhibiting a 3D grating. Later, William H Bragg and William L Bragg formulated Bragg's law as $n\lambda = 2d \sin \theta$ to elucidate the diffraction patterns in ZnS, KCl, and NaCl crystals as reflections of crystal lattice planes (figure 10.1) [1], wherein n is an integer; λ is the wavelength; D is the distance between parallel planes in the crystal lattice; θ is the angle of the incident and reflected beam with the crystal plane. Three integers h, k, l, known as plane indices, define the planes in the crystal lattice [5]. This law correlates the wavelength of electromagnetic spectra to the diffraction angle and the atomic spacing of the lattice in a crystalline sample for being detected, processed, and counted by the x-rays by scanning the sample at 2θ angles and the arbitrary orientation of the powdered sample ensuring all possible directions of diffraction in the lattice. Since, every compound possesses its own set of d-spacings, the transition of spray peaks to d-spacing serves as an identification step for any compound, which is accomplished by comparison of d-spacings to the standard reference models [5].

Thus, in this chapter, we not only elucidate the application of XRD in oncology, antimicrobial activity, macromolecule crystallography, and the pharmaceutical industry but also highlight the instrumentation, sampling, and detection of samples. Moreover, the types of NPs used for XRD and the technique used by XRD for biomedical application are characterized too.

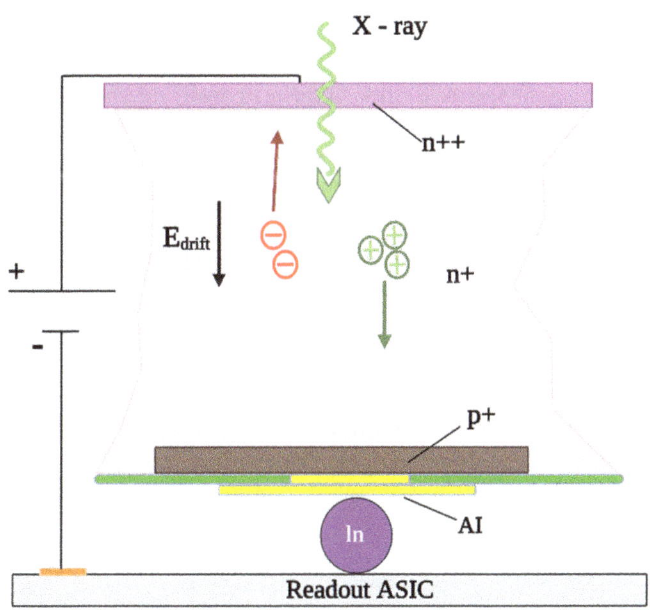

Figure 10.1. Detection of x-rays in a silicon (material based) sensor.

10.2 Instrumentation and sampling of XRD

The cathode ray tube, sample holder, and x-ray detector are the three essential components of an x-ray diffractometer [6]. X-rays originate from the cathode ray tube by heating the filament with a voltage accelerating the electrons and bombarding the target material with electrons, causing enhanced threshold energy to release electrons from the internal shell of copper and thus generating characteristic x-ray spectra of the specific wavelengths for each of the target materials [5]. The filtering of these generated x-rays with a foil or a crystal monochromator is required for the production of monochromatic rays, which are then collimated to the sample and the intensity of the reflected beam is recorded as the sample and detector are rotated [5]. The sample is subjected to x-ray incidence in compliance with Bragg's law to cause constructive interference and an intensity peak. The detector of the diffractometer records and analyzes the x-ray signal, converting it to a count rate wherein the output is received in the printer and computer monitor [5]. Correct powder sample preparation is one of the key criteria for analysis using XRD as materials containing fine colloids are poor x-ray reflectors and are difficult to characterize by XRD. The preparation of the sample not only includes the right samples for the removal of unwanted substances but also the right techniques for obtaining the desired particle size, orientation, and thickness. XRD powder analysis requires extremely fine grains to obtain a good signal-to-noise ratio by avoiding intensity variations, and minimizing the preferences for orientation [1]. Moreover, the reduction of powders in fine particles makes sure of sufficient participation of particles in the diffraction process. The recommended sizes are between 1 and 5 μm for quantification of the different phases targeted [7, 8]. For conventional qualitative assessment of mineral components, the samples are routinely processed to pass through a 325 mesh sieve (45 μm), where grinding is done mechanically, side-stepping the effect of excessive grinding which includes distortion of the lattice and the formation of an amorphous Beilby layer surrounding the grains [1].

The collimated beam of x-rays with a wavelength equivalent to atomic distance is irradiated upon the sample, scattering in all possible directions, generating a diffraction maxima which appears in a specific direction during the collision of dispersed x-rays with the intermittent spots in the lattice of molecules or atoms, liquid crystals, polymers, colloids [9]. When a monochromatic x-ray beam interacts with an ordered 3D crystal, it causes x-ray waves to diffract in specific directions and phases, following the diffraction pattern. The defining vectors of a unit cell dictate the orientations of the diffracted waves and the diffraction spots on the detector which characterizes the periodicity of the crystal. The amplitudes and phases of the crystallized macromolecule reflect its molecular structure which is determined from the generated electron density map. The data collection experiments are used for evaluating the intensity of the diffracted beam, proportional to the square of the diffracted wave amplitude. The phases of these waves are experimentally inaccessible, requiring the use of specialized phasing methods to extract this information [10].

10.3 Data collection and detection of XRD

The data collection technology of XRD causes enhanced improvement in data-acquisition rates through the spectrum of macromolecules via sophisticated equipment such as an x-ray generator, x-ray detector, and a stepping motor system (Goniometer). It usually holds the crystal on the capillary tube of glass or quartz using plasticine and then sets it into an x-ray [11]. Diffracted x-rays are detected by diffractometers, and photographs are used on oscillation and precession cameras for a 2D diffraction pattern causing digital output without wet development and subsequent digital scanning (figure 10.2) [11].

Pixel array detectors permit a massively parallel count of single photons by multiple million circuits with indicators [12]. The emission photoelectrons from the surface of the detector are dependent on the energy of photons, hence spectral imaging is offered by these detectors. The device response is usually calibrated on a per pixel basis using a statistical model for spectral imaging. Moreover, the calibrated sensor was used in two monochromatic pictures to separate dual-energy diffraction measurements. Furthermore, multi-wavelength diffraction is used for the applications of protein structure determination and XRD imaging [12]. Thus, the probability density function of the estimated voltage following x-ray absorption is a challenging function involving both full as well as partial counts [12]. The accomplishment of energy-dispersive spectral detection is dependent on the count rate as a function of threshold value set on a digital counter, which eventually records an initial current plume generated by x-ray absorption together with an image through the number of counts per pixel [13]. The number of photoelectrons in the initial current plume and the peak of the accompanying voltage are affected by x-ray energy during the estimation of recorded counts as a function of a threshold voltage [13].

The direct detector, quantum detector, photon-counting detector, and photon processing detector are the new generation of x-ray detectors developed to process and count x-ray photons as individual quanta by enabling low-noise imaging and energy extraction from the x-ray beam [14]. Medipix-2 is one of these detectors which includes thresholds set for recording only photons within a certain energy

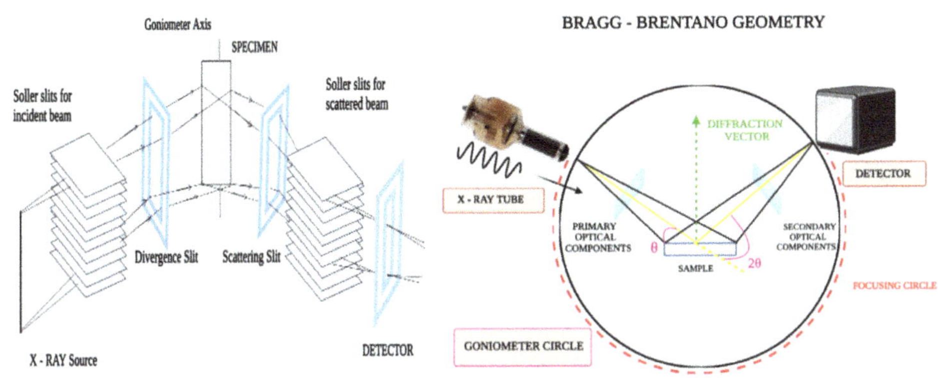

Figure 10.2. Schematic illustration of the instrumentation and geometry of Bragg–Brentano diffractometer.

range and possessing varied thresholds for several counters within each pixel, allowing for comprehensive spectral imaging [15]. Spectral x-ray imaging with single-photon processing detectors is gaining popularity for a variety of applications. The contrast to noise ratio and spectral response as a function of the substance are explored as fundamental parameters [2]. The amount of incident and absorbed photons in the object influences the CNR while the range of useful photon energy is limited due to the pre-requisite of significant absorption by the object. When photons of higher energy are removed from the spectrum, the CNR usually improves causing the layers of materials to be separated and uniquely identified by a considerable variation in their spectral x-ray absorption [2].

Compared to conventional diffractometers using scintillation counters, which detect one single reflection, area detectors are more efficient and at the same time provide the *x*–*y*-coordinates of the x-rays incident over a large part of the diffraction pattern [11]. These advantages are significantly obvious in the XRD of the macromolecular object. The uncertainty in phase complicates structure estimation from diffraction pattern measurements [16]. Although the intensity of each diffraction pattern is measured, the Fourier transform correlations to structural diffraction possessing the ability of inversion depend on the phase of each of the known or assumed diffraction points [12]. The most common method for determining the phase of specific atoms or molecules in the lattice is comparing diffraction patterns and distant from absorption edges. When the diffraction peaks close to resonance possess a shift in their phase, it affects the diffracted intensity pattern, influencing the conditions of interference for multiple wavelength anomalous dispersion (MAD) by on-phase support of diffraction pattern inversion and retrieving the structure of the macromolecule [12]. Despite their widespread use, the MAD is often afflicted by inaccuracies from x-ray damage, causing inappropriate $1/f$ noise, along with the dose-dependent losses of macromolecular crystals, and degradation of resolution [17]. The data interpretation is complicated when MAD measurements are done consecutively with varying exposures at each wavelength. MAD phasing is a novel diffraction technique used for unknown protein structure determination and the blue copper protein isolation from cucumber seedlings via crystallographic phases by several wavelength measurements. Thus, making it physically viable by combining strong, polychromatic synchrotron radiation with precise information collection via multiwire electronic area detectors to allow the easiest solution of the phase problem by solving protein structures which necessitate several isomorphous derivatives and coordinates of analogous structure for molecular replacement. MAD phasing is effective for establishing small- to medium-sized metalloprotein structures when isomorphous derivatives are difficult to obtain, offering a new light on redox and spectroscopic properties of the most prevalent form of metalloproteins, the blue copper proteins [18].

10.4 Types of nanoparticles used in XRD

Metal nanoparticles (Me-NPs) have been intensively investigated due to their astonishing physicochemical properties, which include catalytic properties, antimicrobial activities, optical, magnetic, and electronic properties owing to the enhanced

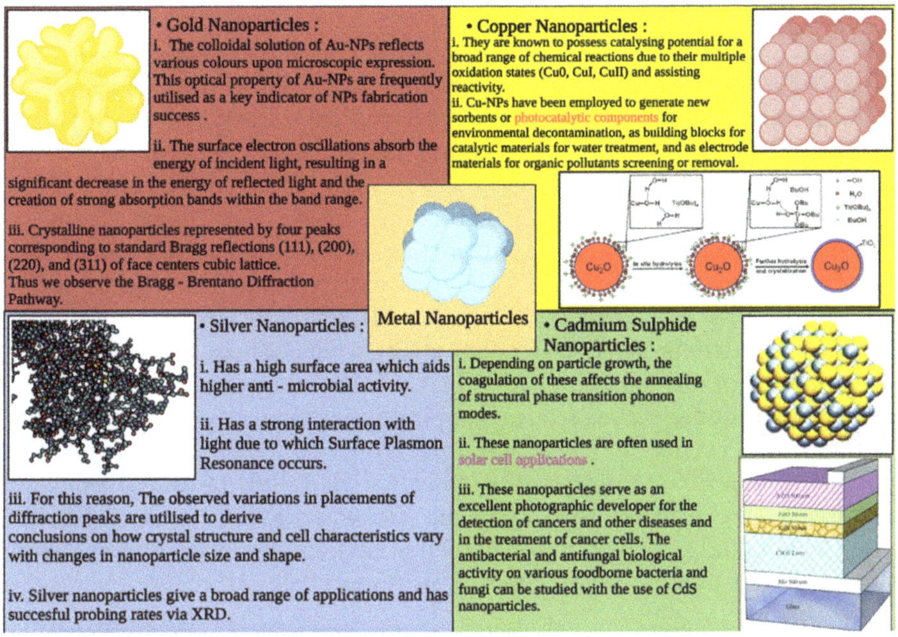

Figure 10.3. Types of nanoparticle used for XRD.

surface activities due to an increased number of surface atoms, allowing more surface area for reactivity. The synthesis of noble Me-NPs is gaining attention because of its wide range of applications [19]. The stability along with minimal resistivity of gold, as well as the great thermal conductivity of silver, is becoming the focus of study for noble metals (NMs) [20]. Me-NPs or nanostructures with different morphologies exhibit higher absorption for different wavelengths of light while expressing non-ideal optical characteristics (figure 10.3) [20].

10.4.1 Silver nanoparticles

Ag-NPs have been known to possess inhibitory and bactericidal properties similar to other Me-NPs. When compared to bulk silver metal, Ag-NPs are predicted to possess a high specific surface area which is the major characteristic of Me-NPs for high antibacterial activity [21, 22]. The small size of Ag-NPs allows for a wide range of novel applications in a variety of industries. They are extremely efficient in absorbing and scattering light with various colors depending on the dimensions and structure of the particles. The excitation at specified wavelengths causes Ag-NPs to interact strongly with light allowing the conduction electrons on the metal surface to undergo a collective oscillation, intended for enhanced scattering and absorption properties via surface plasmon resonance (SPR) [19]. NPs are in solution attached to their surfaces following a bilayer of charge formation by stabilizing the particles and preventing them from aggregating [19]. Ag-NPs are efficient against anaerobic as well as aerobic microbes causing bacterial cellular proteins to precipitate via disruption of the respiratory chain system [23–25].

The correlations of plasmonic properties with Ag-NP structures were investigated by HRTEM, XRD, optical absorption, and EXAFS. The structural parameters of Ag K-edge EXAFS spectra were averaged over ionic and neutral states of Ag. The metallic atomic structure of Ag-NPs poses challenges such as point symmetry variation in the NPs core, Ag–Ag bond length, and the near-surface region structures [26]. EXAFS has been used to investigate the modifications of Ag-NP structures in soda-lime glass [27]. Moreover, EXAFS is more accurate than HRTEM for investigating the characteristics of the lattice structure of Ag-NPs implanted in silicate glasses [28]. The thermal expansion coefficient of glass-embedded Ag-NPs was evaluated over a wide temperature range and thermal expansion mismatching via EXAFS that enables the changes in bond lengths and stress condition of the particles [29]. SAXS offers clear quantitative knowledge about the correlations of localized surface plasmon resonance (LSPR) behavior with the aggregation events in PVA stabilized Ag-NPs [30]. SAXS explained the production of mass fractal aggregates in Ag–Cu alloy NPs produced using copper and silver nitrates in water with hydrazine (reductant) and starch (sol-stabilizing agent). The bimodal size distribution exhibited smaller and larger aggregates in Ag-rich compositions and Cu-rich compositions respectively [31].

10.4.2 Gold nanoparticle

Au-NPs possess exceptional optical and plasmonic capabilities, and when coupled with ligands, they provide immense research potential [32, 33]. Functionalized Au-NPs pose varied applications as biological detection tools, sensors, and drug delivery systems. Au-NP and gold blocks were employed extensively in a variety of sectors because of their stability [20, 33]. For Au-NPs the SPR lines broaden uniformly, whereas non-uniformity in particle size causes inhomogeneous broadening. The particle size of Au-NPs increases with the size effect causing a red-shift in the spectrum absorption peak [20]. Several investigations depicted that real-time WAXS/SAXS/UV–Vis measurements are the accurate way to illustrate the formation of Au-NPs through concentration, temperature, ligand ratio, and solvent type affecting the nucleation as well as growth kinetics of Au-NPs [31]. Luo *et al* designed a chiral Au-NP by transferring the chiral of peptides to Au-NPs. Peptide-orientation produces asymmetric gold nano-polyhedrons with strong circular dichroism coupling. Some compounds possess poor self-fluorescence enhancement efficacy during the synthesis of functional NPs but are improved by conjugating them with Au-NPs. Local SPR of Me-NPs improves the incident light absorption, influencing the fluorescence radiation from close molecules into the far-field in metal-enhanced fluorescence (MEF). This impact is supported by expertise having a significant affect in fields like optics, biology, and medical diagnostics [20]. The energy of incident light is absorbed by the surface electron oscillations, for a considerable reduction in the energy of reflected light, leading to the formation of intense absorption bands within the range. The colloidal solution of Au-NPs reflects various colors upon microscopic expression. This optical property of Au-NPs is frequently utilized as a key indicator of NPs fabrication success [20]. Moreover, XPS is used to investigate the interaction of L-cysteine and Au-NPs to get spectroscopic evidence for kinetic theories of catalyst inhibition and analyze the effect of low-coordinated Au-NPs [34]. XPS and liquid-based particle sizing techniques are used to investigate protein functionalization on the surface of Au-NPs. Thus, it is a reliable method for studying proteins and peptides adsorbed at Au surfaces quantitatively, and successfully characterize the Au-NPs molecular interaction [35].

10.4.3 Copper nanoparticles

Cu-NPs are known to possess catalyzing potential for a broad range of chemical reactions due to their multiple oxidation states and assisting reactiveness. Cu-NPs offer a wide range of applications in science and technology, including catalytic organic transformations, oxidation–reduction, photocatalysis, electrocatalysis [36–38]. The high boiling point of Cu metal allows Cu-NPs to be used in thermophilic and barophilic chemical conditions such as microwave-based reactions, vapor phase reactions, continuous flow reactions, and different organic transformations [39, 40]. Cu and Cu-NPs are ideal for the formation of selective catalytic systems due to their unique characteristics of oxidation state, hence are regarded as a valuable metal. Cu-NPs have been employed to generate new sorbents or photocatalytic components for environmental decontamination, as building blocks for catalytic materials for water treatment, and as electrode materials for organic pollutant screening or removal [41, 42]. Cu-NPs like any other Me-NPs have exhibited various catalytic, electronic, and surface-enhanced plasmonic resonance properties [43, 44], for a wide range of applications in the fields of catalysis, electronics [45]. In the presence of $NaBH_4$, the nitroaromatics undergo reduction due to the catalytic action of Cu-NPs [46]. Until now, there has been little research on the catalytic activities of *in situ* synthesized Cu-NPs in nitroaromatics reduction [47]. During the catalytic reduction of 4-NP in the presence of $NaBH_4$, a precursor, $Cu_2Cl(OH)_3$, was used as a catalyst, which was reduced by $NaBH_4$ to form catalytically active metallic Cu and it is further confirmed by XRD and UV–visible analyses [48].

Cu-NPs may be made using a variety of processes, including sonochemical reduction, metal vapor synthesis, thermal reduction, and chemical reduction owing to the precise control of the nano structural features such as size and shape [49–53]. The crystalline structure of the NP was analyzed via XRD, Bruker D8 using TOPAS 4.2 software exhibiting antimicrobial activity against a gram-negative bacteria *Escherichia coli* and a gram-positive bacteria *Staphyllococcus aureus*. Therefore, the study shows that hydrogels of Cu-NP containing chitosan-pluronic nanocomposite (CPF-CHCu NPs) could be efficiently used in antibacterial applications [54].

10.4.4 Cadmium sulfide

Cadminum sufide (CdS) is a yellow to orange colored crystalline solid with a higher boiling point and it is a common semiconductor material [55]. These CdS crystal photo-cells are extraordinarily sensitive through the full spectrum, ranging from infrared to ultraviolet rays, x-rays, and γ-rays, as well as for corpuscular (α and β) rays. CdS-NPs are characteristically pure with uniformity in their structure, and have either a cubic or hexagonal-shaped structure, or a combination of the two, with the hexagonal or wurtzite phase predominant [55]. Eu [56], Mn [57], and other materials have been employed to dope CdS-NPs in varying concentrations, for luminescence or quenching. These NPs possess a potent application in the decomposition of water by the photocatalytic method [55]. CdS nano-crystals are prepared by different mechanisms: the chemical colloidal method, reverse micellar method, sol–gel method, electrochemical deposition method, Langmuir–Blodgett (LB) method, hydrothermal method, microfluidic method, functionalized chiral method [55]. When NPs are annealed, they tend to agglomerate and produce bigger particles. The coagulation of CdS-NPs influences the annealing of the structural phase to transform phonon modes depending on particle development [58]. Inorganic heterojunction photovoltaic devices commonly incorporate CdS nanoparticles to optimize effectiveness [55] while CdS nanorods are often used in solar cell applications. Many sensor technologies already take advantage of the unique features of structures based on CdS-NPs. The utilization of CdS-NPs in biological applications has made significant progress, allowing fluorescent nanoparticles associated with biological molecules for microscopic sensing devices [55]. Because of the extended fluorescence lifetime and higher fluorescent quantum yields, CdS-NPs exhibit a narrow, symmetric emission spectrum and are photochemically durable. The CdS-NP probes are brighter and more resistant to photobleaching. CdS nanostructures having different exclusive characteristics are coupled with a variety of organic, inorganic, and biological elements for the generation of new materials and technologies with a wide range of applications. CdS-based nanoscale structures, devices, and systems have been widely exploited to demonstrate their potential for bringing revolutionary solutions in electronics, optoelectronics, photovoltaics, sensors, and security [55]. EXAFS is used to investigate metal chalcogenides in CdS-NPs and contrast to XRD, EXAFS, on the other hand, does not simply count on long-range order, making it more suitable for CdS-NP analysis. It was discovered that stabilizing CdS-NPs with a diameter of 1.3 nm–12 nm affected the average bond length of CdS [59]. XPS and SEMEDX (energy-dispersive x-ray spectroscopy) are used for the characterization of CdS@Ag_2S core/shell, which is synthesized via the AOT–*n*-heptane–water microemulsion process [60]. The sensitivity of XPS provides a unique collection of peaks for the quantification of elements within the range of the spectrum with their respective kinetic energies derived from the energy of photons along with their energy requisite for binding. Moreover, core–shell formation is supported by the XPS and SEMEDX [31]. The characterization of the CdS-NP was done using various techniques via the powder x-ray diffraction technique to determine the crystalline nature of the nanoparticles. The antibacterial and antifungal activity of CdS-NP exhibited using well diffusion techniques against *E. coli*, *Bacillus circus*, *S. aureus*, *Aspergillus flavus*, *Fusarium oxysporum*, and *Penicillium expansum* [61].

10.4.5 Metal oxide nanoparticles

Due to their unique physicochemical properties, metal as well as metal oxide NPs are currently attracting significant attention in a variety of domains of solid-state chemistry and are synthesized using a variety of methods. Similar to Me-NPs, metal oxide NPs (MO-NPs) are also heterogeneous, and the impact of these MO-NPs on animate objects is determined by their shape and size in preference to the chemical characteristics of utilized metal ions [62]. These MO-NPs are effective antimicrobial agents, exhibiting a broad range of applications in different industries. Among MO-NPs, ZnO-NPs possess the most efficient antibacterial properties against all kinds of microorganisms (gram-positive and gram-negative bacteria) [155]. They are capable of producing ROS and also have the ability to accumulate on the surface of microorganisms, allowing sensitivity [62]. The cytotoxicity of MO-NPs is also dependent on their physicochemical aspects in the same way as antibacterial activity. The cytotoxic effects of MO-NPs of identical size but differing compositions are frequently variable. Surface coating is currently used for the functionalization of MO-NPs to reduce toxicity and, depending on the original surface qualities of the coating, the toxicity effect may intensify or diminish [63]. The final toxicity is most likely a result of physicochemical changes caused by coating, dissolution, changes in aggregation pattern of particle, zeta potential, and release of ionic or free radical into the solution. MO-NPs dissolve partially in aqueous solutions, causing morphological changes and the development of new crystallographic phases, dependent on the composition, structure, and size of the NPs [64, 65]. Aggregation in aqueous solutions is a common feature of MO-NPs [66], possessing the potency to be stabilized by BSA when a protein corona is formed MO-NPs [66]. A combinatorial study of XANES and EXAFS characterizes CuO, Cu_2O/CuO, and CuO/TiO_2 NPs, where the existence of various oxide phases was verified using these techniques, by exploring the atomic structure of those samples [67]. The particle size is determined using SAXS analysis, while the oxidation condition and local structure of iron atoms are determined using XANES analysis. Cerium oxide is used in a variety of applications for the production of hydrogen, optical displays as a catalyst causing varied industrial and biological applications [68]. CeO-Np was investigated by XRD for its crystalline structure and the laser intensity increases the size of the crystals. When *E. coli* is present in its vicinity, the reduction of the Ce^{4+} charge of nanoparticles to Ce^{3+} takes place causing oxidative stress on proteins and lipids that are present on the plasma membrane of the microorganism or during cellular metabolism electron uptake. Another potential method of antibacterial activity is the formation of ROS by metal NPs which causes oxidative stress that alters the functioning of the bacterial respiratory chain. Moreover, CeO-Np expresses more toxicity towards the *E. coli* and is dependent upon pH, shape, size and the concentration of the particle [69].

A combinatorial SANS/SAXS technique is used for the characterization of the ligand shells on ZnO-NPs [67]. Classical *in situ* techniques like UV–Vis along with SAXS are responsive to ZnO core only, whereas SANS uses the sensitivity of neutrons to H_2 for the detection of organic stabilizers in dispersion. Both approaches are used in the current study to determine the size distribution of the ZnO-NP core together with the stabilizer molecule in a native solution [70]. The XRD patterns of calcined ZnO-NPs produced via an aqueous extract of *Cassia auriculata* leaves to match the hexagonal fcc cubic crystal structure. The crystalline nature of ZnO-NP is seen and studied via XRD technique and used to identify bactericidal properties against *Ralstonia solanacearum* (MTCC), *E. coli* (MTCC 7410), *Klebsiella pneumonia* (MTCC 7407), and *Xanthomonas vesicatoria* (MTCC) via agar well diffusion assay and a growth kinetic assay [71].

10.4.6 Magnetic nanoparticle

MNPs with sizes in the range 1–100 nm and high surface area to volume ratio set them apart from the majority of their corresponding materials and attract a lot of attention in catalysis, neurostimulation, data storage, spintronics, and gyroscopic sensors [72–74]. Materials including metals, alloys, and oxides are favored for MNP production. Magnetic properties, specifically magnetic moment and anisotropy constant are dependent on the size and shape of MNPs. Since the surface layer of MNPs is devoid of translational crystal symmetry, its magnetic characteristics are very different from those of the interior region of the molecules, promoting lower saturation magnetizations together with higher anisotropy constants [75]. The dimensions of the core of MNP and particle production possess an impact on the spin-canting effect [76]. Single-domain MNPs are identically oriented internal magnetization for enhanced saturation of magnetization and the highest attainable magnetic moment. Under external magnetic fields, the magnetic flux of a single-domain particle generally rotates at an enormous magnetic moment, whose hysteresis is explained by the Stoner–Wohlfarth model [77]. The ability of the MNPs contrast agent in the enhancement of longitudinal and transverse relaxation rates of nuclear spins in the vicinity is reflected by its magnetic relaxivity [72].

10.5 Techniques used by XRD for biomedical nanotechnologies

Owing to their high surface-to-volume ratio, nanoscale materials frequently possess different properties to their bulk equivalents, which causes exponential increase in their reactivity at the molecular level. Electronic, optical, and chemical properties are among them, while the mechanical features of NPs vary greatly. The crystalline structure, phase nature, lattice parameters, and crystalline grain size are all typically determined by XRD [31]. Herein we have elucidated the various technologies utilized for XRD for varied applications (figure 10.4).

X-ray absorption spectroscopy (XAS) is one such technique of XRD that calculates the x-ray absorption coefficient as a function of the energy of a material. The XAS element selectivity is determined by a set of absorption spectrum lines for each element that correspond to varied binding energies of its electrons. When Mg_2Ge and $GeCl_4$ react, an *in situ* XAS was employed to investigate the kinetics and mechanism of the generation of germanium NPs [78].

Extended x-ray absorption fine structure (EXAFS) is another useful tool utilizing XRD to determine the chemical state of species that exists at very trace levels to obtain XAS spectra. EXAFS investigations obtained from TEM revealed that GeO_2

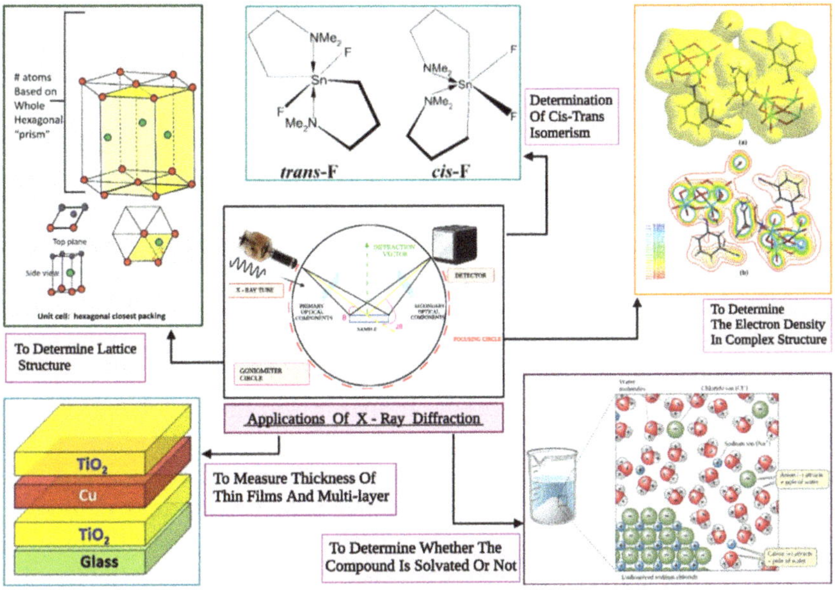

Figure 10.4. Biomedical application of XRD.

NPs were formed with Ge-NPs to reveal a Ge–Ge distance of 2.45 via XRD. Zhang *et al* used the microemulsion method to coat Fe_2O_3-NPs with sodium dodecylbenzene sulfonate, stearic acid, and hexadecyltrimethylammonium bromide surfactants. EXAFS analysis was conducted to study the role of surfactants, and samples tending to increase the Fe–O bond length. All of these compounds possess significant spatial resistance wherein the CTAB molecule possesses the most. The lattice deformation at the interfaces acts as a major stumbling block to rapid NP development [79]. Moreover, EXAFS was used to examine metal chalcogenides, such as CdS-NPs [59]. In contrast to XRD, EXAFS is suited for materials as it does not rely on any long-range order. Lloyd *et al* applied a variety of approaches to track the reduction of Se (IV) to Se(II) by the use of a microbial whole-cell catalyst via EXAFS. The reduction of Se(IV) to Se(II) via an insoluble red amorphous Se(0) phase through EXAFS demonstrates the synthesis of metal selenide both *ex situ* and *in situ* [80]. Sokolov *et al* used x-ray reflectivity, EXAFS, and electron microscopy to evaluate the structural binding of Pd-NPs. When a cuboctahedral fcc structural model of Pd-NP surrounded by thiol was considered, the EXAFS-derived size became less than the TEM-derived size. Both HRTEM and EXAFS detected lattice growth in all types of NPs when compared with bulk Pd [81].

X-ray absorption near-edge structure (XANES) is one of the techniques that uses XRD to characterize NPs for varied biomedical applications. By considering the excitation of an inner shell electron to those states permitted by dipole selection criteria, XANES examines the density of states of empty or partially filled electronic states. Copper cation inversion in Cu–Fe_2O_4 as a function of saturation magnetization is studied using EXAFS. XANES is more useful for determining the absorbing oxidation states, empty orbitals, electronic configuration, and site symmetry of atoms. Both XANES and EXAFS exhibited that Fe ions filled more tetrahedral than octahedral sites, implying that Fe ions occupied more tetrahedral than octahedral sites. Overall, these researchers demonstrated that the analysis on their copper ferrite NPs revealed that these nanostructures had a structure similar to that of the bulk material. The oxidation status of FeO-NPs was investigated using XANES. A combination of XANES and EXAFS to characterize CuO, Cu_2O/CuO, and CuO/TiO_2 NPs. TEM, XPS, and XANES were used to study the nucleation and development of Fe-NPs in SiO_2. Ion implantation caused the creation of dilute cationic Fe^{2+} species in the beginning, but at increasing dissolved iron concentrations, the formation of tiny metallic nuclei was seen, which seeded the nanocluster growth with extended implantation or annealing.

The most extensively used analytical approach for surface chemical analysis is XPS which is used to characterize materials of nanoscale measurements via the photoelectric effect [82]. It is a very efficient quantitative method used for determining the elemental composition, electronic structure, and oxidation states of the material. Functioning in high vacuum conditions it is used to investigate the surface functionalization of the NPs with their ligand exchange interactions and core–shell structures. XPS analyzed the interior heterostructure of the NPs by tuning the environment-dependent crystal structure of metal chalcogenide NPs of different sizes [83]. It aids the analysis of the difference between structures comprising a homogenous alloy and core of NPs. Moreover, XPS determines the interaction of ligands like trioctlyphosphine oxide with a surface of metal chalcogenide NPs. The untapped surface chalcogenide element oxidizes more readily in the presence of air when the TOPO bonds with the surface of metals elements. The composition of the material and the direction of the electron beam are explored by XPS instead of using lateral spatial resolution for detecting elements in a direction vertical to probing electron beams like in TEM and TEM/EELS. An empirical approach detected XPS data of core–shell NPs wherein translating XPS intensities into overlayer thickness is used for spherical NPs [84]. The benefits of XPS would include providing information about the depth, similar to the size of NPs (depth up to 10 nm from the surface) without causing considerable damage to the material. However, the limitations of XPS include the uncontaminated solid dry form used for data interpretation. Moreover, XPS investigated the interaction of naked Au-NPs with L-cysteine, to provide spectroscopic support to kinetic models of catalyst deactivation by Au-atoms of low-coordination present at the edges and corners of NPs [85]. Minelli *et al* used XPS with liquid-based particles to analyze the protein coating present on Au-NPs. XPS functions as a reliable tool for quantitively determining proteins and peptides absorbed on the interface of Au. It also determines the molecular interface in Au-NPs. XPS analysis provides chemical information about the surface of the nanoparticle, used to determine the thickness of the coating of the NP [35]. XPS utilized the Davis method to calculate the size of the Au-NPs in the planar model. The XPS-derived NP estimates were similar to STM data and the degree of similarity was related to the shape of NP [86]. Tunc *et al* demonstrated an approach to detect, locate and identify the charges produced on the surface structures of the NPs in a fully non-contact way by implementing external voltage stress throughout XPS examination of Au–SiO_2 NPs. Therefore, recording the charging and discharging behavior of the NPs, XPS provided information not only about the chemical identification but also regarding the dielectric property of the NPs [87]. XPS with DFT computations and SERS was used to evaluate Ag-NPs functionalizing with gauche tautomer f-taurine. XPS verified the binding of taurine via the sulfonate groups oxygen atoms indicating that 71% of taurine functionalized Ag-NPs were AgO. This procedure yielded a quantitative comprehension upon interaction with Ag-NPs with the aforesaid molecule [88].

Small-angle x-ray scattering (SAXS) is useful for determining the size, particle shape, and distribution of the NPs by providing statistically average data. The development of maghemite NPs in water structurally and chemically by combining time-resolved *in situ* SAXS with XANES. A complicated four-stage formation mechanism including ferric and ferrous chloride with triethanolamine regulated the generation of NPs in solution and modified the qualities of the product formed [89]. Wang *et al* used SAXS to study the structural changes of Pt-NPs as a function of temperature [90]. The size determined by XRD differed from the matching SAXS value at some temperatures as SAXS is more sensitive to the fluctuation zone of electron density whereas XRD exhibits more sensitivity towards the size of the region of long-range order. Also, the particle size is determined by SAXS, whereas the crystallite size is determined by XRD. The differences in the size values between SAXS and XRD are due to the growth mode of the NPs during the thermal treatment. Because SAXS is a low-resolution method, further investigations using XRD or electron diffraction techniques are required for NP characterization. Moreover, SAXS offers better quantitative knowledge of relationships between LSPR behavior with aggregation phenomenon in Ag-NPs. To analyze Ag solutions, present in polymer matrices, a combination of UV–Vis, SAX and QELS was utilized wherein SAXS expressed monomodal scatterer size distribution and multimodal particle size distribution. The cause for the disparity is due to the ability of QELS and UV–Vis to resist large aggregates or particles ranging from the size of 30–60 nm. The detection limitations of SAXS do not include those big particles and aggregates but for smaller particles, all the mentioned approaches are used to determine polydispersity and particle size [91]. SAXS exhibited the production of mass fractal aggregates of NPs constituting Ag–Cu alloy in water with hydrazine. A bimodal distribution with Cu-rich larger aggregates having low mass fraction dimension and Ag-rich smaller aggregates was observed via LSPR spectra of bimodal composition. SAXS is the ideal non-invasive approach for the research since in LSPR studies the length scale of NPs aggregates are subjected to changes. In traditional invasive techniques such as TEM and SEM the solvent dry kinetics and substrate particle interaction affects the nanostructures formed. Therefore, these approaches are not used for the analysis of sol structures or for explaining their LSPR activity [92].

By applying *in situ* time-resolved SAXS, the photoreduction synthesis of palladium and rhodium NPs in PVP/ethanol solution was screened. The metal ion nucleation, particle coalescence, and growth were effectively observed for the formation of the metal NPs [93]. Usually, SAXS aids in simultaneously quantifying the size and the concentration or mass of the NPs as a function of time. The total volume, distribution of size, and the evolution of the size of the Pd and Rh-NPs were determined and quantified via SAXS. SAXS, *in situ* XRD, and XANES was used to investigate the development process of mesostructured Pt-Ru-NPs that have been electrochemically reduced upon a microemulsion lyotropic liquid-crystalline template. These approaches in combination with measurements of EDS, FE-TEM, and SEM helped researchers better understand the process leading to the mesostructured formation of the NPs [94]. The long-range order of the structure and its symmetry depicts the phase of the lyotropic liquid crystal in SAXS. Furthermore, SAXS is an effective tool for estimating the bilayer thickness and structural organization on the hydrocarbon chain of an unsupported lipid membrane [9]. X-ray scattering is useful for investigating the effects of medicinal compounds or peptides on the bilayer. Using an in-house x-ray beamline or a synchrotron source to generate SAXS and wide-angle x-ray scattering (WAXS) provides information on the short-range order system or the packing of the lipid acyl chains [9]. X-rays are produced by moving electrons at high-speed inside the synchrotron ring subjected through a monochromator and the energy of x-rays by focusing the target sample. A temperature control unit should be attached to the sample environment and the distance between sample and detector is determined 'q' range to record diffraction pattern using a CCD camera. Some synchrotron beamlines feature two detectors, allowing both SAXS and WAXS data to be recorded at the same time. The WAXS detector is placed on top of the sample chamber, while the SAXS detector is located further from the sample covering a broad 'q' range. The detector is placed such that half of the diffraction pattern falls on the detector which would allow both the small and broad angles to be recorded [9]. Radiation damage is one of the biggest problems for SAXS and to minimize this damage, samples are measured in a capillary wherein a fresh solution is exposed to the beam [95]. Based on fundamental physical parameters, the optimal diameter of the capillary for a specific wavelength is estimated. Capillaries possessing smaller diameters, allow for better handling of the radiation-sensitive sample, providing high-quality SAXS data for pure biological macromolecules [95].

In 1962, Blake and Phillips carried out the first systematic study of the effect of x-rays on protein crystals of myoglobin at room temperature and concluded that damage and dose were proportional to each other, for each 8 keV x-ray photon absorbed, 70 molecules were disrupted, and 90 more were slightly disordered [96]. The empirical model offered for diffraction decay could not explain all of the observed changes, which implies that there is a probability of possessing small significant changes in the intensities of diffractions due to some structural effects of the irradiation [96].

10.6 Protein crystallography of XRD

X-ray crystallography, neutron crystallography, NMR spectroscopy, and electron crystallography are used to determine varied protein structures and different features of polypeptide structure at high resolution. Structural changes caused in protein specimens by the incident radiation are recorded by XRD patterns in crystallography (figure 10.5). The damage caused by these rays should be minimized to derive a high-resolution structure of the protein [97]. Protein kept at 100 K in advanced x-ray cryo-crystallography suffers from damage like electron diffraction and imaging and is encountered with synchrotron x-ray beams [11, 95]. In recent years, there has been an increase in the application of x-ray crystallography for solving low-resolution structures of PDB [98]. Previously, such data sets were not considered, however, the coincidence of expanding reports of low-resolution data and advances in experimental along with computational approaches for structure determination has made this information more acceptable [99].

About 85% of all known protein structures elucidated as the primary method for determining protein structures is determined by x-ray crystallography for their various applications in the field of biomedicine, biotechnology, and drug designing. Furthermore, x-ray crystallography offers benefits providing pure, stable, and homogenous protein crystalline solutions. Crystal structure determination using x-rays requires purified protein (>95%) in quantities to initiate crystallization testing via enhanced diffraction for the collection of a complete set of data for structural determination. In small steps, the crystal is rotated during x-ray collection to record reflection from various levels of the lattice [100].

Protein crystallography is a relatively new field, publishing the first protein structure, myoglobin, in 1958 [101]. Even though the original model was derived at low resolution (6 Å), better crystals were created two years later, and the model was upgraded at a resolution of 2 Å [102]. Single crystals generated by crystallization procedures are required for the structural determination of proteins using XRD

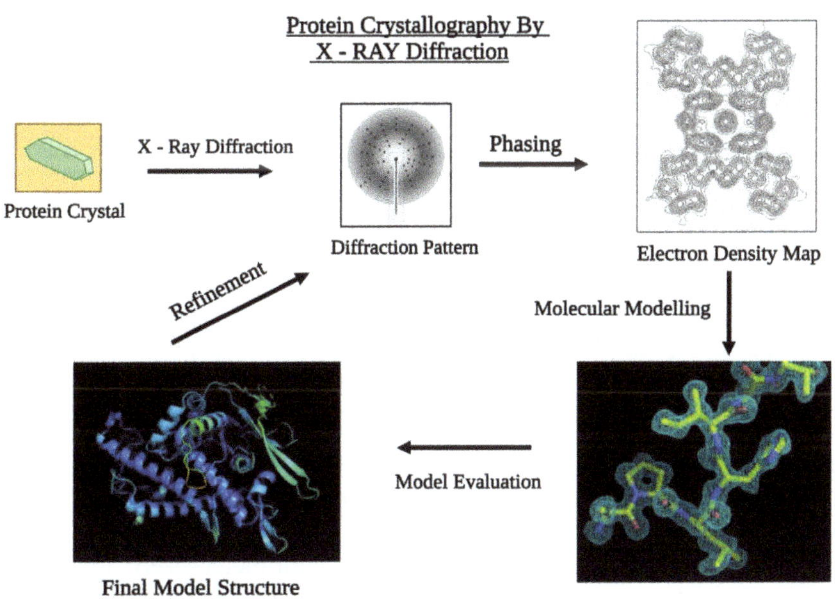

Figure 10.5. Schematic illustration of protein crystallography through the application of XRD.

techniques. Diffraction data of great quality and resolution is collected, ensuring the precision of the 3D structure determination in the ultimate atomic model. Post-crystallization treatments are preferable to increase the crystal quality of the protein. Following the processing and scaling of the collected data, phasing is performed using either molecular replacement or MAD/SAD/MIR [103]. The density modification and model building are carried out pre-refinement and validation of the obtained protein structure [103].

There exist some important differences in protein crystallography using x-rays and electrons. There are at least five fundamental changes in the setting of radiation damage that cause substantial practical implications for application in crystallographic protein structure studies, (i) the dimensions of the crystals; (ii) the number of crystals required; (iii) the method used to cryo-protect protein samples; (iv) the availability of imaging with a potency of the derivation of the native structure of non-crystalline proteins; and (v) the mechanisms employed for phase determination [97]. Despite these practical differences, there exist numerous similarities between the actual technique for both the radiations [97]. The proteins for study are 3D crystals with sizes of around 10 μm, produced due to scattering in XRD. A liquid or gaseous cryogen is typically used on protein specimens for cooling and causing cryo-protection against radiation damage. To avoid structural damage during water crystallization, thick crystals should be treated with a cryo-protectant before cooling [97].

Advances for using x-rays from free-electron lasers or synchrotrons with holography or diffractive imaging are able to provide x-ray images of protein specimens that have suffered radiation damage [104]. The measurements of dispersion caused by XRD are determined from scattered atoms constituted inside the polypeptides of each unit cell through phasing via the production of heavy-atom derivatives or the fusion of modified selenomethionine into recombinant polypeptides [97]. The damage induced by the electron beam is specimen damage and is either primarily caused due to interactions of incident electrons and atoms with polypeptides or the matrix surrounding them or secondary damage by the interaction between protein specimens and free radicals [97]. The damage by radiation causes diffraction spots to fade away and heavy-atom sites become disoriented prior to its detection by signal. During data collection, the former is easy to spot, whereas the latter is more subtle. Furthermore, the precise chemical alterations generated are able to cause structural alterations that differ from the biologically relevant form, leading to incorrect assumptions regarding function. Thus, XRD is the experimental technique, providing structural information on model membranes (Angstrom length scales) lipid mesophases, while the x-ray scattering experiments are suitable for looking into structural and dynamic changes of lipid membranes in response to temperature, pressure, pH, ionic strength [9]. However, using x-rays to determine non-periodic nanoscale structures is far more difficult as direct imaging methods possess limited resolution [105] and there is an inherent loss of phase data in the measurement of diffused x-ray intensity [106]. The sample is placed behind a mask possessing a micrometer-sized aperture with a nanometer-sized hole, focusing a beam based on the scattering of x-rays and direct Fourier inversion of the interference pattern [104]. This Fourier transform holography technique is used for a diverse range of samples and appears to be scalable to a certain limited resolution, even though it is used benificially in ultrafast single-shot imaging [107].

10.7 Macromolecule crystallography by XRD

For more than a century, crystallography has become a multidisciplinary science essential in a substantial part of the scientific study of matter [10]. Crystallography has emerged as a prominent sector in integrated structural biology with the multiscale investigation of chemical biology via mechanistic understanding of biological problems in the recent decade. Due to continuous synchrotron improvements, macromolecular crystallography depicts the potential of an essential element of biological sciences. Even though it has come a long way since the early days, and many sophisticated automatic programs solve crystal structures of complex systems successfully [108, 109]. For the past few decades, macromolecular crystallography has been the primary source of information for biological macromolecular structures and has evolved into the most successful tool for atomic-level investigation of enzyme processes and molecular interactions [103]. It is a common method for determining the 3D structure of biological macromolecules like polypeptides, nucleic acids, or nucleotides in a crystal. This machinery aids in the understanding of the intricate mechanisms of macromolecules for a crucial understanding of their biological importance, following the downstream applications in drug design. Recent technology with methodological advances in macromolecular crystallography has made it possible to solve structures that were previously thought to be impossible to solve, which includes the structures of large macromolecular compounds with atomic or subatomic resolution, and structures assemblies with low resolution [103, 109]. These breakthroughs aid in the synthesis of 3D macromolecule structures derived from twin crystals. This approach, along with cryo-electron microscopy in addition to neutron crystallography, has recently produced a high level of precision in large macromolecular machine structures, acknowledging a better understanding of their functional mechanisms [103]. Crystallography and XRD are generally perceived as one of the analytical approaches used by researchers who are interested in macromolecules structure but are not well-versed in the procedures of structure determination for unprecedented accomplishment (figure 10.6) [109].

Crystallography using x-ray is currently a significant technology intended for studying the folding mechanism of macromolecules and complexes for the structure-based novel therapies [110] by growing high-quality crystals detecting the directions of diffracted beams with their intensities, obtaining the solution of phase problem for molecular model development through optimization of the structure of a protein using XRD techniques. Repetitive cycles are common throughout the process for refining or phasing [103]. Despite the fact that 90% of macromolecules structures are unexplored, there have been several advances in macromolecular x-ray crystallography using cryo-methods for crystal durability enhancement and eradication of dynamic disorder [111, 112]. Aside from high-brilliance, high-precision detectors with the least divergent synchrotron radiation, computational analytical tools are persistently evolving to meet the demand for faster and more comfortable automated structure determination

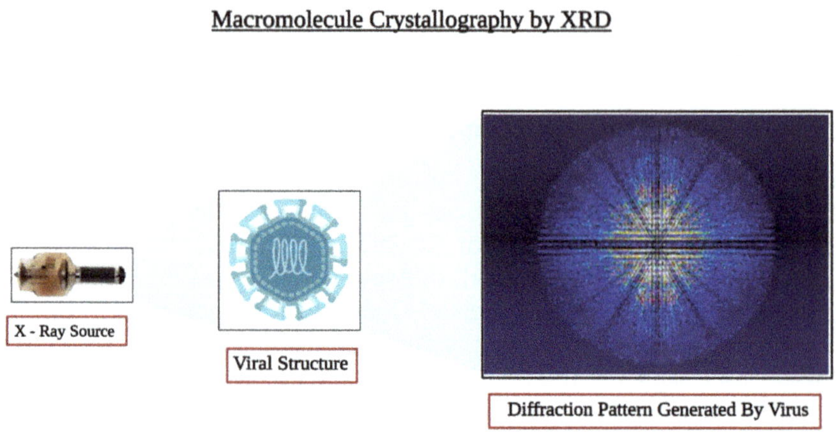

Figure 10.6. Mechanism of XRD for macromolecular crystallography.

techniques, owing to structural genomics programs [103]. Thus, experimental computational methods have been developed to extract as much information as possible from low-resolution diffraction data [103].

The inconsistency in the electron density map is responsible for the limitation of main-chain tracing along with side-chain allocation. The number of solved structures with substantial biological significance is rapidly increasing at resolutions lower than 3.5 Å and many multi-component assemblies diffract x-rays with resolutions below 3.5 Å [99, 113]. Since crystals of such enormous components often exhibit diffraction at resolutions less than 4 Å, low-resolution approaches are required; even though some high-resolution components of macromolecular assemblies are present in the complex due to the requirement of a high-resolution starting structure. To establish such complex structures, the number of unique diffraction intensities with a resolution better than 5 Å generally surpasses the degrees of freedom [113]. A structure derived from low-resolution diffraction data possess quality similar to a high-resolution structure and their analysis of weakly diffracting crystals utilizing x-ray micro-diffraction [109, 114–116].

X-ray crystallography produces the electron density map upon interacting with electrons causing its localization in a time-dependent spatial arrangement of molecules present in the asymmetric unit of the crystal. Extremely flexible molecules are not found in the final model because of their association with poor electron density in low molecular weight ligands [10]. X-ray crystallography generally fails to differentiate between carbon, nitrogen, oxygen, and sometimes even sulfur, because of their similar electronic configuration. Furthermore, because of their single electron, hydrogen atoms are barely detectable by this method. The occupancy is defined as the fraction of the atom occupying a particular point while identifying its position using the coordinates of the atom. It is more precisely expressed as the fraction the atom spends at dynamics disorder of the unit cell in the crystals where the atom is easily available at this place (static/statistic disorder), or a combination of both [10].

10.8 Drug discovery by XRD

For various drug discovery processes, medicinal chemists utilize extensive structural information for drug screening hits [10]. Thus, x-ray crystallography and XRD are proven to be important tools, revealing extremely detailed structural information on ligand interaction with a pharmaceutical target. X-ray crystallography acts as a potent screening tool with the ability to yield structural information on complexes comprising low molecular weight chemicals despite weak binding affinities, as fragment-based drug development in recent years. Since the small number of compounds are required in a fragment library compared to the hundreds of thousands found in drug-like compound libraries, it is now possible to screen an entire fragment library using x-ray crystallography, revealing structural details aiding the fragment for drug conversion process [10]. The significance of the XRD study grew to the point where the rational drug design cycle was developed [117]. A drug is rationally designed and optimized using the knowledge provided by the structure determination of its complex through XRD with the macromolecular target causing drug optimization and chemical optimization [10, 118]. The structural determination of the verified pharmacological target is usually the first step in the traditional workflow of a rational drug design project. The most common technology for this task is x-ray crystallography, but NMR and cryoEM are also important participants [119, 120].

Drug design is investigated via fragment-based drug discovery (FBDD) as an effective approach for identifying ligands, with low affinity. The detection of binding in such molecules requires sensitive approaches, and x-ray crystallography has proven to be particularly effective in identifying weak binders with affinity as low as a few mM. In most cases, x-ray crystallography can be used to screen fragment libraries of a few hundreds of molecules, yielding dozens of complicated structures [121].

10.9 Impact of XRD on oncology

A comparison study using XRD was conducted on blood serum from cancer patients and healthy people for diffraction patterns of pure water. Healthy blood serum was found to be identical to that found in pure water via the strong interaction of water molecules due to non-polar amino acid side chains in healthy blood serum stabilizing its structure, while those found in cancer patients were different. The increased interactions of water with polar molecules of conformationally changed protein in cancer patient samples causing the structure of water in blood serum to be disrupted. Thus, the application of XED in oncology acts as a cancer diagnostic tool and depicts that the presence of cancer-affected protein has a detrimental impact on the structure of water in human serum [122]. The blood serum constitutes 90% water and the remaining serum components (proteins) [122]. The agreement between the experimental x-ray scattering intensity curve and the corresponding theoretical course calculated validated this structure. The occurrence of a side maximum producing a hump at 9° on the right shoulder of the main maximum is a distinguishing feature of the angular distribution of x-ray radiation scattered in pure water [18, 102, 104]. Proteins are macromolecules that are a few tens of the length of the x-ray radiation being examined. The primary x-ray intensity maximum cannot be the result of scattering on distances of the order of the size of protein macromolecules because the method used was normal and not small-angle diffraction. The appearance of maximum angular distributions of x-ray radiation intensity curves reflects water molecule ordering. Disturbance of order, induced by an increase in protein content causes diseases by influencing the shape, position, and height of the maximum [123].

The application of paclitaxel-loaded gelatin NMs for the treatment of superficial bladder cancer utilized XRD. The desolvation process used to synthesize paclitaxel-loaded gelatin NPs and the physicochemical and biological features of the NPs were studied utilizing wide-angle XRD to characterize NPs. More than 1000 NPs were analyzed for particle size distribution utilizing SEM images, which had been taken from four–six fields. Scintag PAD-V diffractometer was used to obtain the spectra wide-angle x-ray diffraction of pure paclitaxel, combinations of paclitaxel and blank gelatin NPs, and paclitaxel-loaded NPs. The entrapped paclitaxel was analyzed using x-ray diffraction to check whether the less water-soluble crystalline state was present in the more water-soluble amorphous state [124].

Ag-NPs in the size range 1–1000 nm are extremely useful for cancer diagnosis and treatment, potentially leading to the development of a new discipline called nano-oncology. Transmission electron microscopy and XRD (Shimadzu 7000 XRD, Japan) with a DRON 2.0 diffractometer with Cu tube via K radiation was used to measure the dimensions and structural characterization of the Ag-NPs for tumor regression [125].

Folic acid, also known as pteroylglutamic acid, possesses an open chemical structure and the closed chemical formula ($M_w = 441.4$ Da) for targeted anti-cancer therapy by conjugating with Au-NP and chemotherapeutics [126]. Folate-Au-NP conjugate possesses promising qualities of non-immunogenicity and cancer selectivity via an endocytic pathway that bypasses the clathrin-coated pathway to endosome or lysosome by transporting through the intracellular vesicle into the cytosol. Folate-4Atp-Au-NP, as well as Folate-MH-Au-NP, were compared *in vitro* by conjugating Au-NP with folate using 4-amino thiophenol (4Atp) and 6-mercapto-1-hexanol (MH) via Bruker D8 Advance XRD at room temperature with wavelengths of 0.154 06 nm (CuK) radiations [127, 128].

Cobalt oxide is one of the most fascinating chemical elements used as NPs for biomedical applications because of its uniqueness for size and shape-dependent properties in pigments, electrochemistry, catalysis, sensors, magnetism, and energy storage. Expert Pro (Phillips) XRD was used to determine the phase formation and crystalline state of cobalt oxide NPs by employing CoK radiation (0.178 nm). Moreover, a Brookhaven 90 Plus particle size analyzer was used to measure the hydrodynamic size of the cobalt oxide NPs aggregates [129, 130].

MNPs hyperthermia is considered a promising cancer treatment wherein cancer tissues are subjected to heating at temperatures between 41 °C and 45 °C via XRD. It is demonstrated as a simple and successful approach to treating cancer when used in conjunction with well-established therapies like irradiation and chemotherapy

[131, 132]. Hyperthermia causes the activation of heat-shock proteins, which decrease the expression of HSP70 by preventing the action of the heat-shock transcription factor 1 (HSF1), making the tumor cells more sensitive [133].

Iron sulfides are now acknowledged as sophisticated inorganic materials with non-traditional applications, which include high-energy-density batteries, diagnostic materials, superconductor precursors as well as photoelectrolysis materials. A co-precipitation method was used to develop greigite (Fe_3S_4) to generate magnetic hyperthermia for the treatment of cancer. To detect the synthesized greigite phase, XRD was utilized as the principal approach [134]. The XRD patterns were generated by the samples and recorded with the Rigaku diffractometer model, which operated at 40 kV and 40 mA and applied a nickel-filtered Cu Ka1 as the radiation source (with wavelength $k = 1.5406$). The powder diffractions of the samples were recorded at a scan rate of 4° min^{-1} throughout 2 h, ranging from 10 to 90.

10.10 Influence of XRD on pharmaceutical industry

XRD has aided in the study of crystal structure and therefore has helped to analyze the physicochemical properties of pharmaceutical materials. Its non-destructive property with a requirement for minimal sample preparation provides an edge over techniques of analysis. Thus, it can be used for analyzing completed dosage solid forms [135].

Each crystalline form of a substance possesses a distinct x-ray powder pattern used to identify it. The strongest 10 reflections observed in single-phase x-ray powder lies in the range of 0°–40° 2θ and is recommended by the USP. In the case of the same crystal form, between reference and the sample, agreement in the 2θ diffraction angles occurs within 0.2°, whereas due to favored orientation effects, relative intensities between reference and specimen differ significantly [136]. The patterns of PXRD provide essential information for the composition of multi-component dosage forms comprising formulation excipients and API. An Allegra tablet with multiple phase formulation was feasible to detect and measure amorphous, nano-crystalline, and crystalline (excipients and API) phases to obtain lower detection thresholds or quantify materials with considerable pattern overlap, data processing approaches such as partial least squares, whole pattern matching, Rietveld analysis, and spectral subtraction. The application of SR allows for greater sensitivity for the measurement of considerably lower amounts of various crystal forms in a therapeutic product. A technique has been patented that detects samples from a mixture of polymorphs and trace levels of a single polymorph with a LOD of 0.005% w/w. The integration of an HPC detector with synchrotron XRD and fine-tuning the optics, in an ad hoc pharmaceutical combination for improved LOD from 0.1% to 0.01% [137]. PXRD is also used to analyze dosage forms other than capsules and tablets as in the case of ethylcellulose microsphere wherein the amount of crystalline tolnaftate was detected by this method. The chemical analysis revealed a larger total amount of drug in the microsphere, which led to the understanding of the drugs dissolved in the polymer matrix [138]. While verifying whether a product is counterfeit an XRD pattern of the sample was compared to the reference tablets

[139]. The energy-dispersive XRD is very efficient since it penetrates through the packaging materials of the tablets [140]. A technique based on micro-diffractometry employing imprinting agents falls under the GRAS category to generate barcodes and are detectable by x-ray on the tablets [141].

The determination of the polymorphic form of a substance is another significant application of XRD. The molecules are initially screened for activity against a specific target and a fraction of the active molecules are subjected to lead optimization. These lead molecules are screened for toxicology based on the purity of the material and the drug safety margin of the compound (analyzed by exposing the compound in animal models). Thus, the compound is subjected to salt and finally produces adequately bioavailable and chemically stable crystalline forms [142]. A 96-well titer plate is used for high throughput polymorph and salt screening via a combinatorial chemistry approach leading to its crystalline structure via XRD [143]. The application of a typical point detector for the analysis of samples is challenging as the specifications of an ideal infinitely thick, flat sample possessing a particle size less than 10 μm cannot be used due to the restricted sample amount. Thus, for quicker data collection a collimated x-ray beam in conjunction with an area detector is utilized [144]. As compared to the conventional detector the average diffraction intensity was collected via a considerable portion of the diffraction ring for better results [144]. The beam of the x-ray is subjected to a sample from 10 to 100 μg for around 5–60 s [145] after that the sample gets automatically changed. Despite possessing a variety of different approaches for characterization of polymorphs [146], demonstrating non-equivalent structure by using powder or single-crystal XRD is the best method for confirming its purity in pharmaceutical applications (figure 10.7) [147].

In μ-XRD, the mapping of heterogenous samples by using a combination of a 2D area detector and a collimated circular beam [135]. Even though a 2D projection image with the lateral resolution is provided by the mapping approaches, they fail to provide depth resolution [148]. Imaging via XR-CT involves aiming x-ray from multiple orientations at an object and then measuring the drop in the intensity by linear pathways. Beer's Law correlates a drop in intensity as a function of path length, material linear attenuation coefficient, and x-ray energy. A special algorithm was used for the distribution of x-ray attenuation over a re-constructed sample leading to the formation of a 3D image. The distribution of density over pharmaceutical tablets is measured by this technique. The local x-ray attenuation is proportionated with the density of the material through the cross-sectional images by this technique. XR-CT is used for analyzing the density distribution of the ribbons produced via roller compaction responsible for the strength of granules and particle size distribution [149]. For segregating molecules and profiling binary mixtures in a quantitative manner, synchrotron x-rays are utilized [150]. XRD-CT is a combination of CT and XRD and a multi-dimensional imaging technique used for the discrimination of tissues in biological samples and the characterization of material [151]. X-rays are directed towards the sample material from various orientations like in XR-CT. 2D diffraction frames are gathered and merged in a linear collection of diffraction patterns for each position Y and sample rotation ω.

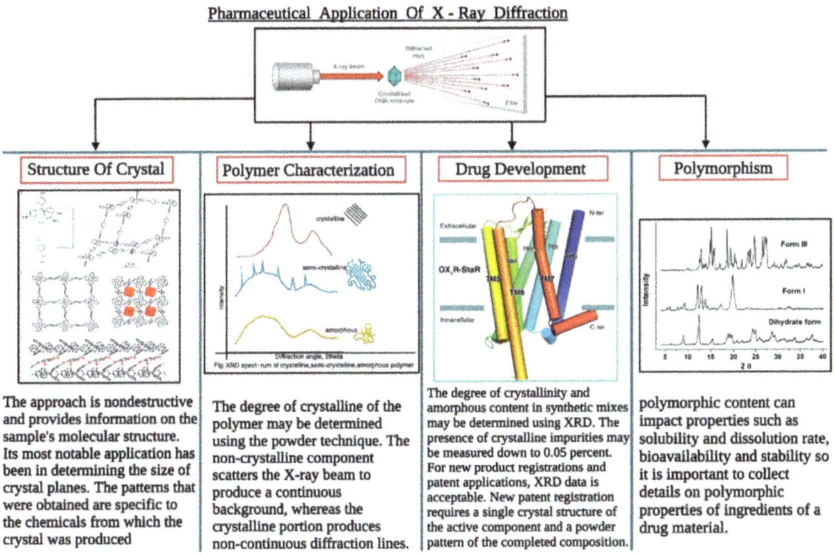

Figure 10.7. Application of XRD in pharmaceutical industry.

The tomographic angle ω, position Υ along with 2θ is the diffracted angle used to convert the ensemble images into a 3D-dataset. The 1D sum pattern is constituted out by summing the linear diffraction pattern across ω and Υ applied to identify phases. The 2θ integration of linear diffraction pattern as a function of Υ and ω to create a global sinogram applied for the reconstruction of the whole diffracted intensity. XRD-CT is effectively used for phase mapping of unidentified and powder nanocrystalline particles in a pellet by employing high-energy synchrotron x-ray beam with a 2D detector [148].

PXRD was formerly thought to be solely useful for identifying and quantifying crystalline phases and provided no application in characterizing amorphous materials in the pharmaceutical industry. Because of the advances in instruments like the accessibility of hybrid photon detectors via high-energy sources, the preferred orientation error and duration of data collection are considerably reduced. PXDR by converting regular x-ray data acts as a strong developing technology for gaining structural insights into nanocrystalline and amorphous materials. This method brings up novel opportunities in predicting macroscopic amorphous pharmaceutical systems by using trends at the atomic and nano-meter levels or by using structural signals. The computed tomography PDF technique is a tool used to spatially map the local structure in 3D objects. The method is used to characterize drugs in intact dosage forms like lyophilized products, and complicated systems of drug delivery like that of implants, comprising of nanocrystalline and amorphous components [152, 153].

In class II and IV drugs in a biopharmaceutical, one of the significant material properties of the formulation exhibited is the particle size and distribution of API.

Moreover, 2D XRD is a Υ profile-based method used as a non-destructive approach for assessing the crystallite size of the API present in compressed tablets [154]. The distribution of diffraction intensity in Υ-direction is utilized for the characterization of material by using a similar technique. Preferential orientation generates fluctuation in the intensity in Υ-direction and 2θ shift (as a function of Υ) caused by residual stress. In pharmaceutical structures, several components of the Υ profile have not been examined and additional research is required to link material performance with this information. Since x-ray FEL with atomic spatial precision and temporal resolution are used to comprehend the method of recrystallization and polymeric phase change. The nucleation during the synthesis of API with the polymorphic outcome from the nucleation is studied via this approach. Counterfeit pharmaceuticals are kept under control in worldwide trades through the development of portable and handheld technologies. The comparison of the diffraction pattern of the genuine drug and sample provided is useful in detecting counterfeit medicinal products [135].

The FDA in September 2004, provided guidelines on the use of process analytical technologies in pharmaceutical industries. Process analysis techniques and methods provided guidelines required to understand and regulate the process of manufacturing as well as on-line/in-line monitoring of the product parameters that assures the consistency with the quality of the product. XRD is a suitable technique for change in the physical structure of API, size of the particle, monitoring homogeneity of in-line content because of the ongoing advancements in data collection and analysis in non-destructive XRD and minimal sample preparation. Faster data capture with greater resolution is a result of the advancements in high-energy sources of XRD for powerful and sophisticated software, better optics, and sensitive detectors. Thus, PXRD is no longer simply used for identifying and quantifying crystalline phases as it is becoming a useful tool for learning about the structure of nanocrystalline and amorphous materials. A 3D image construct used by XRD-CT maps the phases of excipient or API in the perfect dosage form. The local information of a system is amorphously obtained via total scattering PDF. Information regarding the crystallite size of an API is obtained by integration in Υ-direction of 2D XRD pattern [135].

10.11 Conclusion

XRD provides accurate tools for non-destructive analysis of materials such as metals, minerals, polymers, medicines, and semiconductors. A wide range of application software is available to complement the diffraction systems for determining the properties of materials and their application in phase analysis, lattice parameter determination, strain determination, texture and orientation analysis, and order–disorder transformation. In summary, we have discussed the role of XRD in the characterization of nanoparticles for biomedical applications. Moreover, we have also elucidated the instrumentation of XRD and techniques used by XRD for its application in oncology, antimicrobial activity, pharmaceutical industry, protein crystallography, and macromolecule crystallography.

References

[1] Bunaciu A A, UdriŞTioiu E G and Aboul-Enein H Y 2015 X-ray diffraction: instrumentation and applications *Crit. Rev. Anal. Chem.* **45** 289–99

[2] Fröjdh C, Norlin B and Fröjdh E 2013 Spectral X-ray imaging with single photon processing detectors *J. Instrum.* **8** C02010

[3] Roessl E and Proksa R 2007 K-edge imaging in x-ray computed tomography using multi-bin photon counting detectors *Phys. Med. Biol.* **52** 4679

[4] Ballabriga R, Campbell M, Heijne E, Llopart X and Tlustos L 2007 The Medipix3 prototype, a pixel readout chip working in single photon counting mode with improved spectrometric performance *IEEE Trans. Nucl. Sci.* **54** 1824–9

[5] Bunaciu A A, Udriştioiu E G and Aboul-Enein H Y 2015 X-ray diffraction: instrumentation and applications *Crit. Rev. Anal. Chem.* **45** 289–99

[6] Unruh D K and Forbes T Z 2019 *Analytical Geomicrobiology: A Handbook of Instrumental Techniques* ed D S Alessi *et al* (Cambridge: Cambridge University Press) pp 215–37

[7] Mos Y M, Vermeulen A C, Buisman C J and Weijma J 2018 X-ray diffraction of iron containing samples: the importance of a suitable configuration *Geomicrobiol. J.* **35** 511–7

[8] Klug H P and Alexander L E 1974 *X-Ray Diffraction Procedures: For Polycrystalline and Amorphous Materials* (Hoboken, NJ: Wiley)

[9] Tyler A I, Law R V and Seddon J M 2015 *Methods in Membrane Lipids* (Berlin: Springer) pp 199–225

[10] Maveyraud L and Mourey L 2020 Protein X-ray crystallography and drug discovery *Molecules* **25** 1030

[11] Garman E F 1996 Modern methods for rapid x-ray diffraction data collection from crystals of macromolecules *Methods Mol. Biol.* **56** 87–126

[12] Muir R D, Pogranichniy N R, Muir J L, Sullivan S Z, Battaile K P, Mulichak A M, Toth S J, Keefe L J and Simpson G J 2015 Spectral X-ray diffraction using a 6 megapixel photon counting array detector *Proc. SPIE – Int. Soc. Opt. Eng.* **9401** 940109

[13] Muir R D, Pogranichniy N R, Muir J L, Sullivan S Z, Battaile K, Mulichak A M, Toth S J, Keefe L J and Simpson G J 2015 Spectral x-ray diffraction using a 6 megapixel photon counting array detector *Computational Imaging XIII* (Bellingham, WA: International Society for Optics and Photonics) p 940109

[14] Mikulec B, Campbell M, Heijne E, Llopart X and Tlustos L 2003 X-ray imaging using single photon processing with semiconductor pixel detectors *Nucl. Instrum. Methods Phys. Res.* A **511** 282–6

[15] Ballabriga R *et al* 2013 The Medipix3RX: a high resolution, zero dead-time pixel detector readout chip allowing spectroscopic imaging *J. Instrum.* **8** C02016

[16] Clifton I, Duke E, Wakatsuki S and Ren Z 1997 [23] Evaluation of Laue diffraction patterns *Methods Enzymol.* **277** 448–67

[17] Holton J M 2009 A beginner's guide to radiation damage *J. Synchrotron Radiat.* **16** 133–42

[18] Guss J M, Merritt E A, Phizackerley R P, Hedman B, Murata M, Hodgson K O and Freeman H C 1988 Phase determination by multiple-wavelength x-ray diffraction: crystal structure of a basic 'blue' copper protein from cucumbers *Science* **241** 806–11

[19] Abbasi E, Milani M, Fekri Aval S, Kouhi M, Akbarzadeh A, Tayefi Nasrabadi H, Nikasa P, Joo S W, Hanifehpour Y and Nejati-Koshki K 2016 Silver nanoparticles: synthesis methods, bio-applications and properties *Crit. Rev. Microbiol.* **42** 173–80

[20] Fan J, Cheng Y and Sun M 2020 Functionalized gold nanoparticles: synthesis, properties and biomedical applications *Chem. Rec.* **20** 1474–504

[21] Durán N, Marcato P D, De Souza G I, Alves O L and Esposito E 2007 Antibacterial effect of silver nanoparticles produced by fungal process on textile fabrics and their effluent treatment *J. Biomed. Nanotechnol.* **3** 203–8

[22] Cho K-H, Park J-E, Osaka T and Park S-G 2005 The study of antimicrobial activity and preservative effects of nanosilver ingredient *Electrochim. Acta* **51** 956–60

[23] Barreiro E, Casas J S, Couce M D, Sánchez A, Seoane R, Sordo J, Varela J M and Vázquez-López E M 2007 Synthesis and antimicrobial activities of silver (I) sulfanylcarboxylates. Structural isomers with identically or unequally coordinated Ag centers in an Ag4S4 ring *Dalton Trans.* **28** 3074–85

[24] Thomas V, Yallapu M M, Sreedhar B and Bajpai S 2007 A versatile strategy to fabricate hydrogel–silver nanocomposites and investigation of their antimicrobial activity *J. Colloid Interface Sci.* **315** 389–95

[25] Leaper D J 2006 Silver dressings: their role in wound management *Int. Wound J.* **3** 282–94

[26] Heinz M, Srabionyan V V, Bugaev A L, Pryadchenko V V, Ishenko E V, Avakyan L A, Zubavichus Y V, Ihlemann J, Meinertz J and Pippel E 2016 Formation of silver nanoparticles in silicate glass using excimer laser radiation: structural characterization by HRTEM, XRD, EXAFS and optical absorption spectra *J. Alloys Compd.* **681** 307–15

[27] Srabionyan V V, Bugaev A L, Pryadchenko V V, Makhiboroda A V, Rusakova E B, Avakyan L A, Schneider R, Dubiel M and Bugaev L A 2013 EXAFS study of changes in atomic structure of silver nanoparticles in soda-lime glass caused by annealing *J. Non-Cryst. Solids* **382** 24–31

[28] Lindau I, Martensson N, Arvanitis D and Karis O C 2005 *Proc. 12th X-Ray Absorption Fine Structure Int. Conf. (XAFS12)(23–27 June 2003)* Malmo, Sweden-Foreword *(Bristol)* (Bristol: IOP Publishing Ltd)

[29] Dubiel M, Brunsch S and Troger L 2001 Temperature dependence of thermal expansion coefficient of silver nanoparticles and of bulk material determined by EXAFS *J. Synchrotron Radiat.* **8** 539–41

[30] Singh M, Sinha I, Singh A and Mandal R 2011 Correlating SAXS analysis with LSPR behavior: poly (vinyl alcohol)-stabilized Ag nanoparticles *J. Nanopart. Res.* **13** 4387–94

[31] Mourdikoudis S, Pallares R M and Thanh N T 2018 Characterization techniques for nanoparticles: comparison and complementarity upon studying nanoparticle properties *Nanoscale* **10** 12871–934

[32] Jain P K, Lee K S, El-Sayed I H and El-Sayed M A 2006 Calculated absorption and scattering properties of gold nanoparticles of different size, shape, and composition: applications in biological imaging and biomedicine *J. Phys. Chem.* B **110** 7238–48

[33] Eustis S and El-Sayed M A 2006 Why gold nanoparticles are more precious than pretty gold: noble metal surface plasmon resonance and its enhancement of the radiative and nonradiative properties of nanocrystals of different shapes *Chem. Soc. Rev.* **35** 209–17

[34] Caprile L, Cossaro A, Falletta E, Della Pina C, Cavalleri O, Rolandi R, Terreni S, Ferrando R, Rossi M and Floreano L 2012 Interaction of L-cysteine with naked gold nanoparticles supported on HOPG: a high resolution XPS investigation *Nanoscale* **4** 7727–34

[35] Belsey N A, Shard A G and Minelli C 2015 Analysis of protein coatings on gold nanoparticles by XPS and liquid-based particle sizing techniques *Biointerphases* **10** 019012

[36] Wang J, Li H, Zhang D and Bai J 2019 Amorphous Cu0 on carbon nanofiber as recyclable heterogeneous catalyst for N-arylation reactions *Chem. Res. Chin. Univ.* **35** 256–60
[37] Schlichter S, Rocha M, Peixoto A F, Pires J, Freire C and Alvarez M 2018 Copper mesoporous materials as highly efficient recyclable catalysts for the reduction of 4-nitrophenol in aqueous media *Polyhedron* **150** 69–76
[38] Svintsitskiy D, Chupakhin A, Slavinskaya E, Stonkus O, Stadnichenko A, Koscheev S and Boronin A 2013 Study of cupric oxide nanopowders as efficient catalysts for low-temperature CO oxidation *J. Mol. Catal. A: Chem.* **368** 95–106
[39] Gawande M B, Goswami A, Felpin F-X, Asefa T, Huang X, Silva R, Zou X, Zboril R and Varma R S 2016 Cu and Cu-based nanoparticles: synthesis and applications in catalysis *Chem. Rev.* **116** 3722–811
[40] Shaygan Nia A, Rana S, Döhler D, Jirsa F, Meister A, Guadagno L, Koslowski E, Bron M and Binder W H 2015 Carbon-supported copper nanomaterials: recyclable catalysts for Huisgen [3+ 2] cycloaddition reactions *Chem. Eur. J.* **21** 10763–70
[41] Nasrollahzadeh M, Sajadi S M, Rostami-Vartooni A, Bagherzadeh M and Safari R 2015 Immobilization of copper nanoparticles on perlite: green synthesis, characterization and catalytic activity on aqueous reduction of 4-nitrophenol *J. Mol. Catal. A: Chem.* **400** 22–30
[42] Kushwaha A, Moakhar R S, Goh G K and Dalapati G K 2017 Morphologically tailored CuO photocathode using aqueous solution technique for enhanced visible light driven water splitting *J. Photochem. Photobiol.* A **337** 54–61
[43] Yang X, Zhong H, Zhu Y, Jiang H, Shen J, Huang J and Li C 2014 Highly efficient reusable catalyst based on silicon nanowire arrays decorated with copper nanoparticles *J. Mater. Chem.* A **2** 9040–7
[44] Zou X, Tao Z and Asefa T 2013 Semiconductor and plasmonic photocatalysis for selective organic transformations *Curr. Org. Chem.* **17** 1274–87
[45] Deka P, Borah B J, Saikia H and Bharali P 2019 Cu-based nanoparticles as emerging environmental catalysts *Chem. Rec.* **19** 462–73
[46] Kaur R, Giordano C, Gradzielski M and Mehta S K 2014 Synthesis of highly stable, water-dispersible copper nanoparticles as catalysts for nitrobenzene reduction *Chem. Asian J.* **9** 189–98
[47] Sun Y, Xu L, Yin Z and Song X 2013 Synthesis of copper submicro/nanoplates with high stability and their recyclable superior catalytic activity towards 4-nitrophenol reduction *J. Mater. Chem.* A **1** 12361–70
[48] Deka P, Deka R C and Bharali P 2014 In situ generated copper nanoparticle catalyzed reduction of 4-nitrophenol *New J. Chem.* **38** 1789–93
[49] Abiraman T, Ramanathan E, Kavitha G, Rengasamy R and Balasubramanian S 2017 Synthesis of chitosan capped copper oxide nanoleaves using high intensity (30 kHz) ultrasound sonication and their application in antifouling coatings *Ultrason. Sonochem.* **34** 781–91
[50] Mott D, Galkowski J, Wang L, Luo J and Zhong C-J 2007 Synthesis of size-controlled and shaped copper nanoparticles *Langmuir* **23** 5740–5
[51] Ohde H, Hunt F and Wai C M 2001 Synthesis of silver and copper nanoparticles in a water-in-supercritical-carbon dioxide microemulsion *Chem. Mater.* **13** 4130–5
[52] Ponce A A and Klabunde K J 2005 Chemical and catalytic activity of copper nanoparticles prepared via metal vapor synthesis *J. Mol. Catal. A: Chem.* **225** 1–6

[53] Zhang Q and Hua Y J 2014 Electrochemical synthesis of copper nanoparticles using cuprous oxide as a precursor in choline chloride–urea deep eutectic solvent: nucleation and growth mechanism *Phys. Chem. Chem. Phys.* **16** 27088–95

[54] Jayaramudu T, Varaprasad K, Reddy K K, Pyarasani R D, Akbari-Fakhrabadi A and Amalraj J 2020 Chitosan-pluronic based Cu nanocomposite hydrogels for prototype antimicrobial applications *Int. J. Biol. Macromol.* **143** 825–32

[55] Hullavarad N, Hullavarad S and Karulkar P 2008 Cadmium sulphide (CdS) nanotechnology: synthesis and applications *J. Nanosci. Nanotechnol.* **8** 3272–99

[56] Sadhu S, Chowdhury P S and Patra A 2007 Understanding the role of particle size on photophysical properties of CdS:Eu^{3+} nanocrystals *J. Lumin.* **126** 387–92

[57] Costa V C, Shen Y and Bray K L 2002 Luminescence properties of nanocrystalline CdS and CdS:Mn^{2+} doped silica-type glasses *J. Non-Cryst. Solids* **304** 217–23

[58] Sivasubramanian V, Arora A, Premila M, Sundar C and Sastry V 2006 Optical properties of CdS nanoparticles upon annealing *Physica* E **31** 93–8

[59] Rockenberger J, Tröger L, Kornowski A, Vossmeyer T, Eychmüller A, Feldhaus J and Weller H 1997 EXAFS studies on the size dependence of structural and dynamic properties of CdS nanoparticles *J. Phys. Chem.* B **101** 2691–701

[60] Hota G, Idage S and Khilar K C 2007 Characterization of nano-sized CdS–Ag_2S core–shell nanoparticles using XPS technique *Colloids Surf.* A **293** 5–12

[61] Shivashankarappa A and Sanjay K R 2020 *Escherichia coli*-based synthesis of cadmium sulfide nanoparticles, characterization, antimicrobial and cytotoxicity studies *Braz. J. Microbiol.* **51** 939

[62] Chaudhary R G, Bhusari G S, Tiple A D, Rai A R, Somkuvar S R, Potbhare A K, Lambat T L, Ingle P P and Abdala A A 2019 Metal/metal oxide nanoparticles: toxicity, applications, and future prospects *Curr. Pharm. Des.* **25** 4013–29

[63] Stankic S, Suman S, Haque F and Vidic J 2016 Pure and multi metal oxide nanoparticles: synthesis, antibacterial and cytotoxic properties *J. Nanobiotechnol.* **14** 1–20

[64] Misra S K, Dybowska A, Berhanu D, Luoma S N and Valsami-Jones E 2012 The complexity of nanoparticle dissolution and its importance in nanotoxicological studies *Sci. Total Environ.* **438** 225–32

[65] Baumann S O, Schneider J, Sternig A, Thomele D, Stankic S, Berger T, Gronbeck H and Diwald O 2015 Size effects in MgO cube dissolution *Langmuir* **31** 2770–6

[66] Keller A A, Wang H, Zhou D, Lenihan H S, Cherr G, Cardinale B J, Miller R and Ji Z 2010 Stability and aggregation of metal oxide nanoparticles in natural aqueous matrices *Environ. Sci. Technol.* **44** 1962–7

[67] Sharma A, Varshney M, Park J, Ha T-K, Chae K-H and Shin H-J 2015 XANES, EXAFS and photocatalytic investigations on copper oxide nanoparticles and nanocomposites *RSC Adv.* **5** 21762–71

[68] Phokha S, Pinitsoontorn S, Chirawatkul P, Poo-Arporn Y and Maensiri S 2012 Synthesis, characterization, and magnetic properties of monodisperse CeO_2 nanospheres prepared by PVP-assisted hydrothermal method *Nanoscale Res. Lett.* **7** 1–13

[69] Abid S A, Taha A A, Ismail R A and Mohsin M H 2020 Antibacterial and cytotoxic activities of cerium oxide nanoparticles prepared by laser ablation in liquid *Environ. Sci. Pollut. Res. Int.* **27** 30479–89

[70] Schindler T, Schmiele M, Schmutzler T, Kassar T, Segets D, Peukert W, Radulescu A, Kriele A, Gilles R and Unruh T 2015 A combined SAXS/SANS study for the *in situ*

characterization of ligand shells on small nanoparticles: the case of ZnO *Langmuir* **31** 10130–6
[71] Prasad K S, Prasad S K, Ansari M A, Alzohairy M A, Alomary M N, AlYahya S, Srinivasa C, Murali M, Ankegowda V M and Shivamallu C 2020 Tumoricidal and bactericidal properties of ZnONPs synthesized using *Cassia auriculata* leaf extract *Biomolecules* **10** 982
[72] Wu K, Su D, Liu J, Saha R and Wang J-P 2019 Magnetic nanoparticles in nanomedicine: a review of recent advances *Nanotechnology* **30** 502003
[73] Haun J B, Yoon T J, Lee H and Weissleder R 2010 Magnetic nanoparticle biosensors *Wiley Interdiscip. Rev. Nanomed. Nanobiotechnol.* **2** 291–304
[74] Hajba L and Guttman A 2016 The use of magnetic nanoparticles in cancer theranostics: Toward handheld diagnostic devices *Biotechnol. Adv.* **34** 354–61
[75] Wu K, Tu L, Su D and Wang J-P 2017 Magnetic dynamics of ferrofluids: mathematical models and experimental investigations *J. Phys.* D **50** 085005
[76] Darbandi M, Stromberg F, Landers J, Reckers N, Sanyal B, Keune W and Wende H 2012 Nanoscale size effect on surface spin canting in iron oxide nanoparticles synthesized by the microemulsion method *J. Phys.* D **45** 195001
[77] Stoner E C and Wohlfarth E 1948 A mechanism of magnetic hysteresis in heterogeneous alloys *Phil. Trans. R. Soc.* A **240** 599–642
[78] Pugsley A J, Bull C L, Sella A, Sankar G and McMillan P F 2011 XAS/EXAFS studies of Ge nanoparticles produced by reaction between Mg_2Ge and $GeCl_4$ *J. Solid State Chem.* **184** 2345–52
[79] Liu T, Guo L, Tao Y, Hu T, Xie Y and Zhang J 1999 Bondlength alternation of nanoparticles Fe2O3 coated with organic surfactants probed by EXAFS *Nanostruct. Mater.* **11** 1329–34
[80] Pearce C I, Coker V S, Charnock J M, Pattrick R A, Mosselmans J F W, Law N, Beveridge T J and Lloyd J R 2008 Microbial manufacture of chalcogenide-based nanoparticles via the reduction of selenite using Veillonella atypica: an *in situ* EXAFS study *Nanotechnology* **19** 155603
[81] Sun Y, Frenkel A I, Isseroff R, Shonbrun C, Forman M, Shin K, Koga T, White H, Zhang L and Zhu Y 2006 Characterization of palladium nanoparticles by using X-ray reflectivity, EXAFS, and electron microscopy *Langmuir* **22** 807–16
[82] Lu L T 2011 Water-dispersible magnetic nanoparticles for biomedical applications: synthesis and characterisation *PhD Dissertation* University of Liverpool
[83] Sarma D, Santra P K, Mukherjee S and Nag A 2013 X-ray photoelectron spectroscopy: a unique tool to determine the internal heterostructure of nanoparticles *Chem. Mater.* **25** 1222–32
[84] Shard A G 2012 A straightforward method for interpreting XPS data from core–shell nanoparticles *J. Phys. Chem.* C **116** 16806–13
[85] Caprile L *et al* 2012 Interaction of L-cysteine with naked gold nanoparticles supported on HOPG: a high resolution XPS investigation *Nanoscale* **4** 7727–34
[86] Smirnov M Y, Kalinkin A V, Bukhtiyarov A V, Prosvirin I P and Bukhtiyarov V I 2016 Using X-ray photoelectron spectroscopy to evaluate size of metal nanoparticles in the model Au/C samples *J. Phys. Chem.* C **120** 10419–26
[87] Tunc I, Demirok U K, Suzer S, Correa-Duatre M A and Liz-Marzan L M 2005 Charging/discharging of Au (core)/silica (shell) nanoparticles as revealed by XPS *J. Phys. Chem.* B **109** 24182–4

[88] Maiti N, Thomas S, Debnath A and Kapoor S 2016 Raman and XPS study on the interaction of taurine with silver nanoparticles *RSC Adv.* **6** 56406–11

[89] Kabelitz A, Guilherme A, Joester M, Reinholz U, Radtke M, Bienert R, Schulz K, Schmack R, Kraehnert R and Emmerling F 2015 Time-resolved *in situ* studies on the formation mechanism of iron oxide nanoparticles using combined fast-XANES and SAXS *Cryst. Eng. Comm.* **17** 8463–70

[90] Wang W, Chen X, Cai Q, Mo G, Jiang L, Zhang K, Chen Z, Wu Z and Pan W 2008 In situ SAXS study on size changes of platinum nanoparticles with temperature *Eur. Phys. J.* B **65** 57–64

[91] Bulavin L, Kutsevol N, Chumachenko V, Soloviov D, Kuklin A and Marynin A 2016 SAXS combined with UV–vis spectroscopy and QELS: accurate characterization of silver sols synthesized in polymer matrices *Nanoscale Res. Lett.* **11** 1–8

[92] Singh M, Sinha I, Singh A, Mandal R J C, Physicochemical S A and Aspects E 2011 LSPR and SAXS studies of starch stabilized Ag–Cu alloy nanoparticles *Colloids Surf.* A **384** 668–74

[93] Harada M, Tamura N and Takenaka M 2011 Nucleation and growth of metal nanoparticles during photoreduction using *in situ* time-resolved SAXS analysis *J. Phys. Chem.* C **115** 14081–92

[94] Liang Y-C, Juan Y-W, Lu K-T, Jeng U-S, Chen S-A, Chuang W-T, Su C-J, Liu C-L, Pao C-W and Lee J-F 2012 Formation process of mesostructured PtRu nanoparticles electrodeposited on a microemulsion lyotropic liquid crystalline template as revealed by *in situ* XRD, SAXS, and XANES *J. Phys. Chem.* C **116** 26649–55

[95] Schroer M A, Blanchet C E, Gruzinov A Y, Gräwert M A, Brennich M E, Hajizadeh N R, Jeffries C M and Svergun D I 2018 Smaller capillaries improve the small-angle X-ray scattering signal and sample consumption for biomacromolecular solutions *J. Synchrotron Radiat.* **25** 1113–22

[96] Hendrickson W A 1976 Radiation damage in protein crystallography *J. Mol. Biol.* **106** 889–93

[97] Massover W H 2007 Radiation damage to protein specimens from electron beam imaging and diffraction: a mini-review of anti-damage approaches, with special reference to synchrotron X-ray crystallography *J. Synchrotron Radiat.* **14** 116–27

[98] Berman H M, Westbrook J, Feng Z, Gilliland G, Bhat T N, Weissig H, Shindyalov I N and Bourne P E 2000 The Protein Data Bank *Nucleic Acids Res.* **28** 235–42

[99] Karmali A M, Blundell T L and Furnham N 2009 Model-building strategies for low-resolution X-ray crystallographic data *Acta Crystallogr.* D **65** 121–7

[100] Papageorgiou A C, Poudel N and Mattsson J 2021 *Protein Downstream Processing* (Berlin: Springer) pp 377–404

[101] Kendrew J C, Bodo G, Dintzis H M, Parrish R, Wyckoff H and Phillips D C 1958 A three-dimensional model of the myoglobin molecule obtained by x-ray analysis *Nature* **181** 662–6

[102] Bodo G, Dintzis H, Kendrew J C and Wyckoff H 1959 The crystal structure of myoglobin, V. A low-resolution three-dimensional Fourier synthesis of sperm-whale myoglobin crystals *Proc. R. Soc.* A **253** 70–102

[103] Hernandez-Santoyo A 2012 Difficult macromolecular structures determined using X-ray diffraction techniques *Protein Pept. Lett.* **19** 770–7

[104] Eisebitt S, Lüning J, Schlotter W, Lörgen M, Hellwig O, Eberhardt W and Stöhr J 2004 Lensless imaging of magnetic nanostructures by X-ray spectro-holography *Nature* **432** 885–8

[105] Chao W, Anderson E, Denbeaux G P, Harteneck B, Liddle J A, Olynick D L, Pearson A L, Salmassi F, Song C Y and Attwood D T 2003 20-nm-Resolution soft x-ray microscopy demonstrated by use of multilayer test structures *Opt. Lett.* **28** 2019–21

[106] Miao J, Charalambous P, Kirz J and Sayre D 1999 Extending the methodology of X-ray crystallography to allow imaging of micrometre-sized non-crystalline specimens *Nature* **400** 342–4

[107] Neutze R, Wouts R, Van der Spoel D, Weckert E and Hajdu J 2000 Potential for biomolecular imaging with femtosecond X-ray pulses *Nature* **406** 752–7

[108] Förster A and Schulze-Briese C 2019 A shared vision for macromolecular crystallography over the next five years *Struct. Dyn.* **6** 064302

[109] Dauter Z and Wlodawer A 2016 Progress in protein crystallography *Protein Pept. Lett.* **23** 201–10

[110] Canduri F and de Azevedo W F 2008 Protein crystallography in drug discovery *Curr. Drug Targets* **9** 1048–53

[111] Hope H 1990 Crystallography of biological macromolecules at ultra-low temperature *Annu. Rev. Biophys. Biophys. Chem.* **19** 107–26

[112] Garman E F and Owen R L 2006 Cryocooling and radiation damage in macromolecular crystallography *Acta Crystallogr.* D **62** 32–47

[113] Dyda F 2010 Developments in low-resolution biological X-ray crystallography *F1000 Biol. Rep.* **2** 80

[114] Schröder G F, Levitt M and Brunger A T 2010 Super-resolution biomolecular crystallography with low-resolution data *Nature* **464** 1218–22

[115] Hartshorn M J, Murray C W, Cleasby A, Frederickson M, Tickle I J and Jhoti H 2005 Fragment-based lead discovery using X-ray crystallography *J. Med. Chem.* **48** 403–13

[116] Fattori D, Squarcia A and Bartoli S 2008 Fragment-based approach to drug lead discovery: overview and advances in various techniques *Drugs R* D **9** 217–27

[117] Hol W G 1986 Protein crystallography and computer graphics—toward rational drug design *Angew. Chem. Int. Ed. Engl.* **25** 767–78

[118] Fitzpatrick P A, Steinmetz A, Ringe D and Klibanov A M 1993 Enzyme crystal structure in a neat organic solvent *Proc. Natl Acad. Sci.* **90** 8653–7

[119] Cavasotto C N and Phatak S S 2009 Homology modeling in drug discovery: current trends and applications *Drug Discov. Today* **14** 676–83

[120] Sivakumar K, Kannappan S, Vijayakumar B, Jithendran K P, Balasubramaniam S and Panigrahi A 2021 Molecular docking study of bio-inhibitors extracted from marine macroalga *Ulva fasciata* against hemolysin protein of luminescence disease-causing *Vibrio harveyi Arch. Microbiol.* **7** 1–16

[121] Kirsch P, Hartman A M, Hirsch A K and Empting M 2019 Concepts and core principles of fragment-based drug design *Molecules* **24** 4309

[122] Mikusinska-Planner A and Surma M 2000 X-ray diffraction study of human serum *Spectrochim. Acta* A **56** 1835–41

[123] Berg J M, Tymoczko J L and Stryer L 2002 *Biochemistry* (New York: WH Freeman)

[124] Lu Z, Yeh T-K, Tsai M, Au J L-S and Wientjes M G 2004 Paclitaxel-loaded gelatin nanoparticles for intravesical bladder cancer therapy *Clin. Cancer Res.* **10** 7677–84

[125] El-Deeb N M, El-Sherbiny I M, El-Aassara M R and Hafez E E 2015 Novel trend in colon cancer therapy using silver nanoparticles synthesized by honey bee *J. Nanomed. Nanotechnol.* **6** 265

[126] Mansoori G A, Brandenburg K S and Shakeri-Zadeh A 2010 A comparative study of two folate-conjugated gold nanoparticles for cancer nanotechnology applications *Cancers* **2** 1911–28

[127] Dixit V, Van den Bossche J, Sherman D M, Thompson D H and Andres R P 2006 Synthesis and grafting of thioctic acid–PEG–folate conjugates onto Au nanoparticles for selective targeting of folate receptor-positive tumor cells *Bioconjugate Chem.* **17** 603–9

[128] Manohar S, Rayavarapu R, Petersen W and van Leeuwen T G 2009 Cell viability studies of PEG-thiol treated gold nanorods as optoacoustic contrast agents *Photons Plus Ultrasound: Imaging and Sensing 2009* (Bellingham, WA: International Society for Optics and Photonics) 71772D

[129] Chakraborty S P, Sahu S K, Mahapatra S K, Santra S, Bal M, Roy S and Pramanik P 2010 Nanoconjugated vancomycin: new opportunities for the development of anti-VRSA agents *Nanotechnology* **21** 105103

[130] Chattopadhyay S, Chakraborty S, Laha D, Baral R, Pramanik P and Roy S 2012 Surface-modified cobalt oxide nanoparticles: new opportunities for anti-cancer drug development *Cancer Nanotechnol.* **3** 13–23

[131] Falk M and Issels R 2001 Hyperthermia in oncology *Int. J. Hyperth.* **17** 1–18

[132] Moroz P, Jones S and Gray B 2002 Magnetically mediated hyperthermia: current status and future directions *Int. J. Hyperth.* **18** 267–84

[133] Wang J-H, Yao M-Z, Gu J-F, Sun L-Y, Shen Y-F and Liu X-Y 2002 Blocking HSF1 by dominant-negative mutant to sensitize tumor cells to hyperthermia *Biochem. Biophys. Res. Commun.* **290** 1454–61

[134] Chang Y-S, Savitha S, Sadhasivam S, Hsu C-K and Lin F-H 2011 Fabrication, characterization, and application of greigite nanoparticles for cancer hyperthermia *J. Colloid Interface Sci.* **363** 314–9

[135] Thakral N K, Zanon R L, Kelly R C and Thakral S 2018 Applications of powder x-ray diffraction in small molecule pharmaceuticals: achievements and aspirations *J. Pharm. Sci.* **107** 2969–82

[136] Pappa H 2009 Characterization of crystalline and partially crystalline solids by x-ray powder diffraction (XRPD) *Pharm. Forum* 731–40

[137] Gozzo F 2018 The power of synchrotron X-ray powder diffraction for the characterization of pharmaceuticals *Pharmaceut. Technol.* **42** 18

[138] Dash A, Khin-Khin A and Suryanarayanan R 2002 X-ray powder diffractometric method for quantitation of crystalline drug in microparticulate systems. I. Microspheres *J. Pharm. Sci.* **91** 983–90

[139] Maurin J K, Pluciński F, Mazurek A P and Fijałek Z 2007 The usefulness of simple X-ray powder diffraction analysis for counterfeit control—the Viagra® example *J. Pharm. Biomed. Anal.* **43** 1514–8

[140] Crews C, Kenny P S, O'Flynn D and Speller R D 2018 Multivariate calibration of energy-dispersive X-ray diffraction data for predicting the composition of pharmaceutical tablets in packaging *J. Pharm. Biomed. Anal.* **151** 186–93

[141] Musumeci D, Hu C and Ward M D 2011 Anticounterfeit protection of pharmaceutical products with spatial mapping of X-ray-detectable barcodes and logos *Anal. Chem.* **83** 7444–50

[142] Elder D P, Patterson J E and Holm R 2015 The solid-state continuum: a perspective on the interrelationships between different solid-state forms in drug substance and drug product *J. Pharm. Pharmacol.* **67** 757–72

[143] Morissette S L, Almarsson Ö, Peterson M L, Remenar J F, Read M J, Lemmo A V, Ellis S, Cima M J and Gardner C R 2004 High-throughput crystallization: polymorphs, salts, co-crystals and solvates of pharmaceutical solids *Adv. Drug Deliv. Rev.* **56** 275–300

[144] Stephenson G A 2005 Applications of X-ray powder diffraction in the pharmaceutical industry *Rigaku J.* **22** 2–15

[145] D'Amico K 2001 System and methods for the high throughput screening of polymorphs *Google Patents*

[146] Hilfiker R and Von Raumer M 2019 *Polymorphism in the Pharmaceutical Industry: Solid Form and Drug Development* (New York: Wiley)

[147] Food U and Administrative D 2007 *Guidance for Industry-ANDAs: Pharmaceutical Solid Polymorphism, Chemistry, Manufacturing, and Controls Information* (Washington, DC: US Department of Health and Human Services)

[148] Bleuet P, Welcomme E, Dooryhée E, Susini J, Hodeau J-L and Walter P 2008 Probing the structure of heterogeneous diluted materials by diffraction tomography *Nat. Mater.* **7** 468–72

[149] Miguélez-Morán A M, Wu C Y, Dong H and Seville J P 2009 Characterisation of density distributions in roller-compacted ribbons using micro-indentation and X-ray micro-computed tomography *Eur. J. Pharm. Biopharm.* **72** 173–82

[150] Liu R, Yin X, Li H, Shao Q, York P, He Y, Xiao T and Zhang J 2013 Visualization and quantitative profiling of mixing and segregation of granules using synchrotron radiation X-ray microtomography and three dimensional reconstruction *Int. J. Pharm.* **445** 125–33

[151] Harding G, Kosanetzky J and Neitzel U 1987 X-ray diffraction computed tomography *Med. Phys.* **14** 515–25

[152] Jacques S D M, Di Michiel M, Kimber S A J, Yang X, Cernik R J, Beale A M and Billinge S J L 2013 Pair distribution function computed tomography *Nat. Commun.* **4** 2536

[153] Jensen K M, Yang X, Laveda J V, Zeier W G, See K A, Di Michiel M, Melot B C, Corr S A and Billinge S J 2015 X-ray diffraction computed tomography for structural analysis of electrode materials in batteries *J. Electrochem. Soc.* **162** A1310

[154] O'Flynn D, Crews C, Drakos I, Christodoulou C, Wilson M, Veale M, Seller P and Speller R 2016 Materials identification using a small-scale pixellated x-ray diffraction system *J. Phys.* D **49** 175304

[155] Bhattacharjee R *et al* 2022 The emergence of metal oxide nanoparticles (NPs) as a phytomedicine: A two-facet role in plant growth, nano-toxicity and anti-phyto-microbial activity *Biomed. Pharmacother.* **155** 113658

Chapter 11

Scanning electron microscopy for biomedical nanotechnology

Ravikumar B Shinde[1], Shashank S Pawitwar[1] and Ajeet Kaushik

The recent developments in nanotechnology have touched almost every part of science and technology. The biomedical field is not an exception to this. This chapter is focused on advances in scanning electron microscopy (SEM) by application of nanotechnology. Other fields like environmental sciences, medical imaging, and material sciences need microscopic studies, such as electron microscopy. Nanotechnology has particularly helped in improvements in microscopy, such as environmental scanning electron microscopy (ESEM). SEM has furthered the analytical studies in biomedical sciences.

11.1 Introduction

Biomedical nanotechnology is a cutting-edge area of research in medicine, engineering, and science and has several applications for molecular imaging, molecular diagnosis, and targeted therapy. It has revolutionized the field of health sciences. It exploits nanotechnology and nanoscience for health wellness. Hundreds of studies have shown the significance of advanced technologies in studying diseases, tracking its progress and treatment. Increased inclusion of technologies especially, nanotechnology has improved the fields of diagnostics and allowed treatment to be more accurate and accessible (Bhardwaj and Kaushik 2017, Kaushik 2019). A nanoscale platform is the basis of nanotechnology hence highly sophisticated visual aids are necessary to work with it. The International Organization for Standardization (ISO) has defined 'nanomaterial' as a 'material with any external dimension in the nanoscale or having internal structure or surface structure in the nanoscale' (ISO 2010) and 'nanoparticle' as a 'nano-object with all three external dimensions in the nanoscale' where nanoscale is defined as the size range from approximately 1–100 nm

[1] Equal contribution.

doi:10.1088/978-0-7503-3379-5ch11

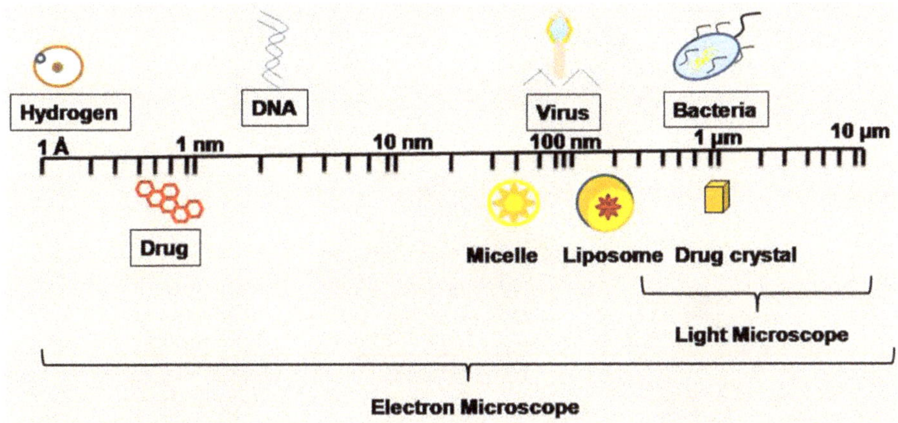

Figure 11.1. Relative sizes of different molecules and nanomaterials showing the application of SEM in visualization (adapted from Panneerselvam and Choi (2014)).

(ISO 2008). Although size is not the only criteria considered in the definition of nano-, the fact is that it is the most important factor. As the size is an important factor in nanoscience, it is a challenge too. Optical microscopes have limitation in nanotechnology applications and hence the electron microscopy is of great help in all developments of nanotechnology (figure 11.1).

The appropriate inputs from various subjects like chemistry, biology, physics, and mathematics has been helpful in addressing various issues in medical sciences. The development of medical devices, instruments for image capture and processing, implants are the processes to solve these issues. This task needs very meticulous efforts with high precision. SEM is the most robust tool for these kinds of studies. These research fields address various problems through the development of bionic parts, implants, medical devices and imaging equipment, along with tissue engineering. It involves extremely delicate and very detailed work that requires very high precision. SEMs are very powerful tools for such studies with diverse applications in biomedical fields ranging from orthodontics to tissue engineering. It is one of the classic and effective imaging techniques to understand and explore the surface/interface morphology and microstructural analysis. SEM images the sample surface by scanning it with a high-energy beam of electrons in a raster scan pattern. The primary electron beam, which is produced under high vacuum, is scanned across the surface of a specimen. When the electrons strike the specimen, a variation of the signal produces an image of the surface, or its elemental composition together with energy dispersive x-rays (EDX). It is a popular tool to use in imaging of microstructures of biotic as well as abiotic materials. SEM analysis is useful to confirm surface morphology of a nanostructure, thin film, and biomolecules. Moreover, various bindings among material–materials, materials–cells, and cell–cell has also been studied using SEM. Various applications of SEM are shown in figure 11.2.

It has been nine decades since the development of SEM. However, there have not been many changes in the basic concept and design. Nonetheless, dramatic progress

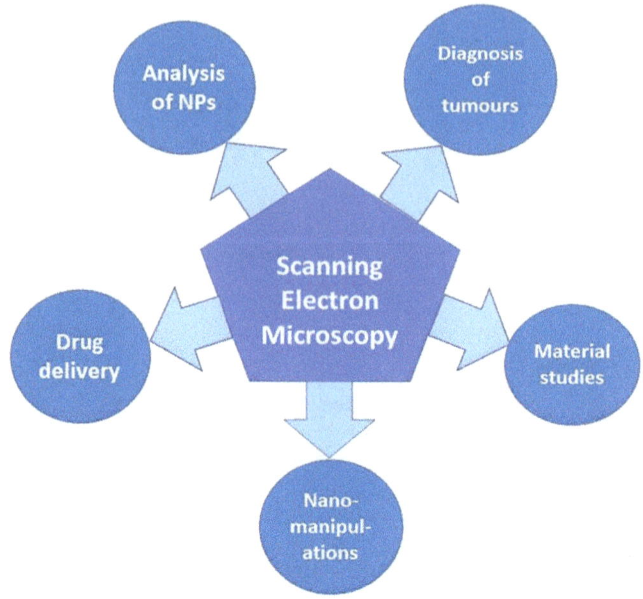

Figure 11.2. Applications of scanning electron microscopy in various fields.

in resolution and power has been witnessed through these decades. In the current decade the biological sciences have enjoyed the resurgence of SEM, especially due to growing applications in biomedical sciences and nanotechnology.

The discovery of electron deflection under magnetic fields led to the development of electron microscopy by using high-energy electron beams. SEM uses collimate and focused electron beams instead of light beams to systematically scan the specimen exterior and produces numerous signals, that are captured by electron detectors as shown in the figure 11.3.

Basically, a high current is passed through a V-shaped tungsten filament that ejects high-energy electron beams through thermioic emission accelerated by applied voltage. The V-shaped tungsten filament helps to collimate the electron beam. These parallel electron beams pass through a series of lenses under vacuum. The vacuum chamber helps electron beam to avoid obstructions, as deflection of electrons by small particles compromise the results. When the electron beam (incident beam) hits the specimen, it emits three kinds of electrons namely primary backscattered, secondary, and Auger electrons. SEM uses primary backscattered and secondary electrons. The detector records the imprint and utilizes that information to generate three-dimensional images.

Unlike optical microscopy, which uses light and glass lenses to illuminate samples to produce magnified images, SEM uses a beam of electrons and electrostatic or electromagnetic lenses to generate images of much higher resolution based on the shorter wavelengths of electrons than visible light photons. The signals emitted from the sample are collected by detectors. The detector signal corresponds to a known location of the beam on the specimen. The signal intensity is used to modulate the corresponding image pixel. The signals collected in series are combined to form an

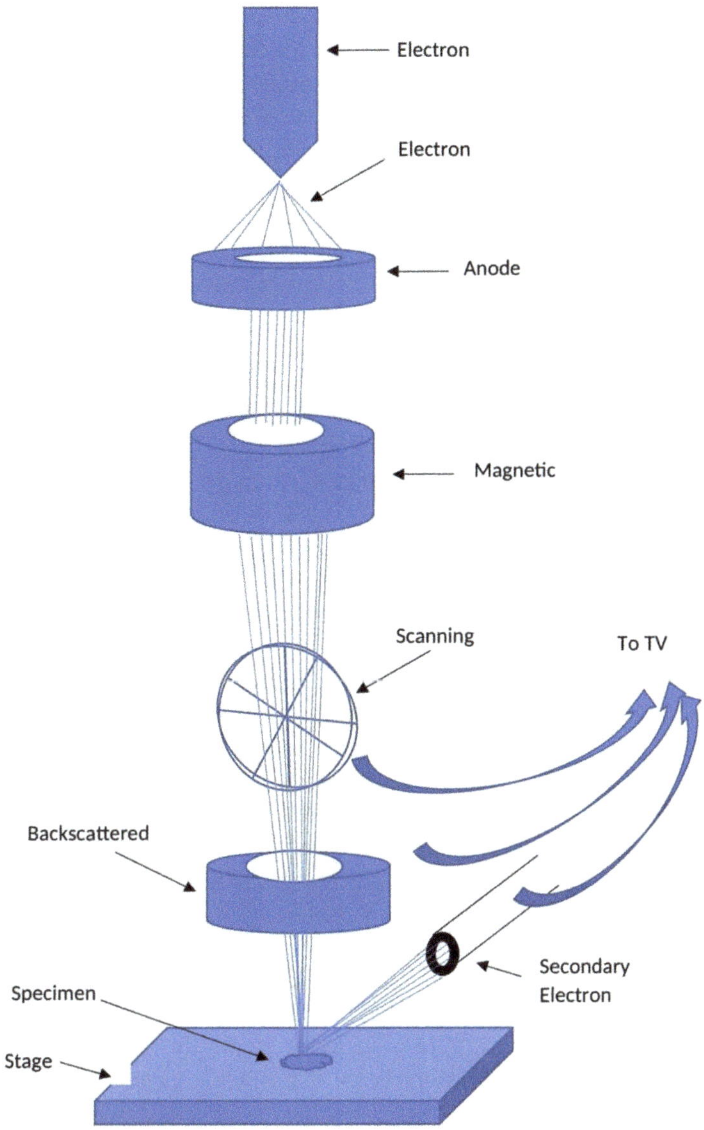

Figure 11.3. Scanning electron microscopy schematic diagram.

image whose dimension distribution depends on the scan pattern chosen. Currently, a resolution of about a few nanometers can be achieved with few Kev. The general arrangement of scanning electron microscopy equipment emphasizes the type of electron source and the main signals resulting from the interaction between the electron beam and the sample.

The new technologies available in scanning electron microscopy equipment for morphological and structural characterization, including wet samples, make it more useful in biological as well as physical sciences. The challenges already being superseded with the use of SEM on the nanoscale for nanofabrication and nanomanipulation. SEM captures images of a samples surface by scanning it with a high-energy beam of electrons in a raster scan pattern (Yan 2010). The beam of electrons produced under high vacuum scan across the specimen surface and the electrons strike the specimen. A signal variation produces an image of the surface. The principles of SEM have been used to develop several functions to gain a better understanding of material surfaces (Yan 2019). Field emission guns SEM (FEGSEM) enable a higher resolution and magnification, which is widely used in nanotechnology and biomedical fields.

Environmental scanning electron microscopy (ESEM) is one of the latest innovations in SEM. It has two novel aspects; first, the introduction of a gaseous environment is allowed in the specimen chamber although the electron gun is kept under the standard SEM high vacuum. And secondly it does not need a coating of carbon or a metallic layer even for samples such as fibers, wood, or polymer which are non-conductive (Muscariello *et al* 2005). SEM images of surfaces have a three-dimensional quality with great resolution and depth of field that offers a visually familiar perspective to many users.

SEM in nanotechnology Several modifications in SEM such as electron back-scattered detection (EBSD), field emission gun, and x-ray element mapping have contributed to enhanced analysis of nanomaterial. Applications of SEM in nanotechnology such as electron beam nanolithography, nanomanipulation, and focused ion beam (FIB) technique have improved *in situ* nanomaterial design and production. SEM is likely to be one of the most versatile tools for the analysis of micro- and nanostructures with a wide range of applications. It provides information on composition as well as surface topography and gives striking pictures of structures. This is mainly due to the ability to produce images with stereoscopic appearance and great plasticity. Second, a high range of variable magnifications from approximately ten times to the range of few nanometers. Third, even information on the composition of the material can be achieved by the selection of signals originating from specific interactions such as characteristic x-ray quanta or backscattered electrons (Patel and Parsania 2018). SEM is a highly useful tool in providing more information about nanomaterials by using a high electron beam probing of samples on a very fine scale. It is fully able to monitor size, size distribution, formation, and morphology of synthesized micro and nano-sizes. It is very handy in describing NP morphology by measurements from histograms. It can be done manually or with the help of specified software. The morphology of nanopowders can be assayed along with its chemical composition energy dispersive x-ray spectroscopy (EDX-SEM) (Mansoureh and Parisa 2018).

11.1.1 Electron backscatter diffraction in SEM

Electron backscatter diffraction (EBSD) provides structural information of most of the inorganic crystalline materials such as metals, minerals, semiconductors, and ceramics. It gives size, boundary character, orientation, texture, and phase identity of grains in the sample under the beam. It can be used to analyze various samples ranging from millimeter sized grains to thin metal films with nanograins. Modern field emission SEMs (FE-SEMs), can be used to measure 20 nm grains with reasonable accuracy. EBSD maps can give the basic characteristics of a material's microstructure along with details about the size and shape of grain.

11.1.2 X-ray analysis in SEM

The important characteristic of x-ray analysis in SEM is that it gives quantitative analytical information about the elemental composition of a specimen. The technique is useful in imaging the three-dimensional variations in composition of a sample as the x-rays are generated when electrons strike the surface of sample (Allen *et al* 2010, Newbury and Ritchie 2013).

11.1.3 Field emission gun scanning electron microscopy

Field emission gun scanning electron microscopy (FEGSEM) is an ultra-high-resolution microscope and is ideal for studying materials on the nanometer scale. The microscope is equipped with energy dispersive x-ray analysis (EDX) and electron backscattered diffraction (EBSD). Lanthanum manganates, a popular ceramic is widely used in oxygen sensors and solid oxide fuel cells EDX analysis is commonly used in elemental detection of the ceramic samples (Shu *et al* 2009, Droushiotis *et al* 2010).

11.1.4 Cryogenic scanning electron microscopy

Life scientists and bioengineers are continuously working on cryogenic scanning electron microscopy (cryo-SEM), which is an ultra-low-temperature technique for visualizing the atomic-level inner workings of samples. Cryo-SEM is the best tool yet for understanding the nanoscale relationships between a biomolecule's natural structure and its function in health and disease. Cryo-SEM is also useful to investigate microstructure development of composite coatings prepared from dispersions of antimony-doped tin oxide (ATO) nanoparticles (~30 nm) or indium tin oxide (ITO) nanoparticles (~40 nm) and latex particles. The cryo-SEM has an advantage over x-ray crystallography as crystallization of some materials is difficult which means there has not been any option to study their fine structures. Apart from biology the cryo-SEM is highly beneficial in material sciences. Cryo-SEM is used to visualize structures and processes that do not lend themselves to other EM techniques. For example, a team at Stanford recently used cryo-EM to observe sensitive lithium-ion battery components and interfaces at the atomic level. Typical lithium-ion batteries contain certain lithium-containing electrode materials, organic electrolytes and solid electrolyte interphases that are structurally unstable under standard transmission EM analysis (Huang *et al* 2019, Luo *et al* 2007).

11.1.5 Low accelerating voltage SEM

Generally, the accelerating voltage can be varied from <1 kV to 30 kV in SEM. Increasing voltage may give a charge effect, less surface details, and sample damage; no doubt it is somewhat dependent on the type of sample. Usually 1 kV–5 kV is considered a low accelerating voltage. Images with better resolution quality can be achieved at lower accelerating voltages. Low kV also gives better image quality of low atomic number (low Z) samples. At low kV the penetration depth of the electrons into low Z materials is much less than higher kV electrons on the same samples. Using low accelerating voltage is a channel to the revelation of new and interesting characteristics of samples. It will help in discovering newer features of nanomaterials, which would be otherwise hidden by the overpowering of high kV (Joy and Newbury 2002, Joy and Joy 1996a, 1996b). Even, very low voltage SEM where the accelerating voltage is below 1 kV has been studied and was found able to give ultra-shallow topographic information virtually decoupled from material (Z-number) contrast in low-dimensional nanostructures (Zarraoa *et al* 2019).

11.1.6 Electron beam (e-beam) lithography integrated SEM

Electron beam (e-beam) lithography is an open lithography method that exploits an electron gun from a SEM to pattern nanoscale features on a substrate surface. Unlike photolithography, the resolution can reach precision levels down to 1 nm with e-beam lithography (Sahin *et al* 2018).

11.1.7 SEM with nanomanipulator

A nanomanipulator is any kind of electromechanical device which can be used for controlled placement of an end effector with better than 100 nm resolution. It is obvious that a nanomanipulator has to be positioned in such a way that the resolution must be conformed to the length scales of the materials to be characterized and/or manipulated. Nanomanipulation under SEM imaging has eased the characterization of nanomaterials and nanostructures and the prototyping/assembly of nanomaterials. Different tasks like electrical probing, cell nanosurgery, pick and place, and assembling can be performed by SEMs with an in-built nanomanipulator (Luu *et al* 2016).

11.1.8 SEM and biomedical applications

SEM is a useful tool to study details at the nanoscale and to push the analyses further. SEMs are highly versatile instruments that are shown to be particularly useful in various biomedical research fields, ranging from orthodontics to bone grafts and tissue engineering (Chen and Liu 2016). SEM has been an important tool for various biomedical fields such as diagnosis; wet-SEM a little modification in conventional electron microcopy was helpful in diagnosis of brain tumors (Barshack *et al* 2004). Advances in SEM-like field emission scanning electron microscope (FESEM) has furthered the resolution and use of SEM in nanoparticle analysis in tissues. The FESEM gives high quality images due to its cold cathode technology

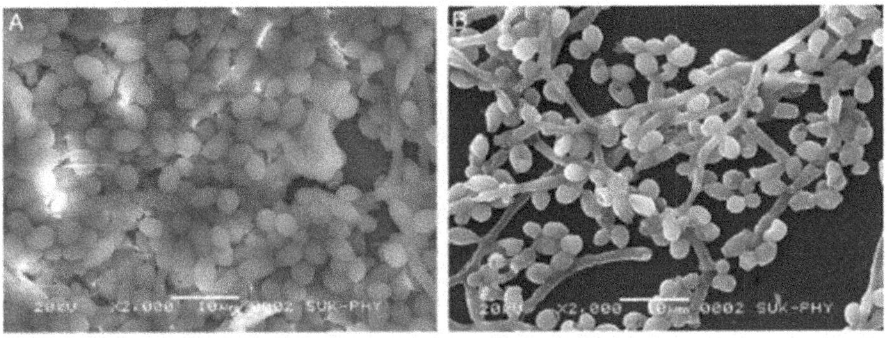

Figure 11.4. A *Candida albicans* biofilm developed *in vitro* on polystyrene. SEM micrograph shows difference in structures of biofilms (A) Untreated and (B) treated with antifungal. Reprinted from Shinde *et al* (2013) with permission from Elsevier.

which makes it more useful in the identification of nanoparticles in tissues (Hubbs *et al* 2013). The diagnosis and identification of infectious diseases can be done with the SEM. Recent improvements in SEM has made it possible to analyze microbial samples without dehydration or fixing which cause shrinkage of microbes during sample preparation (Golding *et al* 2016). Silica nanoparticles have shown promise in drug delivery due to their high drug loading properties. SEM is required to study the porous nature of mesoporous silica nanoparticles (Johansson 2010).

11.1.8.1 Parasitological studies

The systematic study of parasites is an important step in studying their biomedical significance. SEM has been a powerful tool to study life cycles and other related mechanisms of the parasites. Various anti-parasitic studies were done using SEM where the micrographs helped in determining mode of action of drugs (Saini and Rai 2020).

11.1.8.2 Microbial biofilms

A slimy growth of microbes on grafts, implants or transplants is the most common problem in modern surgeries involving transplantations. SEM studies have elucidated the microenvironment of these microbial and help in studying biology and community life of these organisms (figure 11.4).

11.1.9 Comparison of bone grafts

The versatile features of SEM make it a useful instrument in biomedical fields such as dentistry, tissue engineering, and bone grafting. Tumors and trauma cause lesions in bones which are challenging to treat. In a study, xenogenic bone grafts were compared with allografts by using SEM, the images help concluding that the performance of the two materials is equal and confirm the efficiency of highlyprocessedsyntheticgrafts (Kubosch *et al* 2016).

11.1.10 Study of porosity in scaffolds used in tissue engineering

SEM is useful in studying the effect of chemical polishing of scaffolds used in engineering tissues for transplantation. The morphological alterations in scaffolds can also be assessed by using SEM (Wysocki *et al* 2016).

11.1.11 Orthodontic transplants' microscopic study

Continuous contact with saliva and variation in salivary pH may affect orthodontic implants. SEM is useful in studying the corrosive effects of saliva/pH variation in saliva on the dental implants (Hobbelink *et al* 2015).

11.1.11.1 SEM in immunology

Localization of antigens is important in immunological studies. SEMs with electron dense probes are useful in high spatial resolution of macromolecular structures and provides more details of relation of cellular and sub-cellular composition with their functions (figure 11.5).

11.1.11.2 Trauma in lungs and respiratory system

Conditions like acute lung injury or respiratory distress syndrome are the result of inflammation and can be studied effectively using scanning electron microscopy. The properties of surfaces of alveoli such as smoothness and intactness give more details of their damage (Hamlington *et al* 2018).

11.1.12 SEM in nanoscience

Several interdisciplinary research in fields like nanomedicine needs analytical tools and techniques. Often this research may lead to some products like biochips, biomaterials, or some nanodrug delivery systems. Assessment of these end products need powerful tools like SEM (Gould *et al* 2004).

11.1.13 Anatomical studies during surgeries

The human cochlea is a highly sensitive organ of the inner ear. SEM is useful in the assessment of anatomical variations in the cochlea and at the time of insertion of electrodes during cochlear implantation surgeries (Rask-Andersen *et al* 2012).

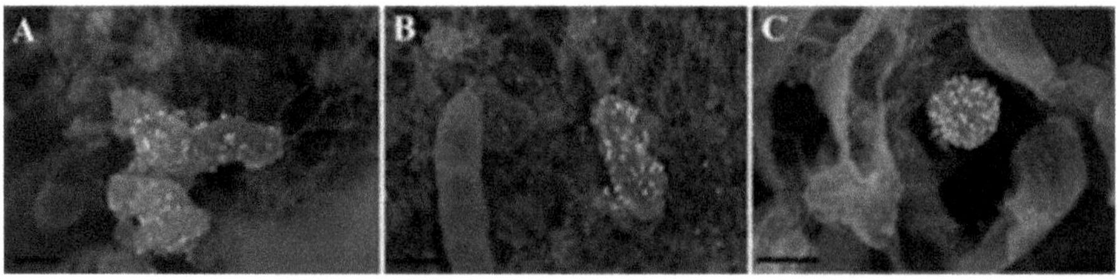

Figure 11.5. Immune-labeled b©acteria demonstrating excessive background labeling in the out of focus regions (A), moderate background labeling (B) or minimal levels of background labeling (C) Fischer *et al* (2012, copyright 2012 John Wiley & Sons, Inc.

11.1.14 Challenges and future aspects

SEM is an important tool in research, diagnosis, nanodrugs, and other medical fields. Structural and anatomical investigation may help in the development of newer diagnostics as well as therapeutics. Of course, the last few decades have enjoyed the strength of SEM in microscopic studies. However, the size and cost of SEMs is one of the important challenges. The technical evolution of SEM is continuing and in the future SEM will become one of the most important analytical tools in biomedical sciences, especially due to the increasing role of nanotechnologies in biomedical sciences. In a study published in *Nature Nanotechnology*, scientists have shown that nanoparticles with various colors would be helpful for multicolor electron microscopy in the near future (Prigozhin *et al* 2019).

11.2 Conclusion

SEM is one of the key factors in the developments in nanotechnology/biomedical nanotechnology. SEM is essential for microscopic analysis in these fields as it makes it convenient and more accurate to analyze the nanomaterials and nanostructures. SEMs with XDS type x-ray analyzers are useful in analysis of local composition and element distribution on surfaces. Specimen preparation and examination is easier in SEM than that of other microscopies. The biomedical field is greatly benefited by SEM. Many direct and indirect applications of SEM in biomedical nanotechnology has been and is being explored. It is one of the best tool for chemical and structural studies at nanoscale. In fact it is a two way process, as SEM is important in studying materials as nanoscale and SEM itself has been revolutionized in several ways by the introduction of different nanotechnologies.

References

Allen L J, Alfonso A J D, Findlay S D, LeBeau J M, Lugg N R and Stemmer S 2010 Elemental mapping in scanning transmission electron microscopy *J. Phys.: Conf. Ser.* **241** 012061

Barshack I, Polak-Charcon S, Behar V, Vainshtein A, Zik O, Ofek E, Hadani M, KopolovicJ and Nass D 2004 Wet SEM: a novel method for rapid diagnosis of brain tumors *Ultrastruct. Pathol.* **28** 255–60

Bhardwaj V and Kaushik A 2017 Biomedical applications of nanotechnology and nanomaterials *Micromachines (Basel)* **2;8** 298

Chen F M and Liu X 2016 Advancing biomaterials of human origin for tissue engineering *Prog. Polym. Sci.* **53** 86–168

Joy D and Newbury D 2002 Low voltage scanning electron microscopy *Microsc. Today* **10** 22–3

Droushiotis N, Doraswami U, Ivey D, Othman M H D, Li K and Kelsall G 2010 Fabrication by co-extrusion and electrochemical characterization of micro-tubular hollow fiber solid oxide fuel cells *Electrochem. Commun.* **12** 792e5

Fischer E R, Hansen B T, Nair V, Hoyt F H and Dorward D W 2012 Scanning electron microscopy *Current Protocols in Microbiology* (Hoboken, NJ: Wiley) ch 2, unit 2B.2

Golding C, Lamboo L, Beniac D and Booth T F 2016 The scanning electron microscope in microbiology and diagnosis of infectious disease *Sci. Rep.* **6** 26516

Gould P 2004 EU firms up funding scheme *Mater. Today* **7** 48–52

Hamlington K L, Smith B J, Dunn C M, Charlebois C M, Roy G S and Bates J H T 2018 Linking lung function to structural damage of alveolar epithelium in ventilator-induced lung injury *Respir. Physiol. Neurobiol.* **255** 22–9

Hobbelink M G, He Y, Xu J, Xie H, Stoll R and Ye Q 2015 Synergistic effect of wire bending and salivary pH on surface properties and mechanical properties of orthodontic stainless-steel arch-wires *Prog. Orthod.* **16** 37

Huang W *et al* 2019 Evolution of the solid–electrolyte interphase on carbonaceous anodes visualized by atomic-resolution cryogenic electron microscopy *Nano Lett.* **19** 5140–8

Hubbs A, Porter D W, Mercer R, Castranova V, Sargent L and Sriram K 2013 Nanoparticulates ed W M Haschek, C G Rousseaux and M A Wallig *Haschek and Rousseaux's Handbook of Toxicologic Pathology* 3rd edn (New York: Academic) pp 1373–419

ISO 2008 ISO International Organization for Standardization *Technical Specification: Nanotechnologies— terminology and Definitions for Nano-objects—Nanoparticle, Nanofibre and Nanoplate (2008)* **ISO/TS 80004** 2–2008

ISO 2010 ISO International Organization for Standardization. (2010) *Nanotechnologies—vocabulary—part 1: Core Terms (2010)* **ISO/TS 80004** 1–2010

Johansson E M 2010 Controlling the pore size and morphology of mesoporous silica *PhD Thesis* (Linköping University)Sweden)

Joy D and Joy C 1996a Ultra-low voltage scanning electron microscopy *Microsc. Today* **4** 12–3

Joy D and Joy C 1996b Low voltage scanning electron microscopy *Micron* **27** 247–63

Kubosch E J, Bernstein A, Wolf L, Fretwurst T, Nelson K and Schmal H 2016 Clinical trial and in-vitro study comparing the efficacy of treating bony lesions with allografts versus synthetic or highly-processed xenogeneic bone grafts *BMC Musculoskelet. Disord* **17** 77

Kaushik A 2019 Biomedical Nanotechnology related grand challenges and perspectives *Front. Nanotechnol.* **1** 1

Luo H, Scriven L E and Francis L F 2007 Cryo-SEM studies of latex/ceramicnanoparticle coating microstructure development *J. Colloid Interface Sci.* **316** 500–9

Luu D K, Shi C and Sun Y 2016 A review of nanomanipulation in scanning electron microscopes ed C Ru, X Liu and Y Sun *Nanopositioning Technologies* (Cham: Springer)

Makhlouf A S H and Barhoum A (eds) 2018 *Emerging Applications of Nanoparticles and Architecture Nanostructures Emerging Applications of Nanoparticles: Current Prospects and Future Trends* (Amsterdam Elsevier)

Mansoureh G and Parisa V 2018 Synthesis of metal nanoparticles using laser ablation technique *Emerging Applications of Nanoparticles and Architectural Nanostructures: Current Prospects and Future Trends* ed A Barhoum and A S H Makhlouf (Amsterdam: Elsevier) ch 19

Muscariello L, Rosso F, Marino G, Giordano A, Barbarisi M, Cafiero G and Barbarisi A 2005 A critical overview of eSEM applications in the biological field *J. Cell Phys.* **205** 328–34

Newbury D E and Ritchie N W M 2013 Elemental mapping of microstructures by scanning electron microscopy-energy dispersive X-ray spectrometry (SEM-EDS): extraordinary advances with the silicon drift detector (SDD) *J. Anal. At. Spectrom.* **28** 973

Panneerselvam S and Choi S 2014 Nanoinformatics: emerging databases and available tools *Int. J. Mol. Sci.* **15** 7158–82

Patel J P and Parsania P H 2018 Characterization, testing, and reinforcing materials of biodegradable composites ed N G Shimpi *Biodegradable and Biocompatible Polymer*

Composites (Woodhead Publishing Series in Composites Science and Engineering) (Cambridge: Woodhead Publishing) pp 55–79

Pednekar P P, Godiyal S C, Jadhav K R and Kadam V J 2017 Mesoporous silica nanoparticles: a promising multifunctional drug delivery system *Micro and Nano Technologies, Nanostructures for Cancer Therapy* ed Ficai A and Grumezescu A M (Amsterdam: Elsevier) pp 593–621

Prighozin M B *et al* 2019 Bright sub-20-nm cathodoluminescent nanoprobes for electron microscopy *Nat. Nanotechnol.* **14** 420–5

Rask-Andersen H, Liu W, Erixon E, Kinnefors A, Pfaller K, Schrott-Fischer A and Glueckert R 2012 Human cochlea: anatomical characteristics and their relevance for cochlear implantation *Anat. Rec.* **295** 1791–811

Raval N, Maheshwari R, Kalyane D, Youngren-Ortiz S R, Chougule M B and Tekade R K 2019 Importance of physicochemical characterization of nanoparticles in pharmaceutical product development *Advances in Pharmaceutical Product Development and Research,Basic Fundamentals of Drug Delivery* ed R K Tekade (New York: Academic) pp 369–400

Sahin O, Ashokkumar M and Ajayan P M 2018 *Micro- and Nanopatterning of Biomaterial Surfaces. Fundamental Biomaterials: Metals* (Cambridge: Woodhead Publishing) pp 67–78

Saini S and Rai A K 2020 Linoleic acid inhibits the release of *Leishmania donovani* derived microvesicles and decreases its survival in macrophages *Front. Cell. Infect. Microbiol* **10** 406

Sampath Kumar T S 2013 Physical and chemical characterization of biomaterials A2 ed A Bandyopadhyay and S Bose *Characterization of Biomaterials* (Oxford: Academic) ch 2

Shinde R B, Raut J S, Chauhan N M and Karuppayil S M 2013 Chloroquine sensitizes biofilms of *Candida albicans* to antifungal azoles *Braz. J. Infect. Dis.* **17** 395–400

Shu Q, Zhang J, Yan B and Liu J 2009 Phase formation mechanism and kinetics in solid-state synthesis of undoped and calcium-doped lanthanummanganite *Mater. Res. Bull.* **44** 649–53

Wysocki B, Idaszek J, Szlązak K, Strzelczyk K, Brynk T, Kurzydłowski K J and Święszkowski W 2016 Post processing and biological evaluation of the titanium scaffolds for bone tissue engineering *Materials (Basel)* **9** 197

Zhou X and Thompson G E 2017 *Electron and Photon Based Spatially Resolved Techniques. Reference Module in Materials Science and Materials Engineering* (Amsterdam: Elsevier)

Yan Y 2019 Tribology and tribocorrosion testing and analysis of metallic biomaterials *Metals for Biomedical Devices* 2nd edn ed M Niinomi (Woodhead Publishing Series in Biomaterials) (Cambridge: Woodhead Publishing) pp 213–34

Yan Y 2010 Tribology and tribo-corrosion testing and analysis of metallic biomaterials *Metals for Biomedical Devices* ed M Niinomi (Woodhead Publishing Series in Biomaterials) (Cambridge: Woodhead Publishing) pp 178–201

Zarraoa L, González M U and Paulo Á S 2019 Imaging low-dimensional nanostructures by very low voltage scanning electron microscopy: ultra-shallow topography and depth-tunable material contrast *Sci. Rep.* **9** 16263

IOP Publishing

Analytical Techniques for Biomedical Nanotechnology

Ajeet Kaushik, Sesha S Srinivasan and Yogendra Kumar Mishra

Chapter 12

Transmission electron microscopy for biomedical nanotechnology

Sayan Mukherjee, Sandeep Kaushik, Poonam Singh, S Shweta and Ishwar Prasad Sahu

The field of nanotechnology is a multidisciplinary fieled that combines knowledge from various disciplines of science, i.e., materials science, applied physics, molecular biology, polymer science, and engineering etc. Nanomaterials measured on nanoscale form the foundation of nanotechnology and, based on their specific characteristics, i.e., size, distribution, composition and morphology, exhibit superior chemical, physical, magnetic, electronic and biological properties. Currently, the nanomaterials exist in a number of potential forms, i.e., nanoparticles, nanofibers, nanorods, nanowires etc making them suitable for various biomedical applications involving tissues and cells. TEM not only provides detailed topological, morphological, compositional information about the materials at nanoscale but also helps in the visualization of biological structures at a higher resolution than that offered by light microscopy. This chapter reviews the latest developments in TEM used for physico-chemical characterization of nanomaterials as well as the progress of nanoparticles of various kinds in the biomedical field.

12.1 Introduction

During the last few years, transmission electron microscopy (TEM) has emerged as an essential tool in the growing field of biomedical research and is widely used for the physical and chemical characterization of materials at nanoscale. The human eye has its own limitations and can reach its limit within a particular range of dimensions. The eye is not even able to distinguish or resolve between closely related points after a certain distance, it is unable to resolve the embedded green splendor of forests at a distance, and the neighboring planets are thus out of reach of the human eye. In order to achieve greater precision, sharpness, and resolution, humans invented hand lenses–the ordinary microscopes, microscopes, telescopes,

doi:10.1088/978-0-7503-3379-5ch12

and are still in the process of upgrading and updating these tools to achieve the highest magnification, resolution, sharpness etc. To observe the celestial bodies we built conical telescopes, and to see microscopic living and physical entities, we built microscopes. The functions of these two are essentially the same: resolution, sharpness, and magnification. While a telescope makes large and far away objects appear nearer and smaller, a microscope makes smaller objects appear larger. Microscopes and telescopes are able to achieve their objectives as they possess a set or series of lenses arranged in a particular pattern which are able to converge and bend the incident light until it forms an image on the retina of the naked eye and, which passes through the other end. However, this chapter is related to the microscope and, in particular, it concerns a type of microscope that converges and distorts not beams of light, but electrons, and is thus known as an electron microscope. A microscope is used to observe objects or structures that are not visible to the naked eye. Normally, our eyes cannot see objects smaller than 0.1 mm, so a microscope is helpful in observing smaller objects than this. The applications of a microscope are found in all spheres of research and result in the broad interdisciplinary perspectives in unraveling the scientific myths and marvels associated with life science, physical science, and chemical science to name just a few. With the help of this we are able to directly study the biological ultra-structure, particle analysis or material characterization, molecular nature and mechanism of disease, determining the structure of bacteria, viruses etc.

12.1.1 Nanotechnology

Nanotechnology or nanoscience, in the field of applied science, is the set of all techniques and related sciences used and studied in the 1–100 nano (i.e., 10^{-9} m) scale. In nanotechnology, fabrication within this range is widely used in interdisciplinary fields, such as applied physics, materials science, semiconductor physics, large molecular chemistry (which focuses on the non-covalent effect of molecules in the field of chemistry), autonomous machines and robotics, chemical engineering, mechanical engineering and electrical engineering. 'Nano' is a Greek word, which literally means very small or minute. Every particle whose size is 100 nm or smaller is considered a 'nanoparticle'. The fineness of a nanoparticle can be estimated from the fact that the diameter of a human hair is 60 000 nm. The term nanotechnology was first used by Norio Taniguchi in the year 1974. Since the beginning of life on Earth, with the continuous changes in nature—constructioon of various nano-particles has been occurring. Nano means substances that are made up of elements of very fine size (billionths of a meter). Nanotechnology is the engineering of molecules and atoms, which integrates disciplines such as physics, chemistry, bioinformatics, and biotechnology. Nanotechnology is growing rapidly in medical and bio-engineering due to its small size, superior capacity, and durability. With the use of nanotechnology, there is less friction in engines, which increases the life of machines. Also fuel consumption is less (Fulden *et al* 2021, Rachel *et al* 2020, Bayda *et al* 2019, Li *et al* 2004).

The 21st century is going to become the nano century. Today there is competition to make the size of objects smaller and stronger. Large scale research is taking place across the world to develop nanotechnology in various fields. Nanotechnology has immense potential in many fields such as electronics, medicine, auto, bioscience, petroleum, forensics, and defense, due to its microscopic size, unmatched strength, and durability. The extremely small size changes the chemical and physical properties of the nanoparticles. For example, when zinc metal nanoparticles are formed, they become transparent (Jadoun *et al* 2021). Nanoparticles are being used in everything from consumer products to medical devices, cosmetics, chemicals, electronics and optics, environment, food and packaging, fuels, energy, textiles and paints, new generation medicines, and plastics etc (Mohanpuria *et al* 2008, Rajan *et al* 2015, Joginder *et al* 2017). Nanotechnology is expanding existing science to the nanoscale, or reshaping existing science into a new modern term. In agriculture, nanoparticles are being used in nano-fertilizers, nano-pesticides/weeds, storage, preservation, product quality improvement, and flavoring, etc (Harpreet *et al* 2021, Kah *et al* 2019, Nazia *et al* 2019). Broadly speaking, nanoparticles can be divided into organic and inorganic substances. Inorganic nanoparticle metals (silver, aluminum, tin, gold, cobalt, copper, iron, molybdenum, nickel, titanium) and their metal oxides are being used extensively. For example, silver nanoparticles are used in refrigerators, clothing, cosmetics, toothbrushes, water filters, etc. Similarly, zinc oxide nanoparticles are used in cosmetic creams. The glass in tall buildings or vehicles can be easily cleaned with the coating of gold nanoparticles. Copper nanoparticles are being used in medicine as fungicides and bactericides. They have the ability to destroy bacteria and fungi (Lucia *et al* 2021, Saba *et al* 2020, Fernando and Sung 2009).

12.1.2 Origin of nanotechnology

The first use of the principles of nanotechnology (but before the name was coined) was Richard Feynman's lecture, 'There's plenty of room at the bottom' during the American Physical Association meeting at Caltech, December 29, 1959. Feynman mentioned a method that suggests the creation of microscopic devices for the quantification of single molecules and granules. He noted the decreasing effect of gravity during this period and the increasing prominence of surface tension and Van der Waals attraction. Professor Norio Taniguchi of the Tokyo University of Science is credited with coining the term nanotechnology. Its definition was described in depth in the 1980s by Eric Drexler, who popularized the science and instruments of the nanoscale with his lectures and in his books. Nanotechnology and nanoscience in the 1980s resulted from two inventions: cluster science and the observational tunneling microscope (STM). With their help, fullerenes were developed in 1986 and carbon nanotubes, and a few years later researchers synthesized semiconductor nanocrystals, which led to the invention of many nanotubes (Sattler 2010).

12.2 Electron microscopy

The first electromagnetic lens was invented by Hans Busch in the year 1926 and he filed a patent for an electron microscope (EM) in 1928, however he did not build the microscope. The first EM was built by Ernst Ruska in the year 1931, a physicist at the University of Berlin, and Max Knoll, an electrical engineer and in the same year, Reinhold Rudenberg, the scientific director of Siemens-Schuckertwerke, acquired the EM patent.

12.2.1 Invention of electron microscope

In 1933, Ernst Ruska further developed an EM developed on the original model that was capable of producing a higher resolution image than optical microscopy (OM). In 1937, Manfred von Arden developed the first scanning electron microscope. In the year 1938, the first commercial EM was released by Siemens-Shakertwerke and from there transmission electron microscopes became more readily available in other regions of the world. The EM was further developed during the Second World War, when the first electromagnetic lens was developed. Its development has led to considerable success in increasing the differentiation potential (Nellist 2008) and since then it has acted as a powerful tool for science and industry.

12.2.2 EM—working principle

The discovery of the EM is based on the fact that the circular electromagnetic field acts on a beam of electrons. It is very similar to the action of a beam of photons on a glass lens. Electron microscopes make use of the magnetic properties of electrons, with Louis de Broglie hypothesized that electrons possess wave properties, taking magnification to a whole new level. Here in case of EM the circular electromagnetic field acts like a lens which is made of several thousand coils of wire enclosed in an iron case. With the passage of a current through the coil, a magnetic field is generated which gives a direction to the movement of electrons froming a beam of electrons having the properties of an electromagnetic wave of very short wavelength. Accelerated by an electric field is the wavelength (λ), 1 V accelerating voltage. This 100 kV accelerating voltage yields a wavelength of 0.04 nm, which is 10 000× less than visible light which increases the resolving power and more useful magnification is obtained (Nellist 2008). An EM can magnify an object up to 5000–10 000 000 times more than that of a light microscope.

12.2.3 Magnification of electron microscope

The magnification of an image produced on a photographic plate depends on two factors: the magnification of a microscope is equal to the product of the magnifications of its eyepiece and objective lenses, namely

Magnification of microscope = Magnification of the eyepiece × Magnification of the objective

Let the magnification of the objective of a compound microscope be 10× and the magnification of the eyepiece is 5×, then the overall magnification of the compound microscope will be $10 \times 5 = 50\times$ (50 times).

12.2.4 Resolving power

The typical electron beam has a wavelength of about 0.005 nm, which is generated by 50 000 V of electricity. Its resolving power is 0.002 11 nm.

Due to the difficulties in making and using magnetic lenses, only 0.1–0.2 nm resolution power is now available.

12.2.5 Uses of electron microscope

(i) Magnification from 20 000 to 100 000 times is possible by electron microscope. Therefore, the cellular organelle can be studied at the molecular level.
(ii) Various bacteria and viruses can be studied in detail with this microscope.
(iii) The distribution of enzymes present in the cell can be studied with an electron microscope.
(iv) The macromolecular level compositions of the cell can be studied.

There are two types of electron microscopes:
SEM—scanning electron microscope
TEM—transmission electron microscope

The images formed by both the SEM and TEM types of microscope and their working principles are completely different from each other.

12.3 Transmission electron microscopy

The field of nanotechnology inovolves life science, material science, physical and biochemical sciences, engineering, and technology of materials in which out of three at least one dimension should be in the range of less than 100 nm (Sattler 2010). Interestingly, the modern concept of nanotechnology was introduced by physicist Richard P Feynman in the 20th century in which nanometer size clusters were proposed as 'computer bits', Williams and Carter 2009, Nellist 2011). The first TEM was created by Max Knoll and Ernst Ruska in 1931 which is a microscopy technique in which a beam of electrons passes through and interacts with a very thin specimen/ sample and the interaction of the electrons with the sample results in forming an image which is magnified and focused on the imaging device such as a fluorescent screen or a photographic film. Subsequently, the sensor of a CCD camera detects this and produces an image. Interestingly, TEM was the most elaborate and powerful technique that was available for the imaging of materials but due to inadequate spatial resolution, the TEM instruments were unable to meet the challenges of imaging 1 nm size atom-clusters and that led to improvements in the spatial resolution of TEM instruments (Williams and Carter 2009).

12.3.1 Advancement in transmission electron microscope

TEM is a very rapidly developing field and spontaneously the scope, applications, its breadth of information in terms of applicability or output, and power of the various types of using TEM techniques to unravel and expand the breadth of knowledge in the field of material science is expanding with advancing time. Interestingly, a modern TEM constitutes a complex characterization facility which is able to collect the diffraction patterns from volumes ranging from a few cubic nanometers in size and imaging samples to the atomic scales. In addition, when the TEM technique is amalgated with tomography, a technique which is able to derive a three-dimensional (3D) information from two-dimensional (2D) images, it becomes possible to know the structure and shape of nanostructures in 3D, even with atomic resolution. Moreover, TEM also allows spectroscopy to be peformed that is capable of analyzing not only the composition of the sample but also the bonding, optical, and electronic structure properties in 2D as well as 3D. Thus, a large number of studies can now be carried out *in situ* in the TEM with simultaneous characterization (Nellist 2011).

12.3.2 Instrumentation of TEM

TEM works on three basic or essential systems:

(a) An electron gun which produces the electron beam and the condenser system which focuses the beam onto the object. Filament or cathode is the main source of electrons and a narrow beam of electrons is emitted from the cathode through the cathode ray tube and the electrons pass through this tube and reach the condenser lens. This lens is a magnetic coil, which condenses electrons into the plane of the object.

(b) The image-producing system consists of the objective lens and a magnetic coil, which produces the first magnified image of the object. This image is of intermediate type, has a movable specimen stage, intermediate and projector lenses, a magnetic coil which magnifies the image produced by the objective lens and which focus the electrons passing through the specimen to form a real, highly magnified image.

(c) The image-recording system, which converts the electron image into an image which can be perceived by the human eye. The photographic plate receives the final image of the object. The object is always to be placed between the condenser lens and the objective lens. The image-recording system usually consists of a fluorescent screen for viewing and focusing the image and a digital camera for a permanent record. Apart from this, a vacuum is also maintained in the path of the electron because transport of electrons is possible only in vacuum (figure 12.1) (Dalip *et al* 2018, Audrey and Peter 2014).

TEMs are capable of producing much higher resolution images than light microscopes, due to the short de Broglie wavelength of electrons. This property

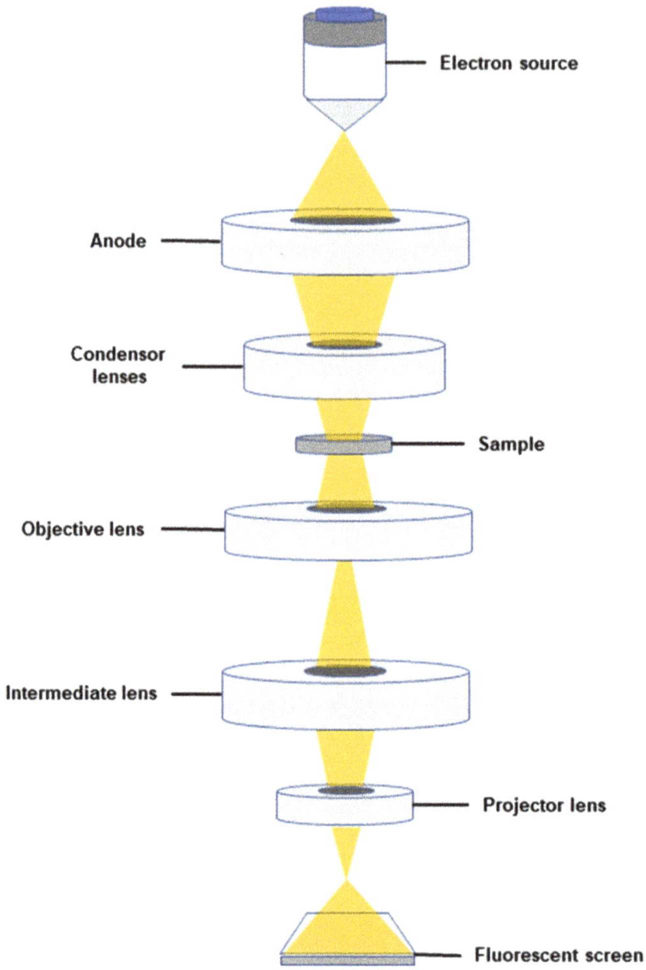

Figure 12.1. Instrumental components of transmission electron microscope.

enables the instrument to make very fine resolutions, even to the depth of a single column of atoms, which is thousands of times less than even the smallest object differentiated by a light microscope. TEM thus plays an important role in the major analysis in both physical and biological sciences, with areas such as cancer research, materials science, virology, pollution, and semiconductor research being important.

12.4 Working principle of transmission electron microscopy

The TEM technique is based upon the principle of electron transmittance and can provide detailed information about shapes, sizes, defects, and structures of nanoparticles through diffraction pattern. It helps in micro-structural examination of materials through high-resolution imaging. Optical and electron microscopes are very similar in producing the image of a specimen, but, the resolving power of the

EM is very large as compared to the OM due to the use of an electron beam of about 10^6 times shorter wavelength in EM than that of a light photon in an OM. Electrons are emitted through the filament or cathode. This electron beam is incident on the object by the condenser lens. These electrons collide with the atomic nuclei of the molecules present in the object. Atomic nuclei of higher molecular weight scatter the electron beam more than atomic nuclei of low molecular weight. The formation of an image in an EM depends on the scattering of electrons. Therefore, atomic nuclei with high atomic mass contribute more to the formation of the image. The electron beam follows a vertical path through the microscope, which is held within a vacuum. The magnetic field generated by the objective and projector lenses focused the electron beam on the photographic plate. The electrons which are scattered by atomic nuclei in the object and flow out through the aperture of the objective lens. The intermediate image of the object is formed by the objective lens. The projector lens further magnifies this image. The magnified image of the object on the photographic plate is due to the electrons scattered by the atomic nuclei of the object (Williams and Carter 2009).

TEM is a commonly used electron microscope. In this microscope an electric field pushes electrons from the negatively charged electrode. Electromagnets generate a magnetic field that focuses electrons on the stained tissue. Many electrons are released directly by penetrating the tissue, but some electrons are absorbed or dispersed by the atoms of metallic stains. Those electrons, which pass through the tissue, are focused by electromagnets on a screen fitted with a phosphorescent material. The electrons hitting the screen excite the phosphorescent material to emit visible light. Electrons that are not transmitted by the tissue leave dark marks on the visible plate. Thus, dark and bright regions in the image formed by TEM show more or less electron density. Electrons can also be focused on the photographic plate (Audrey and Peter 2014).

12.5 Specimen preparation for TEM

Sample preparation of a biological sample. i.e., cells or tissue, in TEM is a multistep process in which each step if not properly followed can virtually degrade the quality of the final electron micrograph. The specimen preparation in TEM consists of the following steps (figure 12.2):

I. **Slicing and cleaning** The first step is to thoroughly clean the surface of the specimen with a suitable buffered solution (physiological pH) so as to get rid of unwanted deposits if any. For cleansing one can also make use of ultrasonic baths but caution is required in order to prevent the sample from being damaged.

II. **Primary fixation** The primary fixation is the most significant and crucial step in the preparation of a biological sample. The fixation steps stabilize and protect the cell structure from changes or damage during subsequent treatments and irradiation. Primary fixation can be carried out using two methods, i.e., chemical fixation and cryofixation.

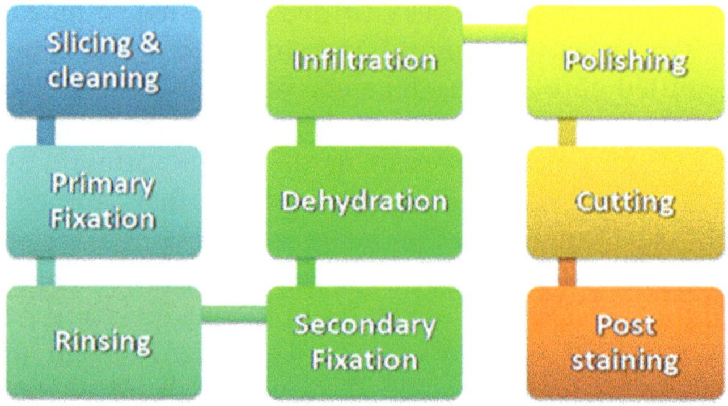

Figure 12.2. Basic steps for specimen preparation in TEM.

Chemical fixation This method is mainly used for stabilization of biological samples and makes use of chemical substances, i.e., glutaraldehyde, paraformaldehyde, acrolein, osmium tetra oxide, etc for irreversible/reversible cross linking of protein molecules with molecules in close proximity.

Cryofixation The modern approach used to immobilize and preserve the cell structure. This method involves rapid freezing of the sample in liquid helium or liquid nitrogen without crystal formation. The water content in the sample thus gets converted into a vitreous ice form.

III. **Rinsing** The fixation step may result in an increase in acidity of the specimen. Therefore, to avoid such a state and to maintain the pH, the specimen should be rinsed thoroughly using a buffer solution such as 0.1 M PBS/cacodylate buffer (pH 7.3).

IV. **Secondary fixation** After chemical fixation, post fixation or secondary fixation of the sample is carried out using osmium tetra oxide to further enhance the quality of the fixation and for increasing the contrast of the microscopic structures inside the sample. In osmium tetra oxide, osmium is a heavy metal that fixes the unsaturated lipids. This process ensures that the phospholipids forming membranes are preserved and are not eliminated during the dehydration step. Secondary fixation is essential to stain the specimen and to protect the specimen during other steps employed such as infiltration and cutting.

V. **Dehydration** Afterwards dehydration or freeze drying of the sample is carried out using an organic solvent (ethanol, acetone, propylene oxide, etc) to replace the water content of the sample with organic solvent having lower surface tension and to embed the sample in an epoxy-type resin that is immiscible with water.

VI. **Infiltration** In this step, epoxy resin is embedded within the cell, to make it hard so that it can bear the pressure of cutting or sectioning. The specimen is first placed in a mold containing epoxy resin and later cured into a hard block using heat or UV light.

VII. **Polishing** After infiltration, some materials undergo polishing to improve the quality of the image. Use of ultrafine abrasives in polishing gives the specimen a mirror-like finish.

VIII. **Cutting** For study under an electron microscope, the specimen should be extremely thin or semi-transparent in nature so that it allows the electron beam to pass through it. Therefore, the sample needs to be cut into semi-thin sections with a glass or diamond knife, using an ultra-microtome. The process of cutting of the specimens into semi-thin and ultrathin sections is also known as ultra-microtomy. These semi-thin and ultrathin sections are then mounted on specimen grids to be viewed under the microscope. The size of each section needs to be within the range 30–60 nm to obtain high resolution.

IX. **Post-staining** For biological specimens staining is usually performed twice, first before the dehydration step and later after sectioning of the sample. In post-staining, heavy metals such as lead citrate, uranyl acetate etc are used to increase the contrast between various structures in the specimen, and to scatter the electron beams (Malatesta 2016).

12.6 Applications of TEM in biomedical nanotechnology

During the last two decades, nanobiotechnology researchers have dramatically upgraded themselves and, in the last few years, the direction of research has progressed in biomedical applications, developing a new field named nanomedicine. TEM is a valuable technique not only for the physico-chemical characterization of newly developed nanoparticles, but also can explore the influences of nanocomposites on biological samples, providing information important for the establishment of efficient diagnostic and therapeutic applications (Malatesta 2016). A superfluity of nanoparticles has been established for different approaches: *in vivo* bio-imaging, drug delivery systems, antimicrobial research, scaffold components for tissue engineering, sensors application, and many other novel uses (Shi *et al* 2010, Nan-Yao *et al* 2019, Liang *et al* 2020). The greatest advantage of nonmaterial in biomedicine is their size (1–100 nm) facilitating their crosstalk with the biomolecular components; in addition, they can assume various conformational shapes (such as shells, rods, dishes, spheres etc), making them suitable for wider applications e.g. surface functionalization can be done for targeting specific cell types. Brief description of recent application of TEM in biomedical nanotechnology researches are provided in below descriptions.

12.6.1 Bio-imaging application

Nanomaterials generally express unique optical, magnetic, and acoustic properties, which manifest as an identical tool in biomedical research such as bio-analytics, biomedical imaging and bio-imaging based therapy (figure 12.3). Light-responsive nanoparticles such as quantum dots, metal nanoparticles, have an edge over others due to their better optical properties, i.e., brighter luminescence, small size, good biocompatibility, easy surface modifications, high sensitivity and higher photo

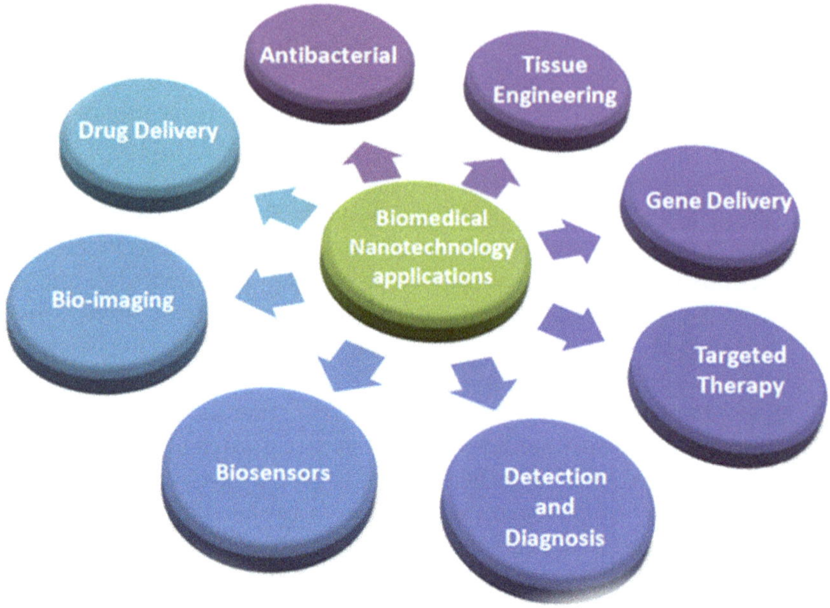

Figure 12.3. Application of nanotechnology in biomedical research.

stability and these characteristic features have thus enabled the sensitive detection of biological samples and the labeling of reporter molecules. TEM images of such nanoparticles are able to demonstrate the nanostructure as well as the size in nanometer scale.

Liang *et al* designed a novel NIR photo-activated photo-sensitizer based on TiO_2 coated UCNP core/shell nanocomposites (UCNPs@TiO_2 NCs) by using water phase transfer to synthesize UCNPs. $NaYF_4$: Yb^{3+}, Tm^{3+} @ $NaGdF_4$: Yb^{3+} core/shell UCNPs can effectively convert NIR light into UV emission, which is matched with the absorption of the TiO_2 shell (Liang *et al* 2020) (figure 12.4). This team had shown the nanostructure and size through TEM imaging.

Das *et al* in a current study, described the bio-imaging property of wire shaped copper nanostructures synthesized via microwave irradiation with single step doping of carbon nanodots (CDs) (Das *et al* 2020). The nanostructure of the CuCs was observed using TEM. The results suggest the wire-like structure of CuNPs in which CDs were observed to be grafted forming CuCs. The selected area electron diffraction (SAED) pattern matches with copper where two major planes (2 0 0) and (2 2 0) were observed to be present in the SAED pattern.

12.6.2 Drug delivery application

The application of nanotechnology in the field of medicine, known as nanomedicine, has the potential to make a useful impact on human health for clinical practice and research. Nanotechnology-based materials offer a variety of new approaches for clinical practices ranging from prevention to treatment and diagnosis of many

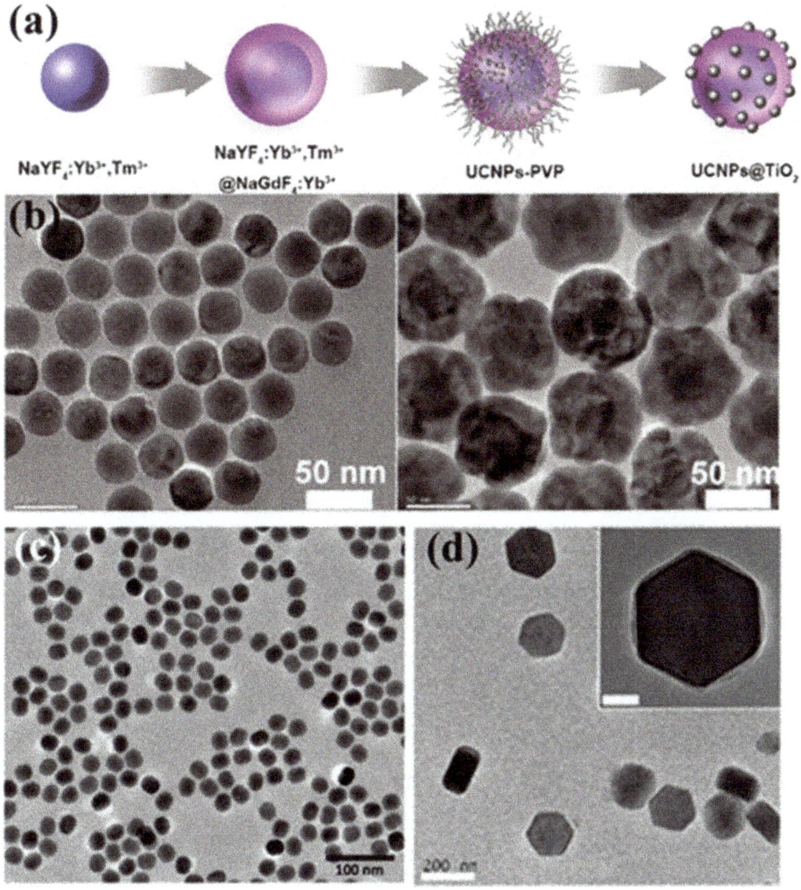

Figure 12.4. (a) Schematic illustration of the hydrothermal preparation synthetic procedure of UCNPs@TiO_2 NCs. (b) TEM images of the original $NaYF_4$:Yb^{3+}, Tm^{3+} cores (scale bar=50 nm). (c) Sol–gel method for synthesized 2-aminoethyl dihydrogen phosphate-stabilized $NaYF_4$:Yb^{3+}, Er^{3+} nanoparticles (scale bar: 100 nm). (d) UPP@ovalbumin was prepared by microemulsion synthesis. Reproduced from Liang *et al* (2020). CC BY 4.0.

diseases and conditions. Herein, we present TEM analysis on nanoparticles focused on drug delivery systems that has been performed in our laboratory.

In the case of radiolabeled nanoparticles, besides nanoparticle characterization, the TEM technique was used to confirm the stability of the nanoparticles after radio labeling. During the last decades a big family of nanostructures that have a surface-acting action, such as nanoparticles (NPs), lipid nanocarriers, and many more, have been developed to be used as drug delivery systems (DDSs) (Petrushevska *et al* 2019). Magnetically assembled drug-loaded nano chains are one of the recent findings in nanocarrier-based delivery technology. The key to controlling the length of the synthesized nano chains is the duration of the reaction mixture's exposure to the magnetic field. The chain length can be optimized depending on the biochemical environment of the target molecule. Through TEM the cluster number and length of these chains can be measured accurately (figures 12.5(a)–(h)) (Kralj and Makovec 2015).

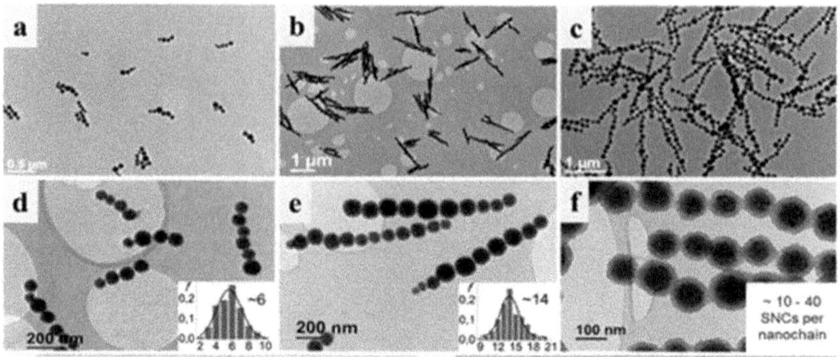

Figure 12.5. (a) and (d) TEM images of the CHAINS 6 composed of around six clusters, (b) and (e) TEM images of the CHAINS 14 composed of approximately 14 clusters, and (c) and (f) TEM images of CHAINS L collected of up to 40 clusters per nanochain. The insets in images (d), (e), and (f) show the length distributions of the nano chains determined by the manual counting of the clusters assembled into individual nano chains. Reprinted with permission from Kralj S and Makovec D (2015). Copyright (2015), American Chemical Society.)

Classical TEM and SEM techniques frequently have to be adapted for an accurate analysis of formulation morphology, especially in the case of hydrated colloidal systems (Malatesta 2016).

12.6.3 Biosensor application

Nanotechnological developments have facilitated the development of nanostructures such as nano optical fibers, nanoparticles, nanowires, and nanotubes, and research on applying these to devices are proving quite successful because these devices can be used to manufacture high-speed, high-density, subminiature sensors, thus enabling the detailed analysis of very small numbers of specimens. Biosensors improved using nanotechnology can prove to be beneficial for minimally invasive diagnosis, point of care, and early disease diagnosis. Such nano biosensors can detect various types of biomolecules such as enzymes, antibodies, antigens, acceptors, and DNA. However, biosensors should also be capable of measuring slight changes at the molecular level from the bond between biomolecules and a specific molecule.

Srijampa *et al* used gold nanoparticles (AuNP) as biosensors to understand the effects of charges on monocyte behavior. TEM images confirmed the morphology of both negatively and positively charged AuNP (AuNP−ve and AuNP+ve), which show a uniform and nearly spherical shape (Srijampa *et al* 2020, Farzadfard *et al* 2020). The average diameters of AuNP−ve and AuNP+ve were found to be 15.7 ± 2.6 nm and 14.8 ± 3.2 nm, respectively (figures 12.6(a) and (b)). Farzadfard *et al* used an electrochemical label-free biosensor designed for the detection of glycated albumin (GA) using reduced graphene oxide/Au nanoparticles (RGO/AuNPs) modified by anti-GA aptamer. TEM images of graphene oxide (GO) and rGO/AuNPs shows the uniform distribution of AuNPs on the surface of graphene sheets, demonstrating the suitable procedure for preparation of rGO/AuNPs with HEPES

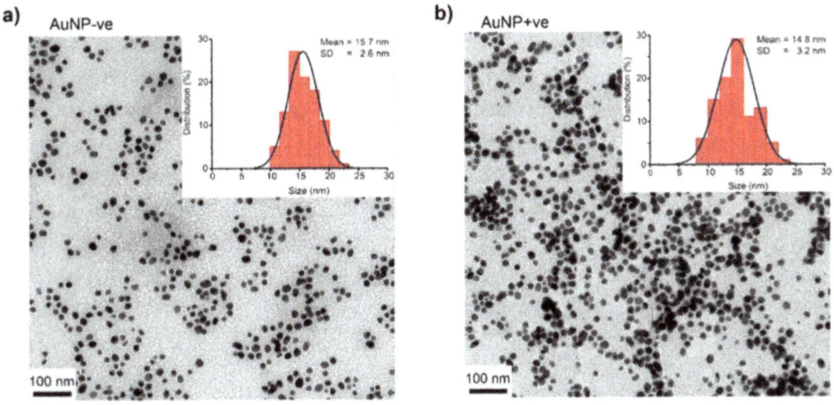

Figure 12.6. TEM images of (a) AuNP−ve and (b) AuNP+ve. Reprinted with permission from Srijampa *et al* (2020) Copyright 2020 American Chemical Society.

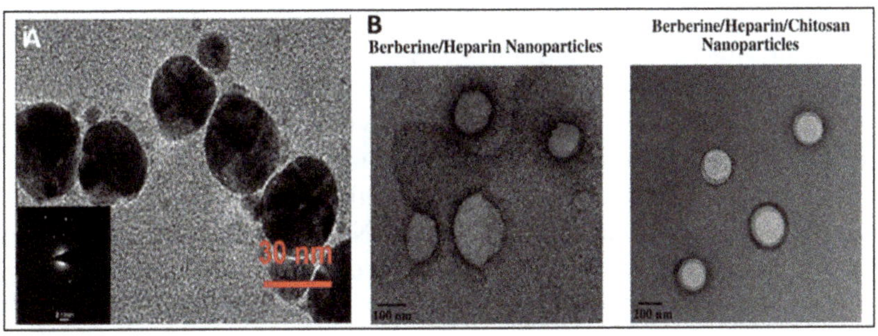

Figure 12.7. (A) The morphology of Ag-NP studied using TEM analysis. Reprinted with permission from Ray *et al* Copyright (2019) American Chemical Society. (B) TEM images of the berberine/heparin nanoparticles and berberine/heparin/chitosan nanoparticles. Reproduced from Patra *et al* (2018) CC BY 4.0.

as a reduce agent. The average diameter of AuNPs decorated on the surface of rGO sheets was 20 nm (Farzadfard *et al* 2020, Ray *et al* 2019).

12.6.4 Tissue engineering application

Tissue engineering is one of the most prominent examples of an interdisciplinary field, where scientists with different backgrounds work together to boost the quality of life by addressing critical health issues. Tissue engineering, in particular, has benefited immensely from nano- and microtechnology. For example, porous nanomaterials have led to highly efficient drug delivery systems because of their high affinity for target cells and tissues (Shafiee and Atala 2017). Ray *et al* demonstrated a facile and unique route to fabricate a hierarchical nanobiocomposite with effective loading of ZnO/silver nanoparticles (AgNPs) in order to attain excellent bactericidal efficacy with good and sustainable release profile (figure 12.7(A)) (Ray *et al* 2019).

Newman *et al* demonstrated that following intravenous administration, 2D graphene oxide (GO) nanosheets were largely excreted via the kidneys; however, a small but significant portion of the material was sequestered in the spleen (Newman *et al* 2020). Herein, they also interrogate the potential consequences of this accumulation and the fate of the spleen-residing GO. Through analyses using both bright-field TEM coupled with electron diffraction and Raman spectroscopy, they have revealed direct evidence of *in vivo* intracellular biodegradation of GO sheets with ultra-structural precision (Newman *et al* 2020). The alkaloid extracted from the barberry plant is named berberine. Researchers have developed a heparin/berberine nanocomposite, suppressing the growth of *Helicobacter pylori* and as well as reducing the cytotoxic effects in infected cells (figure 12.7(B)) (Patra *et al* 2018).

12.6.5 Antimicrobial application

Currently hybrid nanomaterials, consisting of both organic and inorganic components, are implemented for drug delivery, gene therapy, and phototherapy in addition to tissue regeneration, antibacterial, biomolecules detection, and imaging probes. This hybrid nanomaterial not only retains the properties of inorganic and organic constituents but also helps in tuning the properties of hybrid material through the combination of functional components (Goeun *et al* 2021, Xinmin *et al* 2021, Yawei *et al* 2020, Manoswini *et al* 2021).

Manoswini *et al* reported antibacterial and cytotoxic activities for hybrid AgNPs. From TEM images successful loading of Ag nanoparticles within the microgel was confirmed. High contrast AgNPs were uniformly dispersed in low contrast microgels. Also, the amount of encapsulation of AgNPs on the surface of microgels was comparatively higher in comparison to the core of microgels. In order to understand the interaction of gold nanoparticles with bacterial colony, Verma *et al* analyzed the TEM images captured for different bacteria–nanoparticle combinations (figure 12.8). They also described, the complete coverage of *Staphylococcus aureus* and *Enterococcus faecalis* with nanospheres, nanostars, and nanocubes. Furthermore, having a higher degree of polyanionic teichoic acids *S. aureus* has shown multilayer deposition as compared to *E. faecalis*. The cationic nanoparticles mostly aggregated around gram-negative bacterias due to the presence of the lipopolysaccharides and phospholipids (Verma *et al* 2015).

12.7 Challenges and future perspective of TEM

An electron scattering event can be either elastic or inelastic. In a TEM, when the incident high energy electrons interact with the thin TEM specimen, the scattered electrons carry abundant information of the targeting specimen, leading to a variety of operating modes by collecting different signals with different energy or momentum and bringing in comprehensive information about the phase, atomic structure, and chemical composition of the specimen. The correction of aberrations in the EM removes the major barrier to resolution that has existed since its invention.

The greatly improved sensitivity and signal to noise ratio is expected to allow single atom detection not only in imaging but also in spectroscopy, perhaps even in

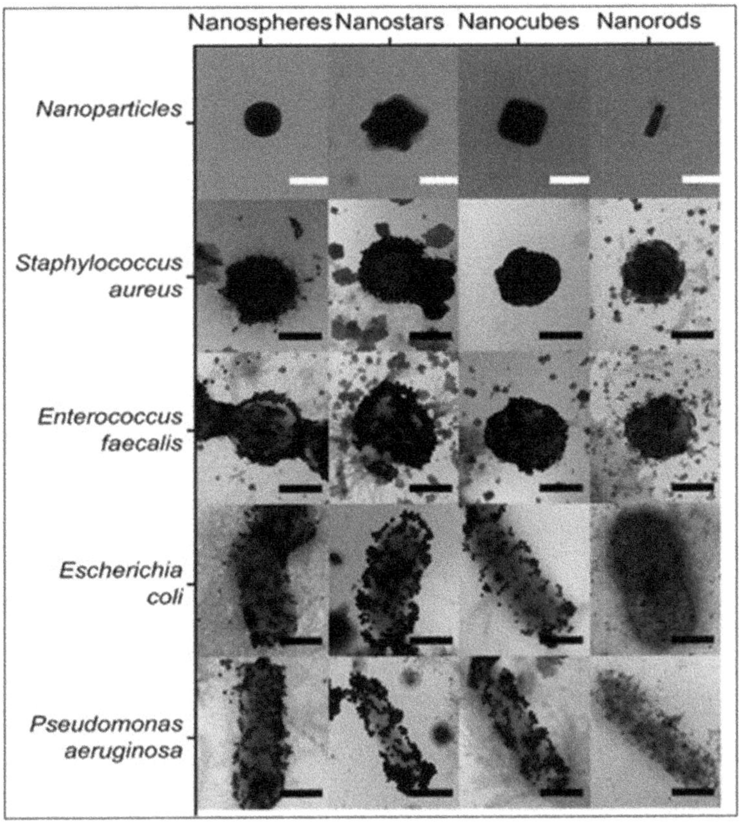

Figure 12.8. TEM images of each of the different shapes of nanoparticles aggregating around various Gram-positive and Gram-negative bacteria. Reproduced from M S Verma *et al* (2015) CC BY 4.0.

three dimensions. Despite its ability to produce highly magnified images of the object, it has some drawbacks of its own. Since electron microscopes are sensitive to vibration and electromagnetic fields they therefore need to be housed in an area that isolates them from possible exposure. Also, as a complete vacuum is required to study an object, it is difficult to study living specimens (Pennycook *et al* 2003). Additionally, sample analysis is limited to materials that are electron transparent in nature.

It is clear that the world of probing matter with electrons will experience revolutionary growth in capabilities in the next decade from ultra-small to ultra-fast and to multi-dimensions. Probing materials' functionalities *in situ* with high spatial- and temporal-resolution will continue to be a main theme. Although enabling instrumentation is often specific for scientific opportunities, there are cross-cutting areas include developing bright electron sources, fast detectors, and dedicated spectrometers. As modern science moves from the understanding of structure and ground states to dynamics and functionalities, such developments would result in transformative advances within fields of science or engineering that allow us to better address our national and international needs.

12.8 Conclusion

Nanoparticle size characterization represents a key step in nanotechnology research and development and quality control. During the development phase especially in the pharmacy industry, electron microscopy is one of the most powerful tools for determining these critical performance defining attributes. This is in detail reflected by the US Food and Drug Administration's (FDA) recommendation of the technique in identifying and demonstrating the efficacy and safety of innovator and generic drug submissions. Transmission electron microscopy provides detailed morphological, topological, compositional information about the nanomaterials, thereby acting as an efficient tool for the characterization of nanomaterials. Additionally, the necessity for ultra-structural analysis demonstrates the potential of TEM in the field of nanomedicine. Hence, the long-established and well-known TEM has been only partially exploited and offers researchers very detailed images of specimens at microscopic and nanoscale.

References

Audrey M G and Peter R 2014 *Lewis Biological Specimen Preparation for Transmission Electron Microscopy* (Princeton, NJ: Princeton University Press)

Bayda S, Adeel M, Tuccinardi T, Cordani M and Rizzolio F 2019 The history of nanoscience and nanotechnology: from chemical–physical applications to nanomedicine *Molecules (Basel, Switzerland)* **25** 112

Choi J, Shin D, Song H, Lee D and Kim K 2016 Current achievements of nanoparticle applications in developing optical sensing and imaging techniques *Nano Converg.* **3** 30

Das B, Dadhich P, Pal P, Thakur S, Neogi S and Dhara S 2020 Carbon nano dot decorated copper nanowires for SERS-fluorescence dual-mode imaging/anti-microbial activity and enhanced angiogenic activity *Spectrochim. Acta* A **227** 117669

Farzadfard A, Shayeh J S, Habibi-Rezaei M and Omidi M 2020 Modification of reduced graphene/Au-aptamer to develop an electrochemical based aptasensor for measurement of glycated albumin *Talanta* **211** 120722

Fernando and Sung 2009 *Nanotechnology Applications in Coatings* (ACS Symposium Series) (Washington, DC: American Chemical Society)

Foulkes R, Man E, Thind J, Yeung S, Joy A and Hoskins C 2020 The regulation of nanomaterials and nanomedicines for clinical application: current and future perspectives *Biomater. Sci.* **8** 4653–64

Fulden U-K, İkuru C and Kuşat K 2021 The usage of composite nanomaterials in biomedical engineering applications *Biotechnol. Bioeng.* **118** 2906–22

Goeun C, Sanoj Rejinold N, Piao H and Choy J-H 2021 Inorganic–inorganic nanohybrids for drug delivery, imaging and photo-therapy: recent developments and future scope *Chem. Sci.* **12** 5044–63

Goodhew P J, Humphreys J and Beanland R 2000 *Electron Microscopy and Analysis* (Boca Raton, FL: CRC Press)

Harpreet S, Sharma A, Bhardwaj S K, Kumar S A, Bhardwaj N and Khatri M 2021 Recent advances in the applications of nano-agrochemicals for sustainable agricultural development *Environ. Sci.: Process. Impacts* **23** 213–39

Jadoun S, Arif R and Jangid N K *et al* 2021 Green synthesis of nanoparticles using plant extracts: a review *Environ. Chem. Lett.* **19** 355–74

Joginder S D, Kumar R, Kumar N, Kaur P, Nehra K and Duhan S 2017 Nanotechnology: the new perspective in precision agriculture *Biotechnol. Rep.* **15** 11–23

Kah M, Tufenkji N and White J C 2019 Nano-enabled strategies to enhance crop nutrition and protection *Nat. Nanotechnol.* **14** 532–40

Kralj S and Makovec D 2015 Magnetic assembly of superparamagnetic iron oxide nanoparticle clusters into nanochains and nanobundles *ACS Nano* **9** 9700–7

Kwon S G, Kwon Y W and Lee T W *et al* 2018 Recent advances in stem cell therapeutics and tissue engineering strategies *Biomater. Res.* **22** 36

Li H, Wang J, Liu H, Yang C, Xu H, Li X and Cui H 2004 Sol–gel preparation of transparent zinc oxide films with highly preferential crystal orientation *Vacuum* **77** 57–62

Liang G, Haojie Wang H S, Haitao Wang M Z, Aihua Jing J L and Li G 2020 Recent progress in the development of upconversion nanomaterials in bioimaging and disease treatment *J. Nanobiotechnol.* **18** 1–22

Lucia S, Morelli L, Ochoa E and Labra M 2021 The emerging role of nanotechnology in skincare *Adv. Colloid Interface Sci.* **293** 102437

Malatesta M 2016 Transmission electron microscopy for nanomedicine: novel applications for long-established techniques *Eur. J. Histochem.* **60** 8–12

Manoswini *et al* 2021 Antibacterial and cytotoxic activity of polymer-metal hybrid nanoparticle *Adv. Nat. Sci.: Nanosci. Nanotechnol.* **12** 025003

Mohanpuria P, Rana N K and Yadav S K 2008 Biosynthesis of nanoparticles: technological concepts and future applications *J. Nanopart. Res.* **10** 507–17

Nan-Yao L, Wen-Chien K and Po-Ren H 2019 Nanoparticles in the treatment of infections caused by multidrug-resistant organisms *Front. Pharmacol.* **10** 1153

Nazia Tarannum D and Yogendra K G 2019 Facile green synthesis and applications of silver nanoparticles: a state-of-the-art review *RSC Adv.* **9** 34926–48

Nellist P D 2008 Science of microscopy 2007 *Sci. Microsc.* **91** 1–68 papers2://publication/uuid/E114CDB9-EEE5–4142-AABE-B50E75A78A7C

Nellist P D 2011 The principles of STEM imaging *Scanning Transmission Electron Microscopy* ed S J Pennycook and P D Nellist (New York: Springer) pp 91–115

Newman *et al* 2020 Splenic capture and *in vivo* intracellular biodegradation of biological-grade graphene oxide sheets *ACS Nano* **14** 10168–86

Patra J K, Das G and Fraceto L F *et al* 2018 Nano based drug delivery systems: recent developments and future prospects *J. Nanobiotechnol.* **16** 71

Pennycook S, Lupini A, Albina B, Maria V, Yingquan P, Nellist P, Duscher G, Buczko R and Pantelides S 2003 Transmission electron microscopy: overview and challenges *AIP Conf. Proc.* **683** 627–33

Petrushevska M, Pavlovska K, Laskova J, Zdravkovski P and Dodov M G 2019 Transmission electron microscopy: novel application of established technique in characterization of nanoparticles as drug delivery systems *Prilozi* **40** 67–72

Rajan A, Vilas V and Philip D 2015 Studies on catalytic, antioxidant, antibacterial and anticancer activities of biogenic gold nanoparticles *J. Mol. Liq.* **212** 331–9

Ray S S and Bandyopadhyay J 2021 Nanotechnology-enabled biomedical engineering: Current trends, future scopes, and perspectives *Nanotechnol. Rev.* **10** 728–43

Ray P G, Shreya Biswas T R, Saptarshi Ghosh D M, Piyali Basak S R and Dhara S 2019 Sonication assisted hierarchical decoration of Ag-NP on zinc oxide nanoflower impregnated eggshell membrane: evaluation of antibacterial activity and *in vitro* cytocompatibility *ACS Sustain. Chem. Eng.* **7** 13717–33

Saba H, Kamangar S A, Ahmeda A, Mahdi Zangeneh M and Zangeneh A 2020 Application of copper nanoparticles containing natural compounds in the treatment of bacterial and fungal diseases *Appl. Organomet. Chem.* **34** e5465

Sattler K 2010 *Handbook of Nanophysics, Volume I: Principles and Methods* (Boca Raton, FL: CRC Press)

Shafiee A and Atala A 2017 Tissue engineering: toward a new era of medicine *Annu. Rev. Med.* **68** 29–40

Shi J, Votruba A R, Farokhzad O C and Langer R 2010 Nanotechnology in drug delivery and tissue engineering: from discovery to applications *Nano Lett.* **10** 3223–30

Srijampa S, Buddhisa S, Ngernpimai S, Leelayuwat C, Proungvitaya S, Chompoosor A and Tippayawat P 2020 Influence of gold nanoparticles with different surface charges on localization and monocyte behavior *Bioconjugate Chem.* **31** 1133–43

Verma M S, Chen P Z, Jones L and Gu F X 2015 Controlling 'chemical nose' biosensor characteristics by modulating gold nanoparticle shape and concentration *Sens. Bio-Sens. Res.* **5** 13–8

Verma D S, Khan L U, Kumar S, Khan S B and Sharma S K 2018 *Handbook of Materials Characterization* (Berlin: Springer International Publishing)

Williams D B and Carter C B 2009 Front matter *Transmission Electron Microscopy* (Berlin: Springer)

Xinmin Z, Zhang P, Fu Z, Meng S, Dai L and Yang H 2021 Applications of nanomaterials in tissue engineering *RSC Adv.* **11** 19041–58

Yawei R *et al* 2020 Photoresponsive materials for antibacterial applications *Cell Rep. Phys. Sci.* **1** 100245

IOP Publishing

Analytical Techniques for Biomedical Nanotechnology

Ajeet Kaushik, Sesha S Srinivasan and Yogendra Kumar Mishra

Chapter 13

Energy dispersive spectroscopy for biomedical nanotechnology

Pooja Rawat, Shraddha Dorlikar, Vidhu Malik, Parshant Kumar Sharma and Jong Soo Rhyee

13.1 Introduction

Energy dispersive spectroscopy is an analytical technique used for the elemental analysis of a material and tissues, used as an attachment to electron microscopy, and analysis is based on the emission of characteristic x-rays [1–3]. However, a quick element identification with a high resolution well below 1 μm is feasible with advanced high-sensitivity energy dispersive spectroscopy (EDS) systems. In energy dispersive spectroscopy, the sample under investigation is bombarded with a high-energy beam of light which causes excitation of the inner shell electron ultimately ejecting it and forming a hole or vacancy. When a sample is exposed to a light beam a continuous and characteristic x-ray is emitted. The hole is filled by the electron from a higher energy shell. The electron from thehigher energy shell drops down and fills the hole with a release of energy in the form of an x-ray. The energy released is equal to the difference between the higher energy shell and the ejected electron's shell. The energy dispersive analyzer detects the x-rays, plots them and labels the peak with the elements producing them [4, 5]. It provides the subcellular structure's chemical composition, and helps in the analysis of near-surface elements and also their quantity at different sites providing a map of the sample [6]. The microscopy produces a higher energy electron and the energy of the electron is high enough to remove the electron from the atomic shell of the element. The distinctive x-ray of the specific element generated is dependent on which shell the electron is removed from, and from which shell the electron came to fill the vacancy. The x-ray generated an initial name of the shell from which the electron is ejected is written followed by the number of the shell from which the electron falls to fill the vacancy. The number of the shell above the vacant shell from which the electron is ejected is labeled as α, β, γ, δ, etc. For instance: K_α indicates that the electron is ejected from the K-shell and the

doi:10.1088/978-0-7503-3379-5ch13

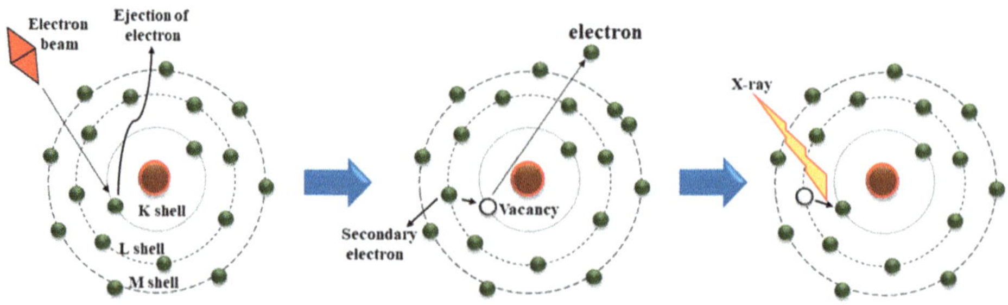

Figure 13.1. Schematic representation of the characteristics of x-ray emission.

electron which fills the hole is from the L-shell (figure 13.1) [7, 8]. In K_{β}, β indicates the electron is from the M-shell. Each element has specific transitions that are possible and are unique. It provides quantitative and qualitative information about the element and compositional data about elements. Therefore, it is possible to identify the element depending on the peak, the bigger the peak the higher the concentration of the element [7].

Since, the ESD can tell which elements are present in the sample under examination, it has use in the biomedical field to study tissue and material. It helps to identify the elements in materials and tissues as according to its principle every element has a unique emission spectrum. It can be used to study nanoparticles and drug delivery, to detect environmental pollutants, and can also be used to detect the accumulation of heavy metals in tissue and also for the characterization of nanoparticles [9]. Due to rapid industrialization environmental pollution has increased. The effluent from factories and industries, from agriculture has led to the accumulation of heavy metals in soil. Since they are not degradable their accumulation in the environment is hazard for the ecosystem. When this heavy metal enters the human body and accumulates in high concentrations it causes various health problems. The accumulation of metals such as mercury and cadmium are responsible for cardiovascular diseases and disorders in children like mental retardation, neurocognitive disorders, behavioral disorders, respiratory problems. These heavy metals can be mutagenic in nature, or may interfere in the biological process. In their study Scimeca *et al* used EDS to detect the accumulation of heavy metals in lung tissues in non-small cell lung cancer and found the presence of elements such as Mn, Co, Pb, and Cr in the lung tissue. Pytlakowska and his group also worked on the detection of heavy metals using MoS_2 decorated grapheme by the energy dispersive x-ray fluorescence spectrometry technique (figure 13.2) [10]. The dispersive micro solid phase extraction (DMSPE)/energy dispersive x-ray fluorescence (EDXRF) procedure might be applied to monitor metal ions in various water samples due to low detection limits varying from 0.07 ng ml^{-1} for Zn(II) to 0.12 ng ml^{-1} for Co(II) and very good precision [10].

Their findings have shed light on the effectiveness of EDS in the study of the composition of tissues and different human organs. EDS analysis was also used to get information about calcification. Calcium is a vital mineral in the human body which is required for various functions, from communication among different

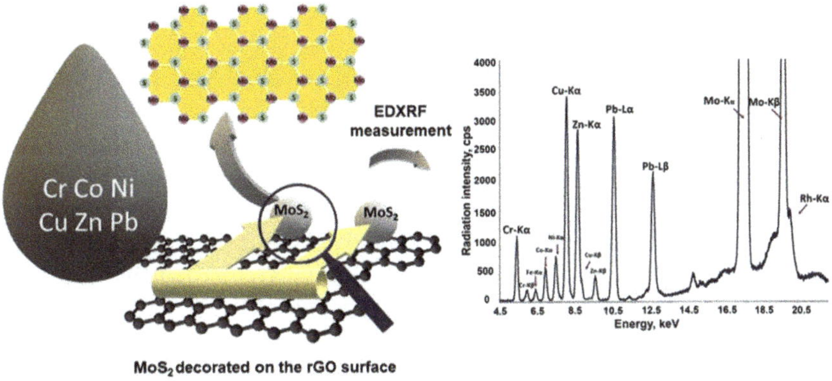

Figure 13.2. Schematic representation of EDXRF measurement for heavy metal ions. Reprinted from [10], Copyright (2020), with permission from Elsevier.

body tissues to maintaining homeostasis. Deposition of this mineral in tissues and organs can lead to various diseases and abnormalities. Calcification is reported to occur in organs such as kidneys, heart, breast, gastrointestinal tract, lungs, stomach, etc [11–13]. EDS analysis was found to be useful to perform elemental analysis of calcification. For instance, Gourgas, *et al* used ESD in their study to confirm whether differences exist in the elemental composition of aortic valve calcification in men and women and found the presence of C, N, O, Ca and P in all the test samples [14].

Nanotechnology is a newly emerging technology which has wide range of applications in various fields, from bio-imaging to drug delivery, in test kits, in food industries, in pharmaceutical industries and in biomarker diagnosis [15, 16]. Nanoparticles have sizes ranging from 1 to 100 nm. The use of nanoparticles has increased in the biomedical field, and by altering their surface properties various nanoparticles can be produced with distinctive applications in biological systems, among these, magnetic nanoparticles have received substantial attention [17, 18]. Nanoparticles are made using organic and inorganic metal liposomes. The nanoparticles made from Ag and Au are widely used in the biomedical field. Au NPs are used in cancer cell imaging and drug targeting and AgNPs are widely used against various microbial infections due to their antimicrobial activity. Due to their small size they can easily gain deep access inside the cell. The use of nanoparticles can cause some harmful effects on living bodies if they accumulate in the body tissue and exceed the safe concentration limit or if they are non-biodegradable. The small size of these particles can have a hazardous effect in the living organism. The toxicity of nanoparticles is dependent on the size, the smaller the size greater the toxicity. The smaller nanoparticles easily gain access to the cell, interfere in normal cellular function and accumulate, ultimately causing toxicity [19, 20]. EDS could have useful application in the biomedical field as it may help to characterize the synthetic NPs and allow the study of the elemental composition as well as obtaining quantitative information of nanoparticles (NP). Gul *et al* synthesized cobalt oxide and cobalt–aluminum oxide nanocrystals and used EDS for their characterization and elemental composition [21]. Hebeish *et al* used EDS in their work where they developed the CMC (carboxy-methyl cellulose) matrix entrapping Ag nanoparticle [22]. Ag nanoparticles are used in various clinical applications as it shows antimicrobial activity but they also show dermal toxicity. They used EDS for qualitative and quantitative elemental analysis. Chen *et al* used EDS to characterize the calcific nodules forms on the valve during calcific aortic valve disease, a cardiovascular disorder [23]. Nanoparticles are widely used for targeted drug delivery in most cancer treatments. Targeted drug delivery using nanoparticles avoids any harm to surrounding normal cells and requires a lower amount of the therapeutic drug. Elbialy *et al* studied *in vivo* targeted drug delivery using magnetic gold nanoparticles loaded with Doxorubicin [24]. In his study he used EDS for elemental analysis of nanoparticles to assure the presence of both iron and gold metals. There are many metals which show toxicity which can be use in beneficial ways. Li *et al* studied the comparative toxicity of Ag and Au nanoparticles and Ag–Au bimetallic nanoparticles on *Daphnia magna* [25]. The toxicity of this nanoparticle, its half-life and concentration inside the body and accumulation is dependent on its shape, size and elemental composition. They used the varying concentration of nanoparticles to check toxicity. In this study, EDS is used for elemental mapping and elemental composition of nanoparticles. Sarecka-Hujar *et al* used EDS for the elemental analysis of pharmaceutical products to investigate their chemical composition and for the presence of the impurities [5]. Ladeira *et al* in their study used EDS to check that the preservation method used to preserve biological samples can also alter the elemental composition of biological tissues [26]. There are various applications in biomedical nanotechnology. In this chapter, all of the fundamental and the applied aspects of EDS analysis in biomedical nanotechnology are briefly discussed.

13.2 General instrumentation

EDS works on the principle that when x-rays fall on a crystal system then they are ionized and free electrons are induced inside the crystal. Thus the crystal becomes conductive and produces an electrical charge separation. Thereby individual x-rays convert into an electrical voltage and produce electrical pulses which give characteristic peaks of every element which are detected by the detector (figure 13.3).

Although EDS analysis does not require any special instrument, typically it is integrated into a scanning electron microscope (SEM) or electron probe micro analysis (EPMA) instrument. It includes an x-ray detector, a Dewar filled with liquid nitrogen for cooling, and software which collects and analyses the energy dispersive spectra.

13.2.1 Detector and its working

As discussed above EDS detectors are integrated with the main instrument (such as SEM or EPMA) and mounted at the end of a long arm inside the sample compartment. In the past decades, EDS detectors were made up of silicon and lithium crystals which were operated at low voltage to achieve results with high

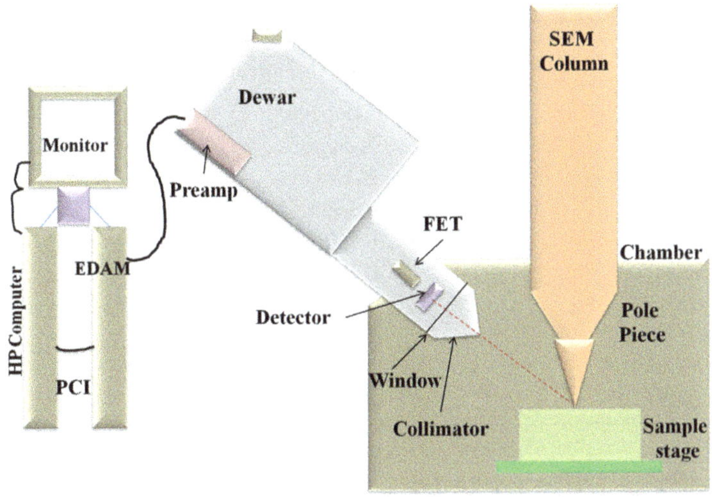

Figure 13.3. Schematic representation of an EDS instrument.

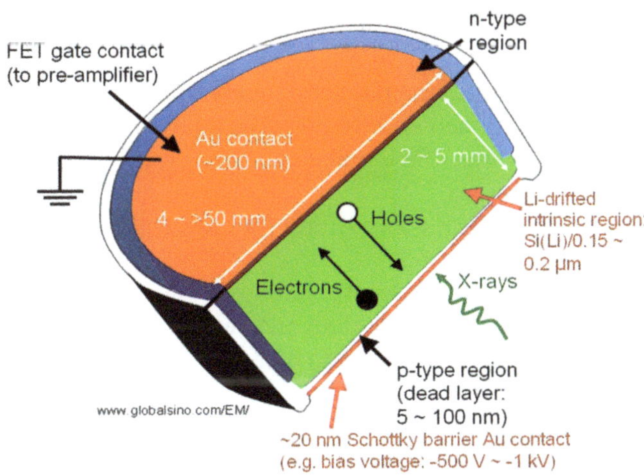

Figure 13.4. Schematic illustration of a lithium-drifted silicon EDS detector (lithium-drifted silicon diodes and Si (Li) EDS detectors practical electron microscopy and database).

sensitivity and also requires liquid nitrogen for cooling purposes (figure 13.4). But nowadays silicon drift detectors are usde since they operate at a high count rate and also do not require liquid nitrogen [25].

Redus *et al* has made a comparative study related to three types of EDS detectors, which are named as follows: (1) silicon drift detector (SDD), (2) silicon photodiode (Si-PIN), and (3) cadmium telluride detector (CdTe) [28]. A combined detector made up of silicon and CdTe is applicable to provide EDS spectra with high resolution for lighter as well as heavier elements [29]. The silicon drift detector

Table 13.1. Characteristic properties of EDS analysis taken from EAG Laboratory instrument.

EDS characteristics	
Primary excitation	Electrons
Detected secondary	X-rays
Elemental range	B-U
Lateral resolution	0.1 μm for SEM-EDS, 1–2 nm STEM-EDS
Detected depth	0.1–3 μm
Detection limit	0.1%–1%
Quantitative?	Yes
Depth profile?	No
Analyze insulator?	Yes
Identify organics?	No

energy dispersive spectrometer (SDD-EDS) works approximately 10 times faster than the usual EDS spectrometer. This detector can detect very high counts (up to 100 000 cps) which is highly recommended for thin biological samples as it will reduce radiation damage [30].

- **Strong points of EDS spectroscopy**:
    1. It provides a full elemental spectrum within few seconds by using 'spot mode'. The obtained spectrum can be analyzed quickly with the help of available software which makes it a great tool for elemental analysis of unidentified phases.
    2. It provides chemical composition (or chemical formula) by operating in 'semi-quantitative mode'.
- **Weak points of EDS spectroscopy**:
    1. In an EDS spectrum more than one peak merges at one point, especially those occurring by the emission of x-rays from K, L, and M shells. These merged peaks can be solved only by de-convoluting the EDS spectrum.
    2. EDS method is insufficient to detect the lightest elements. Especially those that have atomic numbers below carbon (C). Only the polymer-based thin windows can help to detect the lighter elements.
    3. In comparison with EDS, wavelength-dispersive method (WDS) provides results with greater accuracy and precision in chemical elements.

13.2.2 Sample preparation

Generally, all the synthesized samples are associated with a small or large quantity of exogenous and endogenous macromolecules, small molecules and salts. These entities interfere with the spectral analysis, so removal of these extra entities is necessary which requires sample preparation. In particular, EDS does not require any special sample preparation other than SEM or TEM qualitative analysis. However, quantitative analysis in SEM requires a flat, and polished sample.

Although there are several specifications that one should bear in mind for SEM, TEM quantitative analysis which are as follows.

13.2.2.1 Cleaning and drying

Firstly, the sample must be dried and degreased to eliminate surface adsorbed water and organic contamination before measurement. To remove impurities the sample can be washed with volatile solvents as well as with water. Samples should be ultrasonically cleaned when volatile solvents such as methanol, isopropanol, and acetone are used for washing. Whereas samples should always be dried in a hot air oven, after being washed with water.

13.2.2.2 Sample handling

Samples should never be touched without wearing gloves, sample holders, sample exchange tools, and sample stubs. All of the sample tools should be kept on a clean paper during sample preparation.

13.2.2.3 Sample mounting

There are various specifications as different types of sample need different sample mounting and preparation techniques which are employed as follows.

13.2.2.3.1 Case 1: conductive powder samples

Mounting of powder samples is not easy, they require special mounting techniques otherwise they may become loose and fly off under the vacuum and electron beam. One method is that a very small amount of the powder sample can be dispersed in a volatile solvent and a few drops of the suspension can be drop-cast on a neat and clean substrate and dried completely. Another way, is that a large amount of the sample is compressed into a small disk before mounting. The use of carbon or copper conducting adhesive tapes is necessary to mount the powder samples. The sample must be spread with the help of a spatula and it should be pressed very lightly to seat it. Then the sample holder is tilted a little and is tapped to remove the loose material.

13.2.2.3.2 Case 2: less conductive powder samples

In case of less or non-conducting samples, due to the charge effect, drift in images may occur [29]. Therefore, in order to reduce the charge effect one should apply a low acceleration voltage or for the complete removal of the charge effect the sample must be coated with a conductive coating. Coating should be done using a sputtering coater with a thickness of several nanometers. Finally, at the end the sample must be mounted on a sample holder using conductive carbon, copper tapes, or silver paints.

13.2.2.3.3 Case 3: biological samples

1. **Nanoparticle samples:** Drying of nanoparticles is quite tedious since during the drying process surface tension increases and facilitates aggregate formation. Therefore, the use of volatile solvents (such as ethanol) under

sonication is a better approach for fast-drying and to notice individual nanoparticles.

2. **Hydrogel samples:** The sample preparation of hydrogels requires a freeze drying process which is known as 'lyophilization'. This is a low temperature drying process [32].
3. **Bacterial samples:** Preparation of biological or biomedical samples requires appropriate buffers or distilled water to clean the samples. For vigorous cleaning of the samples a surfactant can also be used [27].
4. **Plant samples:** To identify plant sample we should cut a leaf approx 1 mm × 1 mm or 5 mm × 5 mm, i.e., as small as possible and then it should be kept on a metallic sample holder using double sided adhesive electric conducting carbon tape [33].

   Note: if a white color image is observed under SEM measurement then it is due to charge effect and the measurement conditions should be varied as follows:

   (i) electron beam can be reduced
   (ii) magnification can be made smaller
   (iii) move the electron beam position nearer to the edge of leaf

   By applying the above measurement conditions charging from the sample can be reduced or removed. If still there is some charging, then few drops of the diluted ionic liquid can be used but there is no need to apply any carbon or gold coating [27, 33].
5. **Agrochemical samples:** Analysis of agrochemicals adsorbed on plant surfaces is very tedious. It first requires the testing of organic and inorganic pesticides using fruit cuticles then a few droplets are deposited on the plant surface and subjected to EDS analysis (0.5–1.0 μl) [36].
6. **Soil samples:** To observe the chemical and mineralogical changes in soil, first one should take samples from the surface, and then a size variant slide should be prepared by embedding the samples into resin. Only then a full picture of the material can be seen which will provide good qualitative and quantitative information of the sample [37].

The major problem in the EDS analysis of biological samples is its three-dimensional nature, as EDX can only sit at one position in the microscope chamber. The curved or uneven sample arrangement causes artificial shadows in the EDS region and this results in lower count rates compared to normal sample analysis. Use of low accelerating voltage and reducing the beam-sample interaction will be beneficial to avoid sample damage.

According to the sample specification, the *in situ* preparation of the sample can be controlled. The extended low temperature method (ELTM) in an environmental scanning electron microscope for the *in situ* plant sample preparation enables monotonous topographical and material analysis at a higher resolution in the vacuum or low gas pressure conditions of an environmental scanning electron microscope (figure 13.5) [38].

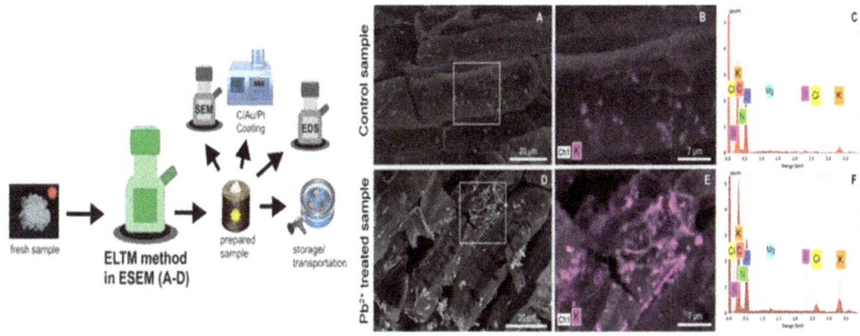

Figure 13.5. Schematic representation of ELTM method and SEM-EDX analysis of cells of cannabis roots cultivated in a heavy metal-free medium as well as exposed to Pb^{2+} ions. Reproduced from [38]. CC BY 4.0.

The SEM image quality and EDS analysis are strongly dependent on the working conditions; however, a high irregularity of environmental scanning electron microscopy (ESEM) parameters, such as freezing velocity, temperature, and humidity can be found and arranged. Although this process has many limitations, like the surface microstructure is well protected with the least artefacts and without any time consuming and expensive chemical treatments. ELTM provides an effective, fast, and economical *in situ* biological sample preparation which allows repetitive observation and elemental analysis.

13.3 EDX result analysis for some biological identities

Energy dispersive x-ray spectroscopy (EDX) microanalysis is a surface technique based on the characteristic x-ray emission of the sample by the incident of a beam of electrons [1–3]. It can scan the surface structure of the respective material at nano and micro scale depending on the typeof material such as inorganic materials (minerals, chalcogenides, heavy elements, ceramics, composites) and organic materials (membrane, polymers, tissues, cell, enzymes) [39]. Although the EDX technique requires standardization using a standard specimen is complicated to achieve. So, very few groups are using this technique for identification and analysis of the elemental composition of a given sample. In the case of biological specimens, the high moisture content requires very extensive studies on sample preparation so that it can resist the high vacuum conditions during scanning electron microscopy-energy dispersive X-ray spectroscopy (SEM-EDX) analysis. The three-dimensional nature of biological samples complicates the collection of EDS data as EDS detectors only sit to one side of the microscope chamber [9, 40]. The curved or rough surface samples create an artificial shadowing where the emitted x-rays aside from the detector are likely to be absorbed by the sample and it leads to a decrease in the electron count rates as compared with the side facing the detector. This will result in artefacts in the elemental maps of the sample, especially for elements with low energy x-rays. A best sample option is a flat surface to get superior quality EDS analysis. Indeed, for sample preparation in biological samples, other difficulties are linked with the cytostatic technique.

In this section, we will explore both outputs of capturing image and scanning EDX by taking different examples of biological samples for qualitative and quantitative analysis, respectively. Biological samples having heavy elements give high detection limits because of the higher background. There are a variety of examples related to EDX detection of biological samples, but here our focus is on the application of EDX analysis on tissue engineering, heavy elements detection, and in nanotechnology.

13.3.1 Application of EDS analysis in tissue engineering for element detection

There are three main points used in tissue engineering, the first is that there are certain requirements fulfilled by the scaffolds made up of biomaterials, second, stimulating signals from cells, and third, growth, which are known as the triad of tissue engineering [41, 42]. EDX is one of the most valuable techniques in tissue engineering and is related to detection of pathologically deposited materials. Petechia *et al* show the SEM mapping with EDX analysis to demonstrate the presence of calcium deposits in a BM-hMSCs sample [43]. The homogeneous distribution of elements like calcium (B), phosphorus (C) and overlapped calcium–phosphorus (D) shown in the EDX mapping relative to the picture in (A) is shown in figure 13.6.

The abnormal deposition of tissue calcium, iron salt or any other mineral salt is defined as a pathologic calcification. These primary changes in the tissue may occur in various part of the body like the breasts [44, 45], joints [46], cartilage [47], cardiac valves [45, 48], brain [44, 50], gallbladder [51], thyroid [52, 53] and many others which affect new borns, adults, and fetuses [54]. Thus, it is necessary to interpret all the physicochemical processes involved in the abnormal deposition of material and

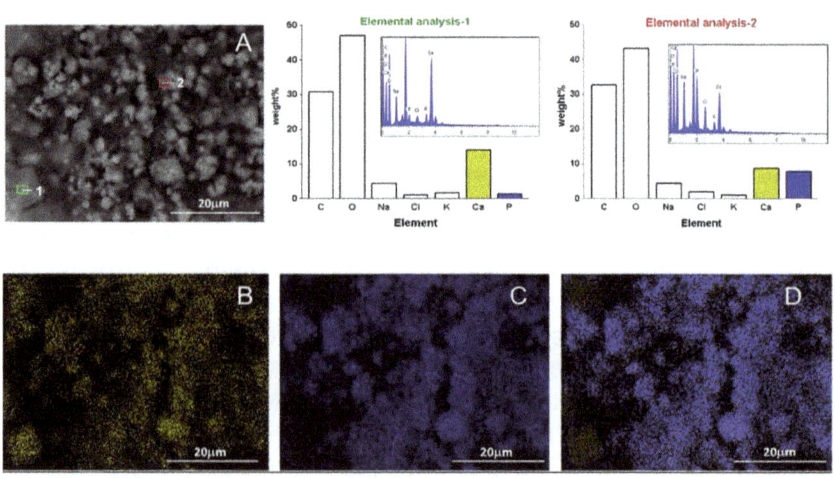

Figure 13.6. SEM image present different Ca^{2+} source deposits in BM-hMSCs treated with ODM (ODM^{+}/PEMF−) for 27 days. Elemental analyses 1 and 2 represent the area emphasized in image (A), respectively regarding small amorphous particle and big crystal-like particles. The percentage weights of each element of the spectra are summarized in the related histograms, Reproduced from [43]. CC BY 4.0.

the detection of these minerals is also necessary. In this regard, the application of EDX microanalysis for elemental detection of different calcification isotypes provides extra information about linkage between disease and calcification.

Other than this EDX also possesses noteworthy advances on the calcification effect and the knowledge of molecular process. Sonou *et al* using the SEM-EDX for the first time reported the exact chemical composition analysis of aortic medial calcification. The best part of this research is that before this study there was no report related to the exact composition determination of medial calcification [55]. To establish a fruitful relationship with diseases, different aspects of such calcifications must be taken into account. The SEM-EDX results of Marra *et al* showed the same chemical composition of the interior as well as of the mineral deposit [56]. Schmid *et al* reported that carbonates (9%), apatite (71%), and a high percentage of protein (15%) were present in the plaque calcifications [57]. Lara *et al* studied the genesis and composition of calcium deposits in atheroma plaques.

In particular, they used the SEM-EDX as the first and foremost step to establish the genesis of these deposits by determining the mineral and organic constituents of atheroma [58]. In other reports, EDX has also been applied during postembryonic and embryonic growth for the examination of bone matrix calcification [43]. In the same direction, Okata *et al* used a standardized rat calvarial bone defect model and investigated the process of calcification during bone healing. Because of the EDX analysis, it is possible to examine the rat's calvarias at 1, 2, 4, and 8 weeks, demonstrating that calcification of bone healing was not completed but that it proceeds gradually [59]. EDX microanalysis can also be applied for the identification of micro-HA crystal obtained from osteoblast cultures [60].

Recently, first time TEM-EDX microanalysis analyzed the elemental detection of micro calcifications and explained the presence of magnesium-substituted HA (Mg-HA) in breast micro calcifications [61]. It should be considered and underlined that the calcification complex form (HA and Mg-HA) are strongly related to malignant lesions whereas benign lesions mainly reported CO. Mg-HA micro calcifications were mostly recognized in breast cancers. All these reports enable the significance of EDX microanalysis to be interpreted in the study of many pathologies related to the calcification process.

13.3.2 Role of EDS analysis in nanotechnology

In the last decade, the controlled synthesis of nanoparticles has enabled the use of nanoparticles in various applications like drug delivery, diagnostic tests, biomedical engineering, etc. The premier food and drug controller agencies like the united states FDA (Food and Drug Administration) has also approved several nanoparticle-based products. Thus, it has become essential to understand the biological response of nanoparticles in order to ascertain their safe use limits [62].

In particular, nanoparticles of silver (Ag NPs) and gold (Au NPs) are being explored for a wide range of applications. The Ag NPs are found to be advantageous for applications in textiles, wound dressing, etc owing to their antimicrobial properties. Ag NPs have also been explored for applications in the food industry,

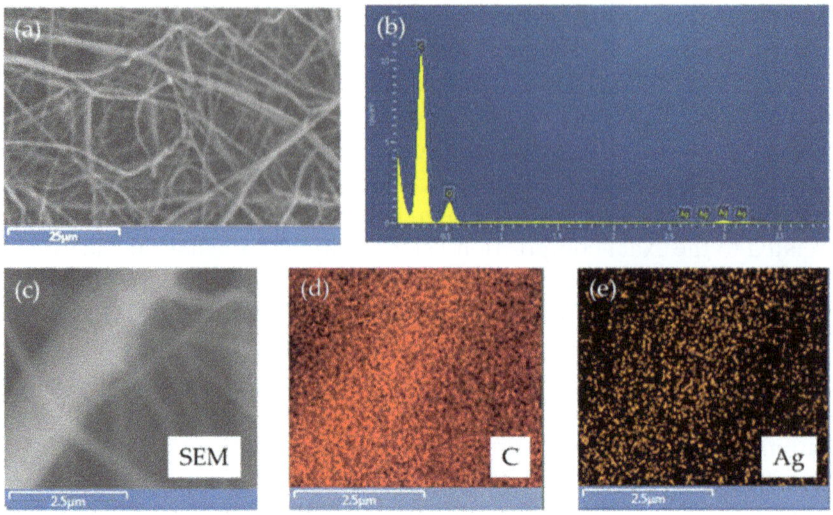

Figure 13.7. (a) SEM image, (b) EDS analysis, (c–e) SEM and elemental mapping of Ag-coated PCL samples measured at 5 kV operating voltage. Reproduced from [69]. CC BY 4.0.

foils and containers with incorporated AgNPs for the packaging and processong of food, or kitchenware coated with AgNPs, and use in health supplements, etc [63, 64]. Au NPs, are being explored for biological diagnostics [65], cell tracers [66], drug delivery [67] and cell imaging [68]. The addition of Ag in poly caprolactone (PCL) scaffolds by sputtering deposition provides successful antibacterial properties. SEM-EDS results show the deposition of Ag nanoparticles on polymer fibers without undergoing any morphological changes in the fiber after the deposition process (figure 13.7) [69].

Nanoparticles have also been found to be advantageous for use in drug delivery and vaccines because they provide protection of payloads from metabolism and also because of their target specificity [70].

For their potential biomedical applications, the toxicity analysis of nanoparticles must first be performed and the biocompatibility ascertained and understood in detail. Also, the process by which cells internalize the nanoparticles needs to be understood. For this, Motskin *et al* used the SEM/EDX to study the sequestration of HS NPs by human monocyte-macrophages in a compartment that allows free diffusion with the extracellular environment [71]. Similarly, Walczak *et al* used the SEM/EDX to characterize the morphology and elemental composition and investigated the behavior of 60 nm Ag NPs and Ag^+ ions obtained from $AgNO_3$ in an *in vitro* model of human gastrointestinal digestion [72]. Jimeno-Romero *et al* investigated the cell and tissue distribution, bioaccumulation, and biological effects of disodium laureth sulfosuccinate (DSLS)-stabilized TiO_2 NPs in marine mussels (*Mytilus galloprovincialis*) by using ultrastructural observations and EDX micro-analysis [73]. In another interesting study, by using the SEM/EDX, Brule *et al* demonstrated that the oral exposure of Ag NPs with human relevant doses can induce microbial alterations in the human gut [74]. The EDX analysis was fundamental for all these investigations.

13.3.3 Detection of heavy elements in biological samples

The growth of industrialization at a rapid rate in the recent past has also increased the environmental pollution due to the release of toxic materials [75]. The heavy metals which are generally released from industries are non-biodegradable and can easily accumulate in ecological systems. Even, trace amounts of some heavy elements have been found to be lethal and toxic with teratogenic, mutagenic, endocrine features. The heavy metals have been also shown to induce behavioral and neurological disorders among children and infants [76, 77]. Among the heavy elements, cadmium (Cd), chromium (Cr), copper (Cu), lead (Pb), nickel (Ni), and zinc (Zn) are highly relevant pollutants due to their increasing presence in the environment, non-degradability, and toxicity [78].

Tszydel *et al* reported the EDX analysis of heavy metals in anal papillae of *Hydropsyche angustipennis* larvae [79]. Using EDX analysis they investigated the morphological abnormality in the anal papillae of *H. angustipennis* because of heavy metal pollution in urban areas. In the laboratory, before heavy metal evaluation, larvae were photographed for anal papillae morphological comparisons. As the contamination increases, papillae start to generate and begin to appear outside as white or pale finger-shaped structures (figure 13.8). The presence of heavy metal was

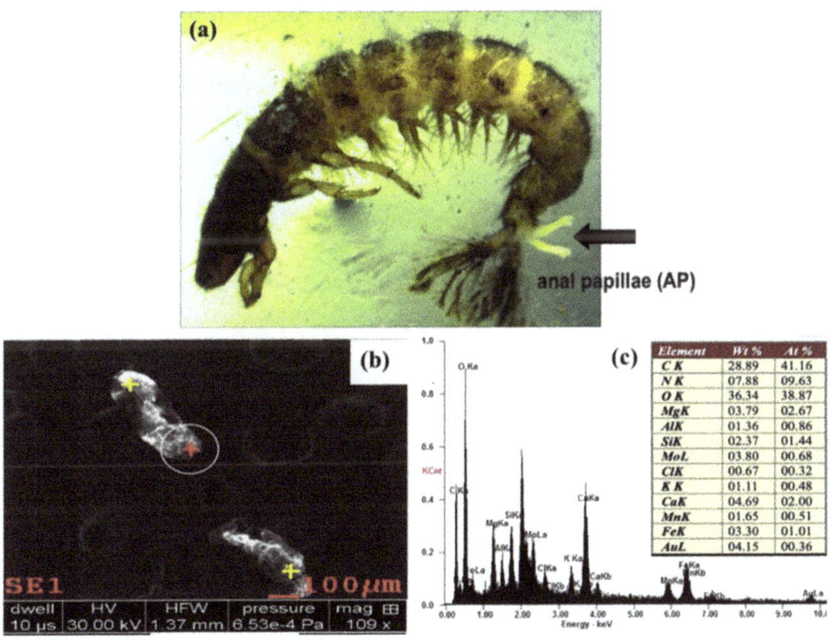

Figure 13.8. (a) Location of anal papillae, (b) SEM photomicrographs and (c) EDX analysis of *H. angustipennis* anal papillae. Reproduced from [79].

monitored by using EDS analysis of *H. angustipennis* anal papillae (figures 13.8(a) and (b)).

The accumulation of heavy metals in tissues can be investigated by EDX microanalysis. Also, EDX is useful in forensic sciences to detect the presence of metals or powders that settle on the clothing or skin. The morphological and chemical examinations of the primer residue particles from firearm discharge can be performed with SEM/EDX analysis [78]. Ferraro *et al* investigated the impact of heavy metal sediment particles from the Reconquista river (RR-PM, one of the most polluted watercourses in Argentina), on the respiratory system of BALB/c mice. The authors studied how this pollution induces lung inflammation in mice [81]. The identification of these toxic elements in lung tissues *ex vivo* can provide detailed insights into the environmental impact on lung carcinogenesis.

In a study, Scimeca *et al* reported whether the accumulation of heavy metals in bone tissues is a reason behind the change in an osteoporotic patient's architecture and bone metabolism. They demonstrated the accumulation of Pb, Cr, and Cd in trabecular head biopsies by using SEM/EDX microanalysis [82]. The EDX microanalysis is widely used for the investigations into heavy metal pollution and its effects on living organisms and the environment. In urban air quality, the presence of Fe, CrMn, and Mn in higher concentrations than the average are detected by SEM/EDX microanalysis [79].

13.3.4 EDX analysis of living (wet) plants and animal using the 'NanoSuit' method

NanoSuit is defined as a simple surface modification which prevents evaporation of liquids or gases present in small biological samples under high vacuum conditions in a field emission-scanning electron microscope (FE-SEM) [83]. Using this method, multicellular species can be kept alive/wet by encasing them in a thin, vacuum-proof membrane within an electron microscope under a high vacuum [84]. The method uses the native extracellular substance (ECS) or any mimicking ECS substance to polymerize a membrane using electron beam or plasma irradiation. The NanoSuits used for the prevention of living organism bodies by a dense and flexible surface also called the 'surface shield enhancer' (SSE). It works like a tiny spacesuit with sufficient electron conductivity for an SEM analysis. Thus, the NanoSuit method allows high-resolution imaging of a wet specimen, both living and fixed using SEM spectroscopy. Takatu *et al* studied the EDS analysis of a wet sample of a living drosophila larva and aloe arborescent using the conventional method and the NanoSuit method presented in figure 13.9 [85].

However, to achieve a high resolution in EDS requires multistage scanning of the sample. Thus a dynamic EDS analysis has not been reported until now. If the specimen moves at the time of measurement, a blurred region appears on the obtained image. Because of this, species with no movement during experimentation give good EDS analysis results. A high intense oxygen peak in the NanoSuit protected sample compared with the conventionally prepared sample results from the presence of water in living organisms.

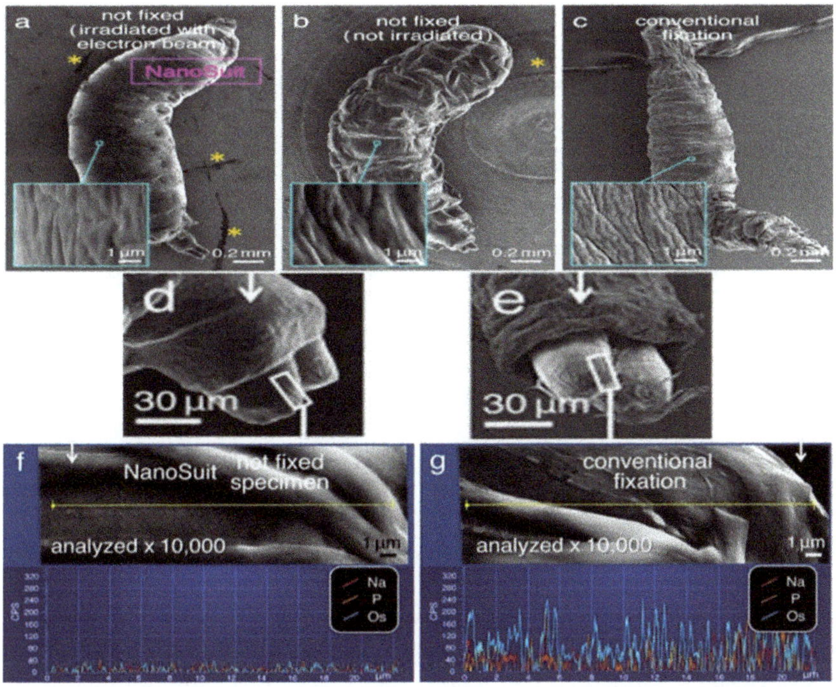

Figure 13.9. (a–c) SEM image of *Drosophila* sample prepared by, (a) living larva examined by the NanoSuit method using electron beam radiation for 60 min, (b) living larva sample without electron beam radiation, (c) sample prepared by conventional fixation method, (d–g) EDX line scan analysis for two different types of sample preparation. Reproduced from [85]. CC BY 4.0.

Takehara *et al* tested in the presenec of a NanoSuit layer formed on living petals using SEM analysis. These samples were placed for 20 min in the SEM observation chamber under an identical vacuum level, but without electron beam radiation [86]. The results suggest that, with the help of electron beam energy, living petals show the ability to allow high vacuum environments, assuming the outer surface substance of petals turn into a NanoSuit in the same way as animal ECS. There is no weight loss for the specimens made by conventional methods during SEM observations, as already 80% weight lost during sample preparation. Thus, the NanoSuit method represents a novel approach that will advance the field of histology.

13.4 Conclusion and future prospects

In this chapter, the basic principle of EDS analysis has been outlined. EDS detects the unique x-rays for analysis. EDS analysis can be useful tool

1. To identify different calcification isotype and give information on how it is related to the disease.
2. To detect heavy metals and minerals as well as mineral impurity in the biological sample such as in tissues and in different body organs.

3. To analyze the pharmaceutical products for their chemical composition and impurities.
4. To study the nanoparticles, their toxicity, and their biocompatibility.

Acknowledgement

The authors thank their respective universities for supporting their work. Pooja Rawat thanks the Brain Pool Program through the National Research Foundation of Korea (NRF) funded by the Ministry of Science and ICT (NRF-2019H1D3A1A01070741).

References

[1] Baydar S V, Oztel O N, Koc R B and Candayan A 2017 *Nano-Biomaterials Science, Development and Evaluation, Evolution Techniques* (Amsterdam: Elsevier) pp 211–32

[2] Echlin P 2009 *Handbook of Sample Preparation for Scanning Electron Microscopy and X-Ray Microanalysis* (New York: Springer)

[3] Avula A, Galor A, Blackwelder P, Carballosa-Gautam M, Hackam A S, Jeng B and Kumar N 2017 Application of scanning electron microscopy with energy-dispersive X-ray spectroscopy for analyzing ocular surface particles on schirmer strips *Cornea* **36** 752–6

[4] Goldstein J 2003 *Scanning Electron Microscopy and X-Ray Microanalysis* (Berlin: Springer)

[5] Sarecka-Hujar B, Balwierz R, Ostrozka-Cieslik A, Dyja R, Lukowiec D and Jankowski A 2017 Scanning electron microscopy and X-ray energy dispersive spectroscopy – useful tools in the analysis of pharmaceutical products *IOP Conf. Ser.: J. Phys.* **931** 012008

[6] Yesilkir-baydar S, Oztel O N, Cakir-koc R and Candayan A 2017 Evaluation techniques *Nano-Biomaterials Science, Development and Evaluation* (Amsterdam: Elsevier) pp 211–32

[7] Wyroba E, Suski S, Miller K and Bartosiewicz R 2015 Biomedical and agricultural applications of energy dispersive X-ray spectroscopy in electron microscopy *Cellular Molecul. Biol. Lett.* **20** 28

[8] Morita M 2018 Scanning electron microscope energy dispersive X-ray spectrometry *Compendium of Surface and Interface Analysis* (Berlin: Springer) pp 557–61

[9] Scimeca M, Bischetti S, Lamsira H K, Bonfiglio R and Bonanno E 2018 Energy dispersive X-ray (EDX) microanalysis: a powerful tool in biomedical research and diagnosis *Eur. J. Histochem.* **62** 2841

[10] Pytlakowska K, Kocot K, Hachuła B, Pilch M, Wrzalik R and Zubko R 2020 Determination of heavy metal ions by energy dispersive X-ray fluorescence spectrometry using reduced graphene oxide decorated with molybdenum disulfide as solid adsorbent *Spectrochim. Acta* B **167** 1–12

[11] Georg S, Ralf W, Vincent B and Markus K 2007 Inhibitors of calcification in blood and urine *Semin. Dial.* **20** 113–21

[12] Francis H 1918 Extensive calcification of the lungs as a distinct disease *Arch. Intern. Med.* **1** 139–46

[13] Urena T P A and Marc D B 2012 Calcium-sensing receptor, calcimimetics, and cardiovascular calcifications in chronic kidney disease *Kidney Int.* **82** 19–25

[14] Gourgas O, Khan K, Schwertani A and Cerruti M 2020 Differences in mineral composition and morphology between men and women in aortic valve calcification *Acta Biomater.* **106** 342–50

[15] Sharma P K, Dorlikar S, Rawat P, Malik V, Vats N and Sharma M *et al* 2021 *Nanotechnology and Its Application: A Review, Nanotechnology in Cancer Management* (Amsterdam: Elsevier) pp 1–33
[16] Mishra S, Kim E-S, Sharma P K, Wang Z-J, Yang S-H, Kaushik A K, Wang C, Yang L and Kim N-Y 2020 Tailored biofunctionalized biosensor for the label-free sensing of prostate-specific antigen *ACS Appl. Bio Mater.* **11** 7821–30
[17] Issa B, Obaidat I M, Albiss B A and Haik Y 2013 Magnetic nanoparticles: surface effects and properties related to biomedicine applications *Int. J. Mol. Sci.* **14** 21266–305
[18] Ramos A P, Cruzl M A E, Tovani C B and Ciancaglini P 2017 Biomedical applications of nano-technology *Biophys. Rev.* **9** 79–89
[19] Voinov M, Paga´n J O S, Morrison E, Smirnova T I and Smirnov A I 2010 Surface-mediated production of hydroxyl radicals as a mechanism of iron oxide nanoparticle biotoxicity *J. Am. Chem. Soc.* **133** 2011
[20] Bahadar H, Maqbool F, Niaz K and Abdollahi M 2015 Toxicity of nanoparticles and an overview of current experimental models *Iran. Biomed. J.* **20** 1–11
[21] Gul I, Khan S M, Mehmood T, Ahmad Z, Badshah H and Shah H 2020 Characterization of cobalt oxide and calcium–aluminum oxide nano-catalyst through scanning electron microscopy, X-ray diffraction, and energy dispersive X-ray spectroscopy *Microsc. Res. Tech.* **83** 1124–31
[22] Hebeish A, Hashem M, Abd El-Hady M M and Sharaf S 2013 Development of CMC hydrogels loaded with silver nano-particles for medical applications *Carbohydr. Polym.* **92** 407–13
[23] Chen J, Peacock J R, Branch J and Merryman W D 2015 Biophysical analysis of dystrophic and osteogenic models of valvular calcification *J. Biomech. Eng.* **137** 020903
[24] Elbialy N, Fathy M M and Khalil W M 2015 Doxorubicin loaded magnetic gold nanoparticles for *in vivo* targeted 2 drug delivery *Int. J. Pharm.* **490** 1–10
[25] Li T, Albee B, Alemayehu M, Diaz R, Ingham L, Kamal S, Rodriguez M and Bishnoi S W 2010 Comparative toxicity study of Ag, Au, and Ag–Au bimetallic nanoparticles on *Daphnia magna Anal. Bioanal. Chem.* **398** 689–700
[26] Ladeira L C M, Santos E C, Valente G E, Silva J D, Santos T A and Maldonado I R S C 2019 Could biological tissue preservation methods change chemical elements proportion measured by energy dispersive X-ray spectroscopy? *Biol. Trace Element Res* **196** 168–72
[27] Wyroba E, Suski S, Miller K and Bartosiewicz R 2015 Biomedical and agricultural applications of energy dispersive X-ray spectroscopy in electron microscopy *Cell. Mol. Biol. Lett.* **20** 488–509
[28] Redus R H, Huber A C, Pantazis J A and Pantazis T J 2011 Enhanced energy range thermoelectrically cooled silicon X-ray detectors *2011 IEEE Nuclear Science Symp. Conf. Record* pp 580–5
[29] Redus R and Huber A 2012 Figure of merit for spectrometers for EDXRF *X-Ray Spectrom* **41** 401–9
[30] Strüder L, Fiorini C, Gatti E, Hartmann R, Holl P, Krause N and Lechner P *et al* 1998 High resolution non dispersive X-ray spectroscopy with state of the art silicon detectors *Mikrochim. Acta Suppl* **15** 11–9
[31] Khan M S I, Oh S W and Kim Y J 2020 Power of scanning electron microscopy and energy dispersive X-ray analysis in rapid microbial detection and identification at the single cell level *Sci. Rep.* **10** 2368

[32] Sakatoku S, Imashuku S and Kawai J 2012 Effect of charging on EDX spectra in SEM-EDX analysis *Adv. X-Ray. Chem. Anal* **43** 453–7

[33] Swerts J, Espen P V and Geladi P 1993 Partial least squares techniques in the energy-dispersive x-ray fluorescence determination of sulfur-graphite mixtures *Anal. Chem.* **65** 1181–5

[34] Imashuku S, Kawakami T, Ze L and Kawai J 2012 Possibility of scanning electron microscope observation and energy dispersive X-ray analysis in microscale region of insulating samples using diluted ionic liquid *Microsc. Microanal.* **18** 365–70

[35] Ansari I, Sundararajan M, Kumar R, Sharma S and Arora C 2020 SEM-EDX: a potential tool for studies medicinal plants *Essential Techniques for Medical and Life Scientists* (Hoboken, NJ: Wiley) pp 124–41

[36] Hunsche M and Noga G 2009 Spatially resolved quantification of agrochemicals on plant surfaces using energy dispersive X-ray microanalysis *Pest. Manag. Sci.* **65** 1352–9

[37] Gutiérrez-Ginés M J, Pastor J and Hernández A J 2012 Integrated approach to assessing the effects of soils polluted with heavy metals on a plant population *Ecotoxicology* **21** 1965–78

[38] Tihlaříková E, Neděla V and Đorđević B 2019 In-situ preparation of plant samples in ESEM for energy dispersive x-ray microanalysis and repetitive observation in SEM and ESEM *Sci. Rep.* **9** 2300

[39] Mishra R K, Zachariah A K and Thomas S 2017 *Microscopy Methods in Nanomaterials Characterization, Energy-Dispersive X-ray Spectroscopy Techniques for Nanomaterial* (Amsterdam: Elsevier) pp 383–405

[40] Pirozzi N M, Kuipers J and Giepmans B N G 2020 Correlative light and electron microscopy IV *Sample Preparation for Energy Dispersive X-Ray Imaging of Biological Tissues* (New York: Springer) pp 90–111

[41] Chan B P and Leong K W 2008 Scaffolding in tissue engineering: general approaches and tissue specific considerations *Eur. Spine J.* **17** S467–79

[42] Lanza R, Langer R, Vacanti J P and Atala A 2020 *Principles of Tissue Engineering* 4th edn (New York: Elsevier Academic)

[43] Petecchia L, Sbrana F and Utzeri R *et al* 2015 Electro-magnetic field promotes osteogenic differentiation of BM-hMSCs through a selective action on Ca^{2+}-related mechanisms *Sci. Rep.* **5** 13856

[44] Henrot P, Leroux A, Barlier C and Génin P 2014 Breast microcalcifications: the lesions in anatomical pathology *Diagn. Interv. Imaging* **95** 141–52

[45] Trenson S and de Ceuninck M 2014 A calcified left ventricular mass *Acta Cardiol.* **69** 316–8

[46] Ando M, Bando H, Endo T, Ichihara S, Hashimoto E and Hyodo K *et al* 2008 Refraction-based 2D, 2.5D and 3D medical imaging: stepping forward to a clinical trial *Eur. J. Radiol.* **68** S32–6

[47] Gutierrez M, Di Geso L, Salaffi F, Carotti M, Girolimetti R and De Angelis R *et al* 2014 Ultrasound detection of cartilage calcification at knee level in calcium pyrophosphate deposition disease *Arthritis Care Res. (Hoboken)* **66** 69–73

[48] Okada Y 2013 Surgical management of mitral annular calcification *Gen. Thorac. Cardiovasc. Surg.* **61** 619–25

[49] Betsholtz C and Keller A 2014 PDGF, pericytes and the pathogenesis of idiopathic basal ganglia calcification (IBGC) *Brain Pathol.* **24** 387–95

[50] McCartney E and Squier W 2014 Patterns and pathways of calcification in the developing brain *Dev. Med. Child Neurol.* **56** 1009–15

[51] Chen M Y, Bechtold R E, Bohrer S P, Zagoria R J and Dyer R B 1999 Abnormal calcification on plain radiographs of the abdomen *Crit. Rev. Diagn. Imaging* **40** 63–202

[52] Wang Z, Zhang H, Zhang P, He L and Dong W 2014 Diagnostic value of ultrasound-detected calcification in thyroid nodules *Ann. Acad. Med. Singap.* **43** 102–6
[53] Lee J, Lee S Y, Cha S H, Cho B S, Kang M H and Lee O J 2013 Fine-needle aspiration of thyroid nodules with macrocalcification *Thyroid* **23** 1106–12
[54] McCarty M F and Di Nicolantonio J J 2014 The molecular biology and pathophysiology of vascular calcification *Postgrad. Med.* **126** 54–64
[55] Sonou T, Ohya M, Yashiro M, Masumoto A, Nakashima Y and Ito T *et al* 2015 Mineral composition of phosphate-induced calcification in a rat aortic tissue culture model *J. Atheroscler. Thromb.* **22** 1197–206
[56] Marra S P, Daghlian C P, Fillinger M F and Kennedy F E 2006 Elemental composition, morphology and mechanical properties of calcified deposits obtained from abdominal aortic aneurysms *Acta Biomater.* **2** 515–20
[57] Schmid K, McSharry W O, Pameijer C H and Binette J P 1980 Chemical and physiochemical studies on the mineral deposits of the human atherosclerotic aorta *Atherosclerosis* **37** 199–210
[58] Lara M J, Ros E, Sierra M, Dorronsoro C and Aguilar J 2014 Composition and genesis of calcium deposits in atheroma plaques *Ultrastruct. Pathol.* **38** 167–77
[59] Okata H, Nakamura M, Henmi A, Yamaguchi S, Mikami Y and Shimauchi H *et al* 2015 Calcification during bone healing in a standardized rat calvarial defect assessed by micro-CT and SEM-EDX *Oral Dis.* **21** 74–82
[60] Scimeca M, Salustri A, Bonanno E, Nardozi D, Rao C and Piccirilli E *et al* 2017 Impairment of PTX3 expression in osteoblasts: a key element for osteoporosis *Cell Death Discov.* **8** e3125
[61] Scimeca M, Bonfiglio R, Montanaro M and Bonanno E 2018 Osteoblast-like cells in human cancers: new cell type and reliable markers for bone metastasis *Future Oncol* **14** 9–11
[62] De Jong W H and Borm P J A 2008 Drug delivery and nanoparticles: applications and hazards *Int. J. Nanomed.* **3** 133–49
[63] Bouwmeester H 1, Dekkers S, Noordam M Y, Hagens W I, Bulder A S and de Heer C *et al* 2009 Review of health safety aspects of nanotechnologies in food production *Regul. Toxicol. Pharmacol.* **53** 52–62
[64] Rai M, Yadav A and Gade A 2009 Silver nanoparticles as a new generation of antimicrobials *Biotechnol. Adv.* **27** 76–83
[65] Storhoff J J and Mirkin C A 1999 Programmed materials synthesis with DNA *Chem. Rev.* **99** 1849–62
[66] Yi H, Leunissen J L M, Shi G M, Gutekunst C A and Hersch S M 2001 A novel procedure for pre-embedding double immunogold-silver labeling at the ultrastructural level *J. Histochem. Cytochem.* **49** 279–83
[67] Voskerician G, Shive M S, Shawgo R S, von Recum H, Anderson J M and Cima M J *et al* 2003 Biocompatibility and biofouling of MEMS drug delivery devices *Biomaterials* **24** 1959–67
[68] Sharma P, Brown S C, Bengtsson N, Zhang Q, Walter G A and Grobmyer S R *et al* 2008 Gold-speckled multimodal nanoparticles for noninvasive bioimaging *Chem. Mater.* **20** 6087–94
[69] Valerini D, Tammaro L, Vitali R, Guillot G and Rinaldi A 2021 Sputter-deposited Ag nanoparticles on electro spun PCL scaffolds: morphology, wettability and antibacterial activity *Coatings* **11** 345
[70] Glass J J, Yuen D, Rae J, Johnston A P, Parton R G and Kent S J *et al* 2016 Human immune cell targeting protein nanoparticles – caveospheres *Nanoscale* **8** 8255–65
[71] Motskin M, Müller K H, Genoud C, Monteith A G and Skepper J N 2011 The sequestration of hydroxyapatite nanoparticles by human monocyte macrophages in a compartment that allows free diffusion with the extracellular environment *Biomaterials* **32** 9470–82

[72] Walczak A P, Fokkink R, Peters R, Tromp P, Herrera Rivera Z E and Rietjens I M *et al* 2013 Behavior of silver nanoparticles and silver ions in an *in vitro* human gastrointestinal digestion model *Nanotoxicology* **7** 1198–210
[73] Jimeno-Romero A, Oron M, Cajaraville M P, Soto M and Marigómez 2016 Nanoparticle size and combined toxicity of TiO_2 and DSLS (surfactant) contribute to lysosomal responses in digestive cells of mussels exposed to TiO_2 nanoparticles *Nanotoxicology* **10** 1168–76
[74] Van den Brule S, Ambroise J, Lecloux H, Levard C, Soulas R and De Temmerman P J *et al* 2016 Dietary silver nanoparticles can disturb the gut microbiota in mice *Part. Fibre Toxicol.* **13** 38
[75] Wang P, Zhang Q, Li Y, Matsiko J, Zhang Y and Jiang G 2017 Airborne persistent toxic substances (PTSs) in China: occurrence and its implication associated with air pollution *Environ. Sci. Process. Impacts* **19** 983–99
[76] Savabieasfahani M, Ali S S, Bacho R, Savabi O and Alsabbak M 2016 Prenatal metal exposure in the Middle East: imprint of war in deciduous teeth of children *Environ. Monit. Assess.* **188** 505
[77] Pathak A K, Yadav S, Kumar P and Kumar R 2013 Source apportionment and spatial temporal variations in the metal content of dust collected from an industrial area adjoining Delhi, India *Sci. Total Enviorn.* **443** 662–72
[78] Sun R and Chen L 2016 Assessment of heavy metal pollution in topsoil around Beijing metropolis *PLoS One* **11** e0155350
[79] Tszydel M, Błońska D, Jóźwiak P and Jóźwiak M 2021 SEM-EDX analysis of heavy metals in anal papillae of *Hydropsyche angustipennis* larvae (Trichoptera, Insecta) as a support for water quality assessment *Eur. Zool.* J **88** 718–30
[80] Brożek-Mucha Z 2014 On the prevalence of gunshot residue in selected populations – an empirical study performed with SEM-EDX analysis *Forensic Sci. Int.* **237** 46–52
[81] Ferraro S A, Curutchet G and Tasat D R 2012 Bio-accessible heavy metals-sediment particles from Reconquista River induce lung inflammation in mice *Environ. Toxicol. Chem.* **31** 2059–68
[82] Scimeca M, Feola M, Romano L, Rao C, Gasbarra E and Bonanno E *et al* 2017 Heavy metals accumulation affects bone microarchitecture in osteoporotic patients *Environ. Toxicol.* **32** 1333–42
[83] Kawasaki H, Itoh T, Takaku Y, Suzuki H, Kosugi I, Meguro S, Iwashita T and Hariyama T 2020 The NanoSuit method: a novel histological approach for examining paraffin sections in a nondestructive manner by correlative light and electron microscopy *Lab. Invest.* **100** 161–73
[84] Takaku Y, Suzuki H, Ohta I, Ishii D, Muranaka Y and Shimomura M *et al* 2013 A thin polymer membrane, nano-suit, enhancing survival across the continuum between air and high vacuum *Proc. Natl Acad. Sci. USA.* **110** 7631–35
[85] Takaku Y, Takehara S, Suzuki C, Suzuki H, Shimomura M and Hariyama T 2020 In situ elemental analyses of living biological specimens using 'NanoSuit' and EDS methods in FE-SEM *Sci. Rep.* **10** 14574
[86] Takehara S, Takaku Y, Suzuki H, Ohta I, Shimomura M and Hariyama T 2018 A 'NanoSuit' successfully protects petals of cherry blossoms in high vacuum: examination of living plants in an FE-SEM *Sci. Rep.* **8** 1685

Chapter 14

Atomic force microscopy for biomedical nanotechnology

Chinmaya Mahapatra

Atomic force microscopy (AFM) is a three-dimensional topographic technique with high-resolution features used to measure surface properties, mainly roughness at the nanoscale. Significant efforts have been made to develop AFM of improved performance to study the various phenomena of materials science, biomedical research, and optimizing materials for targeted biomedical research. AFM provides useful and necessary information at the nanoscale, for example, the quantification of a single molecule. AFM has been frequently useful to develop nano-enabled drug delivery systems, and examinations of tissues. The basic and applied aspects of TEM will the topic of this chapter.

14.1 Introduction

Atomic force microscopy (AFM) is a three-dimensional (3D) topographic technique with high-resolution features used to measure surface properties, mainly roughness at the nanoscale. Significant efforts have been made to develop AFM of improved performance to study the various phenomena of material science, biomedical research, and optimizing materials for targeted biomedical research. Even individual bioconjugated nanostructures can be physically manipulated using AFM with the added advantage of label free monitoring of bioconjugates dynamics. Nanoscale imaging of biological specimens has included microorganisms [1], living mammalian cells [2], cell organalles [3], RNA [4]/RNA nanoparticle [5], DNA/protein–DNA complex [6], and lipid films [7] representing a powerful tool to understand and manipulate biological materials covering vast domains of bioscience. AFM provides useful and necessary information at the nanoscale, for example, the quantification of a single molecule, and recently contributing to single-cell nanomechanics (imaging of intracellular structures) [3]. In the larger context the biological importance of

doi:10.1088/978-0-7503-3379-5ch14

AFM could be evaluated by its critical role in understanding biomolecular interactions with DNA that is leading to the development of new cancer therapeutics [8]. Remarkably AFM is emerging as a tool for studying infectious viruses such as severe acute respiratory syndrome coronavirus 2 (SARS-CoV-2) that has emerged as the recent pandemic by its ability to image nanoscale 3D morphology of native infection versus inactivated virions [9].

Thus, AFM has been significantly developed to compete with optical microscopes largely to create 3D topological maps of surfaces and imaging in various physiological conditions (air/liquid or in interface). Thus, basic and applied aspects of AFM will the topic of this chapter.

14.2 Basic working principal

The flexible nature of AFM in probing, imaging, and also manipulating biological specimens at nano and sub-nano resolution was an amazing invention in 1986 with the ability to measure forces as small as 10–18 N [10]. The intriguing convergence of fundamental science and mathematics in AFM makes it truly interdisciplinary in nature, evident from its evolution to study structure–function properties of single molecules to surfaces. The imaging capabilities of AFM are very diverse from the molecular scale to very hard and soft surfaces, including viscoelastic soft biological structures. Today AFM imaging can be performed irrespective of medium of analysis (air, liquid), optical properties, and electrical conductivity.

AFM imaging in liquid is of special relevance to the study of biological samples or living cells in their native environment by maintaining their osmalarity and pH.

Changes in the scanning environment also significantly affect the composition of the probes, e.g., for scanning in air the probes are made of silicon, but for scanning in liquid silicon nitride tips are used that are gold coated. Variations in the elemental composition of the tips is with respect to their environment, e.g., for scanning in air stiff conical shape tips (the radius of the tip apex is usually 10 nm) are used that provide sharp and defined images. However, such stiffness would be a drawback in a liquid environment preventing semi-light contact-based imaging, thus silicon nitride tips having low spring constant are preferred as this provides semi-contact mode and contact scanning.

14.2.1 Cantilever tip shape

It has been long understood that the shape of probes has a great affect on the resolution of the AFM image and its capability as a manipulating tool. Although colloidal probes (<10 μm diameter) have been used widely in the mechanical characterization, spherical colloidal probes (5.2 μm diameter) have been found to be ideal for studying cellular stiffness such as cellular cytoplasm, nucleus, and cell–cell junctions reliably [11]. The major advantage of using spherical colloidal probes is to avoid damage to cell structure [12]. Apart from this there is no difference in the values obtained when sharp probes like conical or pyramidal tips were used, however, such values could be inconsistent, due to presence of cell cortex increasing the modulus when probed by a sharp tip [13, 14]. In contrast studies with sharp probes (pyramidal) have also shown no damaging effect to the probing cell even during persistent probing [15, 16].

Several studies in this regard have consistently demonstrated that sharp tips yield twice the elastic modulus in comparison to a spherical tip as observed in case of alveolar epithelial cells [17] and chondrocytes [18], in respect to indentation ranging from ($\delta < 400$ nm) [17, 19].

14.2.2 Cantilever stiffness for biological samples

Various parameters dictate the choice of probe with different stiffness, generally for soft biomatter lower stiffness probes are used and for stiff biomatter higher stiffness probes are used. In the case of viscoleastic materials, that covers most of cell and tissue matter, large end radius probes are preferred [20]. Major improvements in imaging biomatter was achieved by Mueller-Falcke *et al* in designing an in-plane switchable stiffness probe between 0.01 and 0.1 N m^{-1} [21, 22] (figure 14.1).

Various other switchable probes were also reported such as resonance tuning of cantilevers by using gains of the oscillation, by moment of inertia or by using a piezoelectric actuator to dynamically change the length of cantilever thereby modulating the stiffness [23, 24]. More recently an advanced optomechanical AFM probe with a very high frequency (130 MHz), based upon an actuator driven harmonic mechanical resonator is set to revolutionize the sub-picometer measurement, that would be of great interest to enable understanding of inaccesable biological phenomenon [25].

Another parameter that is very important in deciding on the type of probe is the probe tip-substrate adhesiveness. In this case if ultra-soft cantilevers are used, they could remain bound to the adhesive samples even during the retraction cycle leading to a non-flat approach curve. Such issues could be addressed by using high tip velocity and longer ramps (larger cantilever sample distance), ultimately to correct the drag artifact when imaging in an aqueous environment [26]. In addition, imaging of alveolar and bronchial epithelial cells demonstrate viscoelastic features that are dictated by cell organization, making the modulus range from elastic to soft glassy materials hence making the choice of probe critical in analysis [27].

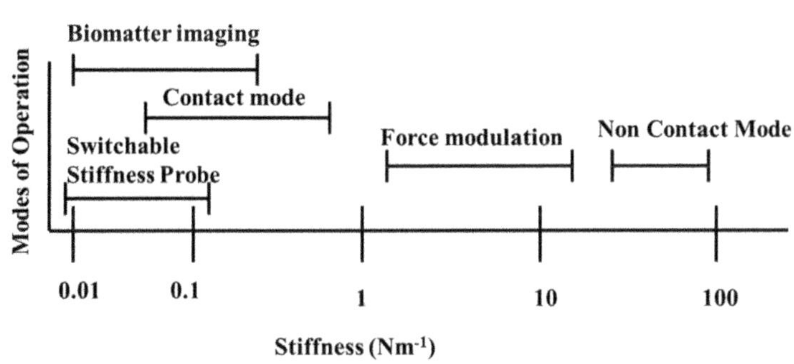

Figure 14.1. The stiffness range for the AFM cantilever from 0.01 to 100 N m^{-1} including the switchable probe that was in the range of 0.01–0.1 N m^{-1}.

The friction and adhesion relationship between the tip and substrate can be traced all the way down to their molecular interaction. In a study with various functionalized groups (thiols and silanes) on tip/substrate has demonstrated decrease in order of COOH/COOH > CH_3/CH_3 > $COOH/CH_3$. Thus the presence of functional groups on the tip/substrate dictates the performance of AFM imaging, and that in aqueous solution increased ionic strength results in lower adhesive interaction [28].

14.3 Calibration

Cells and tissues are viscoelastic in nature and the resultant modulus largely depends on the ramped frequency of the cantilever. With the wide range of ramping frequency, up to 2 kHz, the calibration of all the components of the AFM is critical to obtain reproducible results. The first step is to calibrate the photodiode sensitivity to the cantilever bending and the resultant signal output. Before scanning the probe on the viscoleastic biomatter, the cantilever is ramped against a stiff substrate such as glass, thus the inverse of the linear slope part will provide the calibration factor needed. In the case of cantilever stiffness calibration, the thermal fluctuations method is widely followed as stiffer cantilevers will have smaller deflections as the water molecules collide with the cantilever [29]. Calibration should be performed with samples of known moduli ranging from low to high stiffness.

The spring constant of the cantilever is the most important part to be calibrated, the most commonly used method is the thermal method. The deflection caused due to oscillation in liquid due to thermal movement of water molecules provides the basis of this calibration. Studies have shown that variation in the spring constant depends upon the length of cantilever as observed in the case of a 60 μm cantilever the variation is approximately 15% and for a 225 μm cantilever the variation is approximately 50% [30] (figure 14.2).

Importantly, to avoid the erroneous result of getting a combined viscoelastic value of sample and cantilever, the resonance frequency of the cantilever should be kept larger than the probe frequency.

14.3.1 Calibration of cantilever stiffness

To directly translate the obtained force from the cantilever using Hooke's law the stiffness of the cantilever should be predetermined to get accurate date, as the nominal stiffness of cantilevers are based on their shape and composition [31]. It is important to calibrate before the start of every AFM session, as there are several direct or indirect methods to do so including lateral and normal force calibration [32].

The preferred method is thermal fluctuations as it can be quickly performed in various liquids with the most accurate calibration of the cantilever deflection sensitivity. The most important phenomenon to take into account is that in the thermal difference method water molecules in the solution are colliding with the cantilever surface with respect to the packing density causing some disturbance that should be accounted for the error [33].

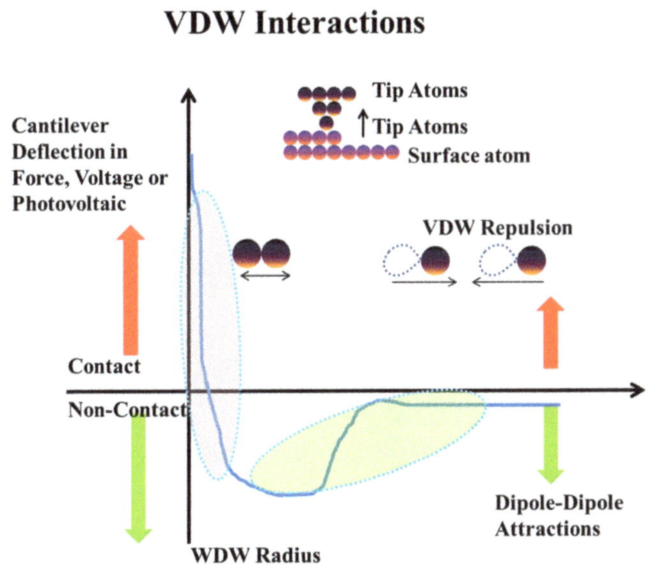

Figure 14.2. Various physical forces that come into play during AFM–probe interaction with the surface of the sample. VDW (Coulombic and van der Waals) based repulsion with relation to (WDW) van der Waals radius.

14.4 Forces in aqueous solution

During cantilever movement in aqueous solution that is typical of the BioAFM working environment various physicochemical interactions take place. Namely, these are H bonding like: RO–H, RS–H, RN–H, ionic interactions, hydrodynamic forces, viscous damping, compression and repulsive force, viscoelasticity, air–liquid interface, surface thermal fluctuations, smooth and rough surfaces, and liquid order packing (figure 14.3).

The laminar and the turbulent flow can significantly affect the drag on the AFM cantilever movement that has been considered via simulation based on the Reynolds-averaged Navier Stokes (RANS) formula.

The behavior of the cantilever is a central part of the AFM working principal, specifically changes in its deflection (or amplitude of oscillation). This begins from the calibration of the cantilever deflection and corresponding photodiode signal output. The reflection of light, therefore, greatly depends on the light matter interaction, including the liquid optical behavior affecting the light amplification by stimulated emission of radiation (LASER) reflectivity from the gold coating on the back of the cantilever. Furthermore, recalibration is highly recommended not only on the change of the medium but also for every new experiment.

14.5 Models for cell mechanic's study

Most commonly the Hertzian models used exclude the attractive/adhesive forces present between the tip and the sample, considering only repulsive forces present between the tip and the sample until it proceeds contact and indents the sample.

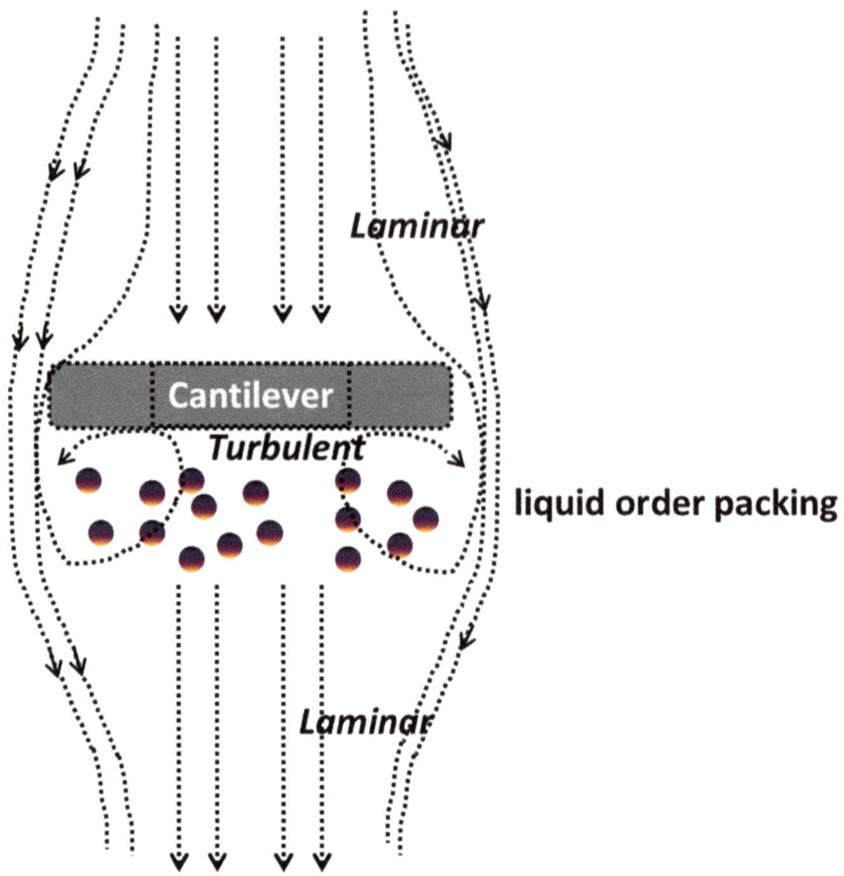

Figure 14.3. The laminar, turbulent flow and liquid order packing density-based drag to the cantilever movement.

Imaging using different shapes of probes have been solved using a Hertz model such as spherical [11, 34], conical [35], or pyramidal [36].

In another attractive force interactions between the tip and sample are studied either using the N,N-Dimethyltryptamine (DMT) model [37] or the Johnson–Kendal–Roberts (JKR) model (usually for soft matter) [11, 38].

14.5.1 Tip/probe interaction with biological material

As previous described the AFM cantilever material can be chosen according to sample stiffness to either consist of either silicon (hard substrate) or silicon nitride (soft substrate) (figure 14.4).

Furthermore the tips are gold coated to maintain inter-environment and to have minimal reaction with the surface, further the coating also significantly improves the tip-enhanced Raman spectroscopy by two orders of magnitude [39] (figure 14.5). Further, the choice of tip dimensions also determines the relationship to the spring constant, k, as defined by the equation:

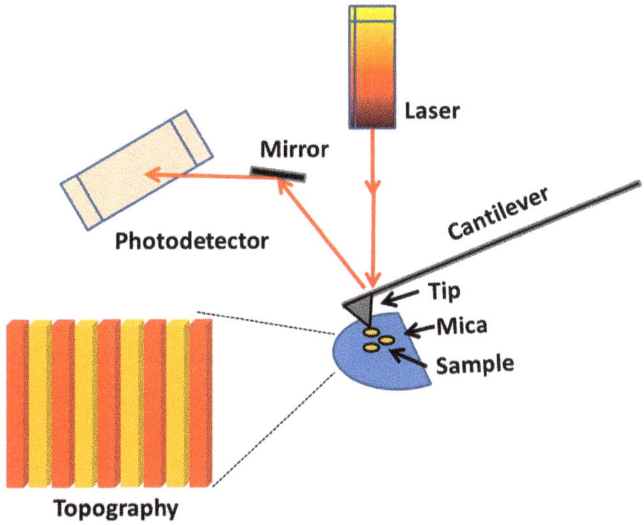

Figure 14.4. Cantilever tip/probe for biological sample analysis demonstrating attractive and repulsive forces.

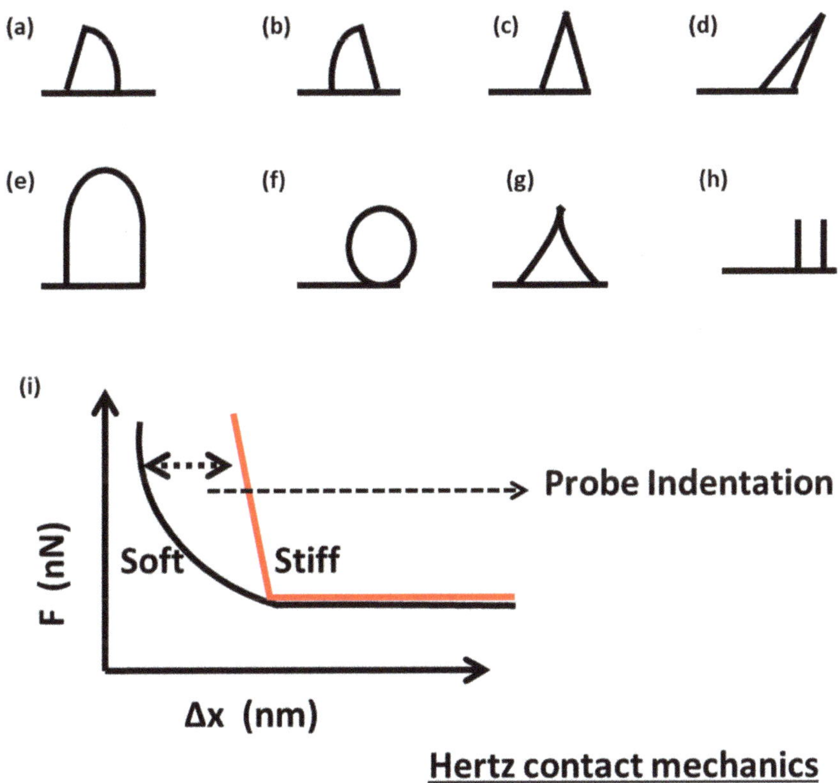

Figure 14.5. Shapes of various probes/tips for analysis of the biological specimen (a–h) and (i) probe indentation in respect to soft and stiff material.

$$k = Ewt^3/4L^3$$

where E = Young's modulus of the cantilever material, w = cantilever width, t = cantilever thickness, and L = cantilever length.

14.6 Basic preparation of biological samples

To obtain the best results tuning of the AFM is needed to analyse the biological samples by correctly setting the proper sample preparation, set point, amplitude, scanning speed and various parameters taken into account during analysis in a liquid environment [40]. The proper scanning amplitude is dependent on the height of the surface features. Higher features on the scanned samples demand higher amplitude in a bid to manage the sensitivity versus the scanning speed, generally for stable samples approximately 40 nm amplitude is recommended as a starting point [41].

Feedback gain is another parameter to consider when imaging the sticky or non-sticky samples, if it is too high it can oscillate too much causing smaller details on the sample surface to be missed [42, 43]. Also sticky or adhesive samples have a tendency for the surface of tip to stick during slow scanning (greatly increases during single-cell scanning), in order to prevent that, if the speed of cantilever is increased it can only prevent sticking at the cost of resolution [44].

Based upon the above understanding preparation of the biological sample (possible adhesive or sticky nature) is of high importance in best performance of AFM.

14.6.1 Viruses

The increasing number of infectious diseases and the threat to public health leading to pandemic, has motivated the investigation of viruses by AFM to precisely predict the structure and develop antiviral modalities. Kuznetsov *et al* reported important protocols to visualize fixed retroviruses. In detail the virus and virus harboring cells were fixed in 0.05% of glutaraldehyde and postfixed with OsO_4 (osmium tetroxide) followed by stepwise dehydration in ethanol [45]. The visualization of human immunodeficiency virus (HIV) was finally performed by adhering it on the poly-L-lysine coated coverslips, however to visualize the disrupted structure of HIV the samples were washed with detergent and HIV protease inhibitor to distinguish between and immature and mature forms. The imaging was performed through tapping mode using silicon nitride cantilevers which have low spring constant as it minimizes the cantilever tip and the viral surface contact to lower lateral forces when imaging in liquid. In contrast to imaging in liquid media, when imaging in air the stiffer cantilever made from silicon with high spring constant (50 N m^{-1}) was used [46].

Lyonnais *et al* recently devised the protocol to visualize the highly infectious virus (SARS-CoV-2). In detail the procedure involves taking the infected cell supernatant followed by sufficient adsorption on appropriate AFM surface like glass or mica coverslip. For efficient adsorption of the virus on the glass or mica surface it was coated with poly-L-lysine with prior surface modification with alkyl silane providing a hydrophobic surface domain. With the binding time of 2–3 min enough for visualization of the virus on the mica, roughly ellipsoidal and spherical type particles were visualized under the approach/retract speed of 10 μm s^{-1} at *z* range of 100 nm, while keeping the applied force at 150 pN [9].

14.6.2 Bacteria

Like viruses the visualization of bacteria is performed both in the fixed and live condition. Both methods could visualize the same sample at almost the same accuracy, but the viscoleastic nature and observation of living cell processes could be lost during the fixation process. In the case of live bacteria imaging (*Escherichia coli, Pseudomonas putida, Agrobacterium tumefaciens* and *Bacillus subtilis*) Huang *et al* reported the protocol wherein the ultrasound cleaned coverslip was used to image the biofilm formation on mineral surfaces after incubating the bacteria on a coverslip for the respective growth time. Similarly bacterial–mineral aggregates in appropriate media were immobilized on a mica surface after drying for 5 min to be observed both in ScanAsyst-Air cantilevers mode with spring constant 0.4 N m^{-1} and tapping mode using spring constant 40 N m^{-1} [47]. The beauty of live bacteria imaging is that it allows understanding of the dynamic nature of the bacterial structural organization such as cell wall remodeling through visualization of peptidoglycan porosity [48]. Various glass functionalizations have been used to immobilize the bacteria such as gelatin, poly-L-lysine, Cell-Tak™ and Vectabond® [49]. However, in many cases fixing of the bacterial cell is required to understand the time dependent processes and also to thoroughly study the intricate structures. In that case as reported by Liu *et al* bacteria are fixed overnight in 2% glutaraldehyde in 0.2 M PBS followed by rinsing in 1mM Tris buffer [50].

14.6.3 Cells

Visualization of cells has always been a matter of discussion as cellular properties change from single-cell to a cell line. Further, cell fixing versus live status including the immobilization, depends on the method which largely determines the AFM outcomes. Adherent cell lines are much easier to immobilize as they could be grown directly on a glass cover slip treated with suitable growth substrate like polylysine or laminine. Low spring constant and non-sharp silicon nitride gold coated probes are mostly used in the imaging of the cells. Calibration is usually performed by first scanning the blank glass coverslip followed by the tapping on the various sides of cells, i.e., extreme edge, side, and middle section of cells. Great care should be taken while performing the modulus analysis of various regions of the cells, strongly agreeing with the Hertz simulation model. With respect to this, in a recent study Kumar *et al* demonstrated the modulus of nanofiber mesh supporting the keratinocytes to evaluate the capability of developed structure in inducing stronger cell–cell junctions in contact mode. Spherical probes were used for this study in order not to rupture the soft cell membrane of epithelial cells, further the spherical probes allowed access to the stiffness of nucleus, cytoplasm, and cell–cell junctions

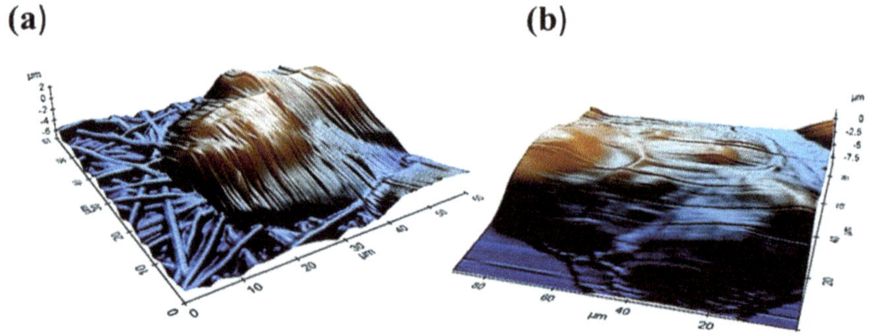

Figure 14.6. AFM images of live HaCaT (keratinocytes) cells grown on (a) nanofiber versus (b) culture plate probed by spherical probe. Reproduced from [11] CC BY 3.0.

respectively. Furthermore, non-linear increase in the resistance force was observed for cells cultured on the nanofiber demonstrating the bulk modulus also varied from 0.0314 to 1.37 as cells are grown from culture plate to nanofiber materials [11] (figure 14.6).

However, sometime the soft viscoelastic cells need to be fixed in order to image the specific proteins and lipids in the cell's membrane. In that case proteins are either fixed by paraformaldehyde and lipid by OsO_4 [51].

14.6.4 Tissue

Tissue surface visualization comprises the majority of samples used in AFM investigations. The tissue comes in various shapes and lateral sizes, including a variation of stiffness, e.g., bone versus adipose tissue. Another limitation with analysis of tissue is keeping the sample throughout in humid condition to prevent dehydration and loss of natural features. In this respect studies on 10 μm sections of human liver and kidney tissue have shown that the fixing method greatly determines its elastic modulus. In detail the elastic modulus in collagen-enriched (CE) areas and collagen-low (CL) areas varied, such as frozen non-fixed (CE 1–8 kPa, CL 0.2–0.8 kPa), frozen fixed (CE 8–11 kPa, CL 1–7 kPa), fixed frozen (CE 8–11 kPa, CL 1–7 kPa), paraffin processed tissue (CE 100–200 kPa, CL 200–400 kPa). The modulus value obtained was by calibrating with the thermal noise method followed by penetration of 1–2 microns keeping the force threshold maximum for paraffin section [52]. Further, Graham *et al* showed that freshly cut 5 μm tissue cryo-sections on glass coverslips can clearly visualize the structural features of the respective tissue, in this case different regions of intervertebral disc [53].

14.6.5 Visualization, probing, and manipulation of RNA, DNA, and proteins

Advancement in AFM has further given the scope to access (visualize or manipulate) the biological micromoleculaes and their related interactions such as individual RNA, DNA proteins, and biomolecules. The AFM imaging capability has also expanded to the visulatization of DNA–protein complexes and protein–protein complexes. However, imaging in all the mentioned biomolecules needs special

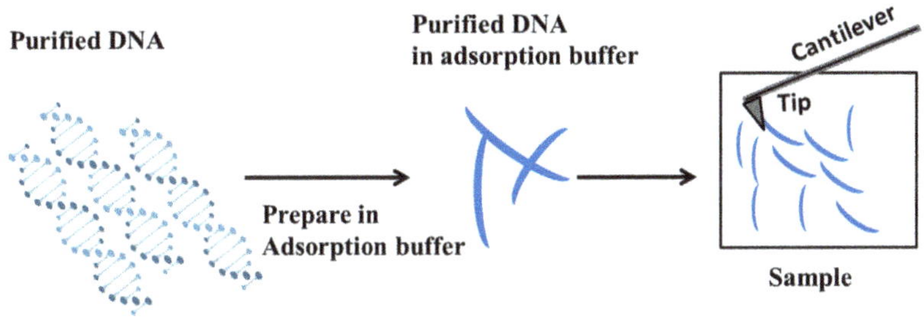

Figure 14.7. Protocol for imaging the individual DNA molecule on mica substrate by AFM.

modification of probe tip, by exploiting the electrostatic interactions between substrate and tip to permit advanced imaging. Shen *et al* in this regard reported simple tunable protocols to *in situ* visualize individual DNA molecules. The AFM imaging was performed in air, briefly diluted DNA solution 5.0 μl in 40.0 mM HEPES buffer with 5.0 mM Mg^{2+} at pH 7.0, was deposited on mica followed by rinsing in ultrapure water and nitrogen drying. In another setup DNA/chitosan complex was made for AFM imaging keeping N/P ratio chitosan-to-DNA charge ratio at 0.05/1.25 and 1.0/25.0 mg l^{-1}. The imaging was performed both in air and liquid using the respective spring constant (in liquid of 2.8 N m^{-1}, scanning rate 1.8 Hz) for air similar to the spring constant for liquid with a 2.2 Hz scanning rate [54] (figure 14.7).

14.6.6 Individual RNA

The folding and unfolding of RNA into various structures has defined biological outcomes (gene regulation to enzymatic catalysis) and functions. This understanding enables understanding of the diverse biological effects and also related effects to central dogma. Walder *et al* understood RNA (folding, unfolding, and refolding) by using single-molecule force spectroscopy (SMFS), in which small RNA hairpins formed between the probe tip and individual RNA leading to stimulated programmed ribosomal frameshifting. The special AFMs with stiffer probes were used to visualize the kinetic trajectories of the HIV RNA hairpin to access the folding characteristics of individual RNA [55].

14.6.7 Proteins

AFM has evolved as a leading tool to measure molecular volumes of protein molecules, elasticity of proteins, etc., either in native or non-native environments. Müller *et al* in this regard studied the native membrane proteins by using AFM, getting the lateral resolution (<1 nm) and vertical resolution (0.1–0.2 nm). An important prerequisite for AFM analysis is immobilization on a flat support such as mica (for hydrophilic) and highly ordered pyrolytic graphite (HOPG) (for hydrophobic) by adsorption. As for imaging in contact mode cantilevers should have softer spring constant kL of 0.05–0.5 N m^{-1} and for dynamic mode a stiffer cantilever was found to be more appropriate (kL > 10 N m^{-1}). For contact mode imaging, cantilevers should have a spring constant kL of 0.05–0.5 N m^{-1}. They should be much stiffer for the dynamic mode (kL > 10 N m^{-1}), depending on the resolution of the deflection sensor [56].

14.6.8 Application in infectious biology—recent update

As discussed above, the immense capability of AFM enables it to also visualize viruses that have emerged as the most infectious agents in human history. In a recent study on the SARS-CoV-2 virus causing COVID-19 by AFM, O'Callahan *et al* have shown the dynamic interaction of a silicon surface that is gold coated with spike proteins of virus. In detail the recombinant trimeric spike (S) proteins diluted in phosphate buffer saline 1.2 mg ml^{-1} were dried under N_2 on Si substrates. Various materials such as Al, Au, Cu, Ce, and Fe were coated on the tip for observing the interaction between metal oxide-coated AFM tips and spike proteins. The observation showed the attractive force order of magnitude, lower for 1–2 nN for iron oxide and CeO_2 and higher 20–25 nN for others including Au. Important conclusions derived from the study indicated certain metal oxide tips (Au) havie specific stronger binding whereas others indicated non-specific binding (Al, Si, Fe, and CeO_2) resulting in an interesting observation in tip–sample contact mechanics of infectious samples [57] (figure 14.8).

Simple sample preparation, wide sample formats, and high resolution imply a stronger direct virus imaging option by AFM. As discussed above SARS-CoV-2 spike protein S1 adsorption at two different (Al_2O_3 and TiO_2) oxide surfaces were studied by Xin et al The study revealed the specific preference of the protein towards TiO_2 under various electrolyte conditions, this study specifically demonstrates the importance of the surface on spike protein adsorption, it would be interesting to understand the protein–material interactions in a future study using an AFM based tool [58]. In another study, Pleshakova *et al* visualized the Hepatitis C Virus Core Protein using a specifically aptamer modified AFM chip surface that binds to the core antigen of HCV (HCVcoreAg protein) from human serum samples. The special chip setup thus made it possible to visualize the Hepatitis C Virus in a distributed pattern, corresponding to the qualitative visualization of virus titer [59].

Although the application of AFM is vast in infectious viral research and is rapidly evolving, covering it here is beyond the scope of this chapter.

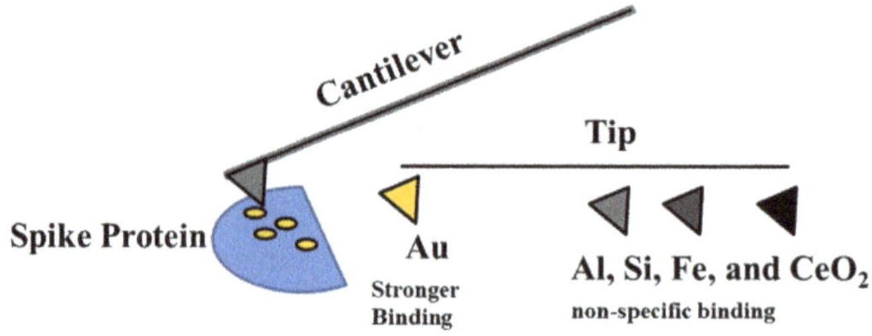

Figure 14.8. Various metal oxide modified tips having specific binding affinity to spike protein.

14.7 Conclusion and future applications

The AFM technique is rapidly evolving with every increasing atomic resolution that has enabled it to provide inaccessible information about various biomolecules and biological structures. Not only is AFM able to provide structural visualization but it also provides information about the modulus of the materials that is invaluable in biomechanics. Advancement in AFM capability to image in liquid medium has provided the opportunity to image samples under their native conditions or in the living state. Furthermore, it is also emerging as tool to manipulate macromolecules including the applicability in single molecule detection, understanding biomolecular interactions and cell–material interactions. In recent years it has opened the window to quantitatively or qualitatively study infectious diseases such as viruses and the recent pandemic SARS-CoV-2. Further advancement of the AFM technique, is expected to provide the thrust to understand inaccessible domains of bioscience, materials science, and other interdisciplinary areas, greatly impacting human life by advancement of knowledge.

References

[1] Van Der Hofstadt M *et al* 2015 Nanoscale imaging of the growth and division of bacterial cells on planar substrates with the atomic force microscope *Ultramicroscopy* **154** 29–36

[2] Shibata M *et al* 2017 High-speed atomic force microscopy imaging of live mammalian cells *Biophys. Physicobiol.* **14** 127–35

[3] Guerrero C R, Garcia P D and Garcia R 2019 Subsurface imaging of cell organelles by force microscopy *ACS Nano* **13** 9629–37

[4] Kuznetsov Y G *et al* 2010 Biophysical and atomic force microscopy characterization of the RNA from satellite tobacco mosaic virus *Nucleic Acids Res.* **38** 8284–94

[5] Sajja S *et al* 2018 Dynamic behavior of RNA nanoparticles analyzed by AFM on a mica/air interface *Langmuir* **34** 15099–108

[6] Lyubchenko Y L, Gall A A and Shlyakhtenko L S 2014 Visualization of DNA and protein–DNA complexes with atomic force microscopy *Methods Mol. Biol. (Clifton, N.J.)* **1117** 367–84

[7] Krapf L *et al* 2011 AFM characterization of spin-coated multilayered dry lipid films prepared from aqueous vesicle suspensions *Colloids Surf.* B **82** 25–32

[8] Main K H S *et al* 2021 Atomic force microscopy—a tool for structural and translational DNA research *APL Bioeng.* **5** 031504

[9] Lyonnais S *et al* 2021 Atomic force microscopy analysis of native infectious and inactivated SARS-CoV-2 virions *Sci. Rep.* **11** 11885

[10] Binnig G, Quate C F and Gerber C 1986 Atomic force microscope *Phys. Rev. Lett.* **56** 930–3

[11] Kumar P *et al* 2021 A designer cell culture insert with a nanofibrous membrane toward engineering an epithelial tissue model validated by cellular nanomechanics *Nanoscale Adv.* **3** 4714–25

[12] Guz N *et al* 2014 If cell mechanics can be described by elastic modulus: study of different models and probes used in indentation experiments *Biophys. J.* **107** 564–75

[13] Chiou Y-W *et al* 2013 The influence of physical and physiological cues on atomic force microscopy-based cell stiffness assessment *PLoS One* **8** e77384

[14] Vargas-Pinto R *et al* 2013 The effect of the endothelial cell cortex on atomic force microscopy measurements *Biophys. J.* **105** 300–9
[15] Gavara N and Chadwick R S 2016 Relationship between cell stiffness and stress fiber amount, assessed by simultaneous atomic force microscopy and live-cell fluorescence imaging *Biomech. Model. Mechanobiol.* **15** 511–23
[16] HAYDON P G *et al* 1996 Membrane deformation of living glial cells using atomic force microscopy *J. Microsc.* **182** 114–20
[17] Rico F *et al* 2005 Probing mechanical properties of living cells by atomic force microscopy with blunted pyramidal cantilever tips *Phys. Rev.* E **72** 021914
[18] Ng L *et al* 2007 Nanomechanical properties of individual chondrocytes and their developing growth factor-stimulated pericellular matrix *J. Biomech.* **40** 1011–23
[19] Costa K D and Yin F C 1999 Analysis of indentation: implications for measuring mechanical properties with atomic force microscopy *J. Biomech. Eng.* **121** 462–71
[20] Moeller G 2009 AFM nanoindentation of viscoelastic materials with large end-radius probes *J. Polym. Sci.* B **47** 1573–87
[21] Mueller-Falcke C *et al* 2006 A nanoscanning platform for bio-engineering: an in-plane probe with switchable stiffness *Nanotechnology* **17** S69–76
[22] De Laat M L C, Pérez Garza H H and Ghatkesar M K 2016 In situ stiffness adjustment of AFM probes by two orders of magnitude *Sensors* **16** 523
[23] Vitorino M V *et al* 2015 Giant resonance tuning of micro and nanomechanical oscillators *Sci. Rep.* **5** 7818
[24] Kawai Y, Takahito O, Meyer E, Gerber C and Esashi M 2006 Piezoelectric actuator integrated cantilever with tunable spring constant for atom probe *Proc. IEEE Int. Conf. on Micro Electro Mechanical Systems (MEMS)*
[25] Schwab L *et al* 2022 Very high frequency probes for atomic force microscopy with silicon optomechanics *Microsyst. Nanoeng.* **8** 32
[26] Alcaraz J *et al* 2002 Correction of microrheological measurements of soft samples with atomic force microscopy for the hydrodynamic drag on the cantilever *Langmuir* **18** 716–21
[27] Alcaraz J *et al* 2003 Microrheology of human lung epithelial cells measured by atomic force microscopy *Biophys. J.* **84** 2071–9
[28] Noy A *et al* 1995 Chemical force microscopy: exploiting chemically-modified tips to quantify adhesion, friction, and functional group distributions in molecular assemblies *J. Am. Chem. Soc.* **117** 7943–51
[29] Gavara N 2017 A beginner's guide to atomic force microscopy probing for cell mechanics *Microsc. Res. Tech.* **80** 75–84
[30] Proksch R *et al* 2004 Finite optical spot size and position corrections in thermal spring constant calibration *Nanotechnology* **15** 1344–50
[31] Neumeister J M and Ducker W A 1994 Lateral, normal, and longitudinal spring constants of atomic force microscopy cantilevers *Rev. Sci. Instrum.* **65** 2527–31
[32] Palacio M L B and Bhushan B 2010 Normal and lateral force calibration techniques for AFM cantilevers *Crit. Rev. Solid State Mater. Sci.* **35** 73–104
[33] Lévy R and Maaloum M 2001 Measuring the spring constant of atomic force microscope cantilevers: thermal fluctuations and other methods *Nanotechnology* **13** 33–7
[34] Hertz H 2021 Ueber die Berührung fester elastischer Körper *J. Reine Angew. Math.* **92** 156–71
[35] Sneddon I N 1965 The relation between load and penetration in the axisymmetric boussinesq problem for a punch of arbitrary profile *Int. J. Eng. Sci.* **3** 47–57

[36] Bilodeau G G 1992 Regular pyramid punch problem *J. Appl. Mech.* **59** 519–23
[37] Adams G G 2013 The DMT theory of adhesion *Encyclopedia of Tribology* ed Q J Wang and Y-W Chung (Boston, MA: Springer) pp 3560–5
[38] Johnson K L *et al* 1971 Surface energy and the contact of elastic solids *Proc. R. Soc. Lond.* A **324** 301–13
[39] Meng L *et al* 2015 Gold-coated AFM tips for tip-enhanced Raman spectroscopy: theoretical calculation and experimental demonstration *Opt. Express* **23** 13804–13
[40] Zhu J *et al* 2009 Gloss phenomena and image analysis of atomic force microscopy in molecular and cell biology *Scanning* **31** 49–58
[41] Keyvani A *et al* 2017 Minimizing tip-sample forces and enhancing sensitivity in atomic force microscopy with dynamically compliant cantilevers *J. Appl. Phys.* **121** 244505
[42] Yang H *et al* 2007 Application of atomic force microscopy as a nanotechnology tool in food science *J. Food Sci.* **72** R65–75
[43] Braga P C and Ricci D 2004 *Atomic Force Microscopy: Biomedical Methods and Applications* (Berlin: Springer)
[44] Viljoen A *et al* 2021 Force spectroscopy of single cells using atomic force microscopy *Nat. Rev. Methods Primers* **1** 63
[45] Kuznetsov Y G *et al* 2004 Atomic force microscopy imaging of retroviruses: Human immunodeficiency virus and murine leukemia virus *Scanning* **26** 209–16
[46] Kuznetsov Y G *et al* 2001 Imaging of viruses by atomic force microscopy *J. Gen. Virol.* **82** 2025–34
[47] Huang Q *et al* 2015 Atomic force microscopy measurements of bacterial adhesion and biofilm formation onto clay-sized particles *Sci. Rep.* **5** 16857
[48] Dufrêne Y F 2014 Atomic force microscopy in microbiology: new structural and functional insights into the microbial cell surface *mBio* **5** e01363
[49] Benn G *et al* 2019 Imaging live bacteria at the nanoscale: comparison of immobilisation strategies *Analyst* **144** 6944–52
[50] Liu BY Z G, Li X L and Chen H 2012 Effect of glutaraldehyde fixation on bacterial cells observed by atomic force microscopy *Scanning* **34** 6–11
[51] Schaepe K *et al* 2015 Assessment of different sample preparation routes for mass spectrometric monitoring and imaging of lipids in bone cells via ToF-SIMS *Biointerphases* **10** 019016
[52] Calò A *et al* 2020 Spatial mapping of the collagen distribution in human and mouse tissues by force volume atomic force microscopy *Sci. Rep.* **10** 15664
[53] Graham H K *et al* 2010 Tissue section AFM: *in situ* ultrastructural imaging of native biomolecules *Matrix Biol.* **29** 254–60
[54] Shen X-C *et al* 2011 A simple and effective sample preparation method for atomic force microscopy visualization of individual DNA molecules *in situ Mol. Biol. Rep.* **38** 965–9
[55] Walder R *et al* 2018 High-precision single-molecule characterization of the folding of an HIV RNA hairpin by atomic force microscopy *Nano Lett.* **18** 6318–25
[56] Müller D J and Engel A 2007 Atomic force microscopy and spectroscopy of native membrane proteins *Nat. Protocols* **2** 2191–7
[57] O'Callahan B *et al* 2021 Atomic force microscopy and infrared nanospectroscopy of COVID-19 spike protein for the quantification of adhesion to common surfaces *Langmuir* **37** 12089–97

[58] Xin Y, Grundmeier G and Keller A 2021 Adsorption of SARS-CoV-2 spike protein S1 at oxide surfaces studied by high-speed atomic force microscopy *Adv. NanoBiomed Res.* **1** 2000024
[59] Pleshakova T O *et al* 2019 Detection of hepatitis C virus core protein in serum using aptamer-functionalized AFM chips *Micromachines* **10** 129

Chapter 15

Microfluidics system for biomedical nanotechnology

Nitish Sagar, Prosenjit Sen and Saurabh Kumar

This chapter presents an overview of microfluidic systems from a biomedical perspective. The physics of microscale fluid flow and fabrication methods of microfluidic chips are discussed in the first section. Later, we highlight the major applications of such microfluidic devices in biomedical areas of research. The use of microfluidic devices in single-cell analysis, polymerase chain reaction (PCR) study, biosensors integration, and organ-on-chip technology is explained in detail. We understand the vastness of this area and thus it is not possible to cover all aspects of the microfluidic systems in a single chapter. However, this chapter will provide general knowledge to help readers become acquainted with such microfluidic systems used in biomedical research.

15.1 Introduction

The principle of miniaturization of devices that once started in the microelectronics industry has reached the domain of fluid mechanics. With the technological advancements in nano-fabrication techniques, researchers have discussed the many benefits of miniaturization that enhance device performance, reduce power consumption, and integrate several functionalities within a small area. This miniaturization concept has been a boon to fluid research and has given rise to a new area, i.e., *microfluidics*. Microfluidics refers to the science of manipulating fluid volumes in the range of micro- to femto-litres with the help of tens to hundreds of micrometers dimension of channels. The reduction in channel size increases the surface-to-volume ratio, and interestingly, surface forces become dominant. These forces play a significant role in the study of microfluidics. Usually, fluid flow is turbulent in nature; however, in the microfluidics channel, the nature of fluid flow is laminar. This is because viscous forces are predominant over inertial forces.

doi:10.1088/978-0-7503-3379-5ch15

It is important to know how this microscale flow science turned into a technological advancement for several research areas. The area of microfluidics developed from different research domains that require precise fluid flow control. As we know, microanalytical techniques like gas-phase chromatography, high-pressure liquid chromatography, and capillary electrophoresis significantly improved chemical analysis. This quest for compact and microscale methods, led to microfluidic device research. The second development came as part of Defense Advanced Research Projects Agency (DARPA) research programs after the end of the Cold War in the 1990s, aimed at developing a portable device to detect chemical and biological threats. This enhanced academic research in microfluidics. The genomics studies, such as DNA sequencing and other micro-analysis related to molecular biology, gave another boost to microfluidics. It offered high throughput and better sensitivity than that of conventional methods. Another contribution was from the field of microelectronics. The silicon-based and micro-electromechanical systems (MEMS) fabrication techniques such as photolithography were used to develop microfluidic devices. Although later, most microfluidic chip researchers opted for an elastomer like polydimethylsiloxane (PDMS), for its inexpensive, optical transparency and biocompatible nature.

Microfluidics offers several advantages: low sample volume consumption, high throughput, low risk of contamination, parallelization of multiple assays, and the ability to integrate multiple detection techniques with microfluidic devices for real-time testing, thus making it an ideal candidate for point-of-care (POC) and lab-on-chip devices. As mentioned above, the benefits of a microfluidic platform stimulated many biological research areas like single-cell study, point-of-care devices for rapid testing, biosensors, mimicking body physiology on chips to study cancer and its metastasis (organ-on-chip), etc.

In this chapter, we will discuss the physics of micro-scale flows explaining the fluid mechanics and how it is different from the bulk flow. The next section will cover various aspects of device fabrication, such as soft lithography, micromachining, and 3D printing. In the last sections, we will cover several applications of microfluidic platforms such as single-cell analysis, PCR-based study, biosensors integration, and organ-on-chip research.

15.2 Physics of micro-scale fluid flow

Microfluidics deals with fluid phenomena that are quite like bulk fluid mechanics, but the surface forces at the microscale are dominant. Unlike in macroscale flows, fluid is not in turbulent flow regime. But in the microfluidics purview, surface tension and surface engineering play an important role in several applications. There are two types of approach in microchannel-based fluid flow—continuous microfluidics and droplet microfluidics [1]. There is another area of research, popularly known as digital microfluidics [2] (manipulation of discrete droplets on planar patterned substrate). For this, different types of forces such as surface acoustic wave (SAW) [3], magnetic force [4], thermocapillary, optical force, electrical force [5], or a combination are used to carry out droplet manipulation.

This section will start with the general conservation equations (mass and momentum) using the Reynolds transport theorem to explain fluid flow mechanics in microchannels, followed by wettability and surface tension. In the later part, we briefly discuss important non-dimensional numbers and its practical relevance in continuous and droplet microfluidics areas. It is to be noted that several conventional fluid mechanics concepts hold true for microfluidic study, and thus we do not include those in this section.

15.2.1 Reynolds transport theorem and conservation equations

Let us take an example to explain general conservation law. Consider an imaginary box of money in which you stored an amount (this we call 'In'). Later, you take out some of the stored money (this we call 'Out'). Also, consider some interest you get for keeping money in the box (this is 'Generation'). You would like to know the net change in your deposit (this is 'Change'). The general intuitive maths suggests:

In − Out + Gen = Change

Or **rate of (In − Out + Gen) = rate of (change)**

We introduce the 'rate of' to calculate the amount with respect to time. This equation of conservation, from the first principle that we get from simple mathematics, also holds for our conservation equations for mass, momentum, or energy.

However, there is another way to discuss these conservation equations in fluid flow, which is known as the Reynold transport theorem (RTT). This theorem bridges the gap between the Lagrangian and Eulerian approach to fluid mechanics. In the Lagrangian method, fluid flow is described by tracing individual fluid particles, while in the Eulerian method, fluid is described using the control volume approach. As we know that our classical physics laws are defined for a system approach, it is essential to have mathematical modeling of those in the control volume approach to study fluid flow either in differential or integral form.

The Reynolds transport theorem relates the control mass system and control volume approach. The general expression of RTT is given by:

$$\left(\frac{dN}{dt}\right)_{\text{sys}} = \frac{\partial}{\partial t}\iiint \rho n d\forall + \iint n\rho \vec{V}\cdot dA \qquad (15.1)$$

where N is any extensive fluid property, n is the intensive fluid property that is N per unit mass, ρ is the fluid density, $d\forall$ represents elementary volume, and dA represents an elementary area of the control surface. $\vec{V}$ is the velocity property crossing the control surface. The left-hand side represents the rate of property change in the system, while the right-hand side of the equation tells us about its net effect in the control volume method. The first term on the right-hand side represents the rate of change of fluid property in control volume, and the second term gives the rate of (outflow–inflow) of the property from the control surface.

This RTT can get conservation equations of mass and momentum by substituting the 'N' value in equation (15.1). In the mass conservation equation, N is mass 'M' and thus n is '1'. Since the mass of the system is conserved, thus the rate of change of mass of the system, dM/dt is zero that leads to a mass conservation equation as:

$$\frac{\partial}{\partial t}\iiint \rho d\forall + \iint \rho \vec{V} \cdot dA = 0 \tag{15.2}$$

Since the elementary volume choice is arbitrary, the derivative term can be placed within an integral operator in the first term in equation (15.2). Using the Gauss divergence theorem to convert the area integral into volume integral in the second term, we get:

$$\frac{\partial \rho}{\partial t} + \nabla \cdot \left(\rho \vec{V}\right) = 0 \tag{15.3}$$

Equation (15.3) represents the mass conservation equation in differential form.

Let us take an example to elucidate this concept. Consider one-dimension steady flow (velocity and other fluid properties at any location do not change with time) through a variable area channel (figure 15.1).

The corresponding continuity equation is $\nabla \cdot (\rho \vec{V}) = 0$. Integrating it over an elemental volume $d\forall$ and using divergence theorem, we get $\iint (\rho \vec{V}) \cdot \hat{n} dA = 0$ where $\hat{n}$ is a unit normal vector to dA. Since the velocity is zero at all boundaries except at inlet and outlet, the above expression can be written as:

$$\left(\iint (\vec{V}\rho) \cdot \hat{n}\mathrm{dA}\right)_{\mathrm{in}} + \left(\iint (\vec{V}\rho) \times \hat{n}\mathrm{dA}\right)_{\mathrm{tuo}} = 0 \tag{15.4}$$

At inlet, $\hat{n}$ is $-\hat{i}$ and at outlet $\hat{n}$ is $\hat{i}$. With u as x-component of velocity, we can write:

$$-\left(\iint \mathrm{Adup}\right)_{\mathrm{ni}} + \left(\iint \mathrm{Adup}\right)_{\mathrm{tuo}} \tag{15.5}$$

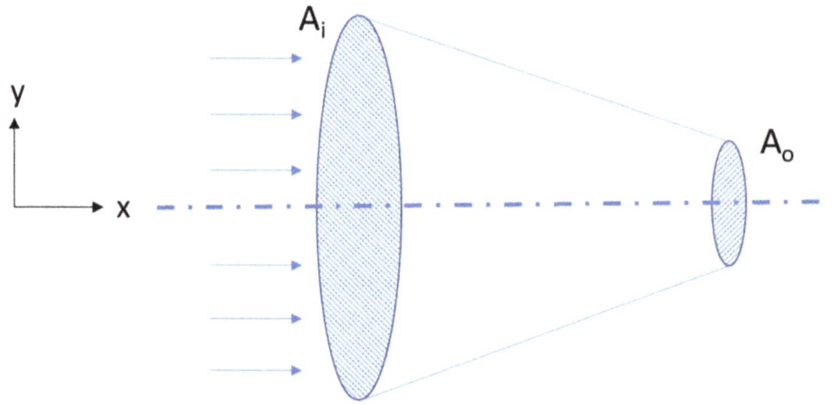

Figure 15.1. Schematic for variable area channel.

For steady state flow, the mass flow rate at inlet and outlet are equal. The average velocity, $\bar{u}$ is an equivalent uniform velocity that could give the same volumetric flow rate as that induced by variable velocity.

$$\bar{\mathbf{u}} = \frac{\iint \mathbf{Adu}}{\mathbf{A}} \tag{15.6}$$

Thus, equation (15.5) can be written in terms of average velocity as:

$$\rho_i \bar{u}_i \mathbf{A}_i = \rho_o \bar{u}_o \mathbf{A}_o \tag{15.7}$$

Equation (15.7) represents the continuity equation in algebraic form that is used to relate the average velocity within variable areas of channel.

The Reynolds transport theorem can be used to get a force balance equation. The momentum conservation equation or Navier–Stokes equation can be written by considering '*N*' as the momentum of fluid 'mV'. Thus, on the left-hand side of equation (15.1), the rate of change of momentum of the system gives force acting on the fluid, F_{sys}. This force on the system can be body force or surface force. Thus, using RTT from equation (15.1), we get:

$$\frac{\partial}{\partial t} \iiint \rho \vec{V} d\forall + \iint (\rho V) \vec{V} \cdot dA = \mathbf{F}_{sys} \tag{15.8}$$

Applying the Gauss divergence theorem and considering the arbitrary choice of elementary volume, the momentum equation for the *i*th direction can be written as:

$$\frac{\partial}{\partial t}(\rho u_i) + \nabla \cdot (\rho u_i \vec{V}) = \nabla \cdot \vec{\tau}_I + \mathbf{b}_i \tag{15.9}$$

Equation (15.5) is referred to as the Navier equilibrium equation that explains the relationship between the rate of momentum change in control volume and forces acting on it. Here, ***i*** is the stress tensor in the *i*th direction. For Newtonian and isotropic fluid, the constitutive relation between stress and strain rate is given in terms of fluid parameters that can be measured such as velocity and pressure. Substituting that in equation (15.5), in vector form for incompressible flow, we get:

$$\rho \frac{dV}{dt} = -\nabla P + \eta \nabla^2 \mathbf{V} + \rho \mathbf{b} \tag{15.10}$$

This represents the Navier–Stokes equation for incompressible flow. It is important to note that the left-hand side of equation (15.6) is negligible in microfluidic applications. Thus, it is boon for us that the non-linear derivative part itself tends to zero, and thus it becomes easy to get analytical solutions for several microfluidic cases such as flow-through circular microchannel. To illustrate the application of the Navier–Stokes equation in microfluidic analysis, we consider a simple example of fluid flowing through a circular duct. Neglecting body forces, we get balance of pressure force and viscous force. Solving this momentum equation, we get the axial velocity profile for a fully developed laminar flow

$$u = -\frac{\mathbf{R2}}{4\mu}\frac{\mathbf{dp}}{\mathbf{dz}}\left(1-\frac{\mathbf{r2}}{\mathbf{R2}}\right) \tag{15.11}$$

This represents the parabolic velocity profile and its variation with the radius of the duct. This expression can be used to relate pressure drop in the duct and flow rate which is given by:

$$\Delta \mathbf{P} = \frac{\mathbf{128\mu QL}}{\pi \mathbf{D4}} \tag{15.12}$$

where μ is the viscosity of fluid, Q is the volume flow rate, L is the length of the duct, D represents the hydraulic diameter. Thus, being able to get such simple expressions is helpful for first-hand calculations to design the channel dimensions for applications.

15.2.2 Surface tension and wettability phenomenon

Another perspective in the microfluidic study is to investigate the wettability of a surface. It is vital from the development of several applications as well as surface chemistry involving de-wetting and de-icing surface, droplet dynamics, inkjet printing, digital microfluidics, etc. Surface tension or surface energy is defined as the amount of work done to increase one unit's surface area. The SI unit of surface tension is *N/m*. Wetting and de-wetting of the surface depend on this crucial physical property.

Let us consider a sessile drop of liquid on a flat surface, as shown in figure 15.2. The different interfacial tensions are shown at the droplet triple contact line as γ_{lv} (liquid–vapor), γ_{sl} (solid–liquid), and γ_{sv} (solid–vapor). Applying force balance at the contact line, we get:

$$\cos\theta = \frac{\gamma_{sv} - \gamma_{sl}}{\gamma_{lv}} \tag{15.13}$$

This equation is referred to as Young's law where θ represents the contact angle. If the contact angle is less than 90°, the surface is said to be hydrophilic, and if it is greater than 90° surface is hydrophobic in nature.

Now, consider a flat surface. What will happen when you pour a few micro-liters of liquid on it? Does it form a film, or is it stable in the form of a droplet? As we know, if we have a drop in the air (with negligible gravity), it attains a spherical shape at minimum energy configuration. But here we have a solid–liquid interaction

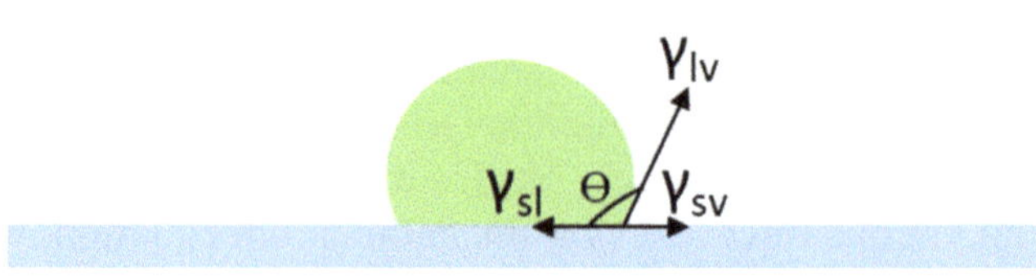

Figure 15.2. Schematic of a sessile drop on a planar substrate.

as well. Figure 15.2 shows that all the three interfacial tensions are essential to define the wetting condition based on its contact angle. Thus, the spreading parameter, S, is defined as the difference of the dry energy state and wet energy state.

$$S = \gamma_{sv} - (\gamma_{sl} - \gamma_{lv}) \tag{15.14}$$

If $S > 0$, we get total wetting, and when $S < 0$, we get partial wetting of the surface in the form of droplets. The low surface energy substrates are hydrophobic in nature and vice versa.

In microfluidics applications, we often require performing surface treatments to convert the hydrophobic surface into hydrophilic and vice versa. Generally, hydrogenated and fluorinated surfaces are used as hydrophobic coatings such as Teflon and PDMS. While in situations like PDMS microchannel, when we need to flow liquid, we plasma treat to hydrophilize the layer.

15.2.3 Non-dimensional numbers and their relevance in microfluidics

To understand the phenomenon occurring in microfluidics scale, it is important to appreciate its associated effects. Usually, in any phenomenon, two or more competing forces play a role and thus, it would better to group them as a non-dimensional form to study its effect.

1. Reynolds number (Re): refers to the ratio of inertial to viscous force. In microfluidics, Re is generally less than unity, thus the viscous force dominates over inertia. Re numbers are used to differentiate between turbulent and laminar flow and help predict different fluid flow patterns. Usually, when the Re number is less than 2000, we assume fluid flow is laminar. However, Re values greater than 2000 are taken as turbulent. In this way, the Re number is useful to control fluid pattern.

$$\mathbf{Re} = \rho \mathbf{VL}/\eta$$

   where ρ is the liquid's density, V is the velocity, L represents the characteristic dimension, and η is the dynamic viscosity.
2. Capillary number: is defined as the ratio of surface tension to viscous force. It is relevant in the case of immiscible liquids such as droplet formations in the continuous immiscible medium. The surface tension affects the free surface dynamics.

$$\mathbf{Ca} = \eta \mathbf{V}/\gamma$$

3. Peclet number: defines the relative importance of convention to diffusion. This is highly important in mixing applications in microfluidics.

$$\mathbf{Pe} = \mathbf{LV/D}$$

   where D is diffusivity.

15.3 Device fabrication

In the previous section, we discussed micro-scale fluid phenomena and the related physics. Going forward, to perform a real experiment, we need a microfluidic device. The microfluidic device was created when progress was made in microelectronics and the MEMS industry combined with biochemical applications. The fabrication of the microfluidic device plays a vital role in its success. The design depends on the application in which it is to be implemented. There are several methods for fabricating microfluidic chips, but most common are soft lithography, micro-machining, and 3D printing. We will discuss each of these to give a complete picture. Depending on the requirements, the user can opt for specific methods.

15.3.1 Soft lithography

This is an important technique for fabricating microchannels and creating micro/nanostructures onto a surface or inside a microchannel. This technique was developed by Whitesides group that involves a soft polymeric mold such as a PDMS replica from a hard master [6]. The master mold is prepared using photolithography on silicon generally. Several polymers are being used to fabricate microfluidic channels such as PDMS (most popular), photocurable perfluoropolyether, photosensitive polymers, and polymerized hydrogels.

An integrated microfluidic device contains a channel layer bonded to either a micro/nanostructured layer or plane surface like glass. To fabricate a channel (figure 15.3), prepolymer PDMS (10:1 silicone elastomer and curing agent, the ratio depends on the stiffness of channel required) is cured on the master mold (generally made of SU8 or Si using photolithography) by keeping it at 70 °C–80 °C for 1 h approximately. After the polymer is fully cured, it is removed from the master mold and bonded with a cleaned glass substrate using plasma treatment. This simple bonding without high temperature or pressure makes multiple layer stacking easier

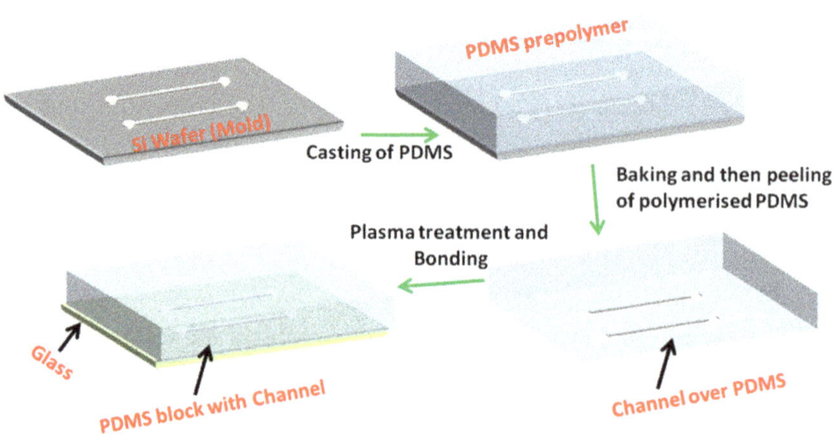

Figure 15.3. Schematic representation of microchannel fabrication with PDMS using soft lithography.

(as in multilayer soft lithography used to create PDMS valves). The important thing to note is that the silicone elastomer ratio to curing agent varies with applications such as multilayer stacking, valves, or pumps. It is also important to note that with multiple uses, device performance reduces due to surface adsorption by some biomolecules from sample or impurities present. To solve this issue, the substrate (the surface to which channel is bonded) is modified using PEG (polyethylene glycol) to prevent biofouling.

There are two soft lithographic methods to create micro/nanostructures on a surface or inside microchannels—contact printing and capillary molding [7]. Contact printing is generally used to generate a chemically modified surface, while capillary molding is used to create topographical-modified physical micro/nanostructures. In contact printing, direct printing is done using an elastomeric stamp, as shown in figure 15.4(a). Once the stamp is cured, it is soaked in the 'ink' to be printed and brought into conformal contact with the substrate where it is to be printed. It is beneficial for low-cost batch production but generally used for 1D patterns. The resolution of such techniques is 500 nm and can go as high as 50 nm with hard PDMS mold. The capillary molding method generates 2D structures on the surface. In this technique, an elastomeric mold (PDMS or PUA) is placed on the polymer surface (figure 15.4(b)). It is then heated above its glass transition temperature due to which capillary force makes polymer flows in the void created between mold and polymer layer. It is also possible with UV curable resin followed by solvent evaporation. The resolution of such a technique is up to 50 nm in PUA mold.

This polymer-based soft lithography process has largely revolutionized microfluidic device fabrication as it enables fast, inexpensive manufacturing with a broad range of polymer materials.

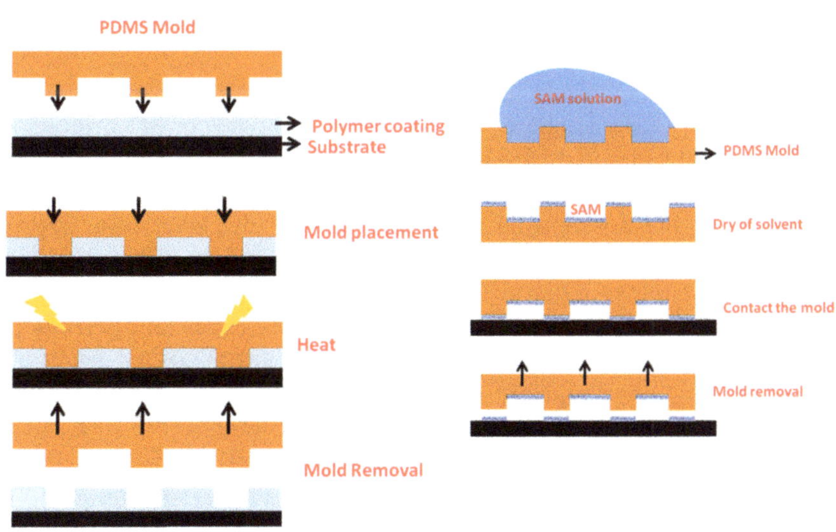

Figure 15.4. (a) Capillary molding and (b) contact printing.

15.3.2 Micromachining

Another approach to fabricate microfluidic devices is the micromachining of glass/Si substrate. There are several advantages of glass and silicon substrates such as thermal stability and solvent resistance, making it an appropriate choice for microfluidic chip fabrication. Typically, micromachining constitutes three steps—photolithography, etching, and bonding.

In the photolithography step, the substrate is cleaned and spin-coated with photoresist (PR). There are two types of PR being used, namely positive and negative. The positive PR is one in which the portion exposed to light becomes soluble to the developer, and in negative PR, the light-exposed part becomes insoluble. The soft bake temperature and duration after the PR coating depends on the type of PR used. After exposure through a photomask (containing microchannel design) in the lithography tool, the pattern is transferred to the PR layer. It is then developed in a photoresist developer to wash away the rest of the PR region. Depending on PR, it is followed by a hard bake. The desired microchannel design is now on the PR coated substrate. This PR layer helps in selective etching the substrate using etchants. Next, PR is inert to the etchant, thus creating microchannels on the substrate. The PR layer is later removed from the substrate. After the etching step, we get an open microchannel on the substrate needed to be bonded to another substrate to close it using thermal or adhesive bonding.

However, the rigidity of substrate, gas impermeability, high cost, and need for cleanroom facilities restrict this method's use for large-scale production.

15.3.3 3D printing

This is a relatively new technique being used. As the structure complexity increases, time and cost of fabrication also go up. It also hinders the automated system for fabrication. Thus, generating 3D structures in a single step is beneficial for rapid and high-throughput manufacturing. In this approach, 3D geometrical information is stored in a computer as a CAD file that runs the attached printer.

Stereolithography (SL) is one of the most popular types of 3D printing used to fabricate microfluidic channels. It polymerizes the photocurable resin layer by layer through laser irradiation. The laser beam is focussed and scanned over the liquid resin's surface for the liquid–solid transformation of the layer, thus creating the structure. The fresh resin is then spread over it, and again light-induced solidification occurs, creating complete 3D structures. There are other 3D printing methods like multi-jet modeling use inkjet printers to create 3D structures and fused deposition modeling in which layers of thermoplastic polymer are deposited using a heated extrude nozzle.

This technique enables fabricating accurate design in one step with acceptable resolution and offers less time and labor cost. Unlike soft lithography and micromachining, 3D printing is an additive manufacturing method that interfaces with an industry grade user interface and embedded control system for large-scale production.

15.4 Biomedical applications of microfluidics

Unil now, we have discussed microfluidics physics and device fabrication methods. One more critical aspect that one should know while developing a microfluidic platform for biomedical applications is the flow control system. Once we fabricate a microchannel say by soft lithography and bond it with the glass substrate, we need to know about flow actuation mechanisms and interfacing with external pumps via tubes.

Flow is generally manipulated using a syringe pump that controls the flow rate. It is a favorable way to actuate liquid as flow rate can be altered directly by changing the stepper motor's speed. It is important to note that it takes a little time for the flow to stabilize when you change the flow rate due to fluctuations in flow rate supplied and pressure [8]. Since the PDMS microchannels are flexible they offer compliance. Researchers have used a flow reduction mechanism to benefit from this case and tried to control the liquid interface movement with high resolution by using feedback control to the input signal. There is another aspect of using elastomeric valves [9] in the microfluidic channel to control the flow rate. Researchers have developed a multilayer soft lithography method to fabricate PDMS check valves where the pneumatics is used to actuate the valves depending on dimensions.

So far, we have chronologically discussed the area of microfluidics explaining its physics and device fabrication methods. However, several specifics need to be discussed as per the applications they are suited to. We will briefly cover such aspects and discuss the role of microfluidics in their respective applications. The design of microfluidic channels depends on the application. This section will discuss some of the major biomedical research areas where microfluidics offers significant experimental advantages over conventional methods to biologists. From fundamental research to the development of a portable diagnostics kit, there is a range of examples from current research to give readers a broad perspective and help them understand the real benefits of microfluidic devices in biomedical applications.

15.4.1 Microfluidics for single-cell analysis

Cells are the basic unit of living organisms. The bulk cell assays provide information, but the average data obtained neglects the differences in intracellular molecular expressions from individual cells due to cell heterogeneity. This leads to the loss of vital data during averaging. The single-cell assays reveal heterogeneities in cell morphology, functions, composition, and genetic performance. However, there are certain challenges in single-cell analysis—owing to the small size of most cells, manipulation is difficult in conventional bulk sample preparation strategies; small concentration of sample demands more sensitive detection methods. With the advances in microfluidics technology, it provides a solution to the above challenges. The micrometer-size channels and physical structures comparable to cells make single-cell manipulation efficient. The microfluidic chips can integrate multiple functionalities such as cell isolation, cell lysis, and cell analysis with detection methods available on-chip.

This section will discuss single-cell manipulation methods on microfluidic chips and applications like characterizing the mechanical and electrical properties of cells.

15.4.1.1 Single-cell isolation

The first step in single-cell analysis is cell isolation. Individuals cells are isolated in an enclosed chamber to separate them. The cell sorting technique should detect cell-type-specific markers, sort cells at single-cell resolution, and maintain cell viability. There are different techniques available such as mechanical traps, droplet traps, and active forces like hydrodynamics trap, DEP trap, magnetic trap and acoustic trap. Figure 15.5 shows trapping of micro/nano scale particle by hydrodynamic forces.

15.4.1.2 Single-cell lysis

Cell lysis occurs when the cell membrane (and/or cell wall) is disrupted, allowing cytoplasm content to be released. There are four methods that are being used for cell lysis—mechanical, chemical, electrical, and thermal. The use of mechanical force is one of the most common ways to puncture the membrane. In microfluidic devices, cells are forced to pass through a filter with an opening too small to pass the whole cell, thus shearing the cell membrane. Another method utilizes a PDMS membrane in a microfluidic channel to crush the cell membrane.

In the thermal cell lysis method, cell samples are heated at high temperatures. This method is generally used in PCR-based assays. In chemical lysis, buffers, or other lytic reagents (surfactants) are used to break the cell membrane. The cell sample flowing in a channel is mixed with cell lysis agents, then made to flow through a sufficient long channel giving it sufficient diffusion time. The mixture is then separated at T-junction, where lysed cells and lytic agents are separated. Exposure of cells to a high electric field is sufficient to cause cell lysis. As the pulse

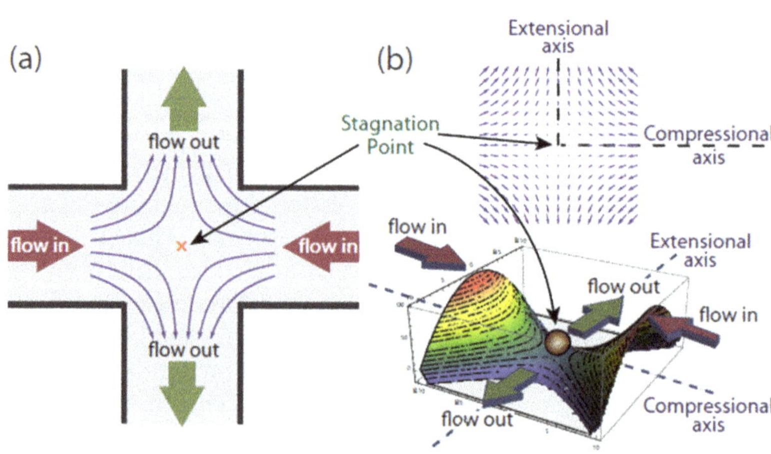

Figure 15.5. Hydrodynamic trap created by two laminar inlet streams which converge at a channel junction and two divergent outlet streams in the opposite direction perpendicular to the inlet. This geometry creates a planar extensional flow which contains a stagnation point or point where velocity is zero (at the center of the channel junction). Reprinted from [10], with the permission of AIP Publishing.

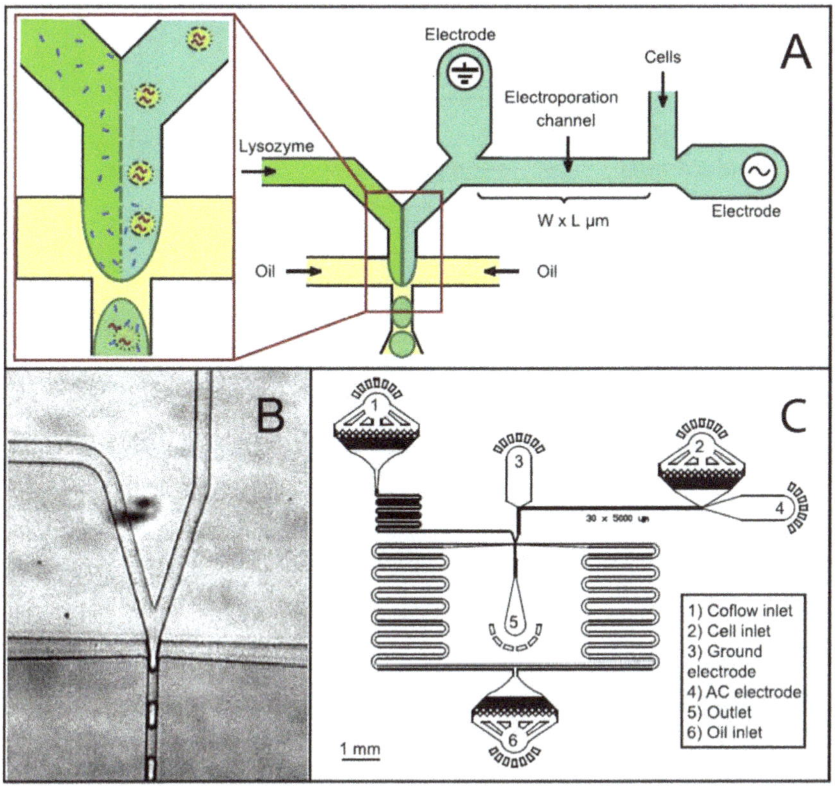

Figure 15.6. The schematic diagram of electrical lysis for droplet screening. (a) Representation of electrical lysis and droplet generation part. (b) Image of the droplet generation. (c) Design of the complete lysis device with electroporation channel having dimensions of 30 µm × 5000 µm. Reprinted from [11], with the permission of AIP Publishing.

length and electric field strength reach a critical value, cells are lysed by dielectric breakdown of the cell membrane (figure 15.6). In microfluidic devices with integrated electrodes, cell lysis can occur at low voltage due to the smaller distance between electrodes and high field strength than a conventional setup requiring 500 V.

15.4.1.3 Mechanical and electrical property of cells

The electrical properties of the cell membrane and cytoplasm and the cytoskeleton's mechanical properties determine the overall biophysical properties of cells [12]. There are different microfluidic devices based on patch-clamp, electro-rotation, and micro-electrical impedance spectroscopy (µ-EIS). The patch-clamp devices characterize cellular ion channel activities by sucking a cell membrane into a micro-pipette to form a high electrical resistance seal. This technique disrupts the cell membrane and hence cannot be used for long-term study. The rotating electric field exerts a force on a suspended cell to rotate due to Maxwell–Wagner polarization

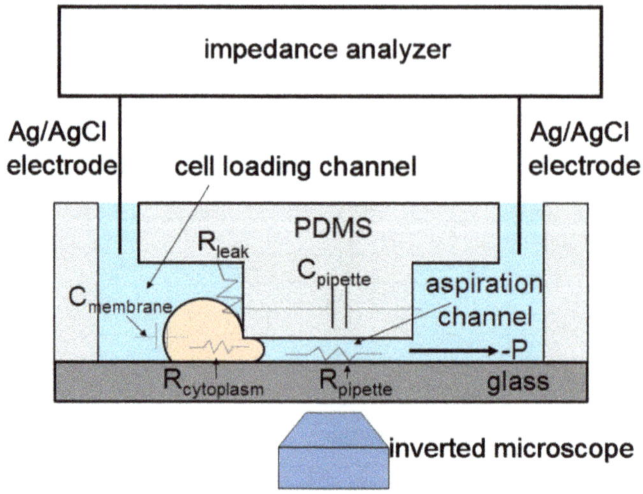

Figure 15.7. Electrical and mechanical characterization of a single cell that is trapped by applying negative pressure. Impedance measurement is conducted by two Ag/AgCl electrodes. Reprinted from [12], with the permission of AIP Publishing.

in electro-rotation devices. In the μ-EIS device, a frequency-dependent signal is applied across a single cell to measure the corresponding current. The microfluidic device with constriction is used to measure the deformability and Young's modulus of cells. Figure 15.7 shows impedance measurement during single-cell entrapment in a constricted micro-channel. Other methods incorporate electro deformation, micro-pipette aspiration, and optical stretcher to measure the mechanical properties of cells.

Apart from mechanical and electrical properties, with the development in microfluidic technology, it is used for studying cell–cell interaction, cell genetic and protein analysis, and diagnosis.

15.4.2 Microfluidics-based PCR devices

Among the microfluidics, the miniaturized PCR instrument (or PCR microfluidics) has become a valuable tool for molecular biology since it can potentially help deoxyribonucleic acid (DNA) amplification. In general, the PCR cycle involves three distinct steps: denaturation, annealing, and extension. In the denaturation step, the temperature rises to ~95 °C; thus, two single strands are denatured from a double-stranded DNA. Next is an annealing step where the primer binds with the target DNA sequence, and the temperature decreases to ~56 °C. Further, in extension steps, DNA polymerase attaches free DNA nucleotides available in solution to template DNA at 72 °C. This activity synthesizes second complementary DNA from free nucleotides in solution. Therefore, the three repetitive steps are necessary to efficiently increase double-stranded DNA concentration. In this context, microfluidics is revolutionizing the way lab-testing procedures are conducted especially for applications accounting in PCR devices. PCR microfluidics of varying design have been developed for effective and fast DNA amplification and are broadly classified as chamber stationary PCR, flow-through PCR, and thermal convection-driven PCR [13]. The chamber stationary PCR works in a conventional manner, that of a normal PCR device, where the solution is kept stationary and the temperature of PCR reaction chamber is cycled between the above mentioned three temperatures. The amplification products upon completion are recovered for either off-line detection or are detected online. Unlike chamber stationary PCR, flow through PCR configures its microfluidics devices with a 'time-conversion concept' wherein the PCR solution is continuously flowing through three different temperature zones necessary for amplification instead of making it stationary. This approach however, is more flexible to change the reaction rate resulting in reduced cycling and heating time. Next, convectively driven PCR microfluidics in its rudimental stages is capable of rapid DNA amplification. The designs for convection-driven PCR devices employs only two temperature zones which facilitates sample flow, resembles flow-through microfluidics to a certain extent. By employing Rayleigh–Benard convection to perform PCR amplification inside a cylindrical cavity measuring 35 μl and continuously shuttling fluid vertically between two temperature zones such that, annealing/extension was above 61 °C and denaturation was below 97 °C. Subsequently, laminar convection comprises a layered PCR which facilitates a cheap reaction chamber with a high reaction speed using a non-contact heating method. PCR microfluidics consists of a chamber with a diameter of 5 mm and thickness of 1 mm heated in the center of the chamber by an infrared source. This design of PCR cycles a volume of 20 μl and achieve a 1 000 000-fold DNA amplification. Convectively driven PCR microfluidics are very simple in their design, have the advantages of cheap fabrication and much faster temperature transition speed.

Further, a polyimide microfluidic device was designed for 30 cycles of PCR with a time ratio of 1:1:2 for denaturation, annealing, and extension step as presented in figure 15.8. Similarly, a design featured 30 cycles of PCR in a polycarbonate substrate using a computer numerical controlled (CNC) vertical milling machine. In this study, however, temperatures were created using two copper heating blocks for denaturation and a combined annealing/extension step. Additionally, to reduce flow resist of these devices, Wu *et al* coated a 0.5 mm inner diameter steel capillary with Norland Optical Adhesive 61 (NOA61) [14]. The above examples implement different materials to simplify the design of these devices and discuss flow resistance optimization. Due to the low cost of plastic devices, they can be disposed of almost immediately in order to avoid cross contamination arising through absorption of DNA onto the channel walls. It is the miniaturization of PCR devices that can offer an opportunity to improve them further in terms of shorter amplification times, higher sample throughput, and by extension result in minimum human/world-to-PCR intervention and contamination. In other words, some advances may contribute to making the operations of these devices simpler and more robust, while others may significantly compromise the purpose of this equipment.

Through a wide array of techniques, microfluidics offers several options for performing digital PCR either by creating droplets or microwells. In comparison, a

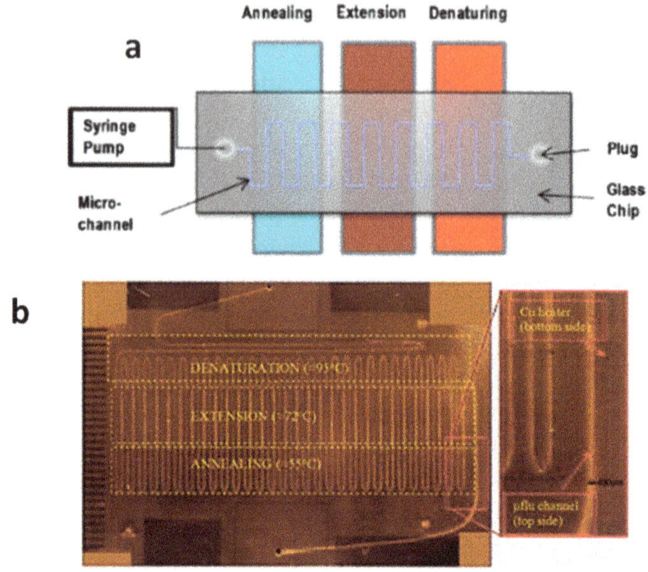

Figure 15.8. (a) Schematic representation of PCR-based microfludics device integrated with heater for denaturation, extension and annealing steps. Reprinted from [15], with the permission of AIP Publishing. (b) A serpentine based microfluidics device using three copper heaters. Reprinted from [16], Copyright (2014), with permission from Elsevier.

droplet of PCR showed a high sensitivity consistent with the standard methods [17]. Additionally, digital PCR spotted minute differences which even the qt-PCR (quantitative PCR) could not detect. For instance, Floren *et al* used digital PCR to identify several different species and were able to correlate tissue samples and the amount of mitochondrial DNA [18]. In another study by Hoshiona *et al* in his quantification of DNA from soil samples, qrt-PCR (quantitative reverse transcription-PCR) underestimated the DNA content due to inhibition, however, digital PCR showed more resilience [19]. Furthermore, isothermal nucleic acid amplification methods show a higher robustness against temperature variations and inhibition compared to conventional PCR. Microfluidics PCR systems for sample preparation and detection avail compartmentalization of DNA molecules into individual volumes from bulk solution. Due to its precise fluid control nature and reduced fabrication costs combination, it can be therefore inferred that isothermal nucleic acid amplifications using PCR microfluidics are providing a pathway for point-of-care applications.

15.4.3 Biosensor integration in microfluidic systems

According to IUPAC, a biosensor is defined as an independent integrated receptor transducer device, which can provide selective quantitative or semi-quantitative analytical information using a biological recognition element. On the other hand, the microfluidic system offers precise control over fluid flow in microscale volume.

Thus, it is another on-going research area to integrate biosensors on the microfluidic chip to achieve reduced sample consumption, portability, multiplexed detection, and low-cost point-of-care devices.

The biosensor has mainly two-components, the biological and physical. The biological components are basically enzymes, nucleic acids, antibodies, etc, that are collectively called bioreceptors and are known for their specific binding capability with analytes/markers. This bioreceptor is immobilized over the transducer surface (physical component), which produces physical and chemical changes after interaction between the bioreceptor and analyte. These signal changes are further amplified, processed, and interpreted also for display in suitable units. As we discuss there are different biological recognition sensing elements such as enzymes, aptamers, and antibodies employed to define selectivity and specificity and decrease the possibility of interference with undesirable substances. Enzymes are proteins that catalyze chemical reactions, typically redox reactions when used as biosensors. Antibody-based biosensors have also become popular after monoclonal antibody technology developed by Kohler and Milstein. Aptamers are amino acid polymers or a single-stranded nucleic acid that can bind to their specific ligands with a dissociation constant in the micromolar to picomolar range. Biosensors can also be classified based on their transduction mechanisms—electrochemical, optical, and mechanical.

15.4.3.1 Enzyme-based biosensor on a microfluidic platform

There have been several efforts to integrate biosensors with microfluidic chips. Glucose and urea levels in the blood have been measured using integrated chips. One such work is in the droplet microfluidics-based electrochemical sensor [20] to sense glucose level in human blood serum.

A platinum-black microelectrode (working electrode) was used for glucose sensors in flowing droplets. As shown in figure 15.9, the tapered capillary tip containing buffer and sample is connected to the PDMS chip. The sample stream is combined with GOx (glucose oxidase) enzyme and substrate glucose.

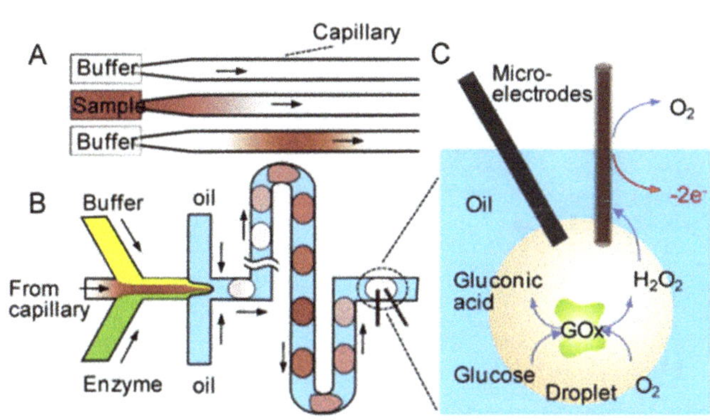

Figure 15.9. Schematic diagram representing the electrochemical sensing of glucose in droplets. Reprinted from [20], Copyright (2014), with permission from Elsevier.

By maintaining a suitable flow rate of mineral oil, the droplet is formed inside the microfluidic channel. The activity of GOx is estimated by measuring H_2O_2 concentration on the Pt-black electrode at the end of the microchannel.

15.4.3.2 Antibody-based biosensor on a microfluidic platform

The integration of a continuous microfluidic device and biosensor using antibodies as the biological recognition element is demonstrated to detect breast cancer using the surface plasmon resonance (SPR) phase imaging method [21]. An automated lab-on-a-chip microfluidic biosensor with multiple channels for the detection of microarray samples is developed (figure 15.10). Since SPR is a temperature-dependent technique, a temperature control unit consisting of micro heaters and temperature sensors to avoid temperature change and variation in the sensing area is used. A regular self-assembled monolayer (SAM) was used to immobilize the anti-rabbit IgG on the modified gold surface. The results showed that the fabricated microfluidic platform, which used SPR phase imaging successfully detected the presence of only IgG in the samples. Similarly, many other applications are reported in the literature on antibody-based biosensor in microfluidics platforms.

15.4.3.3 Aptamer-based biosensor on a microfluidic platform

An on-chip aptamer-based sensor was developed for the continuous detection of transforming growth factor (TGF-β1). The microdevice was fabricated on a glass substrate with gold electrodes and two PDMS layers (figure 15.11). The two PDMS

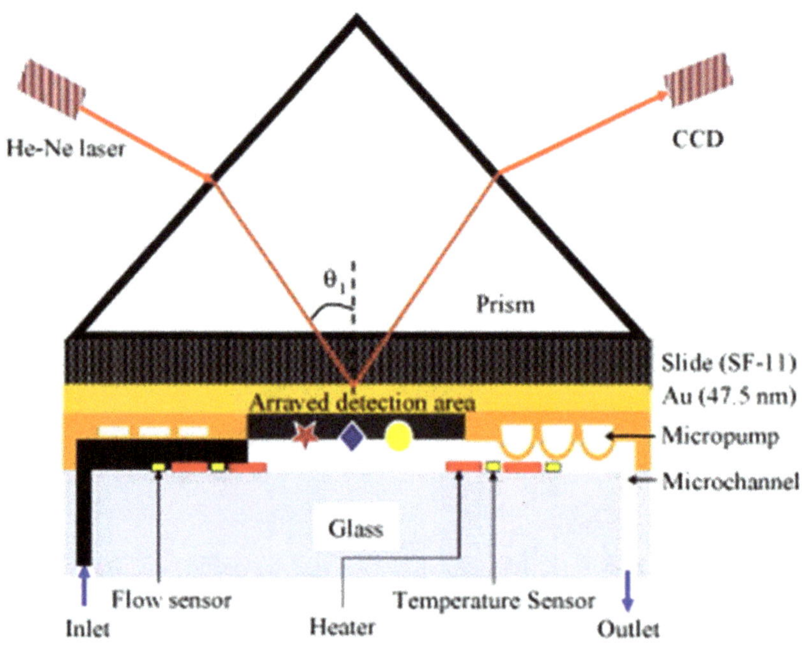

Figure 15.10. Microfluidics integrated SPR imaging system for detection of a microarray immunoassay. Reprinted from [21], Copyright ((2007) with permission from Elsevier.

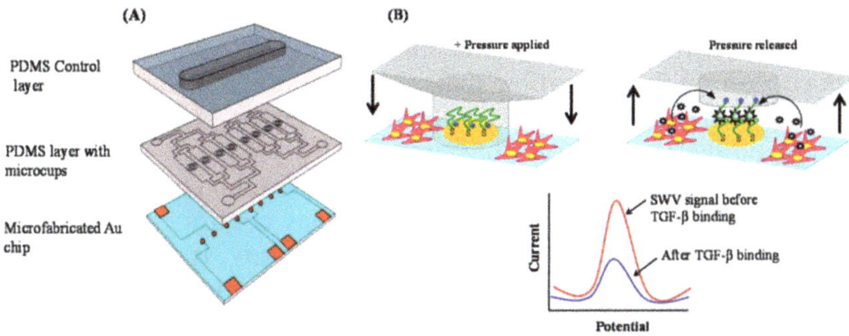

Figure 15.11. Aptasensor integrated microfluidic device for transforming growth factor from liver cells. (a) Schematic of a three layer microfluidic device. (b) Actuation of microcups to protect electrodes during collagen coating. Reprinted with permission from [22]. Copyright (2014) American Chemical Society.

layers were designed so that the first layer contains microchannels and semi-circular microcups, and the second layer was mainly used for pneumatic control. The microcups were raised during the protein secretion by cells which increased protein diffusion toward the sensing area. The microcups were then lowered during the physical separation of cells from the sensing electrode area. Square wave voltammetry (SWV) measurements were used to confirm thc interaction between the cell-secreted protein (TGF-β1) and the specific aptamer. The results showed a decrease in the redox signal, which is proportional to the sample's analyte concentration.

15.4.4 Microfluidics for organ-on-chip technology

Conventionally 2D cell culture is being used to study cell microenvironment and chemicals' effects on cellular response. But it is not very reliable as it does not support tissue-specific functions of cell types and does not mimic *in vivo* conditions. This has led researchers to 3D spheroid-based studies that usually rely on hydrogels, comprised of natural or synthetic polymer extracellular matrix (ECM). It is being used to study cell–cell interactions. However, it also has limitations such as 3D spheroids being variable in size and shape; thus, it is difficult to maintain consistent cell positions for analysis. It also lacks multiscale arrangements of the tissue–tissue interface, such as between vascular endothelium and connective tissues. Fluid flow condition is absent as it is *in vivo* due to circulating blood and the effect of shear stress and interaction with immune cells necessary for healthy body organs. Thus, microfluidic chip-based technique (organ-on-chip) [23] to mimic body physiology offers the possibility to overcome these limitations. It can be referred to as living cells culturing device in continuously perfused chambers to mimic functional level similarities at the tissue and organ level. Researchers have been working in this area with several perspectives like the simulation of cancer model on-chip to study its complex mechanisms for metastasis; vascular-on-chip is another hot area to mimic blood capillaries on a microfluidic chip; development of body-on-chip to recapitulate parts like lungs [24], brain [25], gut, kidney [26], heart [27] on a single platform with a vision for fundamental research and originating the concept of personalized medicine. This section will first discuss the organ-on-chip concept and how it is being used to study organ-level functionalities and physiology, followed by a brief discussion on biocompatible materials as an alternative to PDMS for cell culture. In the later part, we will highlight vasculature-on-chip and cancer-on-chip technologies and their current research status.

With the advent of soft lithography fabrication, microfluidic chips have been seen as a better alternative for cell culture. It provides control over several system parameters that are important in cell culture-based study. It consists of creating a miniaturized perfused channel in which ECM molecules are coated on the surface, followed by the flowing of the cell medium so that cells adhere to ECM coated substrate. Continuous perfusion is being done with the culture medium. The PDMS-based cell culture system being optically transparent, allows real-time optical imaging of cell response to environmental cues. Microsensors can be integrated into the microfluidic chip to analyze cell migrations, tissue barrier integrity, and fluid pressure. Microfluidic devices being a laminar regime flow helps in creating physical and chemical gradients that have assisted researchers in studying directional cell migration, cardiac tissue formation, nerve axon outgrowth, and cell–cell junctional integrity. These devices also offer controlled cell patterning with different types of cells. The ability to integrate a porous substrate between two microchannels (having different cells) has enabled the study of tissue interfaces that mimic vascular endothelium and parenchymal tissues. These microfluidic chips are also useful in creating a complex mechanical microenvironment that can simulate cyclic strain and fluid stresses that are somewhat like what cells experience in breathing and cardiovascular cycling.

Although most organ-on-chip studies are related to established cell lines, it can be used for plant cells or even stem cells study. Researchers have also investigated induced pluripotent stem cells because of the potential to model diseased organs with patient-specific cells. These lines of research are directed towards personalized human-on-chip. Researchers have fabricated chips to study liver, kidney, intestine, heart, lung, skin, blood vessels, brain–blood barrier, bones, and several other disease models like cancer. To provide a better understanding of this research area, we will discuss microfluidic chips for mimicking blood vessels and cancer models.

15.4.4.1 Vasculature-on-chip

The vascular system is found throughout the body, in contact with different organs and tissues. The abnormal functions can lead to several acute diseases like tumor angiogenesis and blood vessels related disease. Thus, it is crucial to develop a vascular system [28] on chip to understand *in vivo* conditions. There are four main methods to fabricate blood vessel-like microchannels on a microfluidic chip.

1. Microfluidics membrane and ECM-based devices: Depending on whether the endothelial monolayer is cultured on a membrane or an ECM, researchers have fabricated two designs. In membrane-based devices, endothelial cells are cultured on a horizontal membrane, which separates two channels, while in an ECM-based device, it is cultured on extracellular matrix sidewalls.

Membrane devices are used to measure the barrier properties of endothelial monolayers. The integration of electrodes in channels assist in the measurement of transendothelial electrical resistance (TEER). The narrow-spaced PDMS pillars are used to confine ECM between two channels. Growth factors can be introduced in channel or ECM directly to create a gradient.
2. 3D template-based models: This involves casting an ECM material around a removable template. A rod is inserted in the PDMS housing, which defines the position for microvessel structures. A solution of ECM (collagen-containing cells) is introduced around the template. Once it is cross-linked, the template is removed. The cylindrical channel network thus formed can be used for perfusion after seeding endothelial cells inside. This technique generates a vessel diameter greater than 50 μm.
3. 3D bioprinting: Liquid droplets containing hydrogels, cells, ECM proteins, and other biochemical cues are dispensed using nozzles to print a vascular array. In direct printing, a solution of ECM material and a suspension of endothelial cells in a dissolvable matrix precursor are required. Gelatin containing ECs is printed as a cylinder in a collagen ECM. The device is rotated and heated at 37 °C to dissolve gelatin. Proliferation and spreading of ECs result in the vessel lumen.
4. Sclf-assembly: The guided capillary self-organization method is used to create a network of capillaries in a microfluidic chamber filled with ECM. In this method, a series of diamond-shaped chambers is connected to establishing chemical and pressure gradients. The design of the microfluidic device allows the pressure difference between the source and sink through ECM. Endothelial cells are mixed in fibrinogen and thrombin ECM and the pipetted into the chamber. Under constant pressure, interstitial flow is initiated and leads to the self-organization of cells in the form of capillaries in about three weeks.

The vasculature-on-chip study is important for studying endothelial dysfunction, cancer, drug screening, and organ regeneration. Endothelial dysfunction causes thrombosis, atherosclerosis, and inflammatory diseases. Tumor angiogenesis and cancer metastasis are two important studies related to blood vessels. Reconstruction of the blood–brain barrier (it regulates the transport system between and brain and blood) and lymphatic system are another aspect of the on-chip vascular study.

15.4.4.2 Cancer-on-chip

This is another hot area of research related to organ-on-chip technology to mimic the tumor microenvironment and study cancer metastasis [29]. Controlling fluid flow, generating biochemical gradients, and incorporating mechanical cues are being done on a microfluidic platform to study different cancer progression aspects. Apart from cancer cells' genetic characteristics, its microenvironment plays an essential role in understanding this deadly disease's fundamentals. Thus, researchers have been investigating mimicking it on a microfluidic chip.

There are four important factors that are essential for developing a cancer model on-chip. They are biochemical cues, other types of cells in the tumor environment, ECM,

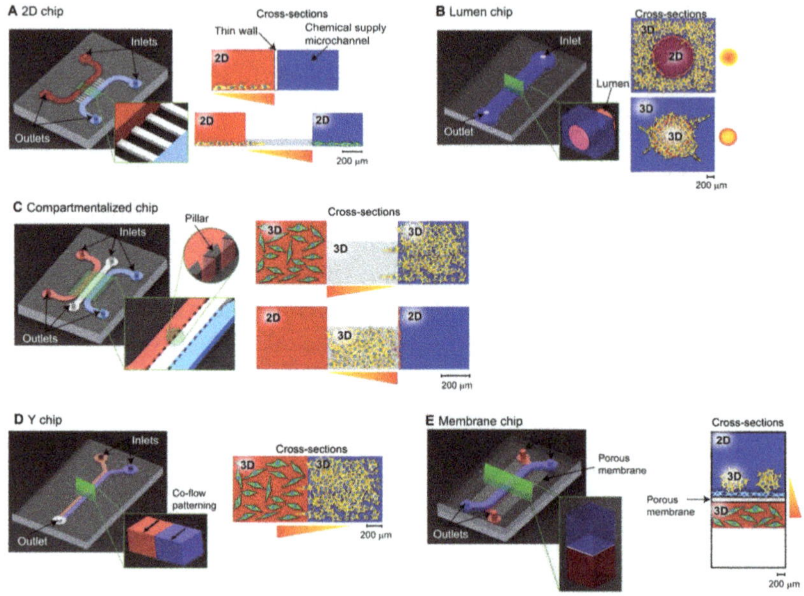

Figure 15.12. Schematic representation of different types of cancer-on-chip designs with different cell culture options [29], adapted under the terms of the CC-BY creative commons license. Copyright 2018 The Company of Biologists Ltd.

and mechanical cues. In short, we can say that these four factors comprise the tumor microenvironment. Researchers have developed different types of cancer-on-chip designs to incorporate the above four factors (figure 15.12). Generally, studies have been made concerning one factor at a time, as it is difficult to fabricate a complete microenvironment device. This is still an on-going research area. Different types of designs like 2D chips, lumen chip, compartmentalized chip, Y-chip, and membrane chip have been fabricated to study cancer-on-chip. 2D chips are single- or multi-chamber 2D culture devices with a controlled solute gradient. In this type of chip, cancer cells are typically exposed to a gradient of a solute, such as oxygen, while their viability or migration is measured. In a lumen chip, a patterned 3D matrix is used to form lumens or tumor compartments. This design is typically used to model blood vessels in tumors, or to tightly pack cancer cells in a cylindrical compartment. Compartmentalized devices use pillars to separate microchannels in which cell culturing is possible in both 2D and 3D. This type of chip is very versatile, allowing the user to pattern different matrix materials and cells in a controlled manner. The Y-chip comprised of parallel matrix compartments patterned by co-flow. This type of chip resembles the compartmentalized chip, as it enables matrix patterning, but is slightly less versatile in its patterning possibilities. In membrane chips, a co-culture device with stacked microchannels is separated by a porous membrane. One of the interesting features of these devices is that a 3D culture is created only in part of the microchannel, with the rest empty to refresh the media. This multi-layered chip type was originally developed to mimic the endo- and epithelial cell layers found in the lung.

15.5 Conclusion

Microfluidics technology has been a boon for several research areas that require fluid manipulation at a small scale. This chapter aims to provide overall knowledge and make readers acquainted with many beneficial applications of microfluidics systems. We have explained the physics of micro-scale flows and wettability effects that are important in microfluidics. We also explained fabrication methods for such microfluidic chips that are being used for several biological applications. In the last section, we have tried to highlight the use of microfluidic devices in single-cell analysis, PCR-based study, biosensor integration, and organ-on-chip technologies. In other words, a microfluidic device can be called a 'lab-on-chip' that perform whole biological assays with reduced sample consumption, enhanced sensitivity, and automation. We understand that it is not possible to discuss every aspect of such platforms in detail in a single chapter; therefore, we have cited respective papers for readers, in case they would like to investigate further in a domain. For the past two decades, microfluidics research has increased tremendously, helping biologists explore and discover a new horizon in biology. However, this technology is still to be utilized to its maximum potential. In the words of renowned physicist Richard Feynman, 'there is plenty of room at the bottom,' and this is true for microfluidic systems as well.

References

[1] Shang L, Cheng Y and Zhao Y 2017 Emerging droplet microfluidics *Chem. Rev.* **117** 7964–8040

[2] Samiei E, Tabrizian M and Hoorfar M 2016 A review of digital microfluidics as portable platforms for lab-on a-chip applications *Lab Chip.* **16** 2376–96

[3] Beyssen D, Le Brizoual L, Elmazria O and Alnot P 2006 Microfluidic device based on surface acoustic wave *Sensors Actuators* B **118** 380–5

[4] Zhang Y and Nguyen N-T 2017 Magnetic digital microfluidics—a review *Lab Chip.* **17** 994–1008

[5] Mugele F and Baret J-C 2005 Electrowetting: from basics to applications *J. Phys. Condens. Matter* **17** R705

[6] Zhao X-M, Xia Y and Whitesides G M 1997 Soft lithographic methods for nano-fabrication *J. Mater. Chem.* **7** 1069–74

[7] Kim P, Kwon K W, Park M C, Lee S H, Kim S M and Suh K Y 2008 Soft lithography for microfluidics: a review *Biochip J.* **2** 1–11

[8] Zeng W, Jacobi I, Beck D J, Li S and Stone H A 2015 Characterization of syringe-pump-driven induced pressure fluctuations in elastic microchannels *Lab Chip.* **15** 1110–5

[9] Unger M A, Chou H-P, Thorsen T, Scherer A and Quake S R 2000 Monolithic microfabricated valves and pumps by multilayer soft lithography *Science* **288** 113–6

[10] Tanyeri M, Johnson-Chavarria E M and Schroeder C M 2010 Hydrodynamic trap for single particles and cells *Appl. Phys. Lett.* **96** 224101

[11] De Lange N, Tran T M and Abate A R 2016 Electrical lysis of cells for detergent-free droplet assays *Biomicrofluidics* **10** 024114

[12] Chen J, Zheng Y, Tan Q, Zhang Y L, Li J and Geddie W R *et al* 2011 A microfluidic device for simultaneous electrical and mechanical measurements on single cells *Biomicrofluidics* **5** 014113

[13] Ahrberg C D, Manz A and Chung B G 2016 Polymerase chain reaction in microfluidic devices *Lab Chip.* **16** 3866–84
[14] Chan K, Wong P-Y, Yu P, Hardick J, Wong K-Y and Wilson S A *et al* 2016 A rapid and low-cost PCR thermal cycler for infectious disease diagnostics *PLoS One* **11** e0149150
[15] Sugumar D, Ismail A, Ravichandran M, Aziah I and Kong L X 2010 Amplification of SPPS150 and *Salmonella typhi* DNA with a high throughput oscillating flow polymerase chain reaction device *Biomicrofluidics* **4** 024103
[16] Moschou D, Vourdas N, Kokkoris G, Papadakis G, Parthenios J and Chatzandroulis S *et al* 2014 All-plastic, low-power, disposable, continuous-flow PCR chip with integrated microheaters for rapid DNA amplification *Sens. Actuators* **B 199** 470–8
[17] Zhu Y, Zhang Y-X, Liu W-W, Ma Y, Fang Q and Yao B 2015 Printing 2-dimentional droplet array for single-cell reverse transcription quantitative PCR assay with a microfluidic robot *Sci. Rep.* **5** 9551
[18] Floren C, Wiedemann I, Brenig B, Schütz E and Beck J 2015 Species identification and quantification in meat and meat products using droplet digital PCR (ddPCR) *Food Chem.* **173** 1054–8
[19] Hoshino T and Inagaki F 2012 Molecular quantification of environmental DNA using microfluidics and digital PCR *Syst. Appl. Microbiol.* **35** 390–5
[20] Gu S, Lu Y, Ding Y, Li L, Song H and Wang J *et al* 2014 A droplet-based microfluidic electrochemical sensor using platinum-black microelectrode and its application in high sensitive glucose sensing *Biosens. Bioelectron* **55** 106–12
[21] Lee K-H, Su Y-D, Chen S-J, Tseng F-G and Lee G-B 2007 Microfluidic systems integrated with two-dimensional surface plasmon resonance phase imaging systems for microarray immunoassay *Biosens. Bioelectron* **23** 466–72
[22] Matharu Z, Patel D, Gao Y, Haque A, Zhou Q and Revzin A 2014 Detecting transforming growth factor-β release from liver cells using an aptasensor integrated with microfluidics *Anal. Chem.* **86** 8865–72
[23] Bhatia S N and Ingber D E 2014 Microfluidic organs-on-chips *Nat. Biotechnol.* **32** 760–72
[24] Huh D, Matthews B D, Mammoto A, Montoya-Zavala M, Hsin H Y and Ingber D E 2010 Reconstituting organ-level lung functions on a chip *Science* **328** 1662–8
[25] Fan Y, Nguyen D T, Akay Y, Xu F and Akay M 2016 Engineering a brain cancer chip for high-throughput drug screening *Sci. Rep.* **6** 25062
[26] Theobald J, Ghanem A, Wallisch P, Banaeiyan A A, Andrade-Navarro M A and Taškova K *et al* 2018 Liver-kidney-on-chip to study toxicity of drug metabolites *ACS Biomater. Sci. Eng.* **4** 78–89
[27] Agarwal A, Goss J A, Cho A, McCain M L and Parker K K 2013 Microfluidic heart on a chip for higher throughput pharmacological studies *Lab Chip.* **13** 3599–608
[28] Kim S, Kim W, Lim S and Jeon J S 2017 Vasculature-on-a-chip for *in vitro* disease models *Bioengineering* **4** 8
[29] Sleeboom J J, Amirabadi H E, Nair P, Sahlgren C M and Den Toonder J M 2018 Metastasis in context: modeling the tumor microenvironment with cancer-on-a-chip approaches *Dis. Model Mech.* **11** dmm033100

IOP Publishing

Chapter 16

Dynamic light scattering (DLS) particle size analysis for biomedical nanotechnology

Vikas Shukla, Karishma Niveria, Poonam Shashidhar and Anita Kamra Verma

The evolution of nanostructures in biomedical application is expanding rapidly. Varied nanostructures are being extensively used for bioimaging, biosensors and as drug/gene carriers because of their biocompatibility, coupled with reduced toxicity. Fundamental parameters like precision, reproducibility, consistency, and robustness are of paramount importance to ensure quality of measurement results and are key factors governing the characterization of nanostructures. The fact that nanoparticles range from 10 nm to 1 μm, with wide variation in optical properties enables their characterization using spectroscopy techniques and microscopy. Unfortunately, practicaly, innumerable challenges exist vis-à-vis the inadequate understanding of dynamic light dispersing (DLS) of the operating procedures dealing with critical issues like preparation of sample and data interpretation. To comprehend these parameters impeccably, DLS photon correlation spectroscopy is used to estimate the particle size and to evaluate their stability with respect to time in suspension, at a diverse range of pH and temperature in terms of their dispersion coefficient and hydrodynamic size. DLS has been accepted as an easy, simple and reproducible tool to determine the size of particle to enable effective understanding of the physico-chemical properties of the prepared nanostructures including size of particle, surface charge, surface modification/derivatization/functionalization, related interactions or loading capacity keeping in mind that these will eventually be used for pharmacokinetics, biodistribution, and targeting. This chapter focuses on light scattering based techniques offering practical guidelines on tackling commonly encountered problems while running DLS to analyze the relevance of this technique from translatory perspective and their application in biomedical nanotechnology.

doi:10.1088/978-0-7503-3379-5ch16

16.1 Introduction

The behavior of nanoparticles (NPs) within the biological *milieu* are dependent on the physico-chemical properties [1, 2]. Therefore, adequate characterization of the NPs is critical to obtain reliable data with high translatory output. The past decades have witnessed the immense contribution of NPs in fields including pharmaceutical, materials science, biology, chemistry, physics, engineering, and computer science [3]. The biomedical applications of nanotechnology have been successfully used as diagnostic tools, detection, drug delivery systems, and implants [4].

A variety of materials are used to formulate nanostructures including inorganic or organic, synthetic or biopolymers, metal, carbon nanotubes, liposomes, and lipids [5]. Hence, estimating tools become relevant owing to safety concerns that are generally attributed to the physico-chemical properties of NPs wherein physical parameters include surface charge [6], particle size [3], shape [5], and chemical parameters include crystallinity [8], impurity [7], surface functionalization with different ligands including PEGylation [6]. Appropriate characterization aids explanation of the NPs under a category of chemical species that are extremely reactive and display unparalleled and unique characteristics when compared to the bulk materials like fluorescence [10], conductivity [9], and magnetism [11].

Nanoparticle formulation requires full physico-chemical characterization of its size, surface charge, shape, and distribution [12]. It is frequently technically challenging to acquire reproducible nanoparticle suspensions with low polydispersity, desired size, and shape. Preparation of a homogeneous suspension of nanoparticles requires precise control of mixing and separation of particles [13]. The nanoparticles have to be robust, only a miniscule of injected dose (<0.7%) manages to reach the target site [14]. It has been observed that the NPs have to negotiate various barriers, such as interstitial fluid pressure, nonspecific distribution, cellular internalization, and drug efflux pumps, to achieve therapeutic efficacy [15].

Dynamic light scattering (DLS) is a robust technique to measure the size and pattern of distribution of particles, that are less than 1 nm in size. DLS is a non-invasive, accurate, and reproducible technique to study agglomeration of particles, that require a small amount of test sample. DLS, is often named photon correlation spectroscopy (PCS) or quasi-elastic light scattering (QELS). It is based on the principle of Brownian motion and correlates with function of motion to the size of the molecules. Brownian motion is known for the erratic motion of the particles, as a result of successive collision by the solvent molecules that surround them. DLS is extensively utilized for measuring the sizes of particles which are suspended in a liquid medium [16]. The DLS technique is frequently used for optimizing the sample preparation, depending on various parameters such as pH-range, ionic strength, concentration, and solvent etc. DLS further serves as a tool to obtain a sample of required characteristics such as particle uniformity and continual stability for advanced structural investigations of macromolecules with respect to x-ray crystallography [17] and illustrating RNA–protein complexes [18].

Several measurement techniques like NMR (nuclear magnetic resonance), spectroscopy, SAXS (small-angle x-ray scattering) and different crystallization setups generally restricted to a monodispersed solution [19], elucidates the total superficial charge on molecules [20] or even permits finite configuration and conformation details to be acquired *in situ* [21–23]. Particularly, in the case of *in situ* DLS instruments, provided with voluntarily adjustable laser probe the calibration of the optics including the super position of lens and laser, that concentrate the dispersed light on receiver fiber should be substantiated to attain optimal performance by means of set of screws with μm precision [23]. This chapter deals with a comprehensive overview with details of DLS and their application in biomedical nanotechnology.

16.1.1 History and background of light scattering

The light scattering detection technique is a utile tool with applications in various scientific fields which is dependent on the source of light and detector to analyze specific molecular characteristics. Initially, the light scattering experiments were carried out by John Tyndall who studied the scattering pattern of colloidal suspensions in the late nineteenth century [24]. The *Tyndall effect* describes the transmission of longer wavelengths, but there were shorter wavelengths that reflected in a diffused manner. Lord Rayleigh further explained the scattering of light from particles that are lower than the wavelength of light. The principle of *Rayleigh scattering* could help explain the color of the blue sky, as it is generated owing to the scattering of light by the atmospheric particles, along the importance of the refractive index of the scattering medium [25, 26].

In contrast to the Rayleigh scattering, Gustav Mie explained the theory of larger particles of relative wavelength. He developed a theory of absorbing and non-absorbing large particles in comparison to the wavelength of light with respect to the particle size and the differences in the refractive index of the medium [27]. The possibility of studying the scattering of the particles independent of size, mass and structure as a function of angle was suggested by Peter Debye which is referred to as *Rayleigh Debye scattering* [28].

The property of light scattering as a technique to designate the diffusion property of the particle led to a series of important discoveries that focused on DLS. DLS focuses on the measurement technique as a function of *Brownian motion* of the particle. A particle suspended in solution is constantly in random fluctuations or exhibits force due to constant interaction with the molecules of the solvent [29]. The concept of DLS differs from static light scattering which provides data on the radius of gyration and molecular weight of the particles as a function of the intensity of light with respect to time. On the other hand, DLS allows the measurement of (D) diffusion coefficient corresponding to the hydrodynamic radius in the solution. The *Stoke Einstein equation* that defines the diffusion coefficient (D) [30] is shown below:

$$D = \frac{k_B T}{6\Pi nrh} \tag{16.1}$$

where,

k_B = Boltzmann constant (1.380×10^{-23} kg m^2 s^{-2} K^{-1})
T = absolute temperature
η = viscosity of the medium

Over the years, various developments have occurred which have allowed measurement of the diffusion coefficient of molecules in solution. These contributions have led to the evolution of the Malvern zetasizer (Malvern, UK) who commercialized the former contemporary DLS equipment trailed by Brookhaven (Long Island, USA) and ALV (Langen, Germany) [23]. In view of the initiation of DLS, it has been verified to be efficient in the measurement of hydrodynamic sizes and behaviors of various biomolecules like nucleic acids, proteins, and viruses in different solvents. They particularly shed light on the aggregation kinetics of the biomolecules in solvents. Studying homogeneity of RNA, proteins and their complexes has become promisingly achievable by DLS technology. A modification of DLS technique, multi-angle dynamic light scattering (MADLS®), has the potential for further enhancing the resolution of DLS and the precision of the DLS technique has been improvized such that the results obtained by size analysis that were known to be independent of angle can now be exploited to improve the sensitivity of the DLS methodology (table 16.1).

Table 16.1. The time-line for the evolution of DLS [31].

Major contributions in development of DLS	Year of discovery
Tyndall effect: Scattering pattern of colloidal suspensions	1868
Rayleigh scattering: Light scattering of particles smaller than the wavelength of light and the importance of the refractive index of the scattering medium	1871
Mie theory: Theory of absorbing and non-absorbing large particles in comparison to the wavelength of light	1908
Brownian motion theory: A particle suspended in a solution is constantly in random fluctuations or forces because of constant interaction with molecules of the solvent	1905
Stokes–Einstein equation: Diffusion coefficient corresponding to the hydrodynamic radius occur in Brownian motion.	1905, 1906
Fluctuation on the theory of light scattering: Phenomenon of critical opalescence related to scattering with density fluctuations	1908, 1910
Rayleigh Debye scattering: Scattering of the particles independent of size, mass, and structure as a function	1915
Brillouin scattering: Inelastic scattering of light in a physical medium by thermally excited acoustical phonons	1941, 1921
Modern light scattering techniques	1964
Development of digital autocorrelator and Doppler shifts in light scattering of pure liquids and polymer solutions	1970

Characterization of polydispersity and distribution function of decay rates	1972
Exponential sampling for polydispersity studies	1981
Improved method for accurate determination of bimodal and broad unimodal distribution	1985
Maximum entropy analysis for quasi electric scattering and photon correlation spectroscopy data	1986, 1989

16.2 Theories of dynamic light scattering

The versatility of the DLS technique has been summarized in the following theories.

16.2.1 Rayleigh scattering

If the particles are tiny with respect to the wavelength of the laser used (generally lower than, $d = \lambda/10$ or roughly 60 nm for a He–Ne laser) then the principle of Rayleigh scattering is applied. The scattering of the particle irradiated through an upright polarized laser shall be in quintessence isotropic, or in other words, identical in every direction. Rayleigh approximation explicated that intensity of light is directly proportional to the sixth power of the diameter of a particle ($I \propto d^6$) while, inversely proportional to fourth power of laser wavelength ($I \propto 1/\lambda^4$) will be essentially isotropic, i.e., equal in all directions. The '*d*' term explains that a 50 nm particle tends to scatter one million- or 10-times increased light when compared to a 5 nm particle. Therefore, a threat exists that the scattered light from larger radiated particles will encompass the dissipated light radiated from the finer particles. The 'd^6' factor also indicates the difficulty of measuring a heterogeneous solution containing 10 nm and 1000 nm particles with DLS, as the net light scattered by ultrafine particles would be negligible. As the λ of used laser decreases an increased scattering intensity is observed explaining the inverse relationship to 4 [32].

16.2.2 Mie theory

Nevertheless, when particle size surpasses the $\lambda/10$ threshold, then Rayleigh scattering is substituted by an anisotropic Mie scattering, where the light shows inelastic scattering, i.e., energy scattered is unequal to the incident light and is angle-dependent (figure16.1) where the scattered light is most intense in the direction of the incident light. Hence, the size of scattering particles will be equivalent to the wavelength of incident ray as a function of minima and maxima in respect to angle (θ) in intensity plot distribution. Where, θ is the angle of scattering particles in the direction of propagation of incident ray. It is the only theory which provides the conversion of intensity distribution into volume by an algorithm assembled into a software (dynamic light scattering software 9kdlsw32 ver. 3.34) from Brookhaven instruments considering both Mie absorption and scattering, stated as:

$$G'V(d) = \frac{GI(d)}{d^3 p(\theta)} \tag{16.2}$$

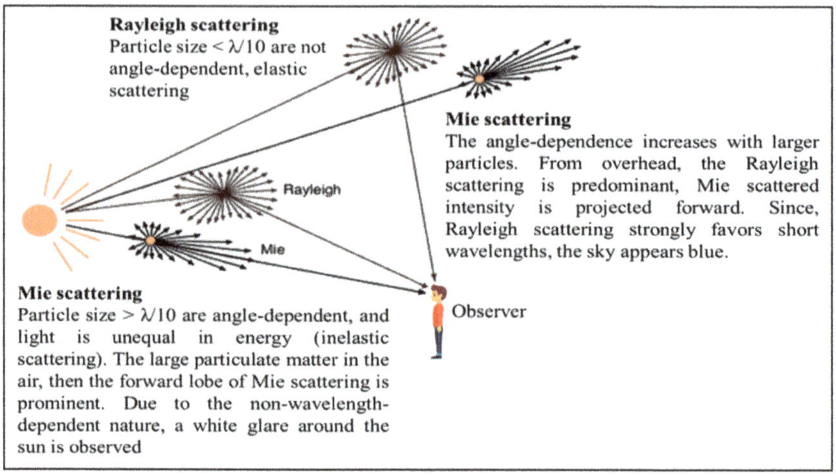

Figure 16.1. Schematic illustration depicting difference between Rayleigh scattering and Mei scattering.

where $G'V$ stands for the size distribution by volume, GI is the size distribution by intensity, d is the scatterer diameter and $P(\theta)$ is the angular part of the Mie theory scattering coefficient. This theory accurately elucidates the minima and maxima in the plot of intensity with angle and finally provides the correct answer considering all angles, sizes, and wavelengths. It is implemented in the Nano software for substituting the intensity distribution into volume (table 16.2) [33, 34].

16.3 Principle of light scattering

As discussed earlier, when a beam of monochromatic light interacts with macromolecules in a solution, light is scattered in diverse directions as a function of the macromolecular shape and size. DLS, also termed as the quasi-light scattering technique is employed to estimate the intensity of light scattered over time [32], measures the Brownian motion and correlates this to the size of the particles. Generally, the particle measurements are done when they are suspended within a liquid. Brownian motion is defined as the random movement of suspended particles caused by bombarding the surrounding solvent molecules. Brownian motion is slower for large macromolecules, while ultrafine particles are jerked further by molecules in the solvent more swiftly. In colloidal systems, particle dispersions exhibit dual phases (dispersed and dispersant), do not settle over time as they are in constant movement due to characteristic Brownian motion of the particles. The surface charge of particles makes the system more complex as the interactions between molecules, their surfaces, and ionic forms create a number of adsorbed layers on the surface of particles. Further, information on accurate temperature is essential for DLS since data on viscosity of the solvent is vital (as the viscosity of the liquid alters with changes in temperature). Also, temperature stability is necessary, or the convection currents within the sample tend to create non-random movements that will affect the interpretation of correct size [34]. The Brownian motion of the macromolecules

Table 16.2. Different scattering techniques applied for various samples.

Scattering techniques	Sample of microorganism	Experimental measurement	Additional information needed	Acquired information
Differential light scattering	(a) Spore	Angular dependence of scattered intensity	—	Refractive index profile of internal structure
	(b) Virus	Angular dependence of scattered intensity	—	Radius of gyration, second virtual coefficient and molecular weight
Quasi-elastic light scattering	(a) Spore	Angular dependence of time resolved intensity fluctuations (TRIF)	—	Intensity structure and asymmetry
		TRIF	—	Translational diffusion coefficient
		TRIF	—	Velocity distribution; effects of environmental conditions
	(b) Motile	microorganism	TRIF	
	(c) Virus		Sedimentation coefficient	Molecular weight
Turbidimetry	(a) Motile	Total loss of intensity by scattering	Increment of refractive index	Effect of environmental conditions on motility
	(b) Any	Total loss of intensity by scattering	Increment of refractive index	Molecular weight

is then related to the hydrodynamic size or the diffusion coefficient (D) [35]. In DLS, the movement of the particles over time is monitored and their specific positions over a range of time helps in interpreting the accurate hydrodynamic size of the particles. For example, larger particles move slowly in a solvent and therefore will not greatly vary from position, whereas smaller particles will move swiftly in a solvent and therefore do not have a specific position. In contrast to Raman spectroscopy, DLS relies on *elastic* electromagnetic scattering of the suspended particles. The electric field is induced in DLS to measure the Brownian motion of the scattering molecule component that are in constant random movement, which diffuse the light intensity of the particle to scatter light varying with time, meanwhile ions which are present in the form of photons have a constant energy. Based on particle movement and smaller particle signal, we can measure the hydrodynamic size of the particles. Usually, samples are used by biochemists to determine protein characteristics. The size of proteins is much smaller than the wavelength of laser ($<0.1\lambda$) incorporated in DLS which allows the light reception and isotropic scattering that follows the *Rayleigh scattering* law [35]. The intensity of scattered light, I depends upon constants like the θ (scattering angle), λ (wavelength), s (distance from scattering particle), n (refractive index of medium), r (radius of particle) which make the formula for the Stoke Einstein equation we can measure the hydrodynamic size of the particles

$$I = I_0 \frac{16\pi^4}{\lambda^4} \frac{1 + \cos^2\theta}{2\, s^2} \left(\frac{n^2 - 1}{n^2 - 2}\right)^2 \tag{16.3}$$

Scattering cross section is the mean value of I obtained by all scattering angles. The scattering intensity depends inversely on the fourth power of λ. Shorter wavelength of light is the key factor to detect fewer scattering molecules. According to the scattered light $I \sim s^{-2}$, the focal length of the lens should be minimized to enhance the scattering intensity, probably by optimizing the fiber cable and the position of the probe. For additional optimization of lenses, materials having lower refractive index like MgF2 coated lenses, can be used to diminish the reflection of the electromagnetic light, i.e., laser light. Background reflections of laser light can further decrease the specificity of the equipment [36, 37]. The intensity of light scattering is based on the sixth power of the size of particles (d). With increase in size, the intensity to scatter light enhances exponentially, that makes DLS sensitive to amass very large molecular size particles or unspecified large molecules. Therefore, larger molecules contribute more to scattering than the smaller molecules. The larger particle diffuse slowly and smaller particles diffuse rapidly so smaller particles decay more easily than the larger particles. When a particle is bombarded, the photon of light recreates the particle size and shape depending on the anisotropic *Mie scattering* distorted in the forward direction [26]. An example of natural light is sunlight scattered through tiny spherical droplets of lipid in diluted milk. While considering the particles much greater than the wavelength, surface reflection becomes more significant, where scattering cross section are the only determinants which shows the amount of light scattered through the particle, and less dependent on frequency of light, which is foremost to help decide a relevant scattering angle for DLS experimental setup. When compared to single-angle dynamic light scattering, mineral liberation analysis (MLA) offers a more accurate, reproducible and robust size distribution of particles. MLA directly measures the molar mass of complexes and macromolecules in solution. By applying MLA in combination with size exclusion chromatography (SEC), along with an on-line concentration detector, the total molar mass and size of biological macromolecules can be estimated [38]. MLA is provided with a refractive index detector and UV absorbance to achieve a precise and improved estimation of the molecular mass (*M*) [39, 40] of unknown larger biological molecules employing scattering intensity *I* and refractive index *RI*:

$$I = \left(\frac{dn}{dc}\right)^2 cM \tag{16.4}$$

$$RI = \frac{dn}{dc} \tag{16.5}$$

16.4 DLS instrumentation

DLS is a state-of-the-art technique that operates on the basic principle of scattering of light to determine particle size assuming the sample solutions like emulsions, suspension, or aerosols show Brownian motion [41]. A typical DLS setup requires laser, sample and light detector, and digital autocorrelator (figure 16.2).

Laser: The incident monochromatic laser light encounters the particles in the solvent undergoing Brownian motion, and gets scattered in all possible directions. The scattered light is then captured by the detector and the scattering intensity is recorded. The incident light undergoes a phenomenon due to the particle motion in the solvent termed 'Doppler broadening' [42]. The Malvern Zetasizer® series of instruments are universally prominent for research purposes. It has raised as an original progression of the Malvern correlator marketed in 1970 [37].

Generally, a He–Ne laser having a wavelength of 633 nm is used in the above-mentioned instrument. As an exception, a few instruments may use diode lasers of 830 nm. Although, other wavelengths such as 532 nm (green) are produced and marketed by Malvern [36]. A laser is a stable source of monochromatic light and its power can be altered with the help of an attenuator (figure 16.2(B)).

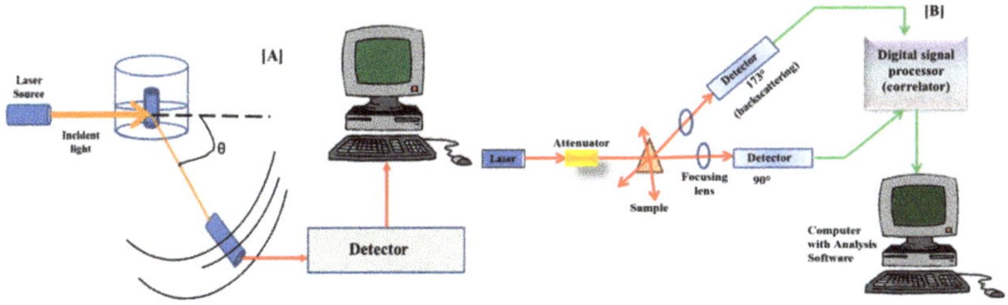

Figure 16.2. Schematic representation of a light scattering setup. Scattering angle θ is obtained by the light dispersed by the particle in a period of time and is focused over a tracking device called a detector or detector-incorporated fiber cable for added downstream processing of data [A]. The advanced instruments have the detectors at 173° angle so as to detect backscattering, although in some older versions (Nano S90, ZS90), the angle is still 90° [B].

Sample: The samples are placed in an optically translucent disposable cuvette/container/capillary. The cuvettes should be clean and square in shape, disposable scratch-free glass or optically translucent plastic (3 × 3 mm, 5 × 5 mm or 10 × 10 mm) are used. To produce good quality data, the sample used for the measurement should be clean, homogenous, transparent or slightly hazy, and without any precipitation.

Detector: The more recent versions of the DLS instruments are equipped with an avalanche photodiode detector (APD), that has a quantum efficiency of over 65% in the red wavelength range, hence a 633 nm He–Ne red laser is used [36]. Advanced DLS instrument (Nano S90, ZS90) has a detector placed at an angle of 173° to detect the backscattered light although some older versions have the detector angle set at 90°. The APD is placed at 173° that allows detection of the backscattered light (backscatter) and also unmasks the scattered light of low intensity [43]. The illumination from the sample obtained is 8-fold higher than that of the detector placed at a 90° angle. The data analysis in DLS is carried out with a help of autocorrelation function. As mentioned earlier, the variation in the intensity of the scattered light is correlated with the intensity of autocorrelation function (ACF) against short decay intervals (τ). The ACF is achieved from monodispersed samples by following the mono-exponential equation:

$$G(T) = 1 + b \cdot e^{-1} D_q^t \qquad (16.6)$$

where D^t is the translational diffusion coefficient, b is the constant that depends upon the equipment optical settings, and q is the scattering vector.

16.5 Correlation function

The correlation function, in general terms, describes the position of a particle with respect to time. Scattered light from the particles and the solvent interaction is recorded over a certain time range by the APD in order to correlate the movement of the particles from their mean position. The scattering light intensity fluctuates with time due to the particle movement. The fluctuation of smaller particles is faster than that of the larger particles in the solution. The larger particles in the solution amplifies the minimum and maximum scattering intensity. This initial intensity is used to trace the further intensities using a correlation function. If the beginning of the correlation function depicts a linear and a constant pattern, it indicates that the particle is at the same initial position. With time, a decay in the correlation function is observed indicating a decreasing trend in the similarity of the positions. A linear behavior is seen again, if there is no similarity in the particle position, which is termed as a baseline.

The correlogram that is generated by the software estimates the RH. The correlogram from DLS measurements performed at 25 °C on monodispersed 100 nm pectin–cisplatin conjugates (PDI 0.241) dispensed in water (100 μg ml^{-1}) in Malvern NanoZS instrument using plastic cuvettes (DTS1070) and analyzed by Zetasizer® (version 7.10) software.

As described earlier, the decay behavior is the time taken by the particles to change their mean position. A faster decay pattern can be observed in the solution

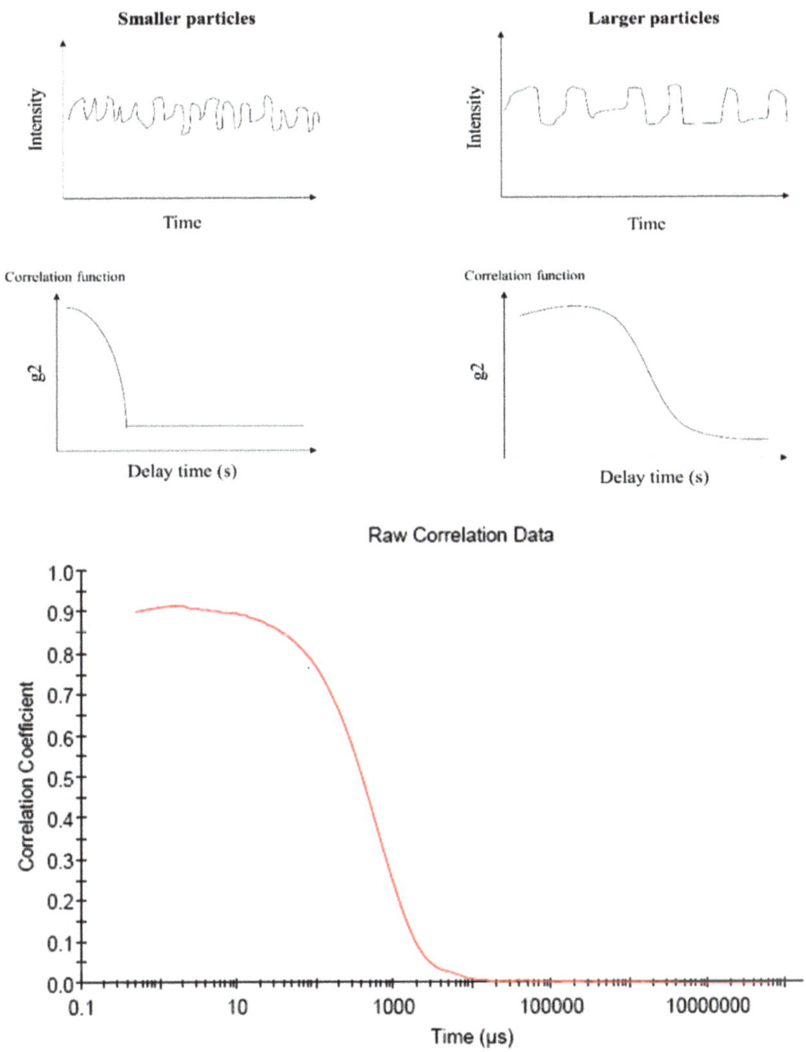

Figure 16.3. Differences in the intensity trace and correlation as a function of size. Reproduced from [38]. Copyright 2009 Biophysical Society. Published by Elsevier Inc.

constituting smaller particles, due to their faster movement. However, the decay pattern in the correlation function is delayed in larger particles [44].

In DLS instruments such as Malvern Zetasizer®, the generated correlogram involves the RCF (raw correlation function) to be plotted (figure 16.3(C)) against delay time (τ). In DLS, the autocorrelation functions [$G2(\tau)$ or $G2(\tau) - 1$] are estimated by fitting the data and then calculating the D_t using equation (16.6). Further, the hydrodynamic radius (R_H) of compact sphere-shaped particles can be predicted by Stokes–Einstein equation:

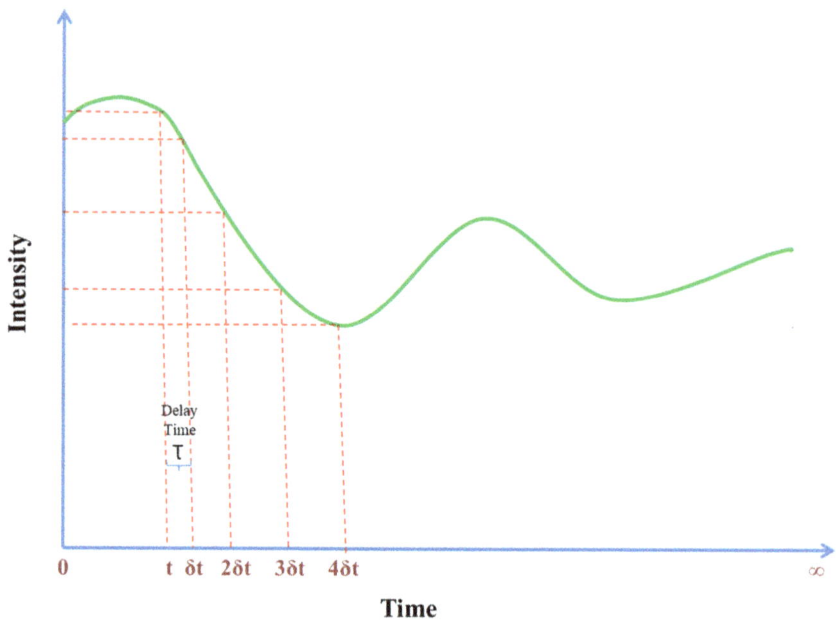

Figure 16.4. Diagram depicting intensity fluctuation of scattered light as a function of time.

$$D_t = \frac{k_B T}{6\pi\eta R_H} \tag{16.7}$$

where R_H = hydrodynamic radius, η = absolute viscosity, T = temperature, and k_B = Boltzmann constant (1.380 648 52 × 10^{-23} J K^{-1}).

Therefore, RH is directly proportional to the inverse of time relaxation of the decay. It is important to note that the hydrodynamic diameter d_h (i.e. d_h = 2 RH) is often preferred to represent the particle size. d_h is represented in nm along with its standard deviation known as polydispersity. Software of the instruments display polydispersity as polydispersity index, or as average percentage of polydispersity. The interrelationship among these three terms is not innate and therefore should be verified. Generally, the percentage polydispersity is equivalent to the root square of the polydispersity index, multiplied by 100 (figure 16.4).

16.6 Analysis and distribution

DLS primarily detects the intensity of scattered incident laser light that has been dissipated by particles in a colloid dispersion. The continuous mobility of the particles within the dispersion causes destructive and constructive interferences and therefore, the intensity of scattered light fluctuates over a period of time. The data can be represented in different ways such as volume and number-based distribution. The Mie theory given by Bohren and Huffman in 1983 defines the transformation of relative distributions of intensity to volume. The conversion necessitates that the refractive indices of all particles in dispersion, that will indicate a higher relational distribution of the contribution of each peak. The concept of distribution profile by intensity, number and volume, can be easily understood by considering a sample having identical numbers of 5 and 50 nm diameter particles. Firstly, according to the DLS techniques, due to the same number of particles the two peaks generated will be of the same relative percentage (1:1 ratio) centered at these sizes. Now if we see according to distribution based on volumes, the peak generated because of the 50 nm particles will have a handout that will be 1000 times larger (1:1000 ratio) in comparison the 5 nm particles because according to the formula of the sphere volume, it is proportional to (diameter). Lastly, according to the Rayleigh theory, the intensity of the dispersed light is equal to (diameter) and the peaks generated due to the intensity of the 50 nm particles is at least 10^6 times higher to that of the 5 nm particles peak (1:10^6 ratio). The average particle diameter can be determined easily in the case of narrow or monodisperse particle size distributions. Considering systems having other than a single range of particle dimensions, Contin algorithm become ideal for analyzing heterodisperse/polydisperse samples. But the investigation of systems along variable particle sizes implying intensity distributions may not efficiently correlate the number of particles in each range [45].

The polydispersity (PDI) of test, is a relevant criterion in DLS evaluation and credibly attained against the diameter of the particle size ranges. Whenever a size distribution curve of the sample in consideration, can be suited to Gaussian distribution. Therefore, PDI corresponds to the following factors—standard deviation (σ) and average hydrodynamic radius (R_{H}) of the particle as per the equation provided below (Koppel 1972) [46]:

$$PDI = \frac{\sigma^2}{R_H^2} \tag{16.8}$$

Consequently, the PDI in straightforward terms is the relative variation whereas the polydispersity resembles the standard deviation (σ). The larger the distribution is, the higher polydisperse the sample, i.e., directly proportional.

16.7 Aspects that impact the DLS results

16.7.1 Preparation of sample

Preparing the sample is critical for accurate DLS measurements. Water and organic solvents like methanol, ethanol, and toluene are used to dissolve the sample or in diluents such as 10% methanol in water [47]. Some solvents like toluene scatter light [48] that may interfere as background noise, but few like dimethylsulfoxide (DMSO) exhibit significant alterations in viscosity with temperature fluctuations [49]. It is important for the sample to be tested in DLS to be homogeneous, clear, and without haze. The base of the cuvette should be checked to ensure no precipitation of solutes. Larger particles tend to precipitate that may be due to meager dispersion, incorrect pH, insufficient sonication, all of which compromise the experimentation. Deionized water is usually not recommended, as the non-ionic state protects long-distance interactions among particles. Therefore, the size of particles in deionized water will be 2–10 nm bigger than the actual size [50]. In PEC, diluting samples with saline water indicated improved data, as the ions are known to protect the particles from long-distance exchanges. Dissolving sample in 10 mM KNO_3 indicated decent results in comparison to NaCl, as the chloride ions are extremely reactive. Samples are filtered by nitrogen extruder to exclude aggregates and dust particles, ensuring narrow size distribution. Using thoroughly cleansed filters having pore sizes that are three times bigger (~5 μm) than the anticipated largest particles within samples can be achieved. An important observation is that the large particles having low density may some on surface of the solvent layer (creaming) [51], that can render DLS ineffective. For powder formulations (e.g., lyophilized samples) stirring vigorously can dissolve the NPs. Sonication requires caution especially when proteins are involved. For polymeric NPs it can take up to 24 h by sonication to obtain a stable and homogeneous dispersion.

16.7.2 Concentration of sample

Multi-scattering occurs when the concentration of NPs is higher, as the scattered light from each NP cross interacts with other NPs prior to reaching the detector thereby losing its intensity [52]. This results in an artifact that is an artificially smaller size of NP. Random agglomerates are formed when the sample is in high concentrations, and surfactants should be used to avoid agglomeration [53]. In contrast, when samples are too diluted, then the generated scattered light is not enough to analyze the results. Hence, it is essential to optimize the concentration of the sample. No general guideline can be provided on the so-called 'ideal concentration' for DLS, as it varies with different aspects related to the laser power, angle of scattering, scattering volume, and detector sensitivity of every instrument [54]; and the molecular weight and the compactness of materials used [55] for NP synthesis. Solid, spherical and more compact NPs scatter more light than dispersed NPs [56]. For example, the manual of the Malvern Zetasizer® states that while running the experiment, to obtain quality data minimum of a million (10^6) residual photons are required to be detected to reduce signal-to-noise (S/N) ratio. Residual photons are estimated as the difference between photons scattered by the solvent and the sample. Brookhaven Instruments, in their manual recommend that the sample concentration should generate counts to a maximum of 600 kcps. As discussed, the S/N in DLS experiments differs as inversely proportional to the square root of photons counted and hence, there is a minimal threshold for photon counts required to achieve good S/N ratio. In practice, it may be necessary to run DLS experiments on serial dilutions to determine the optimal concentration.

16.7.3 Fluorescent samples

Preferably fluorescent and colored samples should not be used in DLS [57]. Fluorescent NPs are being used very often these days since they can be coupled with microscopy. It is essential to run control experiments to exclude the possibility of absorption of light by the fluorophores at the wavelength of the laser. In the case of absorption, the intensity of the scattered light will be lower and hence, artificially smaller sizes for the particles will be estimated [58]. Fluorescent light is non-coherent and recorded as noise. The APD detectors are often not capable of differentiating between various intensities. As a result of fluorescence, the S/N ratio is heightened causing broadening of peaks, resulting in low quality data. Further, most of the prevalent fluorophores show absorbance and emit light at 600–700 nm, which normally interferes with the DLS reading. To minimalize these interferences, few instruments with a narrow band-filter that can filter-out the wavelengths differing from the laser (e.g., 633 ± 2.5 nm) are present. It may further diminish the detected number of photons and therefore necessitate a sample of higher concentrations.

16.7.4 Outcome of agglomeration

NPs have a tendency to agglomerate [59], that are mostly reversible, but often they form reversible agglomerates. Consequently, surfactants are regularly used to make the dispersions stable [60]. Agglomeration in dispersions tends to deteriorate the data quality as the larger agglomerates may scatter more light that may even damage the detector. Too much scattering can mask the low intensity scattered light from smaller particles, broadened peaks emerge while confidence in the data is reduced. Agglomeration is enhanced by increasing concentrations and thus, DLS is reliable only at dilute concentrations (typically 50–100 $\mu g\ ml^{-1}$) that makes it unreliable for many therapeutic formulations as they require higher concentrations (up to few $mg\ ml^{-1}$) [61].

16.7.5 Shape of NPs

Despite the perception, NPs are generally not spherical. For nanotubes, nanorods, DLS provides a RH that hypothetically indicates that in dispersion, the radius of a solid sphere in motion at a similar speed to that of aspherical NPs. Recently, Nair *et al* [62] explained a modified Stokes–Einstein equation, so as to fit the data obtained from cylindrical structures (e.g., nanotubes):

$$Dt = \frac{kBT}{3\pi\eta L}\left[ln\left(\frac{L}{d}\right) + 0{:}32\right] \tag{16.9}$$

where, k_B = Boltzmann constant (1.380 648 52 × 10^{-23} J K^{-1}), T = temperature, η = absolute viscosity, L = length of cylinder and d = diameter of cylinder.

The aspect ratio (L/d) is often known for nanotubes, therefore, D_t for these cylindrical nanomaterials can easily be determined using DLS.

16.7.6 Rotational diffusion of NPs

Typically, in DLS, the translational diffusion coefficient (D_t) is taken into consideration, but the rotational diffusion coefficient (D_r) is often neglected as it remains undetected as the dispersed particles rotate rapidly. However, in colloidal gold, even crystalline and larger NPs, the intensity peaks at smaller sizes (0–10 nm) apparently appear because of the rotational diffusion of NPs [63]. The best way to differentiate these peaks is to compare the DLS spectra of the same sample at both the scattering angles, 90° and 173°. In translational diffusion, scattering of light due to NP rotation is angle-dependent, but in rotational diffusion it is not angle dependent, and therefore, shift for peaks due to rotational diffusion will be not be observed. In contrast, peaks due to translational diffusion shift at different scattering angles.

16.7.7 Cuvette

As far as possible, plastic cuvettes should not be used, when samples are dissolved in organic solvents or if the experiments require a high temperature of ⩾50 °C and above. Even if the area of illumination is very near to its wall in the case of glass cuvettes, then a portion of the laser light reflected from the wall can be detected and recorded as a high intensity light. This is referred to as flaring and characteristically appears as a sharp peak between 1 and 10 μm. To circumvent the flaring, the area of illumination must be shifted near the center of the cuvette with the help of the focusing lens.

16.7.8 Maintenance of the instrument

The DLS instrument must be appropriately maintained to obtain reliable and consistent good quality data from. After switching on the machine, the instrument must not be disturbed for minimum of 30 min for the laser to stabilize. The National Institute of Standards and Technology (NIST) [64], issued guidelines for proper maintenance of the instruments wherein, it needs to be regularly checked with reference to standard NPs of known size with low PDI. Usually, latex beads of diverse sizes (e.g., 100 nm), colloidal gold NPs, bovine serum albumin (BSA) or cytochrome C may be used as references for sizes ⩾20 nm and ⩽20 nm, respectively. The instrument should be calibrated to indicate sizes with ~2% deviation for reference samples is acceptable.

16.8 Application of DLS in biomedical nanotechnology

DLS is routinely used in materials science, biology, pharmaceutical, and engineering laboratories to determine the size distribution and surface charge density of nucleic acids, proteins, and complexes to monitor ligand binding and to detect macromolecular aggregates in solutions. To warrant quantitative data that is reproducible, samples should be prepared with care as protein handling is sensitive to minor changes in experimental conditions such as temperature variation that may cause aggregation giving compromised DLS results that may affect protein activity. Parameters like solvent viscosity, temperature and inter-particle interactions further influence particle size determination. It is very simple to perform with broad range of test buffers, at varying temperatures and concentration. DLS is additionally a non-invasive method that requires a relatively small amount of sample and rapidly provides essential data. Utilizations of DLS to examine the uniformity of bioactive agents such as RNA, protein and their composites are hereby discussed [31].

16.8.1 Detection of protein aggregation

DLS is suitable to determine the wide range of size analysis (R_H) of peptides, protein and their aggregation, polymerization, clustering and amplification in real time solution, which is an utmost concern for the pharmaceutical industry. Milk proteins undergo rapid degradation and aggregation during its processing and storage as milk products. Therefore, DLS enables determination and analysis of its low-resolution constructs, from a pure homogenous sample devoid of aggregation and degradation. Patel *et al* analyzed the physical behavior of Ovalbumin sample lacking degradation, i.e., under 5% of high molecular weight antigen (HMWA), pH-dependent assembly and disassembly of Apoferritin [65], agglomeration of human prion protein (PrP) based on UV irradiation or proteolytic degradation [66, 67], protein crystallization [68] were analysis of the physical behavior of variety of globular protein.

16.8.2 Protein–protein interaction studies

DLS can effectively help study protein–protein interaction/complex (PPC). Single proteins behave erroneously at different concentrations, in context of their uniformity that can be detected through DLS. To evaluate PPC, a low volume of SEC-purified sample are required. PPC measurements realistically predicted the viscosity of HMWA, which is a function of temperature, pH and dispersion medium. For example, interaction of monoclonal antibody (IgG1 and IgG4) and antigen (tumor associated glycoprotein) [69] study protein–protein interaction from dilute to concentrated in acidic medium [70], first-time full-length elucidation of Nidogen-1 devoid of degradation along with its interaction with Laminin in medium was studied [71], Hanlon *et al* [72] worked with inexpensive proteins—α-chymotrypsin and trypsin inhibitor in response to environmental conditions (buffer, salinity and temperature), effect of cations (Mg/Ca) on interaction of Argin (G3 domain) to human IgG together form chimeric protein [73].

16.8.3 Homogeneity of RNA

RNA polymeric molecules degrade rapidly on exposure to ribonuclease, skin contact, and air. DLS is consistently used to analyse the homogeneity of a RNA sample from *in vitro* transcription. The West Nile viral infection exhibits RNA genome flanked by 5′ and 3′ UTR was characterized by a variety of biophysical study [74], D'Amare *et al* [75] determined the crystallization of RNA molecules.

16.8.4 Protein–RNA complex studies

Along with PPC studies, protein–RNA composites can likewise be effectively considered for DLS measurements. Currently, [76] Abd *et al* studied the interaction of RNA fragments of HIV-1 to is precursors $Pr55^{Gag}$ where, DLS effectively helped to characterize the interaction that maintains the RNA assembly. Analogously, host OAS1 protein (41 kDa) and West Nile viral RNA (5′ TR and 3′ TR) were analyzed at different concentrations, and demonstrated that all the particles exhibited extremely monodispersed in preparation [74]. As discussed above, DLS can be a useful technique to consider uniformity of proteins, RNA, and their composites. It has been reported that R_h values can also be utilized to study low-resolution conformations or individual samples and their composites.

In considering the biomedical field of application, nanoparticles act as a cargo/carrier to load biomolecules (nucleic acid, drugs, protein, and carbohydrates) and innumerable diseases can be targeted including cancer, bone disorders, cardiovascular, neurological disorders etc.

16.9 Enhanced DLS measurements using complementary hydrodynamic methods

Besides highlighting the advanced data on homogeneity, the principle of dynamic light scattering can also be enlisted as a corresponding technique to analyze the shape and size of high molecular weight molecules.

16.9.1 Determination of molecular weight

Estimating molecular mass or molecular weight is another prominent parameter for assessing physical characteristics of biomolecules such as proteins, lipids, and nucleic acids. While comparing the sequentially arranged molecular weight of any biomolecules with experimentally measured molecular weight, the functional data related to their degradation, oligomeric conformation, and transition in molecular weight can be interpreted upon interaction with medium or other binding molecules. SEC also helps determine the molecular weight of biomolecules and their associated complexes. Since, it is primarily built on the assumption that DLS depends on molecular weight standard and the spherical shape of the biomolecules; deviation from this shape often results in overestimation of molecular mass through elongated shape. The widely accepted assumption for molecular mass assessment is its integration into the sedimentation velocity information, through an analytical ultracentrifuge coupled with R_h measured by DLS utilizing the Svedberg equation [77],

$$M_w = \frac{6\pi\eta_0 R_h N_A s^0_{20,\,w}}{1 - v\overline{\rho}_0} \tag{16.10}$$

where M_w is the molecular weight, v partial specific volume, η_0 solvent viscosity, R_h hydrodynamic radius and ρ_0: solvent density. R_h data from DLS is a beneficial variable including sedimentation coefficient to provide data related to molecular weight.

16.9.2 Study homogeneity of biological samples with exposure to high-energy x-rays

Structural and functional analysis of macromolecules is facilitated by SAXS, a form of static light scattering system based upon x-ray beam. SAXS information can be acquired either through synchrotron utilizing speedy and higher energy monochromatic x-rays or by an in-house machinery system. Generally, data assortment in remote SAXS (~20 °C) needs 2–4 h x-ray manifestation time for testing the sample, while synchrotron just requiresa a few seconds [78]. In addition, while acquiring SAXS information from a single experimental setup, the users can acquire data for multiple samples and it may take 10 h for some samples. So, to maintain the stability of samples, they were often stored either at ~20 °C for long term intervals or radiation damage might change the homogeneity in the macromolecular arrangement to aggregated/degraded state. The use of DLS to test the homogeneity of samples is regularly done after collecting the SAXS data on RNA, protein, and their composites [73].

Moreover, DLS estimations are a valuable autonomous crosscheck, used to characterize the shape reconstruction of high molecular weight molecules (HMWM) by utilizing SAXS information, an intensely computational program. For the characterization of SAXS in the absence of any inclination, we measure the hydrodynamic constants which include sedimentation coefficient and Rh by utilizing computer program software HYDROPRO [79], and differentiate them with tentatively decide DLS effects and corresponding hydrodynamic procedures. In addition, it is conceivable to consider polysaccharides and nucleic acids utilizing bundles in the HYDRO family [80, 81]. The same practice has been followed for DNA, RNA, proteins, and their composites [82].

As discussed, DLS is frequently used in nanomedicine, under 'batch' mode, that possesses crucial parameters for the analysis of heterogenous/poly-dispersed samples, and is hence considered a low-resolution protocol [18, 83]. In effect, as the outcomes of the scattering intensity on the particle size is to the sixth power, even a slight number of large particles tend to mask the smaller ones. Therefore, DLS is a valuable user-friendly tool to evaluate the integrity and stability of the sample, when exposed to an inappropriate pH, or very high salt concentration, or in plasma [83].

Yet, if the polydispersity of heterogenous samples is measured, it frequently produces results that are misleading. In reality, it is incapable of distinguishing between the polydispersity of the heterogenous samples that has been synthesized having two/three populations of particle that are in comparable size ranges [18, 83], it is further incapable of differentiating between small particles and larger aggregates [36] and is unable to consistently measure the polydispersity of the heterogenous samples when exposed to plasma proteins [18, 84]. Since intensity of scattered light is directly proportional to sixth power of macromolecules, huge agglomeration, even a modest quantity, will influence the estimations. For reproducible results, deionized water should be used, the cuvette must be cleaned thoroughly, and before performing DLS experiment the samples must be filtered. DLS signals are based upon the concentration and size of macromolecules. Consequently, to gain authentic estimations, it is necessary to optimize the concentration ranges. DLS is an intensity weighed methodology, ensemble-based technique that is normally suited for monodispersed samples only. DLS estimations are extremely reliant on temperature and viscosity of the medium. Whilst the assumption that molecular weight determination utilizing DLS is conceivable, the plotting of the scattered light intensity (K^*c/R_θ), here K^* is an optical constant, c its concentration, and R_θ is the Rayleigh ratio as a function of angular dependent light scattering versus concentration as elaborated by

Wyatt [85], is not really authentic and a reproducible strategy. Hence, alternative strategies must be used based on a combination system like static light scattering (SLS) with multi-angle laser light scattering (MALLS) and analytic ultracentrifuge.

16.10 Conclusion

DLS quantifies and correlates the time-dependent variations in the light scattered by the nanoparticles in suspension (autocorrelation function), and helps study the uniformity and inter- and intraspecific interaction of biomolecules. The technique assumes that the object to measure has a spherical shape and necessitates that the solution is of known viscosity. DLS is a non-invasive strategy that gives quick, accurate, and consistent quality results, considering agglomerations in biomolecular preparation and often requiring trace amounts of sample. DLS analysis is economically viable, that does not require a specialist staff. Hence, it is considered to be a preliminary measurement for sizing the particles that is recognized globally by the regulators. To the best of our knowledge, there is not a single sizing technique that can resolve and give all the appropriate information required for pre-clinical studies. Batch mode DLS is suitable to detect major issues with sample integrity and stability at early stages. It has attracted major attention towards academia and small and large-scale industrial research workstations. DLS is a versatile technique with innumerable applications that include size distribution as well as molecular mass determination of milk protein in bovine milk like casein micelles. Molecular mass determination and dimensions computations of molecules in scale of 10 μm to lower than 1 nm and bearing molecular mass lower than 1 kDa is another attractive application. A key benefit of DLS involves the use of very small amounts of sample (<3 μl). It is an acceptable technology for interaction studies of RNA–protein and adapted DLS in-line process systems are designated satisfactory. Conducting experiments on vast scale of sample buffer and wide temperature range is achievable employing DLS.

Acknowledgment

Vikas Shukla is thankful to ICMR Government of India for his Senior Research Fellowship (SRF), Karishma Niveria is thankful to CSIR for her SRF and Poonam Shashidhar is thankful to her in-country fellowship from TERI and Deakin University, Australia.

List of symbols

C	Concentration
I_0/Isca/Idet	Incident/scattered/detected light intensity
kB	Boltzmann's constant (1.380×10^{-23} kg m^2 s^{-2} K^{-1})
T	Absolute temperature
ν	Particle velocity
η	Viscosity of medium
G′V	Size distribution by volume
GI	Size distribution by intensity

d	Scatter diameter
$P(\theta)$	Angular angle of Mie scattering coefficient
θ	Scattering angle
λ	Wavelength
s	Distance from scattering particle
n	Refractive index of medium
r	Radius of particle
τ	Short decay intervals
D^t	Translational diffusion coefficient
q	Scattering vector
PDI	Polydispersity index
σ	Standard deviation
R_H	Average hydrodynamic radius
K	Optical constant
R_θ	Rayleigh ratio function of angular light scattering
k	Debye–Huckel parameter

References

[1] Treuel L, Eslahian K A, Docter D, Lang T, Zellner R, Nienhaus K, Nienhaus G U, Stauber R H and Maskos M 2014 Physicochemical characterization of nanoparticles and their behavior in the biological environment *Phys. Chem. Chem. Phys.* **16** 15053–67

[2] Akbarzadeh A, Samiei M and Davaran S 2012 Magnetic nanoparticles: preparation, physical properties, and applications in biomedicine *Nanoscale Res. Lett.* **7** 1–3

[3] Patra J K *et al* 2018 Nano based drug delivery systems: recent developments and future prospects *J. Nanobiotechnol.* **16** 1–33

[4] Choi Y H and Han H K 2018 Nanomedicines: current status and future perspectives in aspect of drug delivery and pharmacokinetics *J. Pharm. Investig.* **48** 43–60

[5] Liu D, Yang F, Xiong F and Gu N 2016 The smart drug delivery system and its clinical potential *Theranostics* **6** 1306

[6] Favi P M, Gao M, Johana Sepúlveda Arango L, Ospina S P, Morales M, Pavon J J and Webster T J 2015 Shape and surface effects on the cytotoxicity of nanoparticles: gold nanospheres versus gold nanostars *J. Biomed. Mater. Res.* A **103** 3449–62

[7] Kong B, Seog J H, Graham L M and Lee S B 2011 Experimental considerations on the cytotoxicity of nanoparticles *Nanomedicine* **6** 929–41

[8] Selim A A, Al-Sunaidi A and Tabet N 2012 Effect of the surface texture and crystallinity of ZnO nanoparticles on their toxicity *Mater. Sci. Eng.* C **32** 2356–60

[9] Alshehri A H, Jakubowska M, Młożniak A, Horaczek M, Rudka D, Free C and Carey J D 2012 Enhanced electrical conductivity of silver nanoparticles for high frequency electronic applications *ACS Appl. Mater. Interfaces* **4** 7007–10

[10] Shi D, Sadat M E, Dunn A W and Mast D B 2015 Photo-fluorescent and magnetic properties of iron oxide nanoparticles for biomedical applications *Nanoscale* **7** 8209–32

[11] Nealon G L, Donnio B, Greget R, Kappler J P, Terazzi E and Gallani J L 2012 Magnetism in gold nanoparticles *Nanoscale* **4** 5244–58

[12] Oberdörster G 2010 Safety assessment for nanotechnology and nanomedicine: concepts of nanotoxicology *J. Intern. Med.* **267** 89–105

[13] Cosco D, Paolino D, De Angelis F, Cilurzo F, Celia C, Di Marzio L, Russo D, Tsapis N, Fattal E and Fresta M 2015 Aqueous-core PEG-coated PLA nanocapsules for an efficient entrapment of water soluble anticancer drugs and a smart therapeutic response *Eur. J. Pharm. Biopharm.* **89** 30–9

[14] Schmidt C and Storsberg J 2019 Nanomaterials: tools, technology, and methodology of nanotechnology-based biomedical systems for diagnostics and therapy *The Road from Nanomedicine to Precision Medicine* (Boca Raton, FL: CRC Press) pp 335–66

[15] Park W and Na K 2015 Advances in the synthesis and application of nanoparticles for drug delivery *Wiley Interdiscip. Rev. Nanomed. Nanobiotechnol.* **7** 494–508

[16] Schmitz K S 2012 *Introduction to Dynamic Light Scattering by Macromolecules* (Amsterdam: Elsevier)

[17] Jeffries C M, Graewert M A, Blanchet C E, Langley D B, Whitten A E and Svergun D I 2016 Preparing monodisperse macromolecular samples for successful biological small-angle X-ray and neutron-scattering experiments *Nat. Protoc.* **11** 2122–53

[18] Bernacchi S 2020 Dynamic light scattering analysis on RNA associated to proteins *RNA Spectroscopy* (New York: Humana) pp 31–9

[19] Falke S, Dierks K, Blanchet C, Graewert M, Cipriani F, Meijers R, Svergun D and Betzel C 2018 Multi-channel *in situ* dynamic light scattering instrumentation enhancing biological small-angle X-ray scattering experiments at the PETRA III beamline P12 *J. Synchrotron Radiat.* **25** 361–72

[20] Cox R A 1980 *Biophysical Chemistry Part III: The Behavior of Biological Macromolecules* ed C R Cantor and P R Schimmel (San Francisco, CA: Freeman)

[21] Minton A P 2007 Static light scattering from concentrated protein solutions, I: general theory for protein mixtures and application to self-associating proteins *Biophys. J.* **93** 1321–8

[22] Schubert R, Meyer A, Dierks K, Kapis S, Reimer R, Einspahr H, Perbandt M and Betzel C 2015 Reliably distinguishing protein nanocrystals from amorphous precipitate by means of depolarized dynamic light scattering *J. Appl. Crystallogr.* **48** 1476–84

[23] Malvern Instruments. TN101104 Intensity Volume Number. Malvern Instruments Limited. http://malvern.com/en/pdf/secure/TN101104IntensityVolumeNumber.pdf (accessed July 2016)

[24] Tyndall J 1869 On the blue color of the sky, the polarization of skylight, and polarization of light by cloudy matter generally *J. Franklin Inst.* **88** 34–40

[25] Strutt J W (Lord Rayleigh) 1871 On the scattering of light by small particles *Lond. Edin. Dub. Phil. Mag. J. Sci.* **41** 447–54

[26] Strutt J W (Lord Rayleigh) 1871 On the light from the sky, its polarization and colour *Philos. Mag.* **41** 274

[27] Mie G 1908 Beiträge zur Optik trüber Medien, speziell kolloidaler Metallösungen *Ann. Phys.* **330** 377–445

[28] Debye P 1915 Zerstreuung von röntgenstrahlen *Ann. Phys.* **351** 809–23

[29] Carvalho P M, Felício M R, Santos N C, Gonçalves S and Domingues M M 2018 Application of light scattering techniques to nanoparticle characterization and development *Front. Chem.* **6** 237

[30] Kätzel U, Vorbau M, Stintz M, Gottschalk-Gaudig T and Barthel H 2008 Dynamic light scattering for the characterization of polydisperse fractal systems: II. Relation between structure and DLS results *Part. Part. Syst. Charact* **25** 19–30

[31] Stetefeld J, McKenna S A and Patel T R 2016 Dynamic light scattering: a practical guide and applications in biomedical sciences *Biophys. Rev.* **8** 409–27

[32] Lindsay H M, Klein R, Weitz D A, Lin M Y and Meakin P 1988 Effect of rotational diffusion on quasielastic light scattering from fractal colloid aggregates *Phys. Rev.* A **38** 2614
[33] Dynamic Light Scattering (DLS): An Introduction, https://azom.com/article.aspx?ArticleID=16774
[34] Sandhu R, Singh N, Dhankhar J, Gandhi K and Sharma R 2019 Dynamic light scattering (DLS) technique, principle, theoretical considerations and applications *Centre of Advanced Faculty Training in Dairy Processing (2018–19), Nanotechnological and Biochemical Techniques for Assessing the Quality and Safety of Milk and Milk Products* pp 135–7
[35] Bhattacharjee S 2016 DLS and zeta potential—what they are and what they are not? *J. Control. Release* **235** 337–51
[36] Dahneke B E (ed) 1983 *Measurement of Suspended Particles by Quasi-Elastic Light Scattering* (New York: Wiley)
[37] Pecora R (ed) 2013 *Dynamic Light Scattering: Applications of Photon Correlation Spectroscopy* (Berlin: Springer Science & Business Media)
[38] Fernández C and Minton A P 2009 Static light scattering from concentrated protein solutions II: experimental test of theory for protein mixtures and weakly self-associating proteins *Biophys. J.* **96** 1992–8
[39] Graewert M A *et al* 2015 Automated pipeline for purification, biophysical and x-ray analysis of biomacromolecular solutions *Sci. Rep.* **5** 1–8
[40] Minton A P 2016 Recent applications of light scattering measurement in the biological and biopharmaceutical sciences *Anal. Biochem* **501** 4
[41] Falke S and Betzel C 2019 Dynamic light scattering (DLS) *Radiation in Bioanalysis* (Cham: Springer) pp 173–93
[42] Amin S, Barnett G V, Pathak J A, Roberts C J and Sarangapani P S 2014 Protein aggregation, particle formation, characterization and rheology *Curr. Opin. Colloid Interface Sci.* **19** 438–49
[43] Washington C 1992 *Particle Size Analysis in Pharmaceutics and Other Industries: Theory and Practice* (Boca Raton, FL: CRC Press)
[44] Johnson C S and Gabriel D A 2018 *Laser Light Scattering* (Boca Raton, FL: CRC Press)
[45] Raja P M V and Barron A R 2021 Dynamic Light Scattering. https://chem.libretexts.org/@go/page/55841
[46] Koppel D E 1972 Analysis of macromolecular polydispersity in intensity correlation spectroscopy: the method of cumulants *J. Chem. Phys.* **57** 4814–20
[47] Washington C 1992 *Particle Size Analysis in Pharmaceutics and Other Industries: Theory and Practice* (Boca Raton, FL: CRC Press)
[48] Pohl R, Hauser R, Li M, De Souza E, Feldstein R, Seibert R, Ozhan K, Kashyap N and Steiner S 2012 Ultra-rapid absorption of recombinant human insulin induced by zinc chelation and surface charge masking *J. Diabetes Sci. Technol.* **6** 755–63
[49] Finnigan J A and Jacobs D J 1970 Light scattering from benzene, toluene, carbon disulphide and carbon tetrachloride *Chem. Phys. Lett.* **6** 141–3
[50] Noday D A, Steif P S and Rabin Y 2009 Viscosity of cryoprotective agents near glass transition: a new device, technique, and data on DMSO, DP6, and VS55 *Exp. Mech.* **49** 663–72
[51] Guide for DLS sample preparation from Brookhaven instruments, http://brookhaveninstruments.com/pdf/theory/Guide_for_DLS_sample_preparation.pdf

[52] Chanamai R and McClements D J 2000 Creaming stability of flocculated monodisperse oil-in-water emulsions *J. Colloid Interface Sci.* **225** 214–8

[53] Panchal J, Kotarek J, Marszal E and Topp E M 2014 Analyzing subvisible particles in protein drug products: a comparison of dynamic light scattering (DLS) and resonant mass measurement (RMM) *AAPS J.* **16** 440–51

[54] Müller K H, Motskin M, Philpott A J, Routh A F, Shanahan C M, Duer M J and Skepper J N 2014 The effect of particle agglomeration on the formation of a surface-connected compartment induced by hydroxyapatite nanoparticles in human monocyte-derived macrophages *Biomaterials* **35** 1074–88

[55] Zheng T, Cherubin P, Cilenti L, Teter K and Huo Q 2016 A simple and fast method to study the hydrodynamic size difference of protein disulfide isomerase in oxidized and reduced form using gold nanoparticles and dynamic light scattering *Analyst* **141** 934–8

[56] Karow A R, Götzl J and Garidel P 2015 Resolving power of dynamic light scattering for protein and polystyrene nanoparticles *Pharm. Dev. Technol* **20** 84–9

[57] Meng Z, Hashmi S M and Elimelech M 2013 Aggregation rate and fractal dimension of fullerene nanoparticles via simultaneous multiangle static and dynamic light scattering measurement *J. Colloid Interface Sci.* **392** 27–33

[58] Geißler D, Gollwitzer C, Sikora A, Minelli C, Krumrey M and Resch-Genger U 2015 Effect of fluorescent staining on size measurements of polymeric nanoparticles using DLS and SAXS *Anal. Methods* **7** 9785–90

[59] Murdock R C, Braydich-Stolle L, Schrand A M, Schlager J J and Hussain S M 2008 Characterization of nanomaterial dispersion in solution prior to *in vitro* exposure using dynamic light scattering technique *Toxicol. Sci.* **101** 239–53

[60] Liu H H, Surawanvijit S, Rallo R, Orkoulas G and Cohen Y 2011 Analysis of nanoparticle agglomeration in aqueous suspensions via constant-number Monte Carlo simulation *Environ. Sci. Technol.* **45** 9284–92

[61] De Jong W H and Borm P J 2008 Drug delivery and nanoparticles: applications and hazards *Int. J. Nanomed* **3** 133

[62] Zhou C, Qi W, Lewis E N and Carpenter J F 2015 Concomitant Raman spectroscopy and dynamic light scattering for characterization of therapeutic proteins at high concentrations *Anal. Biochem* **472** 7–20

[63] Nair N, Kim W J, Braatz R D and Strano M S 2008 Dynamics of surfactant-suspended single-walled carbon nanotubes in a centrifugal field *Langmuir* **24** 1790–5

[64] Kaszuba M, Connah M T, McNeil-Watson F K and Nobbmann U 2007 Resolving concentrated particle size mixtures using dynamic light scattering *Part. Part. Syst. Charact* **24** 159–62

[65] Jaenicke R 1987 Folding and association of proteins *Prog. Biophys. Mol. Biol* **49** 117–237

[66] Redecke L *et al* 2009 UV-light-induced conversion and aggregation of prion proteins *Free Radic. Biol. Med* **46** 1353–61

[67] Georgieva D, Koker M, Redecke L, Perbandt M, Clos J, Bredehorst R, Genov N and Betzel C 2004 Oligomerization of the proteolytic products is an intrinsic property of prion proteins *Biochem. Biophys. Res. Commun* **323** 1278–86

[68] Schubert R, Meyer A, Baitan D, Dierks K, Perbandt M and Betzel C 2017 Real-time observation of protein dense liquid cluster evolution during nucleation in protein crystallization *Cryst. Growth Des.* **17** 954–8

[69] Neergaard M S, Nielsen A D, Parshad H and Van De Weert M 2014 Stability of monoclonal antibodies at high-concentration: head-to-head comparison of the IgG1 and IgG4 subclass *J. Pharm. Sci.* **103** 115–27
[70] Blanco M A, Perevozchikova T, Martorana V, Manno M and Roberts C J 2014 Protein–protein interactions in dilute to concentrated solutions: α-chymotrypsinogen in acidic conditions *J. Phys. Chem.* B **118** 5817–31
[71] Patel T R, Bernards C, Meier M, McEleney K, Winzor D J, Koch M and Stetefeld J 2014 Structural elucidation of full-length nidogen and the laminin–nidogen complex in solution *Matrix Biol.* **33** 60–7
[72] Hanlon A D, Larkin M I and Reddick R M 2010 Free-solution, label-free protein–protein interactions characterized by dynamic light scattering *Biophys. J.* **98** 297–304
[73] Patel T R, Meier M, Li J, Morris G, Rowe A J and Stetefeld J 2011 T-shaped arrangement of the recombinant agrin G3–IgG Fc protein *Protein Sci.* **20** 931–40
[74] Deo S, Patel T R, Dzananovic E, Booy E P, Zeid K, McEleney K, Harding S E and McKenna S A 2014 Activation of 2′,5′-oligoadenylate synthetase by stem loops at the 5′-end of the West Nile virus genome *PLoS One* **9** e92545
[75] Ferré-D'Amaré A R, Zhou K and Doudna J A 1998 A general module for RNA crystallization *J. Mol. Biol.* **279** 621–31
[76] Abd El-Wahab E W, Smyth R P, Mailler E, Bernacchi S, Vivet-Boudou V, Hijnen M, Jossinet F, Mak J, Paillart J C and Marquet R 2014 Specific recognition of the HIV-1 genomic RNA by the Gag precursor *Nat. Commun.* **5** 1–3
[77] Svedberg T and Pedersen K O 1940 The ultracentrifuge *The Ultracentrifuge* (oxford: Clarendon Press)
[78] Rambo R P 2017 Considerations for sample preparation using size-exclusion chromatography for home and synchrotron sources *Biological Small Angle Scattering: Techniques, Strategies and Tips* (Singapore: Springer) pp 31–45
[79] Ortega A, Amorós D and De La Torre J G 2011 Prediction of hydrodynamic and other solution properties of rigid proteins from atomic-and residue-level models *Biophys. J.* **101** 892–8
[80] Amorós D, Ortega A and García de la Torre J 2011 Hydrodynamic properties of wormlike macromolecules: Monte Carlo simulation and global analysis of experimental data *Macromolecules* **44** 5788–97
[81] Benítez A A, Cifre J G, Baños F G and de la Torre J G 2015 Prediction of solution properties and dynamics of RNAs by means of Brownian dynamics simulation of coarse-grained models: ribosomal 5S RNA and phenylalanine transfer RNA *BMC Biophys.* **8** 1–9
[82] Vadlamani G, Thomas M D, Patel T R, Donald L J, Reeve T M, Stetefeld J, Standing K G, Vocadlo D J and Mark B L 2015 The β-lactamase gene regulator AmpR is a tetramer that recognizes and binds the d-Ala-d-Ala motif of its repressor UDP-N-acetylmuramic acid (MurNAc)-pentapeptide *J. Biol. Chem.* **290** 2630–43
[83] Maguire C M, Rösslein M, Wick P and Prina-Mello A 2018 Characterisation of particles in solution—a perspective on light scattering and comparative technologies *Sci. Technol. Adv. Mater.* **19** 732–45
[84] Hassan P A, Rana S and Verma G 2015 Making sense of Brownian motion: colloid characterization by dynamic light scattering *Langmuir* **31** 3–12
[85] Wyatt P J 1993 Light scattering and the absolute characterization of macromolecules *Anal. Chim. Acta* **272** 1–40

IOP Publishing

Analytical Techniques for Biomedical Nanotechnology

Ajeet Kaushik, Sesha S Srinivasan and Yogendra Kumar Mishra

Chapter 17

Zeta potential measurements and analysis for biomedical nanotechnology

Sanjoy Kumar Das, Soumalya Chakraborty, Rajan Rajabalaya and Bhaskar Mazumder

Complementary to homogeneity and hydrodynamic size, another parameter which is also very important to decode the application of a material in biomedical research is the estimation of surface charge. The surface charge estimation of a nano-system is generally performed using zeta potential measurements via electrophoretic light scattering (ELS). In addition, electrophoretic mobility interpretation of a nano-system can be explained using zeta potential experiments. Currently, this is an essential measurement in colloidal science in order to explore molecule dynamics. Both fundamental and applied aspects of zeta potential technology are described in this chapter.

17.1 Introduction

Zeta potential is a parameter for the measurement of the electrochemical equilibrium at the interface between particles and liquid. It provides an estimate of the electrostatic repulsion/attraction between particles and is considered to be one of the fundamental parameters affecting the stability of colloidal particles. In ancient literature, the Greek letter zeta, Z, was usually used to indicate it, hence it has obtained the name zeta potential, written as Z-potential [1]. The most popular theory for calculating zeta potential was developed by Marian Smoluchowski in the year 1903 [2]. Interestingly, this theory was originally developed for electrophoresis. Later, people started to apply his theory in the calculation of zeta potential. The universality and validity of this theory for dispersed particles of any shape and any concentration make it mostly used in zeta potential literature. However, there still some limitations to this early theory as it was mainly determined experimentally. The main limitations are that Smoluchowski's theory neglects the contribution of surface conductivity and only works for particles that have sizes much larger than

doi:10.1088/978-0-7503-3379-5ch17

the interface layer, denoted as κ ($1/\kappa$ is Debye length and a is the particle radius) [1]. Overbeek and Booth as early pioneers in this area started to develop electrokinetic theories with a more theoretical rather than an experimental foundation, enabling it to incorporate surface conductivity for electrokinetic applications. Modern rigorous electrokinetic theories that are valid for almost any κa are mostly generated by Ukrainian (Dukhin) and Australian (O'Brien) scientists [1].

Zeta potential is a significant physicochemical parameter which affects the stability of the nanosuspension. Extremely positive or negative zeta potential values induce greater repulsive forces, while repulsion between particles with similar electrical charge prevents particle aggregation and thus facilitates redispersal [3]. The zeta potential determination may give helpful insights regarding the nature, behavior, and toxicity of nanomaterials in environmental and biological systems. Zeta potential measurement is recommended as a required nanomaterial characterization parameter in different regulatory and scientific documents. The US EPA (TSCA), the International Organization for Standardization (ISO), proposed the rule for the characterization of nanomaterials. There are several documents describing how to measure zeta potential for engineered nanomaterials (ASTM E2865-12 and ISO 13099-1, -2, and -3), but they contain minimal guidance regarding the reporting protocol of those measurements [4]. It is an important parameter for several applications including the characterization of biomedical polymers, electrokinetic transport of particles or blood cells, membrane efficiency, and microfluidics [5]. It is affected by many factors. The most significant factor affecting zeta potential is the pH of the medium. Other factors include ionic strength, the concentration of any additives, and temperature [6]. The zeta potential of nanocarriers is very important. It is determined by using a Zetasizer or by other means and provides information on the charge of the particles and the tendency of the particles in a formulation to aggregate or to remain discrete [7]. Among the existing methods for zeta potential determination of suspended particles, due to its sensitivity, accuracy, and versatility, ELS is by far the best choice for many applications [8]. Zeta potential, unlike particle size or molecular weight, is a property involving not only the particles but also their environment, e.g., pH, ionic strength, and even the type of ions in the suspension. Therefore, in many instances, even though the zeta potential of suspended particles is measured after dilution to produce high resolution and accurate results, these results would differ greatly from their true values in the original environment and may have little practical use or might even mislead the user [8]. Researchers are currently applying biosynthesized nanoparticles (NPs) for a variety of biomedical detection applications [9]. Zetasizer nano series (Malvern, Worcestershire, UK) has been developed which can be used for the measurement of the size and zeta potential of biogenic nanoparticles (e.g., Ag-nanoparticles) [10]. Recently, Algebaly *et al* biologically synthesized silver nanoparticles for use as antibacterial and cytotoxic potential and they used a Zetasizer device for the measurement of the size of biogenic AgNPs [11]. Moreover, there is an existing research gap regarding the independent impact of zeta potential in the toxic nature of polymeric NP. NP surface charge, which can either be negative or positive (based on the properties and fabrication methods of the material employed), is one of the most critical, influencing functions of NPs. In particular, more attention needs to be paid to nanotoxicity when NPs are designed for biomedical use since nanoscale particles will be directly exposed to bodily fluids, cells, and organs [12].

This chapter discusses the effects of surface charge on nanomaterial performance, a fundamental overview of zeta potential, and the measurement of zeta potential. This chapter also discusses the different techniques and methods used for the measurement of zeta potential and the analysis of zeta potential and its implementation in biomedical nanotechnology.

17.2 Effect of surface charge on nanomaterial performance

Zeta potential measurements provide an important criterion for the stability of a colloid system. But they are still poorly considered in the case of solid surfaces and the investigation of protein adsorption on biomaterials is almost unexplored. To this regard, zeta potential describes the surface charging behavior in contact with water-based electrolytes and gives information about the isoelectric point, the surface charge in the function of pH, but also (indirectly) of the functional groups exposed at the solid–liquid interface, the reactivity of the surface in the test solution and absorption processes [13]. In cell biology, the concept of zeta potential has been used to study cell biological activation, cell agglutination, and cell adhesion which are related to cell surface charge properties. Although zeta potential measurements have been utilized in probing the interaction between cells and biomolecules, it remains an untapped method for studying the interaction between nanoparticles and biological cells [14]. In 2008 Zang *et al* used the zeta potential measurements to probe the surface charge responses of normal breast epithelial cells (MCF10A) and breast cancer epithelial cells (MCF7) during iron oxide nanoparticle and CPMV nanoparticle endocytosis respectively. As observed, after MCF7 and MCF10A cells were incubated respectively with two types of nanoparticle, the significant differences in their surface charge change indicated the potential role of zeta potential as a valuable biological signature in studying the cellular interaction of nanoparticles, as well as specific cell functionality [14]. Zeta potential has been used to diagnose the cellular interaction with charged ions or molecules. It was shown that the presence of negatively charged ions or molecules decreases the surface zeta potential and, in contrast, the presence of positively charged ions increases the surface zeta potential [15].

17.3 Fundamental overview of zeta potential

Most colloidal dispersions in polar (aqueous) media spontaneously carry an electric charge. There are various mechanisms responsible for the development of this charge [16]. These include affinity differences of two phases for electrons, ionization of surface groups, differential ion adsorption from electrolyte solution, differential ion dissolution from a crystal lattice, surface anisotropy, and isomorphous substitution. Despite the fact that electrolytes cannot ionize in fully nonpolar media (solvents with very low dielectric constants of 2, like alkanes), particles dispersed in such a medium can accumulate charge. Electrostatic forces are crucial and play a significant role in stabilizing non-aqueous suspensions, but the charging mechanism differs from that in aqueous dispersions. In that case, sometimes acid–base (or electron donor–acceptor) interactions between the particle surface and the dispersing agent or the existence of traces of polar impurities (water) may be the dominating mechanism for charge generation [17]. The development of this charge at the particle surface affects the distribution of ions in the surrounding interfacial region and ultimately leads to the generation of an electrical double layer (EDL) at the particle–liquid medium interface. The development of the electrical double layer at the particle surface is an instantaneous process and is formed of two layers. A schematic representation of the electrical double layer is shown in figure 17.1. In the inner layer, the so-called Stern layer, is where the oppositely charged particles are tightly coupled to the core of the central particle. The second and outermost layer is a diffusive layer consisting of both opposite and the same charged ions/molecules [18]. Within the diffuse layer, there is a hypothetical boundary inside which the ions and particles form a stable/rigid entity. This boundary is also known as the slipping plane (surface of hydrodynamic shear) [4].

When a particle moves under the application of an electric field, the ions within this boundary translate with the particle, and ions outside the boundary migrate separately in the dispersing fluid [4]. Simply, the zeta potential is the value of the electrostatic potential on the imaginary slipping plane [18, 19]. The zeta potential is a property that all materials possess, or acquire when suspended in a fluid. The sign and magnitude that zeta potential possesses impacts on process control, quality control, and product specification; at the simplest level, it can help maintain a more consistent product and at a complex level, it can improve product quality and performance [17].

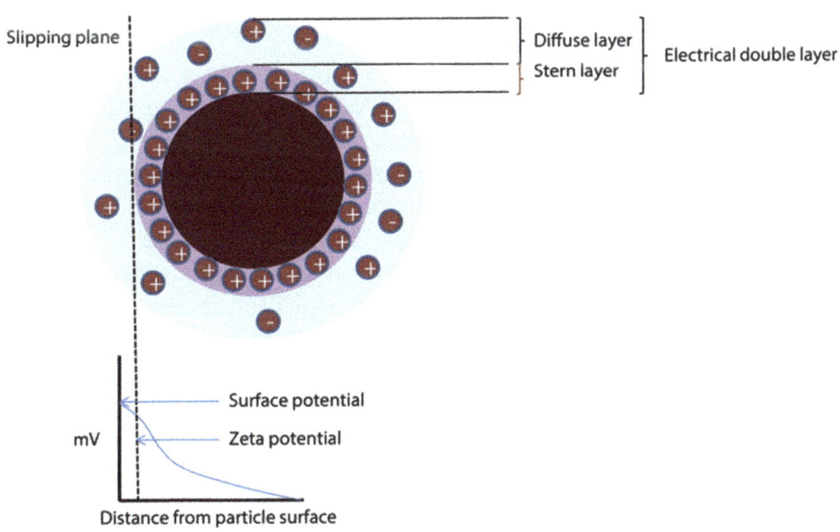

Figure 17.1. Schematic representation of the electrical double layer.

17.4 Measurement of zeta potential

17.4.1 Existing factors and current challenges associated with zeta potential measurement

The zeta potential depends on both nanoparticle and solution properties. Therefore, both the magnitude and sign of the zeta potential are affected by many for a specific nanoparticle. As the basic principle of zeta potential measurement is measuring particle motion under an electric (or acoustic) field, the factors affecting particle motion can affect particle motion as well. There should be minimal interparticle interaction during zeta potential measurement to obtain an accurate result, and thus, strictly, the zeta potential should only be applied to situations approaching infinite dilution. This theoretical consideration must, of course, be balanced by the practical limits of detection of the scattered light. Sometimes in the case of a highly concentrated system, electrophoretic light scattering is not a good choice, rather electroacoustics based methods can be applied. It is significant to note that conductive aqueous phase is necessary for particle mobility in an electrical field. As the deionized water is not sufficiently conductive, the addition of salt (e.g., 0.1 mM NaCl or $NaNO_3$) is necessary, to impart the required conductivity. Sometimes this practice can lead to complications in zeta potential measurement. Some materials, e.g., Ag-nanoparticles may react with added chloride and precipitate as an AgCl layer on particles, ultimately affecting their zeta potential value. A similar kind of complicacy also arises regarding the application of alternating electrical field during zeta potential determination. Most inorganic nanomaterials (e.g., TiO_2 or SiO_2) show stable behavior under an alternating field, but such stability may not be observed in the case of organic and proteinaceous nanoparticles. The presence of both monovalent (e.g., Na^+) and polyvalent ions (e.g., Ca^{2+}) also affects the double layer and alters the electrophoretic mobility, thereby changing the calculated zeta potential [4]. When a nanoparticle is immersed in an aqueous medium, the association/disassociation reactions occur on the surface. This association/disassociation reaction along with the adsorption of ions yields a surface charge as a function of electrolyte concentration and pH [20]. In the case of many nanomaterials like metal oxides and functionalized carbons, the pH of the medium influences the surface charge of the functional groups, ultimately affecting the zeta potential [4]. Also, the existence of surface curvature or roughness on the nanoparticle surface possesses a significant impact on the surface charge density and zeta potential. A predetermined assumption that the ionic distribution on the surface is described by Boltzmann distribution (BD), holds the theoretical foundation for the analytical calculation of electric charge of the surface for an ideal system. However, such an assumption is only valid for zeta potentials smaller than 25 mV and flat surfaces with no curvature and no overlapping electrical double layers [20]. In the case of nanosystems with surface curvature, local variation of the ionic concentration is affected by particle size and surface condition. Thus the resulting zeta potential at the surface also varies. Usually a reduction in particle size leads to an increased curvature effect due to the decreased surface to volume ratio by the decrease in particle diameter. The surface condition also plays an important role by creating a local variation of ionic distribution and causing electrical double layer overlapping [21]. In order to properly calculate the nanoparticle surface charge, first, ionic diffusion must be defined by Poisson–Nernst–Planck (PNP) equations without Boltzmann's assumption [22]. Next, rather than defining a constant surface charge/potential boundary condition, electrical charge at the surface should be calculated as a function of ionic density forming on the surface. In such a case, the development of surface charge and resulting EDL are coupled [23], also called charge regulation (CR). Incorporation of CR in surface charge calculation is highly suggested in that case [20]. Problems such as aggregation [24], low signal-to-noise [25], and blackening of the electrodes [26, 27] can occur at high ionic strength. Aggregation may alter the effective particle size. The most serious problem with aggregation is that the large size of the particles makes them settle from the solution, so the sample either becomes too dilute to achieve a satisfactory signal-to-noise ratio or the remaining dispersed particles are not representative of the agglomerated majority. Moreover, being a dynamic process the effect of aggregation on the zeta potential may change with time. A reduction of particle concentration can decrease the aggregation rate, but this also lowers the signal-to-noise ratio. Thus, trial and error optimization is typically necessary to find the optimal particle concentration for measurements under conditions where particles are aggregating. Conditions that achieve a good signal-to-noise ratio, and where the measured value does not change significantly during the course of the measurement due to loss of particles from the suspension, will typically provide a reliable zeta potential [4]. In some particular instances, especially when the ionic strength of the system is very high or the system contains organic matter (e.g., physiological buffers with glucose and amino acids), a blackening of electrodes is usually observed during measurement. This affects the electric field strength, so measurements of electrophoretic mobility used to determine the zeta potential cannot be made reliably [26]. Polymeric coatings or adsorbed macromolecules, e.g., proteins, polymers, polyelectrolytes on nanomaterial is another important attribute which may alter zeta potential. With such a coating or adsorbed macromolecular layer like protein corona, the slipping plane, and hence zeta potential is located within the polymeric layer. Depending on the nature of the polymer, its presence could decrease the zeta potential by pushing the shear plane outward, thereby decreasing the overall magnitude of the zeta potential, even though the particles are more stable against aggregation [4, 5, 28, 29].

17.4.2 Techniques and methods used for the measurement of zeta potential

17.4.2.1 Electrophoretic light scattering

It is very difficult to measure zeta potential directly. Zeta potential is usually measured indirectly through the laser Doppler electrophoresis instrument by the combination of the principle of electrophoretic light scattering (ELS) with the Doppler frequency shift. From the electrophoretic mobility of charged particles under an applied electrical field, gained through ELS experiment, zeta potential data is acquired with the help of a suitable model (discussed later) [4]. The setup for the measurement of electrophoretic mobility is shown in figure 17.2. In an ELS

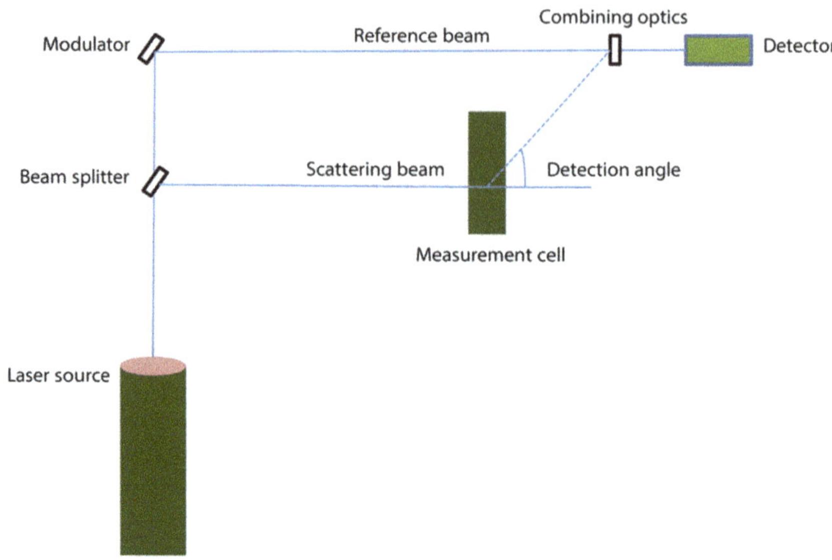

Figure 17.2. Setup for the measurement of electrophoretic mobility.

experiment a laser beam is split into reference and excitation beams. The excitation beam is directed through the sample while an electric field is applied to induce nanoparticle electrophoresis. When charged colloidal particles move toward either the anode or the cathode, the frequency of scattered light from the particles is affected by the Doppler effect. Upon recombination of the scattered and reference beams, a difference frequency (Doppler shift frequency) is produced [28].

Here, the Doppler shift frequency, f_D, of scattered light is related to the particle drift velocity or electrophoretic velocity as [30]:

$$f_D = \frac{2v_z}{\lambda} = \frac{2v \sin\theta}{\lambda}$$

where λ is the laser light wavelength, v is the particle electrophoretic or drift velocity, v_z is that along the incident light axis, and θ is the angle between the velocity vector and the incident light axis [30].

Electrophoretic mobility, μ, is defined from electrophoretic velocity, v, and electric field, E, as [30]:

$$\mu = \frac{v}{E}$$

Zeta potential is estimated by correlating it with electrophoretic mobility with the help of Henry's equation [30]:

$$\mu = \frac{2\varepsilon F\zeta(ka)}{3\eta}$$

where μ is the electrophoretic mobility, ζ is the zeta potential, ε is the solvent dielectric permittivity (or constant), η is the viscosity, and $F(\kappa a)$ is Henry's function (dimensionless), the value of which varies between 1 and 3/2 according to the ratio of the particle size to the Debye length, $1/\kappa$.

Strictly, this equation only applies for isolated particles of zeta potential less than around 25 mV. When $\kappa a \gg 1$ (approximately 100) in a non-polar system and the double layer is thin in comparison to the particle radius, the value of Henry's function becomes 1.5; it is known as the Smoluchowski approximation [16]. Many engineered nanoparticles are much smaller, giving rise to $\kappa a < 1$. For such instances, the solutions of O'Brien and White or Hückel–Onsager equations may be applied. In the case of a polar media (like water) and $\kappa a < 1$ condition, the value of Henry's function becomes 1. It is known as the Hückel approximation [4, 31].

In some typical commercial equipment of electrophoretic light scattering method, an experimental setup is used heterodyne interferometry (e.g., the Mach–Zehnder interferometer arrangement) to extract the Doppler shift frequency of the scattered light, and then, an interference wave between the lasing light and a frequency-shifted scattered light is detected by using a photomultiplier. In this equipment, it is difficult to detect the electrophoretic mobility for the sample containing very low concentrations (below 0.001 wt.%) and high concentrations (above 10 wt.%). The commercial equipment covering a wide concentration range is very expensive (e.g., ELSZ-1000ZS, Photal) [32].

In one of the promising laser Doppler velocimeter (LDV) techniques, namely self-mixing LDV, the laser itself is intensity-modulated by beat signals due to the interference between the lasing field and a frequency-shifted scattered field reinjected into the laser. Thus, the velocity of the moving target can be obtained by observing the intensity-modulated laser light [32, 33].

It should be noted that only the movements caused by the applied external electric field are related to the zeta potential. Unfortunately, many other sources, such as the inhomogeneity of the temperature or the concentration, will also cause the directional movement of the particles [34]. The effect of these movements is the main cause of the noise in the technique of electrophoretic light scattering. To improve the accuracy of the technique, Huang *et al* (2020) proposed a symmetric measurement method to measure the particle velocity from two symmetrical detection points at the vertical arms on both sides of a U-shaped sample pool. A U-shaped sample pool has been widely used in many zeta potential determination procedures, and the measurement point is generally at the bottom of the pool.

Due to the structural symmetry of the sample pool and the uniformity of the external electric field inside the pool, the movement of the particles, influenced by the external electrical field shows an equal velocity of the particles at the vertical arms on both sides, except in opposite directions. This movement pattern is characteristic of the influence by the external electric field and is significantly different from the movements caused by other sources. According to the authors, the symmetric measurement can distinguish the directional movement caused by an external electric field from the others and finally can improve the signal-to-noise of the determination of the zeta potential [35].

In a typical optical configuration used for electrophoretic mobility (and hence zeta potential) measurements, the laser beam has to penetrate the sample for scattered light at a forward angle of 13° to be detected. This optical configuration imparts restrictions on the measurement of the turbidity of the system in terms of the limit of detection of the maximum value. In the case of high sample concentration, the laser beam will become attenuated by the particles. It will cause a reduction of the scattered light that is being detected. At very high concentrations, no scattered light is detected. The upper limit of concentration for zeta potential measurements will depend upon several factors such as the particle size, polydispersity, and optical properties of the particles. One alternative to determine the electrophoretic mobility of a highly concentrated sample is to reduce the path length of the cell, so the transmission of the laser through the sample will also eventually be enhanced. Even though such a cell will allow electrophoretic mobility measurements to be made on concentrated samples, the conversion to zeta potential, and subsequent interpretation of what the results obtained mean, is not straightforward [16].

17.4.2.2 Tunable resistive pulse sensing

Effective theranostic application of nanoparticles requires not only its operation in serum and other complex biological media [29] but also the development of precise high-resolution nanoparticle characterization tools for this challenging environment rather than in their native form or idealized matrices [36]. After the entry of nanoparticles in a biological medium, a coating is formed around the nanoparticle surface due to the absorption of proteins from the surrounding environment. This coating is also called the 'protein corona' [37]. The nature of this coating is dynamic and changes with time until the attainment of equilibrium. In the initial step, the most abundant proteins present in serum, typically albumin, cover the surface of the NPs. However, other higher affinity proteins may displace albumin and become strongly adsorbed to the surface of the NPs over time, a process which is known as the the Vroman effect. NP surface chemistry has been found to influence the nature of protein coronas [38]. In the case of characterization of nanoparticles in complex biological media, measurement of nanoparticle surface charge density, as well as zeta potential, is considered as a very significant parameter as it indicates the aggregation behavior and electrostatic stability of nanoparticles. ELS is the most prominently utilized method for the characterization of zeta potential. But in some particular instances this technique become biased, especially in the case of the subpopulations of particles that scatter light more intensely such as, for example, larger particles. Furthermore, a distribution of surface charge densities is likely to exist within any population depending upon the composition of the adsorbed protein layer. Such variability may correlate with particle size and agglomeration state and therefore light scattering properties, which suggests a potential bias in an analysis by ELS [29]. In such instances particle-by-particle surface charge measurement by the tunable resistive pulse sensing (TRPS) technique can provide a more reliable measurement alternative for zeta potential. Single-particle electrokinetic measurements of nanoparticles using resistive pulse sensing were first shown by Deblois et al Cylindrical nanopores, track-in etched polycarbonate were employed to estimate the electrophoretic mobility of latex spheres and various viruses. From the translocation times of the particulate, particle velocities, and respective electrophoretic mobilities were obtained [39]. Tunable resistive pulse sensing is a recent modification of resistive pulse sensing in which surface charge is estimated by mapping the 'blockade' signals during the passage of the particles through a pore and subsequent calculation of their velocities [40]. A temporary occlusion is created if a particle traverses through a pore on a membrane. As a consequence, a reduction in ionic current across the pore occurs, which is measured in tunable resistive pulse sensing technique in the form of a blockade signal. As the exact geometry of the pore is unknown, a similar measurement is also done for the calibration particles with known properties, and the relative values from the two measurements are compared [41, 42]. The magnitude of the measured blockade signal is directly proportional to the volume of the particle, allowing determination of the particle diameter assuming spherical geometry of the particle. The shapes of the pulse signal of both calibration and sample particles are analyzed to provide information regarding the particle velocity and are used to compute the NP's zeta potential [29]. The technique thus provides an estimate of the statistical distribution of the zeta potential values for a sample and also allows the simultaneous determination of the size and zeta potential of a single nanoparticle [40]. The ability to look at the statistical distribution of the NP surface charge across a sample and correlate it to other parameters, for example, the size, permits a deeper understanding of the nature of a NP sample and therefore could produce more accurate predictions of their behavior in biological environments [29, 43].

17.4.2.3 Electroacoustics based measurement

Electroacoustics spectroscopy provides a simple way to measure zeta potential and has proved to be a powerful tool. The traditional methods of determining zeta potentials suffer from reliability-related drawbacks. In cases of measurements involving very dilute systems, it is very prone to contamination problems, but even in the case of an accurate assessment of the direct current, current estimates of zeta potentials can be in error by as much as 100% or 100 mV in the most unfavorable cases. Electroacoustics overcomes the contamination problem as it allows the measurement of a significant particle concentration. The simultaneous measurement of both size and zeta potential, using the electroacoustic spectroscopy technique, means that the correct average size is used for estimating zeta in polydisperse systems. The use of the entire mobility spectrum, over a range of frequencies, allows one to avoid the ambiguities which can occur with a single point (direct current) measurement [44]. Electroacoustics consists of two types of process. Firstly, a macroscopic potential difference is created due to the passage of a sound wave in a colloidal suspension. It is called the ultrasonic vibration potential (UVP) effect. Secondly, an opposite phenomenon is observed if an alternating electric field is applied to a colloidal suspension, as a consequence a sound wave is generated, which is called the electrokinetic sonic amplitude (ESA). In both cases, the applied field and the response occur at the same frequency. Both UVP and ESA have been exploited for the estimation of zeta potential and sophisticated instruments are

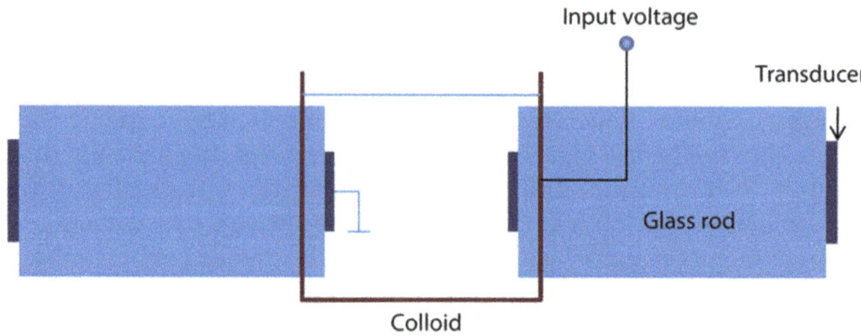

Figure 17.3. Acoustosizer for measurement of zeta potential.

available based on both principles (Matec ESA 8000, could operate in either ESA or CVP mode, but only worked at 1 MHz frequency and requires particle size as the input data). In the case of both CVP and ESA, the parameter ultimately provided is dynamic mobility. The ESA technique provides a direct estimation of this parameter, whereas the alternative route requires not only the CVP but also the complex conductivity. CVP devices only operate at one frequency and the conductivity measurement is performed only in the low-frequency limit, which leads to an inherent error in estimating the dynamic mobility especially for low conductivity systems due to neglect of the imaginary part of the conductivity. For these reasons, ESA techniques are preferred over CVP based techniques [45]. The first theoretical treatment of the ESA effect and its reciprocal relationship with CVP was demonstrated by O'Brien. They also indicated a stepwise procedure for the measurement of zeta potential through the ESA effect. According to the author's simultaneous determination of zeta potential and particle size is a three-step procedure, starting from generation of an ESA spectrum, followed by calculation of a dynamic mobility spectrum from an ESA spectrum, lastly estimation of size and charge density from that dynamic mobility spectrum [46]. Acoustosizer and Acoustosizer II (Colloidal Dynamics USA) works on this principle. A schematic diagram of Acoustosizer is shown in figure 17.3.

Recently, another commercial device for measuring zeta potentials in concentrated suspension has been launched onto the market by Colloidal Dispersions, Mount Kisco, New York, USA. This calculates the zeta potential from the colloid vibration current (CVI) [47].

17.4.2.4 Electroosmotic flow-based measurement

The phenomenon of electroosmosis was first explored by Reuss in 1809 in an experiment where a clay–sand–water mixture in a U-tube was exposed to direct current. Upon the application of an electrical field in a direction parallel to the wall of a capillary, a Coulombic force is experienced by the ions in the diffuse layers and they move toward the electrode of opposite polarity, ultimately creating a motion of the fluid near the wall and transfers momentum via viscous forces into the bulk liquid. So a net motion of bulk liquid along the wall is created and is called electroosmosis flow [48]. Electric current is also generated by this movement. Due to the tangential direction of the applied electrical force to the surface, the resulting ion migration does not impact on the charge density in the electrical double layer. The resulting velocity profile is plug-like, where the velocity is zero at the wall (no-slip condition) and rises to a uniform velocity in the bulk. As the thickness of the electrical double layer is very small (around 30 nm) compared to the microchannel (around 50 mm), to an observer it appears as if the fluid slips by the surface. The velocity at the edge of the EDL is given by the classic Helmholtz–Smoluchowski equation:

$$u_{\mathrm{HS}} = -\frac{\varepsilon_0 \varepsilon_{\mathrm{T}} \zeta E_x}{\eta}$$

where ε_0 and ε_{T} are the dielectric permittivity of a vacuum and the relative dielectric permittivity of the solution, E_x is the tangential electric field and ζ is the zeta potential.

Usually the group of terms, $(\varepsilon_0 \varepsilon_{\mathrm{T}} \zeta / \eta)$, are combined together into a proportionality constant called the electroosmotic mobility (μ) of the solid–liquid interface. Since the velocity only varies in the electrical double layer, the total flow rate is approximated by $Q = u_{\mathrm{HS}} A_{\mathrm{c}}$, where A_{c} is the cross-sectional area of the microchannel. Thus it is possible to determine the zeta potential by measuring the fluid velocity or volume flow rate under electroosmotic flow [49]. It was shown that the electroosmotic flow-based method is not suitable in the case of the oppositely charged surface and tracer particles and also limited to low salinity conditions especially when using polymeric tracer particles. Although in the electroosmotic flow method the formation of a capillary flow channel is not required, it disables a non-destructive surface zeta potential of fragile or valuable samples, such as QCM-D sensors, in comparison to the streaming potential approach [50].

17.4.2.5 Streaming potential based measurement

If the fluid is induced to flow tangentially to the interface of the capillary by a fluid pressure drop (a porous medium can be approximated as an array of parallel capillaries), and then some excess ions within the diffuse layer are transported with the flow, giving rise to a streaming current. This streaming current is balanced by a conduction current, leading to the streaming potential [51]. This phenomenon can be exploited for the estimation of the zeta potential of solid surfaces using the so-called streaming potential technique. A schematic representation of the streaming potential technique to measure zeta potential on the biomaterial surface is shown in figure 17.4.

In a typical experimental apparatus, a capillary is usually connected to a pump using a pipe network and a series of transducers are placed in a special strategic manner to measure the pressure drop, flow rate, streaming potential, and conductivity. The piping network is designed so that the flow direction can be reversed in the microchannels. The potential must be measured with a high impedance electrometer to avoid the generation of the streaming current and therefore the flow

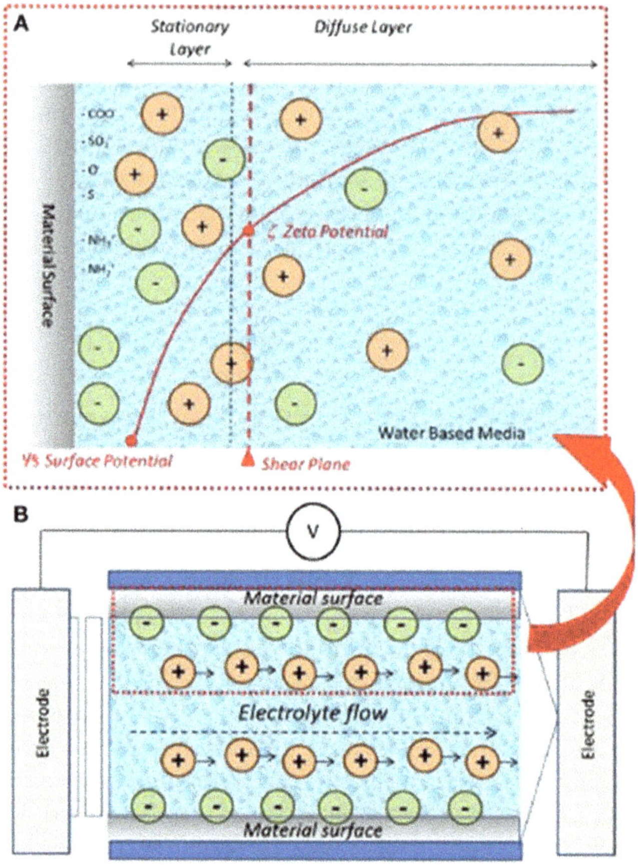

Figure 17.4. (A) Schematic representation of charge development at the biomaterial-water-based medium interface and zeta potential, (B) schematic representation of the streaming potential technique for the measurement of solid surface zeta potential. Reproduced from [13]. CC BY 4.0.

in the microchannel. Also, the characteristics of the electrode should be such that it responds reversibly to current flows (e.g., Ag/AgCl). The slope of the streaming potential plot provides the estimate of zeta potential. To obtain an accurate streaming potential plot, the number of experiments performed must be enhanced (at least 20) [49].

17.5 Analysis of zeta potential and its implementation in biomedical nanotechnology

Zeta potential is regarded as an important characterization parameter for the surface property of nanomaterials and understanding of various factors influencing its values has not been achieved yet [52]. A zeta potential measurement made at a single condition of fixed pH, ionic strength, and solution composition may have a limited scientific value. However, monitoring changes in the measured zeta potential in different systems can be more informative. Most of the information provided by a measured zeta potential value of a system is qualitative [4]. The zeta potential is a key indicator of the stability of colloidal dispersions. The magnitude of the zeta potential indicates the degree of electrostatic repulsion between adjacent, similarly charged particles in the dispersion. For molecules and particles that are small enough, a high value of zeta potential will confer stability against particle aggregation. In the case of the systems with a small zeta potential, attractive forces may exceed this repulsion and the dispersion may break and flocculate. So, colloids with high zeta potential (negative or positive) are electrically stabilized, while colloids with low zeta potentials tend to coagulate or flocculate [53]. The zeta potential of particles typically ranges from +100 mV to −100 mV. Highly dispersed nanoparticles have zeta potential values greater than +30 mV or less than −30 mV. NPs having zeta potential values ranging from −10 to +10 mV are considered to be neutral. This is a general rule of thumb and is not always true in the case of nanomaterials [54]. In the case of a combined electrostatic and steric stabilization, a minimum zeta potential of 20 mV is desirable [55]. Zeta potential is also an important indicator of the alteration of the chemical architecture of the surface of the nanomaterials. An altered value of either the sign or the magnitude of the zeta potential of nanoparticles can play the role of a qualitative diagnostic for changes to the particle surface chemistry, e.g., adsorption of a macromolecule or other ligands onto a nanoparticle, specific interactions with dissolved ions, or a chemical reaction of the particle surface [4]. These properties may have short term and long term impacts on the fate and toxicity profile of the nanomaterials in biological systems in the case of pharmaceutical and biomedical application, which was discussed earlier.

17.6 Conclusion

The pH of the sample, specific adsorption of ions, the surface charge of the particles, size of the nanoparticles, and the concentration of a component used in formulation can play a vital role during the determination of zeta potential. Each of the methods for the determination of zeta potential has its advantages and drawbacks. Now new methods have been developed to overcome the drawbacks for the determination of zeta potential. Although research is being conducted on nanotoxicity, particularly on nanoparticles used in biomedical applications, much more research still needs to be conducted in the near future so that the effect of toxicity on the zeta potential estimation is clearer.

References

[1] Raja P M V and Barron A R 2020 *Zeta Potential Analysis* https://chem.libretexts.org/link?55842 (accesed on 25 June 2020)

[2] Ceylan Z, Meral R, Özogul F and Yilmaz M T 2020 Importance of electrospun chitosan-based nanoscale materials for sea food products safety ed S Gopi, S Thomas and A Pius *Chitin and Chitosan, Volume 1: Preparation and Properties* (Amsterdam: Elsevier) pp 195–223

[3] Honary S and Zahir F 2013 Effect of zeta potential on the properties of nano-drug delivery systems—a review (part 2) *Trop. J. Pharm. Res* **12** 265–73

[4] Lowry G V, Hill R J, Harper S, Rawle A F, Hendren C O, Klaessig F, Nobbmann U, Sayreh P and Rumblei J 2016 Guidance to improve the scientific value of zeta-potential measurements in nanoEHS *Environ. Sci. Nano* **3** 953–65

[5] Ostolska I and Wiśniewska M 2014 Application of the zeta potential measurements to explanation of colloidal Cr_2O_3 stability mechanism in the presence of the ionic polyamino acids *Colloid Polym. Sci.* **292** 2453–64

[6] Lu G W and Gao P 2010 Emulsions and microemulsions for topical and transdermal drug delivery *Handbook of Non-Invasive Drug Delivery Systems* (Amsterdam: Elsevier) pp 59–94

[7] Gupta V and Trivedi P 2018 In vitro and *in vivo* characterization of pharmaceutical topical nanocarriers containing anticancer drugs for skin cancer treatment *Lipid Nanocarriers for Drug Targeting* (Amsterdam: Elsevier) pp 563–627

[8] Xu R 2008 Progress in nanoparticles characterization: sizing and zeta potential measurement *Particuology* **6** 112–5

[9] Tripathi R M and Chung S J 2019 Biogenic nanomaterials: synthesis, characterization, growth mechanism, and biomedical applications *J. Microbiol. Methods* **157** 65–80

[10] Mohammed A E, Al-Qahtani A, Al-Mutairi A, Al-Shamri B and Aabed K F 2018 Antibacterial and cytotoxic potential of biosynthesized silver nanoparticles by some plant extracts *Nanomaterials (Basel)* **8** 382

[11] AlgebalyA S, MohammedA E, AbutahaN and ElobeidM M 2020 Biogenic synthesis of silver nanoparticles: antibacterial and cytotoxic potential *Saudi J. Biol. Sci.* **27** 1340–51

[12] Shao X R, Wei X Q, Song X, Hao L Y, Cai X X, Zhang Z R, Peng Q and Lin Y F 2015 Independent effect of polymeric nanoparticle zeta potential/surface charge, on their cytotoxicity and affinity to cells *Cell Prolif.* **48** 465–74

[13] Ferraris S, Cazzola M, Peretti V, Stella B and Spriano S 2018 Zeta potential measurements on solid surfaces for *in vitro* biomaterials testing/: surface charge, reactivity upon contact with fluids and protein absorption *Front. Bioeng. Biotechnol.* **6** 1–7

[14] Zhang Y, Yang M, Portney N G, Cui D, Budak G, Ozbay E, Ozkan M and OzkanC S 2008 Zeta potential: a surface electrical characteristic to probe the interaction of nanoparticles with normal and cancer human breast epithelial cells *Biomed. Microdevices* **10** 321–8

[15] Mikolajczyk A, Gajewicz A, Rasulev B, Schaeublin N, Maurer-Gardner E, Hussain S, Leszczynski J and Puzyn T 2015 Zeta potential (ζ) for metal oxide nanoparticles: a predictive model developed by nano-QSPR approach *Chem. Mater.* **27** 2400–7

[16] Kaszuba M, Corbett J, Watson F M and Jones A 2010 High-concentration zeta potential measurements using light-scattering techniques *Phil. Trans. R. Soc.* A **368** 4439–51

[17] Fairhurst D 2013 *An Overview of the Zeta Potential—Part 1: The Concept. American Pharmaceutical Review.* https://americanpharmaceuticalreview.com/Featured-Articles/133232-An-Overview-of-the-Zeta-Potential-Part-1-The-Concept/ (accessed on 24 March 2020)

[18] Carvalho P, Felicio M, Santos N C, Goncalves S and Domingues M M 2018 Application of light scattering techniques to nanoparticle characterization and development *Front. Chem.* **6** 1–17

[19] Bhattacharjee S 2016 DLS and zeta potential—what they are and what they are not? *J. Control. Release* **235** 337–51

[20] Alan B O, Barisik M and Ozcelik H G 2020 Roughness effects on surface charge properties of silica nanoparticles *J. Phys. Chem.* C **124** 7274–86
[21] Shi Y R, Ye M P, Du L C and Weng Y X 2018 Experimental determination of particle size-dependent surface charge density for silica nanospheres *J. Chem.* C **122** 23764–71
[22] Polat M and Polat H 2010 Analytical solution of Poisson–Boltzmann equation for interacting plates of arbitrary potentials and same sign *J. Colloid Interface Sci.* **341** 178–85
[23] Huang K D and Yang R J 2007 Electrokinetic behaviour of overlapped electric double layers in nanofluidic channels *Nanotechnology* **18** 115701
[24] Deryabin D G, Efremova L V and Vasilchenko A S 2015 A zeta potential value determines the aggregate's size of penta-substituted fullerene derivatives in aqueous suspension whereas positive charge is required for toxicity against bacterial *Cells J. Nanobiotechnol.* **13** 50
[25] *Limits of Concentrations when Measuring Zeta Potential* https://azom.com/article.aspx?ArticleID=16795 (accessed on 12 April 2020)
[26] *Facilitating the Measurement of Zeta Potential in Proteins* https://azom.com/article.aspx?ArticleID=16096 (accessed on 20 April 2020)
[27] *Zeta Potential Measurements of High Conductivity Colloidal Samples* https://pharmaceutical-business-review.com/wp-content/uploads/2018/07/15f81155-932d-4af3-975f-2e51e3b99012.pdf%0A%0A (accessed on 20 April 2020)
[28] Doane T L, Chuang C, Hill R J and Burda C 2012 Nanoparticle ζ-potentials *Acc. Chem. Res.* **45** 317–26
[29] Sikora A, Shard A G and Minelli C 2016 Size and ζ-potential measurement of silica nanoparticles in serum using tunable resistive pulse sensing *Langmuir* **32** 2216–24
[30] Sudo S, Ohtomo T, Otsuka K, Sudo S, Ohtomo T and Otsuka K 2013 Easy measurement and analysis method of zeta potential and electrophoretic mobility of water-dispersed colloidal particles by using a self-mixing solid-state laser *J. Appl. Phys.* **114** 063106
[31] Delgado A V, González-Caballero F, Hunter R J, Koopal L K and Lyklema J 2005 Measurement and interpretation of electrokinetic phenomenon *Pure Appl. Chem.* **77** 1753–805
[32] Sudo S and Otsuka K 2014 Measurements of liquid surface fluctuations using a self-mixing solid-state laser *J. Appl. Phys.* **115** 233103
[33] Otsuka K, Abe K, Ko J Y and Lim T S 2002 Real-time nanometer vibration measurement with a self-mixing microchip solid-state laser *Opt. Lett.* **27** 13–39
[34] Shit G C, Mondal A, Sinha A and Kundu P K 2016 Two-layer electro-osmotic flow and heat transfer in a hydrophobic micro-channel with fluid–solid interfacial slip and zeta potential difference *Colloids Surf.* A **506** 535–49
[35] Huang G, Xu B, Qiu J, Peng L, Luo K, Liu D and Han P 2020 Symmetric electrophoretic light scattering for determination of the zeta potential of colloidal systems *Colloids Surf.* A **587** 124339
[36] Vogel R, Pal A K, Jambhrunkar S, Patel P and Thakur S S 2017 High-resolution single particle zeta potential characterisation of biological nanoparticles using tunable resistive pulse sensing *Sci. Rep.* **7** 1–13
[37] Lynch I and Dawson K A 2008 Protein–nanoparticle interactions *Nano Today* **3** 40–7
[38] Tenzer S *et al* 2013 Rapid formation of plasma protein corona critically affects nanoparticle pathophysiology *Nat. Nanotechnol.* **8** 772–81
[39] Deblois R W, Bean C P and Wesley R K A 1977 Electrokinetic measurements with submicron particles and pores by resistive pulse technique *J. Colloid Interface Sci.* **61** 323–35

[40] Kozak D, Anderson W, Vogel R, Chen S, Antaw F and Trau M 2012 Simultaneous size and ζ-potential measurements of individual nanoparticles in dispersion using size-tunable pore sensors *ACS Nano* **6** 6990–7
[41] Ito T, Sun L and Crooks R M 2003 Simultaneous determination of the size and surface charge of individual nanoparticles using a carbon nanotube-based coulter counter *Anal. Chem.* **75** 2399–406
[42] Vogel R, Willmott G, Kozak D, Roberts G S, Anderson W, Groenewegen L, Glossop B, Barnett A, Turner A and Trau M 2011 Quantitative sizing of nano/microparticles with a tunable elastomeric pore sensor *Anal. Chem.* **83** 3499–506
[43] Vogel R, Anderson W, Eldridge J, Glossop B and Willmott G 2012 A variable pressure method for characterizing nanoparticle surface charge using pore sensors *Anal. Chem.* **84** 3125–31
[44] Hunter R J and Hunter R J 2006 More reliable zeta potentials using electroacoustics *Prog. Colloid Polym. Sci.* **2004** 1–10
[45] Greenwood R 2003 Review of the measurement of zeta potentials in concentrated aqueous suspensions using electroacoustics *Adv. Colloid Interface Sci.* **106** 55–81
[46] O'Brien R W, Cannon D W and Rowlands W N 1995 Electroacoustic determination of particle size and zeta potential *J. Colloid Interface Sci.* **173** 406–18
[47] Dukhin A S and Parlia S 2014 Measuring zeta potential of protein nano-particles using electroacoustics *Colloid. Surf.* B **121** 257–63
[48] Luong D T and Sprik R 2013 Streaming potential and electroosmosis measurements to characterize porous materials *ISRN Geophys.* **2013** 1–8
[49] Glawdel T and Ren C 2015 Zeta potential measurement ed D Li *Encyclopedia of Microfluidics and Nanofluidics* (New York: Springer) pp 202–26
[50] Plohl O, Zemljic L F, Potrc S and Luxbacher T 2020 Applicability of electro-osmotic flow for the analysis of the surface zeta potential *RSC Adv.* **10** 6777–89
[51] Thanh L D 2019 Streaming potential and zeta potential measurements in porous rocks *J. Geosci. Environ. Prot.* **6** 89–100
[52] Biriukov D, Fibich P and Předota M 2020 Zeta potential determination from molecular simulations *J. Phys. Chem.* **124** 3159–70
[53] Chirayil C J, Abraham J, Mishra R K, George S C and Thomas S 2017 Instrumental techniques for the characterization of nanoparticles ed S Thomas, R Thomas, A K Zachariah and R K Mishra *Micro and Nano Technologies, Thermal and Rheological Measurement Techniques for Nanomaterials Characterization* (Amsterdam: Elsivier) pp 1–36
[54] Barhoum A, García-Betancourt M L, Rahier H and Assche G 2018 Physicochemical characterization of nanomaterials: polymorph, composition, wettability, and thermal stability ed A Barhoum and A S H Makhlouf *Micro and Nano Technologies, Emerging Applications of Nanoparticles and Architecture Nanostructures* (Amsterdam: Elsevier) pp 255–78
[55] Shah M R, Imran M and Ullah S 2017 Nanosuspensions ed M R Shah, M Imran and S Ullah *Micro and Nano Technologies, Lipid-Based Nanocarriers for Drug Delivery and Diagnosis* (Norwich, NY: William Andrew Publishing) pp 139–72

IOP Publishing

Analytical Techniques for Biomedical Nanotechnology

Ajeet Kaushik, Sesha S Srinivasan and Yogendra Kumar Mishra

Chapter 18

Electron paramagnetic (spin) resonance spectroscopy for biomedical nanotechnology

S V Satya Prasad, Kartikey Verma and Subhash Singh

Electron paramagnetic resonance (EPR) or the electron spin resonance (ESR) spectroscopy is used to study the free radicals and paramagnetic species in nano–biomaterials. In the biomedical applications such as oximetry, the EPR is employed to measure the level of oxygen in tissues. The direct detection of transition metal ions such as copper ions or iron ions will allow detection of neurodegenerative diseases due to the formation of amyloid- or amyloid like fibrillary structures. EPR imaging demonstrates an unparalleled tool for the 3D mapping of the spatial distribution of paramagnetic species and reactive oxygen species (ROS) and hence widely applicable to clinical and biomedical research applications. The present chapter focuses on the applications of EPR in the biomedical field especially at nano level.

18.1 Introduction and working of EPR spectrometer

Electron paramagnetic resonance(EPR)/electron spin resonance (ESR) was initially discovered in 1944 by E K Zavoisky. It is the resonance spectroscopy of different systems having unpaired electrons [1]. EPR spectroscopy is a non-destructive technique for the analysis of free radicals, unstable compounds developed *in situ*, and various paramagnetic transition metal compounds such as Cu^{2+}, Fe^{3+}, Mn^{2+}, and $Mo5^{+}$ at a definite state of valency. The compounds exhibiting electrochemical oxidation or reduction are also analysed using EPR [2]. Therefore, covering diverse fields of science and technology, EPR has become the most sought after advanced technique in the current era. ESR measures the spin energy level transitions of electrons which are induced due to the suitable frequency radiation. The strength of the magnetic field determines the frequency of the radiation. In general every EPR spectrometer works in the 9.5 GHz frequency region which is also called the X-band region. The strength of the field in this region is between 0.35 and 1.24 T.

doi:10.1088/978-0-7503-3379-5ch18

The uniqueness of EPR as compared to other conventional spectroscopy techniques lies in the fact that the radiation frequency is kept constant and the magnetic field is varied to get an absorption spectrum. When the energy is absorbed, an electron travels from a lower energy level to a higher one.

The main source of radiation is a klystron, a high powered microwave source with low noise and high sensitivity. The operation of the spectrometer is in the microwave region where the incident radiation can be a continuous wave or in low frequency discontinuous pulses. A resonant cavity is placed at the center of the electromagnet and it houses the sample. The microwaves are sent to the sample along an iris. Weak signals emerging from the sample are amplified by the cavity. Different kinds of solid diodes are responsive to the energy from microwaves. When separation in the energy bands is in parity with the energy from incoming microwaves, absorption lines are shown. For the outer components like the detector, the source is integral to the control of the microwave bridge. Moreover, the instrument's performance is enhanced with the addition of components such as an amplifier, attenuator, and field modulator. Figure 18.1 represents a line diagram of a typical ESR/EPR spectrometer.

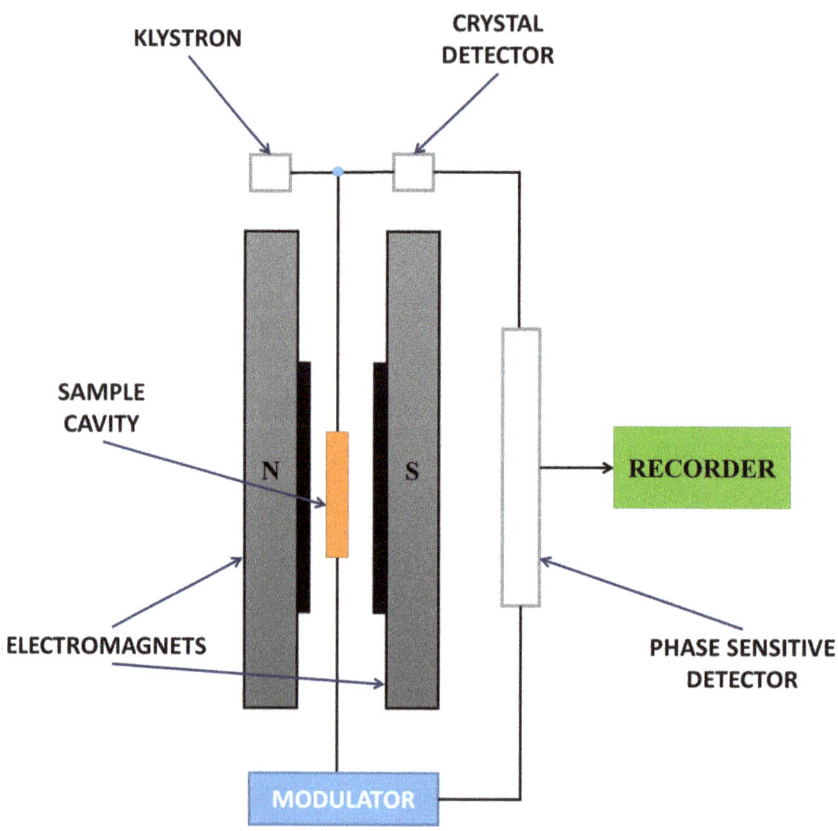

Figure 18.1. Line diagram of an ESR spectrometer illustrating its construction and the major components.

The construction of new age spectrometers is slightly different from that shown in figure 18.1. In the current generation spectrometers, the source of the microwave is from gun oscillators which replace the klystrons. Also, in place of the recorders, there are analog to digital converters or personal computers attached to the phase sensitive detector [3]. The spectroscopy of EPR gives a spectrum of information on the system being analysed for diverse sophistication levels. As a direct method, the EPR spectrum's amplitude (second integral) quantifies the individual paramagnetic systems by making use of the suitable reference samples of identified concentration. This is either time decided or static. For time based systems, the EPR can be used to determine the kinetics of biochemical processes. Moreover, analysis of the EPR spectrum also provides information on the nature of paramagnetic systems and the coordination of the individual metal center inside a molecule can also be known.

18.2 Evolution of biomedical EPR spectroscopy

History has demonstrated that the EPR technique has been successful in the analysis of biological entities. One of the best instances supporting this was the discovery of non-heme iron or the nitrosylated heme in 1960, which incidentally was the first discovery of endogenous NO generated in mammals. This was around 25 years prior to the discovery of endogenous L-arginine/NO [2]. But it was unfortunate that the scientific community did not recognize the significance of this EPR discovery. Therefore, the history of biological EPR dates to the mid-20th century. At this time, large quantities of information were discovered and diverse applications of EPR were suggested or formulated. Therefore, apart from its applications in chemical, physical, and biological structures, EPR spectroscopy also became significant in the biomedical field. Previously the development of biological EPR was restricted to a very few laboratories and the findings were also not as expected. The reason for this might be the complex and expensive technical equipment. Hence, the EPR technique was rare or in some cases unfamiliar in the biomedical area. With the advent of new technology, software and the latest EPR/ESR instrumentation there has been a gradual increase in development. Many endeavors have been put up for precise bioanalytical procedures on a more frequent basis [4].

EPR spectroscopy has become indispensable in biomedicine because the transition metals and the free radicals play a vital role and are the base for many biological activities having relevance in the field of medicine. Some of the evident illustrations are reactive oxygen species (ROS) which are the end products of the conventional metabolism of oxygen. These are integral to the homeostasis and signaling of cells. In adverse conditions, increased ROS levels can significantly harm the cells. As per the *free-radical theory*, these are considered to be primary influencers in the functional decline of aging in an organism. The technique of EPR is constructed on the phenomenon of electromagnetic radiation being absorbed by a single or multiple unpaired electrons (the paramagnetic compounds), in the presence of an external magnetic field. Hence the spectroscopy of EPR is suitable to be applicable for natural paramagnetic compounds such as metallo-enzymes, free radicals or tyrosyl radicals/semiquinones. The metallo-enzymes are nothing but paramagnetic ions of metal and the semiquinones are proteins within the body having radical cofactors. Not only paramagnetic systems, but the spectroscopy of EPR is also applicable for the diamagnetic systems if there is an introduction of paramagnetic reporter species. The biomolecules' dynamics and the structural investigations can be carried out if metal ions that are diamagnetic are replaced with paramagnetic groups [5]. This is possible by introducing spin labels in specified sites of nucleic acids or proteins.

18.3 Different methods of EPR in biomedical nano applications

- **EPR oximetry**

  This is essential to quantify the oxygen present in blood or in various tissues to diagnose and treat a number of diseases linked to the supply or use of oxygen. Due to its higher levels of accuracy or low invasiveness, the EPR oximetry technique has become the most sought after one. Exploring the methods of EPR imaging, information on spatial distribution of the oxygen levels can be gathered. Many of the previous researchers give a broad explanation of the theory of EPR oximetry. The different applications have also been listed in this research [4, 6]. When the naturally triplet molecule of oxygen radical interacts with the paramagnetic in natural spin probes, it is possible to determine the concentrations of oxygen. Also in this case by EPR spectroscopy, the partial pressures of oxygen can also be determined. The spin probes for the molecules of oxygen can be applied in the soluble state or in the solid state. When two electrons show non-vanishing probability such that they localize in a same single orbital of atom or molecule, they exhibit an additional interaction called the Heisenberg *spin exchange*. The interactions of paramagnetic bodies and the Heisenberg spin exchange changes the width of the EPR line. This change in width is proportional to the partial pressures or the concentration of oxygen which accurately quantifies the levels of oxygen.

Some EPR applications are assessing tissue or tumor oxygenation, knowing about the oxidate stress and flow of blood within brain and calculating the cellular respiration by evaluating the quantity of oxygen among cells and mitochondria [7–9]. In some cases insoluble particles of paramagnetic probes are utilized for continuous measurement of oxygen in certain tissues in the process of EPR spectroscopy. Some examples of this are certain kinds of charcoals or substances such as PDMS (bioinert polymer), LiNc-BuO which when coated to certain tissues will enhance the responsiveness to oxygen [10].

- **Direct detection of paramagnetic species**

  Different paramagnetic bodies that play vital roles *in vivo* are stable and hence they can be directly observed by EPR spectroscopy. Some instances are tyrosyl radical which are free radicals of amino acids or semiquinones present within proteins. The paramagnetic Cu^{2+} is also such a body. The paramagnetic species array can be directly identified by the EPR method. The response of the properties of a species to different physicochemical factors can also be determined. An important benefit of the technique is that the paramagnetic species can be analysed in their home environment without disturbing or modifying the tissue. Some of the essential paramagnetic bodies which can be observed directly inside the tissues or cells inside a body with the help of a typical EPR spectrometer (X band) integrated with cryogenic fittings are:

Tissues or cells having high concentrations of exogenous or endogenous NO show EPR signal properties of Hb–NO (heme–NO) in blood. They also exhibit dinitrosyl–Fe complexes at the g value of approximately 2.03 [2]. Ideally it is impossible to discover these significant NO signalling bodies without the existence of the EPR technique. Also the metal chelator (desferal) treated tissues or cells display signal properties that are novel. EPR is a reliable method to determine the pools of chelatable Fe/Cu [11].

Some additional instances of EPR spectroscopy are in dermatology where pathological or conventional tissues such as melanoma and substantia nigra possess polymeric pigments called melanins. These melanins constitute a steady group of free radicals which can be recognized through the EPR techniques. Early tumors such as nevi or melanomas in tissues can be diagnosed through EPR techniques through unequivocal pigment identification in different tissues [12]. EPR spectroscopy has a significant application that is the reflective assessment of the dosage of radiation. When radiating, calcified or solid tissues like bones, fingernails, and tooth enamel produce extremely stable radicals traced by EPR. The EPR signal's amplitude is in proportion to the combined radiation dosage received by the person in the instant. But primarily the disadvantage of the technique lies in the invasiveness because, to accurately estimate the dosage of the radiation, an enamel biopsy (approximately 70 mg) of the tooth needs to be done [13]. In some cases the concentration and the duration of the cexistence of the radicals (ascorbyl, phenoxyl radicals) allows them to be detected under EPR [14].

It has been found out that many ions of transition metals such as Fe^{2+}, Cu^{2+}, Zn^{2+} play a significant part within the nervous system and help in diseases like Parkinson's, prion and Alzheimer's [15]. When these ions are bounded, it leads to misfolding or plaque of various proteins forming for each disease type. In one instance, the concentration of Cu^{2+} within the neocortical parenchyma of a healthy and normal brain is around 70 μM but in cases of patients with Alzheimer's the amyloid plaques have a concentration of around 400 μM which proves the influence of Cu^{2+} in the generation of plaque. Therefore, it is absolutely necessary to understand the influence of such ions in diseases pertaining to the central nervous system. Specifically for the structural properties of sites where ion binding takes place. The consequences in the formation of plaque are also to be studied for developing therapeutic drugs. Not only for Cu^{2+} but even the various paramagnetic metal ions EPR can be directly used to understand the ion coordination with proteins in their respective aggregated forms.

Previous studies of continuous wave EPR suggest that the ion Cu^{2+} in the prion proteins of mammals binds with both the N and C terminal parts and the quantity of binding sites is influenced by the pH of the surrounding environment.

Generally, EPR is a flexible technique. The duration for preparing a sample or obtaining data or the experimental procedure completely depends on the definite application of EPR and is usually in the range of hours or minutes. The experiments of spin trapping are ideally done for live cells inside a capillary with 105–107 cells inside 10–100 μl of medium. The recording of the spectra is done at room temperature. Some of the preparations of live tissues such as vascular tissue strips of lab animals are also done at room temperature (37 °C). For the essential paramagnetic centers such as parts of mitochondria's respiratory chain, the samples of tissues (100–500 mg) are studied by subjecting them to the electron paramagnetic resonance spectroscopy inside the liquid nitrogen at sub cooling temperatures [2].

In the case of multi-organ failure within a body systemic inflammation called sepsis occurs which can eventually lead to death. The exact mechanism behind this has not yet been completely explained but the failure of organs due to sepsis has been associated with mitochondrial dysfunction [16]. An EPR study was conducted on patients suffering from severe sepsis and muscle biopsies were taken [17]. The samples of tissue were obtained from nine diverse sources of the paramagnetic bodies and quantified by adopting the self-developed spectra technique. They were analysed under EPR at low temperature. It was observed that a specific parameter among the nice paramagnetic species recognized as a specific pair of spin-coupled semiquinones. There seemed to be a relationship of the concentration with the mitochondrial complex II redox state. This has a negative correlation with the severity of illness in the patient. Also, the lowered mitochondrial complex I concentration has relationship with mortality. Although further research is necessary in this case, the obtained results closely connect mitochondrial dysfunction and sepsis of complexes I/II in respiratory chain.

- **Spin trapping**

  The conversion of a substance into a paramagnetic condition through a redox reaction or through chemical modification having stable radicals is analysed by the EPR technique. Spin trapping or spin labeling or spin probing is the method in which free radicals that are extremely short lived are intercepted through a special compound known as a spin trap. This enables the formation of steady radicals adduct which can be traced using EPR [18, 19]. The EPR properties of spin adduct are similar to that of the trapped radicals therefore it is easily traceable. Nitrones are the most common spin traps used [20]. Different hydrophilic and hydrophobic iron dithiocarbamate complexes are normally employed to spin trap biological NO in EPR [21]. Cyclic hydroxyl amines are considered as spin probes because they oxidize into paramagnetic NO which are traceable by EPR. Therefore, in cells/tissues the assessment of biological superoxide produced is done by the superoxide dismutase-sensitive oxidation of cyclic hydroxyl amines [22]. The novel pH-sensitive nitroxides may be used for tissue spin probing. The nitroxide-biradicals may also be utilized as probes for the SH group [23]. The spin labeling method is an influential tool for analysing the functional as well as structural changes in membranes or proteins. This technique is also applicable for intact cells in certain conditions.

- **Spin trapping of ROS**

  The ROS are the end products of conventional oxygen metabolism and are vital for homeostasis and cell signalling. But adverse situations such as stress within the environment lead to increase in ROS levels and because of their highly reactive nature, they lead to cell damage. Cardiovascular diseases or ischemic injuries such as heart attacks or strokes increase the ROS levels. As per the *free-radical theory*, ROS primarily influence the functional decline in an organism during aging. Therefore, it is absolutely essential to investigate the ROS. Many researchers have employed EPR along with spin trapping *in vivo*, to detect and quantify ROS and also to evaluate their redox state [24]. Studies were done with the help of spin traps 5,5-dimethyl-1-pyrroline-*N*-oxide (DMPO) and 5-(diethoxyphosphoryl)-5-methyl-1-pyrroline-N-oxide (DEPMPO) to quantify the superoxide anion radicals obtained from human neutrophils *in vivo* when the interaction takes place with *Staphylococcus* bacteria [25]. When isolated human granulocytes were incubated with bacteria (*S. epidermidis* and *S. aureus*) within DEPMPO/DMPO, there was large increase in the level of spin adducts. After considering the duration of spin adduct life along with EPR interpretation the ($O_2^{\bullet -}$) superoxide radical was identified as the main radical product obtained through neutrophils.

Investigation of spin trap by PBN (phenylbutylnitrone) and it was found that in the isolated hearts of rat, radical stimulated lipid peroxidation through post-ischemic reperfusion occurs. In a study carried out for 30 min, alkoxy radicals were generated during the first 15 min of reperfusion. Later, after 10 min, the radical reduced and heart function returned to normalcy which was due to the existence of PBN. Also the recovery rate was higher compared to PBN-free conditions.

Investigations on the influence of calcium channel blocker (CV159) over the hepatic ischemia injury in rats revealed that CV159 directly scavenges HO•. Therefore it can be said that the presence of CV159 effectively minimizes the damage in organs without the activity of radical scavenging [26].

The spin trapping techniques of EPR for quantifying NO• production inside biological bodies have been researched and it can be said that most of the spin traps utilized for this have high NO• affinity.

- **Cancer diagnosis**

  The diagnosis of cancer is done through the EPR spin labeling technique. The products obtained from tumors have the ability to modify the conformation in serum albumin. Therefore with the help of a nitroxide labeled fatty acid such as 16-doxyl-stearic and the EPR, these minute changes can be traced. With the validation of the technique on a large number of patients to date, it was established that in the initial stages of cancer, spectroscopic differences were identifiable. This difference increased with the progress in the tumor [27]. A significant discovery showed that EPR signals produced by sodium nitroprusside at *g* equal to 2.03, distinguished the tumor cells from the healthy cells when it came in contact with the extracellular fluids and tumor cells. This was fortified with various types of tumors in animals. The reason for the differentiation between tumor and normally healthy cells by EPR has been associated with the high reduction conditions over the surface of the tumor cells within the body [28].

- **Spin-immunoassay**

  The spin-immunoassay application of the EPR which is quite interesting has been almost forgotten in the current era. This technique determines certain substances within biological fluids. This provides a sensitive yet a simple and an accurate process which has the basis of binding the compound of interest competitively via the substance model of nitroxide. One of the most ideal instances of spin-immunoassay is the establishment of morphine/drugs in the samples of saliva, blood, or urine [29].

- **EPR in diagnosis and prognosis**

  The diagnosis or prognosis of diseases can be done through EPR oximetry in which tissue oxygenation analysis *in vivo* provides information about the state of the disease. This helps in the process of diagnosis and helps in making decisions about the nature of treatment, disease therapy associated with the supply and use of the oxygen present inside the tissues. Also the EPR techniques for direct and indirect paramagnetic species detection have the potential to diagnose the species included in various pathophysiological processes. EPR dosimetry can quantify the radiation from various redox reactions to process therapeutic approaches. Similarly spin trapping can also diagnose various diseases. But one specific use of EPR is the measurement of stable nitroxide radicals on an extremely sensitive immunoassay of hepatitis B. This technique employs the quantifying of stable nitroxide radical obtained from peroxidase antibody conjugates with EPR spectroscopy. This method proved to be of higher sensitivity than that of the ELISA system in which chromogen is used in the presence of hydrogen peroxide. A stable radical is obtained when p-AP (p-acetamidophenol) and HHTIO (4-hydrazonomethyl-1-hydroxy- 2, 2, 5, 5-tetramethyl-3-imidazoline-3-oxide) are present and this proved to be tenfold more sensitive than ELISA with extremely high results that can be reproduced.

  The follow-up investigation demonstrated that the p-AP/HHTIO technique displayed higher seropositivity antigen when ELISA already turned negative. It proves that this assay gives an extremely high sensitivity technique for diagnosing hepatitis B especially in situations where conventional markers are already negative.

- **EPR imaging**

  EPR imaging is a valuable clinical tool for 3D mapping of spatially distributed paramagnetic bodies. It maps tissue oxygenation as well as free-radical spatial distribution inside big tissues, body parts (hands, feet) in humans and animals which can be easily accommodated in imaging devices. Advancements in the clinical field as well as biomedical applications of EPR have led to the better use of the technique. This includes research of drug delivery, cardiac research, dermatology, infection monitoring, and melanoma research [30–32].

The spin trapping and EPR imaging can be used together for *in vivo* applications to image endogenous NO in live mice abdomen 2.98. EPR projections can be obtained very quickly (10–20 ms) to enable time-resolved imaging. This was demonstrated after the temporal and spatial variations of free-radical distribution in rat hearts [33]. EPR can be used along with various imaging method like EPR/NMR to analyse the influence of smoke from cigarettes in the redox form on lungs, heart, kidneys, liver, and bladder [34].

For *in vivo* studies, when the concentration levels of paramagnetic entities is low, it is difficult to produce an EPR signal that is reliable for analysing data and thereby it becomes difficult to generate an EPR image. Recent studies in the EPR imaging for *in vivo* studies developed a new technique multiharmonic electron paramagnetic resonance imaging was done to enhance the S/N ratio in continuous wave method. Samples of PH1 (0.32 mg [N–Me-Py-$(TCNQ)_2$]), PH2 (2 ml 20 µM 3CP) and PH3 (three tubes of [N–Me-Py-$(TCNQ)_2$]) were employed for *in vivo* analysis in rats [35].

As shown in figure 18.2, the 3D imaging exhibited a S/N ratio that is 60 times higher than first harmonics in comparison to the first derivative for an applied

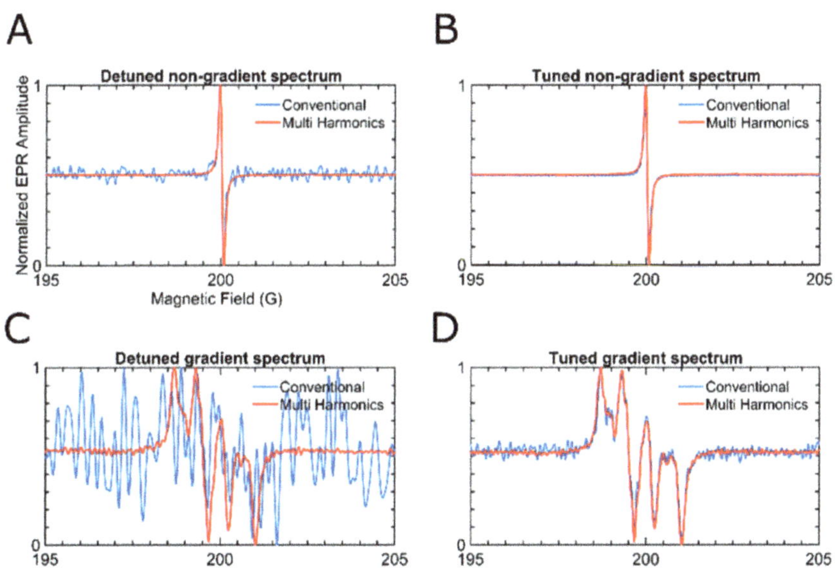

Figure 18.2. Normalized spectra of non-gradient and gradient projections from imaging PH_3. Reprinted from [35], Copyright (2020), with permission from Elsevier.

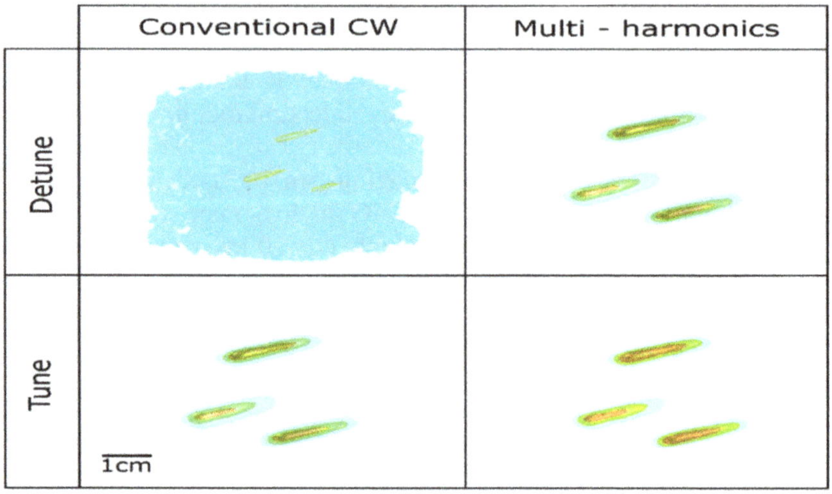

Figure 18.3. Representation of a reconstructed 3D EPR surface images of top and bottom panels of resonator resulting from PH_3. Reprinted from [35], Copyright (2020), with permission from Elsevier.

gradient with extremely low signal. When the signals were strong, the multiharmonic analysis (MHA) had a S/N ratio better by four times. In figure 18.2, parts A, C on the left show the results in detuned conditions. Those on the right (B, D) show the spectra for a coupled resonator. The blue line is the first derivative and the red is the first spectrum that is reconstructed at the time of multiharmonics analysis. Reconstructed 3D image from projections that are detuned exhibited large noise over tuned conditions.

In order to practically implement the multiharmonic method, EPR was performed on a mouse head. The probe PH_3 was employed for *in vivo* EPR imaging.

The reconstructed 3D surface images of top (detuned) and bottom (tuned) panels of resonator conditions rendered from non-over modulated projections by MHA is shown in figure 18.3. The image has been seen at 15% threshold. This is of the PH_3 employed for *in vivo* analysis.

18.4 EPR studies of bionanomaterials

A unique fact related to many nanomaterials is that they facilitate the formation of ROS and are linked to the toxicities of NS [36]. ROS, like singlet oxygen, superoxide, hydroxyl radicals, and hydrogen peroxide in the process of intracellular metabolism occur as by-products. They are extremely important for the physiology of tissues and cells. But excessive ROS has a negative influence as it produces oxidative stress damaging the DNA as well as the resulting response of the pathogens [37, 38]. Nanomaterials have the ability to influence both the levels and types of ROS and also the antioxidant defense system which can prove harmful to the organisms. The EPR spectroscopy technique is ideal for identification and quantification of intermediates that are reactive towards unpaired electrons in a biological environment. It has been established as the most trusted method for identifying and characterizing radical intermediates in relation to these nanomaterials [5, 39].

Hence the increase in the research into bionanomaterials has generated the need for analytical as well as non-destructive spectroscopic techniques that are suitable for characterization of the nanoscale bodies especially the interstitials. Although there are advances in microscopic methods like transmission electron microscopy (TEM), electrostatic force microscopy (EFM), and scanning electron microscopy (SEM) with *in situ* capabilities, most of these are incapable of giving data at the atomic level on molecular dynamics within the interfacial layers or structures, the electrostatic interactions, and hydrophobic effect [40, 41]. These are the primary forces that are the reason for biocompatibility or reactivity of bionanomaterials. Although certain characteristic gaps within bio–nano interfaces can be filled by solid state nuclear magnetic resonance (NMR), its low sensitivity nature restricts its application. To use NMR, the signals need enhancement by the dynamic nuclear polarization [42]. But the sensitivity of EPR is sufficient for the study of the interface of nanoparticle-liquids also at low concentrations [43]. EPR can also be applied to materials that are opaque or even to solutions which cannot be analysed by optical techniques. The extension of EPR is spin trapping which directly recognizes or quantifies what are generated on the surfaces of nano metal oxides which are linked to nanomaterial cytotoxicity [44]. It is the site-directed spin labeling EPR which has emerged as an ideal technique for analysing structures, oligonucleotides, proteins and their complications.

18.4.1 Surface-mediated production of free radicals and radical scavenging properties of nanomaterials

Nanotechnology has made it possible to engineer many novel fabricated nanomaterials (FNMs) along with nanowires/nanotubes, nanoparticles, and substrates with nanostructures. These materials are made to combine with conventional materials to facilitate endocytosis as certain materials are smaller than cells. These fabricated materials have unique characteristics which are very different to the conventional bulky ones. Also FNMs have significantly enhanced surface-to-volume ratio. Therefore, in these fabricated materials, the surface characteristics are dominantly influencing their biological interactions. Some of the reactions lead to the formation of ROS which are the primary reason for oxidative stress in biological surroundings. It is the nano Fe oxides produced by nanomaterials that are widely analysed as they have wide applications pertaining to MRI, magnetic data storing and localized drug delivery. Moreover, multimodal biomedical imaging as well as medical therapy and diagnosis is also included [45, 46]. Even though there are advances in nanotechnology, only in recent times has weight been given to the biosafety of Fe oxides. Cytotoxicity analysis on γ-Fe_2O_3 or Fe_3O_4 has exhibited negative influences for *in vitro* as well as *in vivo* conditions [47, 48]. By surface modification of these nanoparticles with organic ligands, these negative biological effects can be alleviated. This can also be reduced by covering the Fe oxide under layers with inert elements like gold [49].

While the reason behind biotoxicity of this is still under debate, many of the studies have confirmed that in modified nanoparticles, large areas of the surface and enhanced defects are the reason for toxilogical effects [48]. Although there is a theory which supports the influence of metal oxides nanoparticles on oxidative stress, detailed information on the mechanisms of the molecules or their relationship with physicochemical characteristics of the bio–nano interface is not completely understood. The gaps in the data can be filled by EPR spin trapping which forms steady paramagnetic spin adducts through chemical reactions between diamagnetic components and free radicals with a short life. These stable adducts can accumulate within a solution and be easily traced by EPR. Therefore, spin trapping EPR technique directly identifies and quantifies ROS.

One such instance of EPR spin trapping to assess free-radical formation and also of the metal nanoparticles was done using DMPO as a spin trap. The results suggested that γ-Fe_2O_3 generates exceptional amounts of OH_ free radicals in a Fenton reaction driven by superoxide [44]. It was also suggested that catalytic centers on the surfaces of nanoparticles were 50 times more influential than OH_ radical boosters on comparison with Fe^{3+} ions. Conventional techniques for modifying the surfaces like passivating surface with 935 oleate molecules or 18 bovine serum albumin molecules could not suppress the generation of OH_ radicals. Voinov *et al* developed an experimental procedure that is suitable for diverse conditions of reactive free-radical generation. In figure 18.4, the overall spin trapping of EPR seems ideal for producing analytical assays to evaluate the free-radical formation in bionanomaterials in relation to biotoxicity.

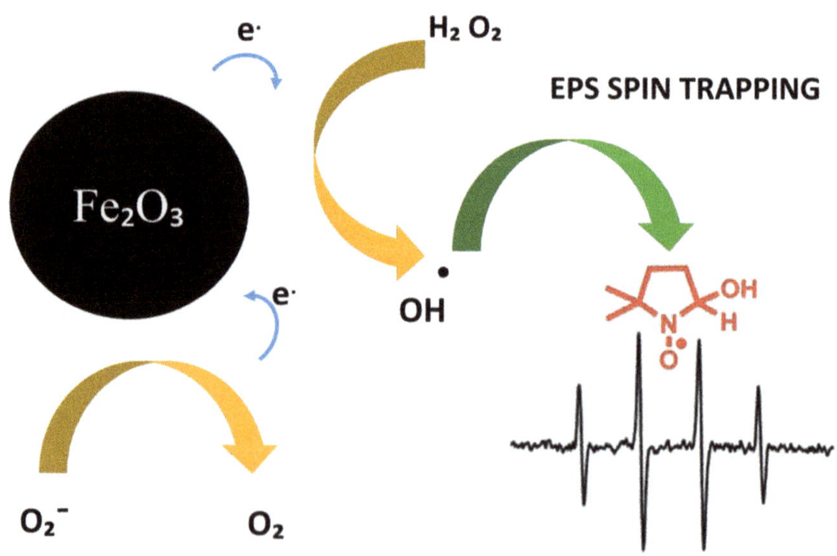

Figure 18.4. Concept of the spin trapping EPR experiment in the characterization of a free-radical formation of metal nanoparticles of Fe_2O_3 under the Fenton reaction. Reprinted from [50], Copyright (2019), with permission from Elsevier.

Some of the metal oxide nanoparticles have a tendency for radical scavenging and can protect oxidative stress [51]. A nanoceria or serium oxide has such anti-oxidative characteristics. Spin trapping EPR by DEPMPO suggested that serium oxide has the ability to scavenge superoxide anions and is considered to be a mimic of SOD (superoxide dismutase). The results obtained by a combination of EPR–XPS and EPR UV–Vis spectroscopy supported that the surface oxidation in serium oxide scavenges superoxide which is in direct relation to cerium (III) concentrations on the nanoparticle's surface [52]. The meager solubility of nanoceria in water and improper tracing techniques has restricted its application even though it exhibited promising effects. This also affected targeted delivery, poor absorption and distribution. But most of these issues pertaining to biocompatibility and water solubility have been eradicated through hybrid bionanomaterials. Literature has focussed on coating the nanoceria with compounds such as chitosan, dextran, glucose, herapin, polyacrylic acid, and polyethylene glycol. Serium oxide which is stable, biocompatible, and soluble in water has been developed by coating it with a combination of glycol chitosan polyhydroxyl and ethylene glycol. It has been described as a robust antioxidant.

18.4.2 Spin labeled EPR to characterize nanoparticles functionalized with ligand

In the past five decades, biomolecule spin labeling has become a vital component for analysing the dynamics and structures of complex macromolecules. The methodology for this technique has been well established and recent advances have also enhanced the focus on biophysical EPR. More specifically, HF EPR and pulsed double resonance techniques have been developed [53]. The newly developed spin labels have given spin labeling EPR (SLEPR) in the analysis of dynamics and structures of soluble proteins, DNA, biological membranes and RNA complexes [54]. Hence to characterize the dynamics and structures of ligand-protected nanoparticles biophysical EPRs have evolved.

Spin labels of diradical disulfide were employed to analyse the place-exchange reactions in gold nanoparticles protected with ligands [50]. The continuous wave EPR in the X band which has the ability to distinguish mono/diradical species was employed for the studies. This is due to the fact that diradicals exhibit stronger interactions of spin exchange. Hence these changes are easily seen on the nanoparticle surface covered by ligand-exchange. It exhibits that ligand-exchange adsorb only disulfide molecule and established it as an ideal technique for thiolate-protected gold nanoparticles. It is the various binding sites on the gold nanoparticle surface that reorganize the aging process and are the reason behind reactive trends.

The SLEPR processes also are familiar with local dynamics inside a ligand shell having nano assemblies. In the earlier cases SLEPR was used for nano assemblies of organic molecules (micelles) on mesoporous surfaces of silica and bicells. That research has also been done for a nano system doped with similar spin labeled molecule (phospholipid) to study the lipid bilayers. The surface of nanoparticles with ligands was grafted by spin labels post nanoparticle synthesis which was done in the case of poly isobutylcyanoacrylate functionalized using the chains of polysaccharide. The spectra analysis exhibited superposition of NO compounds which were in slow as well as fast motion. NO had the highest percentage when linked to the most rigid polysaccharide which happens to be shortest chitosan. Therefore, the conclusion was that SLEPR is influenced by the folding capacity of polysaccharide chains which enable interactions that are hydrophobic [50].

The probes which are pH sensitive have also been employed in SLEPR nanostructural analysis. These probes are the derivatives of imidazolidine and its nitorxide [55]. These NO consist of functionalities of N in heterocyclic ring which results in pH sensitive EPR. This occurs only close to the probe pK_a as there is an extra internal electric field produced by functionality protonation.

This type of EPR analysis on nanostructures was done in which a number of ligands of varying lengths of hydrocarbon bridge were fabricated. The bridge was between sulfur and the pH-sensitive imidazoline NO as seen in figure 18.5. The ligands are named S, M, and L to depict their lengths. The integration of ligands with carboxylate-terminated tiopronin shielded the gold nanoparticles during the

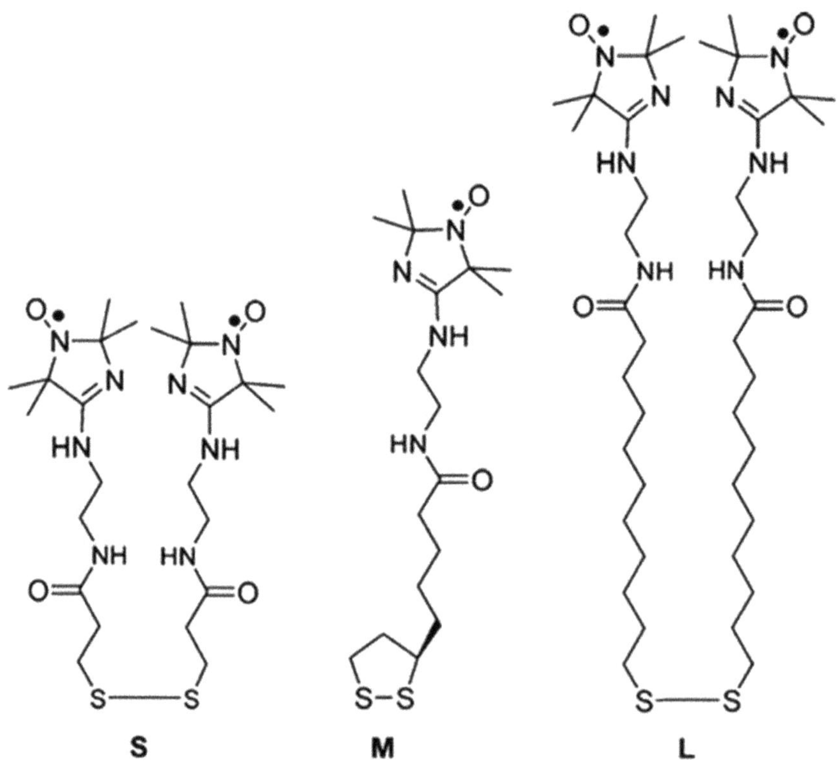

Figure 18.5. The ligand structures which are pH-sensitive and spin labeled to anchor the gold surface. Reprinted from [50], Copyright (2019), with permission from Elsevier.

reactions of ligand-exchange. One spin label for one nanoparticle was the average labeling. This was to eradicate any magnetic spin interactions. The protonation of NO was seen under EPR of the X band for changing isotropic N and the surface's electrostatic potential. This analysis proved that a shift in pK_a is influenced by the spin probe's position with respect to the polar interface of NP [50]. Hence, tailored ligands of NO that are pH sensitive have been employed as probes in gold nanoparticles at the polar interface.

18.4.3 SLEPR for the analysis of nano-confinements in nano- and mesoporous materials

The nanoporous or the mesoporous material form their base as per the anodic aluminum oxide which has wide applications pertaining to the storage and generation of energy, drug delivery matrices, biosensors and photosensors, and catalyst adsorbents for separating the molecules [56]. These materials encounter numerous challenges in the above applications which include, monitoring of the molecular interacting time with surfaces and meeting the chemical characteristics SLEPR and size of nanopores within the target molecules. These challenges can be easily managed using novel approaches by which can give details of either of the biomolecule structures as well as the surrounding interaction within pores. Hence EPR is also suitable for opaque samples with sufficient sensitivity to control the changes within the structures. It can also be used for a monolayered protein adsorbed by the solid surface.

The dynamics of enzymes as well as peptides integrated within mesoporous materials and the influence of nano-confinement on the molecules was studied by Professor Chiang. According to his suggestions, the fluctuations within the side chain are suppressed by the nano-confinements. Also the backbone dynamics were seen clearly in the spectra of EPR. The prion protein peptide inside mesopores and bulk solutions was studied by a continuous wave SLEPR in the X band [57]. The subsequent research culminated double electron–electron resonance (DEER), electron spin echo (ESE), electron spin echo envelope modulation (ESEEM) and EPR with a continuous wave to analyse the polypeptide's interfacial hydration layers within nanochannels filled with water. The density of water surrounding the surface of peptide was heterogeneous and normal. Also within the nanochannels, there were no structural altercations in peptide [58]. Crystalline ice formation was suppressed within the nanopores during the analysis of dynamics in water by EPR through NO soluble in water. The energy of activation in NO influenced the confinement conditions (nano) and it was lower in case of peptide-attached spin label over NO dissolved within the aqueous state of pores.

There are various factors to be considered when there are interactions between the biomolecules and meso-/nanopores. These include chemical selection of pores with respect to the nature of the molecules entering, pore geometry, and chemistry of the surface. It is the electrostatic interactions that primarily influence molecular and surface interactions. Hence, local pH, electro-surface pore characteristics and acid–base properties of inorganic/organic materials are necessary in both basic as well as application based perspectives.

18.5 EPR in drug delivery systems

It is known that the EPR spectroscopy is classified as direct radical measurement, spin labeling, and trapping. This section is dedicated to the drug delivery approaches of EPR systems. Metal ions like Fe^{3+} or Mn^{2+} may be detected to the level of parts per million (ppm). The metal traces can be seen in color pigments or minerals such as manganese II in bentonite and talcum. They are also the impurities in API (active pharmaceutical ingredient) and excipients as seen in figure 18.6. It is seen that bentonite as well as talcum exhibit signals of Fe and Mn but black iron oxide has predominant signals of iron.

These are capable of catalysing the degraded API, therefore, EPR can detect and quantify paramagnetic impurity [60]. At the time of sterilization, gamma radiations can form radicals that have a short life and are stable which are traceable by EPR [61]. EPR is utilized for sterilizing polymer based parental particles like PLG. It is the interaction of radicals and the drug molecules that degrade API. Moreover, polymers can degrade which can result in degradation as well as release kinetics to be altered or produce enhanced intoxicated by-products. Hence the radicals that are induced remain for extremely long durations inside dry solids such as polymers or crystalline drugs. Hence the signals of EPR can be used for tracking the penetration of water within the polymers since the radicals in a wet state have the tendency to disappear [59]. The detection of radicals induced by radiation can find out if the components have discovered the treatment and the radiation dosage is predicted through re-irradiation of defined doses. The intensity of the signal is measured later [62].

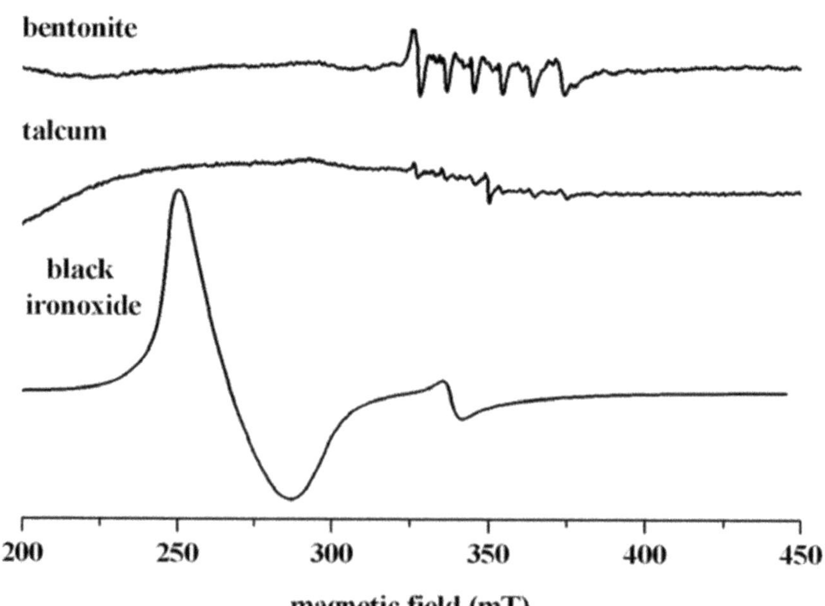

Figure 18.6. The EPR spectra of API with intrinsic EPR active centers in bentonite, talcum, and black iron oxide. Reprinted from [59], Copyright (2010), with permission from Elsevier.

However, EPR cannot detect most of the systems of drug delivery since diamagnetism is their characteristic and there is no existence of paramagnetic molecules. Hence spin probes are needed for detection. It is known that large varieties of nitroxyl radicals that are stable exist having physicochemical properties like values of HLB and hydrodynamic radius. These spin probes have the ability to stimulate the drugs with low molecular weight. There also exist spin probes which link covalently with polymers or proteins which are large molecules. This can be done through spin labeling. Therefore, opaque samples can also be analysed by EPR. Components like tablets, suspension, solids or solutions can also be analysed by EPR spectra and provide details about microacidity or microviscocity, radical concentration and the environment polarity. The spatial distribution is also discovered by EPR imaging.

The research into the delivery of drugs is important to estimate the pH of microenvironments within the systems of drug delivery at the time of release. This is because the stability, solubility, polymer degradation, and release patterns of the drugs are influenced by pH value. Biodegradable polymers like polyorthoesters have monomers that are acidic in nature within their backbones and it is this polymer that is used in common. When incubated inside physiological environment, the polymers hydrolyse into monomer and oligomer that is acidic in nature. The implant of PLGA that is in the process of degradation has exhibited a pH value of two for *in vivo* conditions [63]. The microacidity can also be altered through the hydrolysable drugs that are decomposing [59]. The drug pH is also influenced by low solubility bases and buffer compounds. Previous research suggests the addition of sodium acetate enhanced the pH of degrading PLA [64]. The microacidity can be quantified by EPR by identifying the pH gradients within the polymers that degrade or the tablets for *in vitro* environment. EPR studies have also been carried out to analyse the pH variation within the skin of humans post treating with drugs. The evaluation was done in an *ex vivo* environment. Some other applications include determination of pH in the gut as well as the stomach inside conditions of *in vitro*. One of the important factors influencing the performance of colloidal carriers of drug are their ability to shield its constituents with changing environments. The distribution process dynamics also influence the performance of drug delivery. This ability in the systems of drug delivery is analysed by reduction of ascorbic acid assay because within the aqueous phase ascorbic acid reduces at a rapid manner and is also localized.

In the case of nanocapsules, the reduction of spin probe is influenced by the material of the shell and is quicker for poly (D,L-lactide) PLA in comparison to pegylated PLA [59]. Post the administration, the colloidal systems are diluted *in vivo* as well as *in vitro*. This method of dilution can alter the distribution equilibria and lead to drug relocation. The release of drugs at nanoscale is not easy since the kinetics of their spin probes may be followed easily without sample preparation. This spin probe, when it relocates, will alter the spectral shape. The process controls the distribution kinetics of PLA nanocapsules by spin probe among the oily inner core and water phase on the exterior. It was observed that 10% of the included molecule was diffused within the external aqueous environment in a minute.

The quick distribution is due to the low thickness of the shell which does not block diffusion. Drug distribution *in vivo*, post consumption is affected when fat is digested which influences the rate of absorption directly. The EPR for *in vivo* has the ability to follow the spin probes distribution among oil, micelles, and water in systems that deliver drugs and have self-emulsifying characteristics [59].

18.6 Conclusions

The EPR or ESR spectroscopy is used to study the free radicals and paramagnetic species in nano–biomaterials. The basic strength of EPR lies in its specificity within an experiment. The elimination of background signals as well as greater quantities of extremely fine information obtained within a solution phase along with samples that are solid in nature make EPR an ideal characterization technique in comparison to other methods such as NMR. Generally, EPR is a flexible technique. The duration for preparing a sample, obtaining data, or the experimental procedure completely depends on the definite application of EPR and can usually range between hours or minutes. The EPR spectroscopy is a non-destructive technique for the analysis of free radicals, unstable compounds developed *in situ* and various paramagnetic transition metal compounds such as Cu^{2+}, Fe^{3+}, Mn^{2+}, and Mo^{5+} at a definite state of valency.

In recent years EPR found application in the field of biomedical science. Its application in the biomedical field include EPR oximetry where the oxygen present in blood or in various tissues is quantified to diagnose and treat diseases linked to the supply or use of oxygen. EPR spectroscopy is used to detect various paramagnetic bodies which play a vital role *in vivo*. Early tumors such as nevi or melanomas in tissues can be diagnosed through EPR techniques. The spin labeling method of EPR analyses the functional as well as structural changes in membranes or proteins. The diagnosis of cancer is also possible via the EPR spin labeling technique. The spin-immunoassay application of the EPR determines certain substances within biological fluids such as saliva, blood, or urine to establish the presence of morphine/drugs [29]. EPR oximetry may be used to analyse tissue oxygenation *in vivo* to determine the state of a disease state and make decisions on the nature of treatment or disease therapy. EPR imaging is also possible which facilitates 3D mapping of spatially distributed paramagnetic bodies. Therefore, technological advancements and such applications of the EPR have made it an absolute indispensable asset in the medical field which endorses research of drug delivery, cardiac research, dermatology, infection monitoring, and melanoma research [30–32]. With further advances in nanotechnology, it is absolutely certain that EPR has a bright future in the biomedical field.

References

[1] Kochelaev B I and Yablokov Y V 1995 *The Beginning of Paramagnetic Resonance* (Singapore: World Scientific)

[2] Kleschyov A L and Terekhov M 2013 Electron paramagnetic resonance in a biomedical laboratory *Bioanalysis* **5** 2233–7

[3] Berliner L J 2016 The evolution of biomedical EPR (ESR) *Biomed. Spectrosc. Imaging* **5** 5–26

[4] Klare J P 2012 Biomedical applications of electron paramagnetic resonance (EPR) spectroscopy *Biomed. Spectrosc. Imaging* **1** 101–24

[5] Chiesa M, Giamello E and Che M 2010 EPR characterization and reactivity of surface-localized inorganic radicals and radical ions *Chem. Rev.* **110** 1320–47

[6] Kosaka H, Sawai Y O, Sakaguchi H I, Kumura E I, Harada N O, Watanabe M A and Shiga T A 1994 ESR spectral transition by arteriovenous cycle in nitric oxide hemoglobin of cytokine-treated rats *Am. J. Physiol.-Cell Physiol.* **266** C1400–5

[7] Gallez B, Baudelet C and Jordan B F 2004 Assessment of tumor oxygenation by electron paramagnetic resonance: principles and applications *NMR Biomed.* **17** 240–62

[8] Liu S, Timmins G S, Shi H, Gasparovic C M and Liu K J 2004 Application of *in vivo* EPR in brain research: monitoring tissue oxygenation, blood flow, and oxidative stress *NMR Biomed.* **17** 327–34

[9] Presley T, Kuppusamy P, Zweier J L and Ilangovan G 2006 Electron paramagnetic resonance oximetry as a quantitative method to measure cellular respiration: a consideration of oxygen diffusion interference *Biophys. J.* **91** 4623–31

[10] Meenakshisundaram G, Eteshola E, Pandian R P, Bratasz A, Selvendiran K, Lee S C, Krishna M C, Swartz H M and Kuppusamy P 2009 Oxygen sensitivity and biocompatibility of an implantable paramagnetic probe for repeated measurements of tissue oxygenation *Biomed. Microdevices* **11** 817–26

[11] Cesareo E, Korkina L, D'Errico G, Vitiello G, Aguzzi M S, Passarelli F, Pedersen J Z and Facchiano A 2012 An endogenous electron spin resonance (ESR) signal discriminates nevi from melanomas in human specimens: a step forward in its diagnostic application *PLoS One* **7** e48849

[12] Fattibene P and Callens F 2010 EPR dosimetry with tooth enamel: a review *Appl. Radiat. Isot.* **68** 2033–116

[13] Brustolon M and Giamello E (ed) 2009 *Electron Paramagnetic Resonance: A Practitioner's Toolkit* (Hoboken, NJ: Wiley)

[14] Kozlowski H, Luczkowski M, Remelli M and Valensin D 2012 Copper, zinc and iron in neurodegenerative diseases (Alzheimer's, Parkinson's and prion diseases) *Coord. Chem. Rev.* **256** 2129–41

[15] Viles J H 2012 Metal ions and amyloid fiber formation in neurodegenerative diseases. Copper, zinc and iron in Alzheimer's, Parkinson's and prion diseases *Coord. Chem. Rev.* **256** 2271–84

[16] Brealey D, Brand M, Hargreaves I, Heales S, Land J, Smolenski R, Davies N A, Cooper C E and Singer M 2002 Association between mitochondrial dysfunction and severity and outcome of septic shock *Lancet* **360** 219–23

[17] Svistunenko D A, Davies N, Brealey D, Singer M and Cooper C E 2006 Mitochondrial dysfunction in patients with severe sepsis: an EPR interrogation of individual respiratory chain components *Biochim. Biophys. Acta* **1757** 262–72

[18] Mason R P and Ganini D 2019 Immuno-spin trapping of macromolecules free radicals *in vitro* and *in vivo*—one stop shopping for free radical detection *Free Radic. Biol. Med.* **131** 318–31

[19] Besson E *et al* 2019 Embedding cyclic nitrone in mesoporous silica particles for EPR spin trapping of superoxide and other radicals *Analyst* **144** 4194–203

[20] Hawkins C L and Davies M J 2014 Detection and characterisation of radicals in biological materials using EPR methodology *Biochim. Biophys. Acta* **1840** 708–21

[21] Jackson S K 2019 Applications of electron paramagnetic resonance (EPR) spectroscopy in the study of oxidative stress in biological systems *Redox-Mediated Signal Transduction* (New York: Humana Press) pp 93–102

[22] Dikalov S I and Harrison D G 2014 Methods for detection of mitochondrial and cellular reactive oxygen species *Antioxid. Redox Signal.* **20** 372–82

[23] Fujii H G, Emoto M C and Sato-Akaba H 2019 Brain redox imaging using *in vivo* electron paramagnetic resonance imaging and nitroxide imaging probes *Magnetochemistry* **5** 11

[24] Swartz H M, Khan N and Khramtsov V V 2007 Use of electron paramagnetic resonance spectroscopy to evaluate the redox state *in vivo Antioxid. Redox Signal.* **9** 1757–72

[25] Lundqvist H, Dånmark S, Johansson U, Gustafsson H and Öllinger K 2008 Evaluation of electron spin resonance for studies of superoxide anion production by human neutrophils interacting with *Staphylococcus aureus* and *Staphylococcus epidermidis J. Biochem. Biophys. Methods* **70** 1059–65

[26] Hataji K *et al* 2010 Effects of a calcium-channel blocker (CV159) on hepatic ischemia/reperfusion injury in rats: evaluation with selective NO/pO2 electrodes and an electron paramagnetic resonance spin-trapping method *Biol. Pharm. Bull.* **33** 77–83

[27] Maia L B and Moura J J 2016 Detection of nitric oxide by electron paramagnetic resonance spectroscopy: spin-trapping with iron-dithiocarbamates *Plant Nitric Oxide* (New York: Humana Press) pp 81–102

[28] Kleschyov A L, Sedov K R, Mordvintcev P I and Vanin A F 1994 Biotransformation of sodium nitroprusside into dinitrosyl iron complexes in tissue of ascites tumors of mice *Biochem. Biophys. Res. Commun.* **202** 168–73

[29] Wieser A *et al* 2000 Comparison of sample preparation and signal evaluation methods for EPR analysis of tooth enamel *Appl. Radiat. Isot.* **52** 1059–64

[30] Kuppusamy P and Zweier J L 2004 Cardiac applications of EPR imaging *NMR Biomed.* **17** 226–39

[31] Tsai P, Cao G L, Merkel T J and Rosen G M 2008 Spin labelling of *Bacillus anthracis* endospores: a model for *in vivo* tracking by EPR imaging *Free Radic. Res.* **42** 49–56

[32] Vanea E, Charlier N, DeWever J, Dinguizli M, Feron O, Baurain J F and Gallez B 2008 Molecular electron paramagnetic resonance imaging of melanin in melanomas: a proof-of-concept *NMR Biomed.* **21** 296–300

[33] Chen Z, Reyes L A, Johnson D H, Velayutham M, Yang C, Samouilov A and Zweier J L 2013 Fast gated EPR imaging of the beating heart: spatiotemporally resolved 3D imaging of free-radical distribution during the cardiac cycle *Magn. Reson. Med.* **69** 594–601

[34] Caia G L, Efimova O V, Velayutham M, El-Mahdy M A, Abdelghany T M, Kesselring E, Petryakov S, Sun Z, Samouilov A and Zweier J L 2012 Organ specific mapping of *in vivo* redox state in control and cigarette smoke-exposed mice using EPR/NMR co-imaging *J. Magn. Reson.* **216** 21–7

[35] Gonet M, Baranowski M, Czechowski T, Kucinska M, Plewinski A, Szczepanik P, Jurga S and Murias M 2020 Multiharmonic electron paramagnetic resonance imaging as an innovative approach for *in vivo* studies *Free Radic. Biol. Med.* **152** 271–9

[36] Manke A, Wang L and Rojanasakul Y 2013 Mechanisms of nanoparticle-induced oxidative stress and toxicity *BioMed Res. Int.* **2013**

[37] Li N, Xia T and Nel A E 2008 The role of oxidative stress in ambient particulate matter-induced lung diseases and its implications in the toxicity of engineered nanoparticles *Free Radic. Biol. Med.* **44** 1689–99

[38] Bonner J C 2007 Lung fibrotic responses to particle exposure *Toxicol. Pathol.* **35** 148–53

[39] Wang Z, Ma W, Chen C, Ji H and Zhao J 2011 Probing paramagnetic species in titania-based heterogeneous photocatalysis by electron spin resonance (ESR) spectroscopy—a mini review *Chem. Eng. J.* **170** 353–62

[40] Tyagi A K and Malik A 2010 In situ SEM, TEM and AFM studies of the antimicrobial activity of lemon grass oil in liquid and vapour phase against *Candida albicans Micron* **41** 797–805

[41] Tao F F and Salmeron M 2011 In situ studies of chemistry and structure of materials in reactive environments *Science* **331** 171–4

[42] Rossini A J, Zagdoun A, Lelli M, Lesage A, Coperet C and Emsley L 2013 Dynamic nuclear polarization surface enhanced NMR spectroscopy *Acc. Chem. Res.* **46** 1942–51

[43] Zachary M and Chechik V 2007 Hopping of thiolate ligands between Au nanoparticles revealed by EPR spectroscopy *Angew. Chem. Int. Ed.* **46** 3304–7

[44] Voinov M A, Pagán J O, Morrison E, Smirnova T I and Smirnov A I 2011 Surface-mediated production of hydroxyl radicals as a mechanism of iron oxide nanoparticle biotoxicity *J. Am. Chem. Soc.* **133** 35–41

[45] Gupta A K and Gupta M 2005 Synthesis and surface engineering of iron oxide nanoparticles for biomedical applications *Biomaterials* **26** 3995–4021

[46] Liu Z, Lammers T, Ehling J, Fokong S, Bornemann J, Kiessling F and Gätjens J 2011 Iron oxide nanoparticle-containing microbubble composites as contrast agents for MR and ultrasound dual-modality imaging *Biomaterials* **32** 6155–63

[47] Petri-Fink A, Chastellain M, Juillerat-Jeanneret L, Ferrari A and Hofmann H 2005 Development of functionalized superparamagnetic iron oxide nanoparticles for interaction with human cancer cells *Biomaterials* **26** 2685–94

[48] Lewinski N, Colvin V and Drezek R 2008 Cytotoxicity of nanoparticles *Small* **4** 26–49

[49] Bouchard L S, Anwar M S, Liu G L, Hann B, Xie Z H, Gray J W, Wang X, Pines A and Chen F F 2009 Picomolar sensitivity MRI and photoacoustic imaging of cobalt nanoparticles *Proc. Natl Acad. Sci.* **106** 4085–9

[50] Smirnova T I and Smirnov A I 2019 EPR studies of bionanomaterials *Experimental Methods in the Physical Sciences* vol 50 (New York: Academic) pp 129–59

[51] Yin J J, Liu J, Ehrenshaft M, Roberts J E, Fu P P, Mason R P and Zhao B 2012 Phototoxicity of nano titanium dioxides in HaCaT keratinocytes—generation of reactive oxygen species and cell damage *Toxicol. Appl. Pharmacol.* **263** 81–8

[52] Heckert E G, Karakoti A S, Seal S and Self W T 2008 The role of cerium redox state in the SOD mimetic activity of nanoceria *Biomaterials* **29** 2705–9

[53] Smirnova T I and Smirnov A I 2007 High-field ESR spectroscopy in membrane and protein biophysics *ESR spectroscopy in Membrane Biophysics* (Boston, MA: Springer) pp 165–251

[54] Smirnova T I and Smirnov A I 2015 Peptide–membrane interactions by spin-labeling EPR *Methods Enzymology* vol 564 (New York: Academic) pp 219–58

[55] Voinov M A and Smirnov A I 2015 Ionizable nitroxides for studying local electrostatic properties of lipid bilayers and protein systems by EPR *Methods Enzymol.*

[56] Jani A M, Losic D and Voelcker N H 2013 Nanoporous anodic aluminium oxide: advances in surface engineering and emerging applications *Prog. Mater Sci.* **58** 636–704

[57] Huang Y W and Chiang Y W 2011 Spin-label ESR with nanochannels to improve the study of backbone dynamics and structural conformations of polypeptides *Phys. Chem. Chem. Phys.* **13** 17521–31
[58] Lai Y C, Chen Y F and Chiang Y W 2013 ESR study of interfacial hydration layers of polypeptides in water-filled nanochannels and in vitrified bulk solvents *PLoS One* **8** e68264
[59] Kempe S, Metz H and Mäder K 2010 Application of electron paramagnetic resonance (EPR) spectroscopy and imaging in drug delivery research—chances and challenges *Eur. J. Pharm. Biopharm.* **74** 55–66
[60] Williams H E, Loades V C, Claybourn M and Murphy D M 2006 Electron paramagnetic resonance spectroscopy studies of oxidative degradation of an active pharmaceutical ingredient and quantitative analysis of the organic radical intermediates using partial least-squares regression *Anal. Chem.* **78** 604–8
[61] Desai K G and Park H J 2006 Study of gamma-irradiation effects on chitosan microparticles *Drug Deliv.* **13** 39–50
[62] Basly J P, Basly I and Bernard M 1998 ESR spectroscopy applied to the study of pharmaceuticals radiosterilization: cefoperazone *J. Pharm. Biomed. Anal.* **17** 871–5
[63] Mäder K, Gallez B, Liu K J and Swartz H M 1996 Non-invasive *in vivo* characterization of release processes in biodegradable polymers by low-frequency electron paramagnetic resonance spectroscopy *Biomaterials* **17** 457–61
[64] Rübe A and Mäder K 2005 Electron spin resonance study on the dynamics of polymeric nanocapsules *J. Biomed. Nanotechnol.* **1** 208–13

IOP Publishing

Analytical Techniques for Biomedical Nanotechnology

Ajeet Kaushik, Sesha S Srinivasan and Yogendra Kumar Mishra

Chapter 19

X-ray photoelectron spectroscopy for biomedical applications

Anindita Tarafdar, Hima Sree Buddhiraju and Aravind Kumar Rengan

X-ray photoelectron spectroscopy (XPS) is an extensively used analytical technique for surface analysis of both conducting and insulator materials. Many advances have happened since its invention in 1900 to make it more convenient for use in multiple fields of research. It works on the principle of the photoelectric effect and can provide intricate information about the chemical environment at atomical and elemental level on the surface layers of the specimen. General information about the instrumentation and its data interpretation for different aspects of applications in biomedicine are briefly discussed in this chapter.

19.1 Introduction

X-ray photoelectron spectroscopy (XPS), formerly known as ESCA (electron spectroscopy for chemical analysis), is a widely used analytical technique. The process can be simply explained using the three terms in the name itself—x-ray, photoelectron, spectroscopy. In this technique, x-rays are used to excite a particular material—from which photoelectrons are generated and we achieve a spectrum from these photoelectrons, which is eventually analyzed to determine the overall chemical nature of the material. The spectrum gives us qualitative as well as quantitative information about the elements present on the sample surface. The x-ray induced photoelectron spectrum is presented as a graph of the number of electrons that are being emitted per unit time (count) versus electron binding energy. It is a non-destructive, highly surface-sensitive technique, as photoemission occurs only from the top few atomic layers (~10 nm) because of the small mean free path of electrons in solids [1]. The resulting emission of electrons is from the core orbital shells of atoms of the sample, with discrete kinetic energy which is then correlated with known binding energy for elements and their atomic energy levels. XPS is an

doi:10.1088/978-0-7503-3379-5ch19

essential tool for understanding the surface chemistry of materials as it gives us information about the local bonding environment of a given species [2]. Analysis of the overall spectrum gives us information about (i) elemental composition (relative atomic % of elements), (ii) electronic state of the elements, (iii) chemical/empirical formula—the chemical composition of that particular material [3]. Apart from surface mapping, in many cases depth profiling or the distribution of species up to some vertical distance from the surface plane can also be done in a non-destructive way [4].

Since the 20th century, many scientists worldwide have devoted their careers to the development of and advancements in the principle, instrumentation, and data processing of XPS. Using the early classical techniques, it was possible to get only descriptive information about the physical characteristics of a surface like pore size distributions, surface roughness, and topography. With the advent of modern spectroscopic methods for surface analysis, chemical characteristics like elemental analysis, chemical state information, horizontal and vertical distribution of species, and quantitative analysis like elemental ratios or oxidation state ratios of the same element on the surface layers of a material could also be done. Particularly two Swedish physicists, who happen to be father and son have made noteworthy contributions in this regard. Manne Siegbahn was awarded the 1924 Nobel Prize in physics for his discoveries and research in the field of XPS. He developed equipment and techniques to determine the wavelengths of x-rays more accurately, which was of substantial help to subsequent researchers. His son, Kai Siegbahn, known as the father of XPS, was awarded the 1981 Nobel Prize in physics for developing high-resolution electron spectroscopy [1]. He found that the chemical environment of an element has minute, yet measurable effects on electron binding energies which is reflected in the XPS spectrum and has significantly increased the value of it in surface analysis.

Nanoscale objects are pretty much active all the time, which makes the nanoscale world a constant bustle of activity. So, characterizing these tiny objects at a particular moment of their activity is quite crucial and requires specialized instruments and techniques. Surface layer or composition of the thin film on a surface plays a crucial role in the performance of nanomaterials because of their very high surface-to-volume ratio. Depending upon the variety of applications, nanoparticles often have complex surface designs and functionalization, so XPS plays an important role in understanding their properties and behaviors by quantifying the nature of its surface and thickness of the coatings [5]. In recent years, much research has been done with self-assembled nanocomplexes for more convenient drug delivery, and common techniques like Fourier transform infrared spectroscopy (FTIR) and nuclear magnetic resonance (NMR) studies are unable to provide crucial insights about the molecular interactions within the different components of the nanocomplex which leads to their self-assembly or disintegration depending upon the chemical environment. XPS is being used to study the surface composition as well as types of bonds formed [6, 7]. Some surface modifications with polymers increase the biocompatibility of the biomaterials and implants, and to detect the proper surface enrichment XPS is being regularly used to analyze the chemical composition of the interface [8–12]. Adsorption and chemical interaction studies of biomolecules is also very significant in biosensor research and development, which is performed using some modifications in sample preparation for XPS, so that it is ultrahigh vacuum (UHV) compatible [13]. This technique is also very useful in examining cell and tissue surfaces, which in turn helps in tissue engineering applications.

The surface sensitivity in the range of tens of nanometers along with the specificity in the detection of chemical environment, makes it a unique and popular analytical technique in many fields of research. For the analysis, very small sample amounts are required, which adds to the convenience of this technique. XPS is very effective in the detection and qualitative analysis of all the elements except two elements—hydrogen and helium. It is widely used for mapping the surface composition of a material but compared to other techniques the only drawback experienced is because of the small lateral resolution across a surface. The lateral resolution is limited because of the diameter of x-ray beam, which is generally in the range of millimeters and is comparatively larger than the distance of importance in surface mapping. Also, some limitations occur due the requirement of the sample to be UHV compatible, but with some adaptation in the sample preparation before introducing it into the XPS instrument, it works fine.

19.2 Principle

XPS works on the principle of the photoelectric effect. The photoelectric effect was described by Einstein in 1905, and he was awarded the 1921 Nobel Prize in physics for 'his discovery of the law of photoelectric effect'. The process is initiated by irradiating monochromatic, soft x-ray beams onto the sample, under extremely high vacuum. The incident photons cause photoionization and results in emission of an electron from the inner orbital. Energy of the emitted electrons is proportional to the frequency (ν) of incident radiation and does not depend on its intensity or duration of exposure. But sometimes certain loss of energy occurs because of inelastic collisions undergone by the electrons, which results in reduction of kinetic energy and may also prevent the escape of electrons from the surface. Even though the path length of photons is in micrometers, mean free path of electrons is of the order of tens of angstroms because of the much higher probability of electrons interacting with material and losing its energy. So, even though ionization takes place to depths of few micrometers, the electrons that can leave the solid surface without any energy loss are only those that emerge from depths of tens of angstroms from the surface.

The kinetic energy of the emitted electrons is calculated using the equation:

$$\mathrm{KE} = hv - \mathrm{BE} - \varphi,$$

where KE = kinetic energy of emitted electron,

$h\nu$ = energy of the photon,

BE = binding energy of the atomic orbital fromwhich the electron originates,

φ = spectrometer work function

For photoemission to happen the core–shell electron should be able to overcome the binding energy of the shell and the work function required, which is possible when the energy of the impinging photons from the incident radiation is greater than the sum of them both ($h\nu > \text{BE} + \varphi$).

The incident beam should be monochromatic or monoenergetic x-ray because if the energy of the photons ($h\nu$), in the equation varies then it is very difficult to trace the kinetic energy of the photoelectrons. So, if we know the incident beam energy then the outcoming electron's energies can be easily decided and further correlated to get the exact chemical nature of the element present. Soft x-rays having energy lower than 6 keV, like Mg Kα (1253.6 eV) or Al Kα (1486.6 eV) are mostly used for XPS. The energy analyzer has two plates of concentric hemispherical in shape and a certain bias or negative potential is applied to it for measuring the kinetic energy of the emitted electrons. The measured energies of the detected photoelectrons are compiled into a spectrum with characteristic peaks of each element because of their distinct binding energies.

19.3 Instrumentation

The instrument is typically made up of five parts—an x-ray source, specimen holding stage, a lens system for transfer of extracted electrons, electron energy analyzer, and electron detector. All the components of an XPS instrument are placed within an UHV chamber to avoid surface contamination of the sample and scattering of air molecules by the emitted electrons from the sample in their path towards the analyzer [14]. As it is a highly surface-sensitive technique, any slightest of contamination would also hinder the analysis of the actual chemical composition (figure 19.1).

X-ray source: Mg Kα (1253.6 eV) or Al Kα (1486.6 eV) are mostly used x-rays. A monochromator is used to eliminate the less intense lines and allow only the most intense one, in order to avoid additional peaks in the spectrum due to excitation by multiple energies [15]. Using a monochromator reduces the line width, which helps in XPS spectral resolution but decreases the x-ray flux.

Lens system: several electron optics acting as extraction lenses, together as a system is placed before the analyzer and it plays some significant roles like (i) demarking the surface area from where emitted electrons will be analyzed (ii) decide the acceptance angle of the electrons [14, 15].

Analyzer: the design of the analyzer is concentric hemispherical with two hemispheres at different negative potential, as being applied to them. They are maintained at the required voltage bias in order to allow only those electrons having a certain energy to pass through it to the other end and be detected. The energy resolution of the analyzer depends on its radius, higher radius hemispheres having better resolution capacities.

Detector: they are basically electron multipliers, used in arrays to strengthen the signal received.

There is also an inert gas ion sputtering gun which is used for depth profiling and sometimes when sputter cleaning of sample surface is required. Many new and

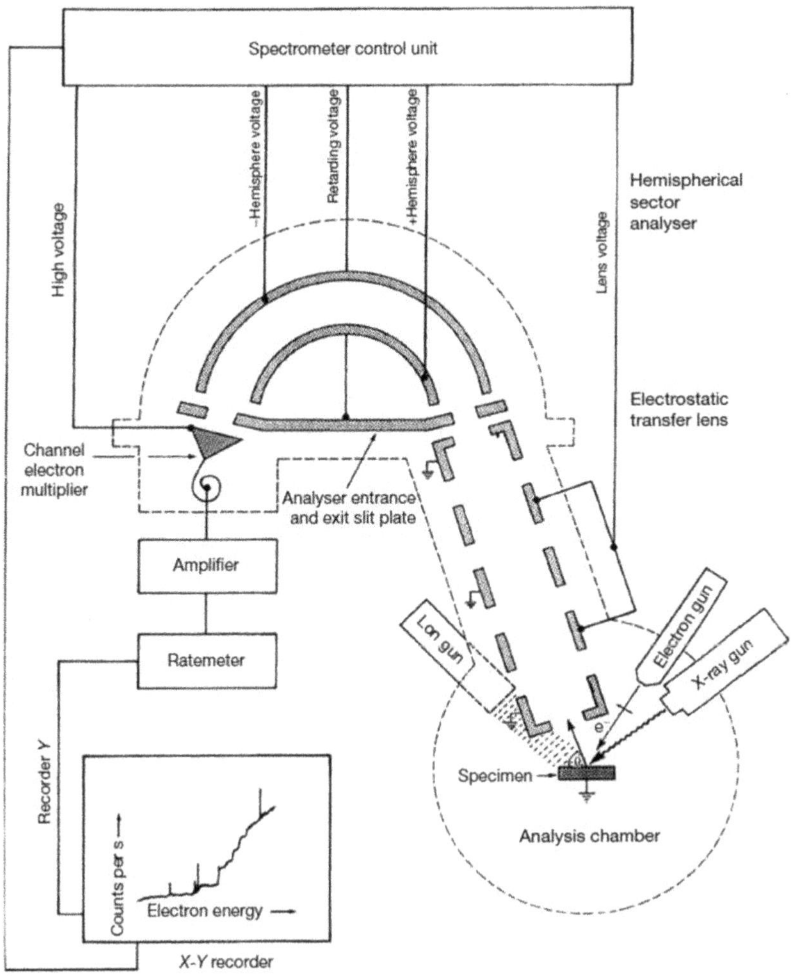

Figure 19.1. Schematic of XPS spectrometer. Reprinted from [14], Copyright (2013), with permission from Elsevier.

upcoming instruments also have some additional features to enhance the application capabilities, like temperature modifications of the sample and some other imaging and detection modifications [2].

19.4 Sample preparation

Generally, the sample should be solid, powder, or thin film, but with certain special modifications even liquid samples can sometimes be analyzed. Compared to other techniques, a very small amount of sample is required for this process. As XPS is a surface-sensitive technique, utmost care must be taken in sample handling to avoid any unwanted contamination or oxidation. Depending upon the type of specimen material like metal, polymer or nanoparticle, conducting or semiconducting in nature, specific sample preparation and handling details are available [5, 6, 16]. Another very important point to keep in mind is that the sample should be vacuum compatible, because the analysis and detection happens within a UHV chamber. So, any kind of volatile material should be avoided or removed before introducing the sample into the specimen holding stage.

19.5 Data interpretation

The XPS spectrum obtained is a plot of intensity (i.e., count of number of electrons emitted per unit time) versus binding energy of a particular element. A characteristic stepped background and peak splitting are obtained in the spectra. The stepped background occurs because the overall intensity at which each electron comes out of the material surface varies from one element to another as it depends on the binding energy of the element and, the electrons coming out of a deeper area lose energy in their path and emerge with reduced energy compared to the ones located nearer to the surface. So peak fitting and baseline subtraction must be done before analysis.

Both qualitative and quantitative analysis of the material can be done from the spectra. First the quantitative analysis is done and all the peaks in the spectra are assigned, to identify the elements present in the material. This is done according to the element specific binding energy, already available in the instrument software. All the orbitals of a particular element present should have same relative intensities in the spectra.

Then quantitative analysis is done to determine the atomic concentrations of a particular element present in the material. It is calculated only after baseline subtraction and peak fitting is done, because the height of a peak and the area under the peak for a particular element is required and is crucial for correct demarcations.

19.6 Features

Sensitivity and specificity: sensitivity of XPS is defined as the depth from which unscattered electron can be detected, the electrons that haev not lost any energy due to inelastic collision and are able to come out of the sample surface [17]. Using Beer's law:

$$I = I_0 \exp\left(-\frac{d}{\lambda}\right)$$

where I = intensity of the emitted electron, I_0 = total number of emitted electrons, d = depth from which electron is emitted, λ = inelastic mean free path, it is found that 95% of the detected electrons come from a depth of 10 nm. So, the sampling depth for XPS, measured normal to the surface is 10 nm, which is not outlying the sample surface.

It is also highly specific as the peaks in the spectrum are according to the characteristic binding energy of an element and its chemical environment.

Orbital splitting: except the s orbital, the p, d and f orbitals with angular momentum quantum number greater than 0 ($l > 0$), split into two peaks in the

XPS spectra. This happens because of the difference in energy level caused by the favorable or unfavorable alignment between the magnetic field of spin of the electron and the orbital angular momentum.

Chemical shift: using XPS the chemical environment of the atoms in the sample can be easily decided from the visible shifts in the peaks. In the XPS spectrum the peaks shift depending on the electronegativity of the nearest neighboring element (the type of bond formed) and the oxidation state of the atom, because as stated by Siegbahn there changes occur in binding energy according to the chemical reaction undergone by the element.

Non-destructive depth profiling: depth profiling without any ion sputtering can also be done by altering the angle at which the beam is being incident on the material surface [4]. In this way by changing the incident angle θ, the sampling depth d can be increased, and detection can be done up to depths of micrometer range.

19.7 Applications

19.7.1 In tissue engineering

Hydroxyapatite ($Ca_{10}(PO_4)_6(OH)_2$), is the fundamental component of human bones, and because of its exceptional properties, the applications of HAP have been extended to orthopedic and dental treatments as bioceramics. In the literature, it has been reported that nano range HAP with adequate morphology, phase purity, higher surface activity and similarity in composition with bone mineral would enhance osseointegration along with improvements in bone tissue growth [18]. A nanocomposite with core–shell made of hydroxyapatite (HAP) and gum acacia (GA) was synthesized by the precipitation method by Padmanabhan *et al* for drug delivery and tissue engineering applications. GA, a naturally occurring polymeric gum from the acacia plant, is a composite combination of polysaccharides and glycoproteins [19]. This gum has exceptional emulsifying and surface-active properties, which helps in the arrangement of HAP nanoparticles/nanocomposites.

Here, to direct the structural features of the nanocomposite XPS is employed. The XPS spectrum of GA-HAP nanocomposite signifies the existence of distinguishing peaks of C, O, Ca, and P which makes up the composite. The binding energy versus intensity graph of C 1s has three major components as shown in figure 19.2. The peak at a binding energy of 284.6 eV indicates the presence of C–C bonds of aromatic carbon. Other peaks at 286.5 and 289.3 eV prove that C–O and C=O exist correspondingly.

19.7.2 In 3D bioprinting

Microbial infections at the site of tissue implants in bone tissue engineering make the healing process delayed or a complete failure. To overcome this, implants with antimicrobial polymers are desirable. In one such method, silver ions were thermally reduced to AgNps and encased by PCL (polycaprolactone). Using PCL/AgNps filaments through 3D printing technique these customized structures were fabricated. Analyzing the XPS spectrum it can be confirmed that the silver ions get reduced to silver nanoparticles and are present in PCL/AgNps composites.

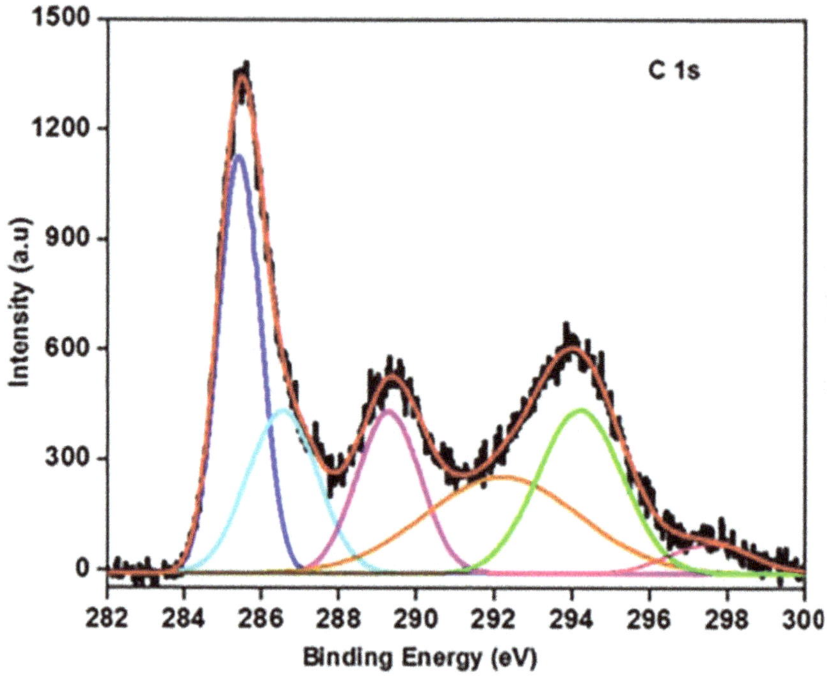

Figure 19.2. XPS spectrum of GA-HAP nanocomposite. Reprinted from [18], Copyright (2018), with permission from Elsevier.

As shown in figure 19.3, the 200–600 eV range was selected to scan the scaffolds. The XPS spectra of C 1s, and O 1s corresponds to PCL. The Ag 3D peaks observed in different concentrations of the silver confirmed the existence of silver in the 3D printed scaffolds. The peak separation of nanocomposite indicates reduction of silver [20].

Biomaterials have been produced and used in a variety of medical specialties, including plastic surgery, ophthalmology, orthopedic and cardiac surgery, urology, and dentistry [21]. Mostly titanium alloys are used because of their mechanical properties, excellent corrosion resistance and high biocompatibility. Despite these advantages, titanium lacks prevention of bacterial adhesion and proliferation [22].

Titanium surface is coated with biomaterials that have antibacterial properties to inhibit or prevent the growth of bacteria and also inhibit the formation of biofilm on the implant surface which is responsible for bacterial infections and implant failure. One such coating material is chitosan, a natural bioactive polymer commonly employed because of its cytocompatibility, antibacterial properties, and biodegradability [23]. It can be formulated into various forms (nanoparticles, gels, fiber's, membranes etc) that are useful in different biomedical applications such as drug delivery, wound healing, tissue engineering, and skin regeneration [24]. XPS is used for the verification of chemical composition and also the presence of different elemental compositions measured at the surfaces of all samples.

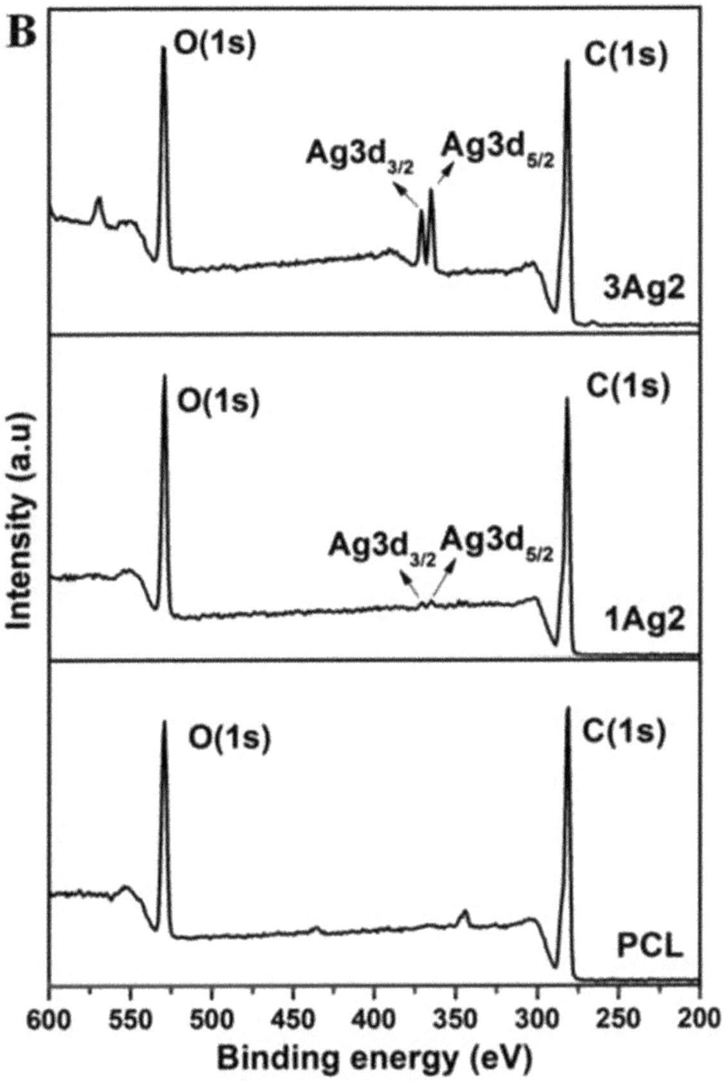

Figure 19.3. XPS spectrum of 3D printed PCL/AgNp scaffold. Reprinted from [20], Copyright (2021), with permission from Elsevier.

19.7.3 Surface nanotopography

Surface nanotopography analysis is an important parameter that influences cellular and physiological processes [25]. Protein adsorption (interaction with the external solid surface) on biomaterials is a major support for various biomedical applications in different areas such as biosensing, microchips/DNA chips, diagnostic devices, 3D bioprinting, and nanotechnology. Protein adsorption must be regulated in the case of medical implants, when there are chances of triggering immune responses and inflammatory reactions due to cell–surface interactions. Consequently, occurrence

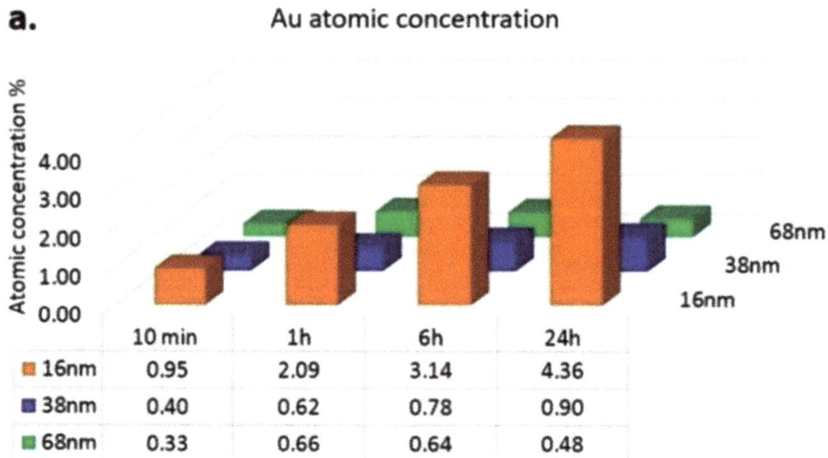

Figure 19.4. Atomic composition of the plasma polymer coated with gold nanoparticles. Reprinted with permission from [26]. Copyright (2017) American Chemical Society.

of protein adsorption must be controlled to enhance the properties of biomaterials for their specific applications. Surface roughness will increase the protein adsorption as it is decided by the roughness height and lateral layout.

To understand the effect of nanoroughness on protein–surface interaction, nano engineered surfaces were formed by gold nanoparticle immobilization (16, 32, and 68 nm) and their outer surfaces were kept constant by a biocompatible film, plasma-deposited polyoxazoline (PPOx) which reacts covalently with the carboxylic acid groups that are present on biomolecules. The plasma polymer coated with and without gold nanoparticles were characterized for detecting surface elemental composition, as well as quantification were determined using XPS (figure 19.4) [26].

19.7.4 Polymers

Polymers are the versatile forms of macromolecules that are used in various biomedical applications based on their biostability and biodegradability properties. Both the natural and synthetic polymers are used in stents, urinary catheters, implants, and in nanoparticles for targeted drug delivery. Some of the polymers include poly (lactic-co-glycolic acid) (PLGA), poly (glycolic acid) (PGA) and poly (lactic acid) (PLA) have been approved by the US Food and Drug Administration (FDA) for certain medical applications apart from natural polymers [27].

Polyvinylidene fluoride (PVDF) is a non-degradable, biocompatible, and also an electroactive polymer. It also exhibits excellent chemical resistance and thermal stability which increases its use or applications not only in biomedical field (implant preparation) but also in electronics (biosensors), environmental, and energy harvesting fields. It also has ferroelectric and piezoelectric properties that are useful in the generation of electric charges on their surface upon excitation with electrical or mechanical stimulus [28]. When PVDF nanofibers that are formed by the

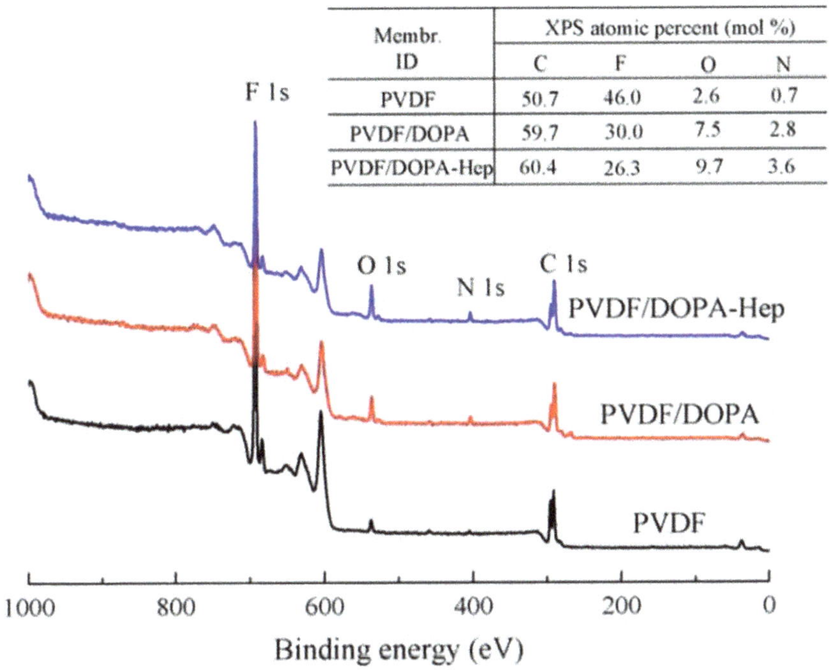

Membr. ID	XPS atomic percent (mol %)			
	C	F	O	N
PVDF	50.7	46.0	2.6	0.7
PVDF/DOPA	59.7	30.0	7.5	2.8
PVDF/DOPA-Hep	60.4	26.3	9.7	3.6

Figure 19.5. XPS spectra of surface functionalized PVDF membrane. Reprinted from [29], Copyright (2009), with permission from Elsevier.

electrospinning technique are doped with different piezoactive materials such as titanium dioxide (TiO_2), zinc oxide (ZnO), barium titanate (BT), barium calcium zirconate titanate, potassium sodium niobate; XPS is used to define the chemical state of the sample elements [28].

PVDF membranes are one of the favourable membranes that are used in hemodialysis, protein filtration, hemapheresis etc. Despite these many advantages, there are some disadvantages like low surface energy and hydrophobic nature. When used in blood filtration, protein and cellular adsorption on these hydrophobic surfaces leads to thrombus formation and other complications. These can be improved by surface modifications of the PVDF membrane. Heparin was surface immobilized onto PVDF membrane through a spacer poly(3,4-dihydroxy-l-phenyl-alanine) (poly(DOPA)), this is called surface heparinization which improves the hemocompatibility of the materials that are in contact with the blood. The surface chemical compositions for the modified and unmodified membranes were analyzed by XPS. As shown in figure 19.5 the contents of the carbon, oxygen, and nitrogen increased after the coating with Poly DOPA on the surface of PVDF [29].

19.8 Conclusion and future scope

The ability to gain complete chemical environment analysis along with the features of depth profiling and surface functionalization/interaction studies makes XPS a very important research tool. It has applications in varied fields like material sciences, life sciences, nanotechnology, electronics, and bioengineering. Proper data interpretation is crucial and should be done with much caution. Developments in easing the step of data interpretation would make it more popular than it is in the present day. To avoid any misleading data proper care and caution should be taken in all the steps, starting from sample preparation to data collection and interpretation. Some of the innovations with this technique like imaging, which are to happen in the near future will be of immense help in biomedical nanotechnology.

References

[1] Briggs D 2005 X-ray photoelectron spectroscopy (XPS) *Handbook of Adhesion* 2nd edn (Hoboken, NJ: Wiley) pp 621–2

[2] Sublemontier O, Nicolas C, Aureau D, Patanen M, Kintz H and Liu X *et al* 2014 X-ray photoelectron spectroscopy of isolated nanoparticles *J. Phys. Chem. Lett.* **5** 3399–403

[3] Watts J and Wolstenholme J 2003 An introduction to surface analysis by XPS and AES *An Introduction to Surface Analysis by XPS and AES* ed J F Watts and J Wolstenholme (New York: Wiley-VCH) pp 224

[4] Sivkov D, Nekipelov S, Petrova O, Vinogradov A, Mingaleva A and Isaenko S *et al* 2020 Studies of buried layers and interfaces of tungsten carbide coatings on the MWCNT surface by XPS and NEXAFS spectroscopy *Appl. Sci.* **10** 4736

[5] Baer D 2020 Guide to making XPS measurements on nanoparticles *J. Vac. Sci. Technol.* A **38** 031201

[6] Korin E, Froumin N and Cohen S 2017 Surface analysis of nanocomplexes by X-ray photoelectron spectroscopy (XPS) *ACS Biomater. Sci. Eng.* **3** 882–9

[7] Techane S D, Gamble L J and Castner D G 2011 X-ray photoelectron spectroscopy characterization of gold nanoparticles functionalized with amine-terminated alkanethiols *Biointerphases* **6** 98–104

[8] Welch N G, Mukherjee S, Hossain M A, Praveen P, Werkmeister J A and Wade J D *et al* 2019 Coatings releasing the relaxin peptide analogue B7-33 reduce fibrotic encapsulation *ACS Appl. Mater. Interfaces* **11** 45511–9

[9] Chan C M and Weng L T 2016 Surface characterization of polymer blends by XPS and ToF-SIMS *Materials (Basel)* **9** 655

[10] Gao G, Lange D, Hilpert K, Kindrachuk J, Zou Y and Cheng J T J *et al* 2011 The biocompatibility and biofilm resistance of implant coatings based on hydrophilic polymer brushes conjugated with antimicrobial peptides *Biomaterials* **32** 3899–909

[11] Thissen H, Gengenbach T, du Toit R, Sweeney D F, Kingshott P and Griesser H J *et al* 2010 Clinical observations of biofouling on PEO coated silicone hydrogel contact lenses *Biomaterials* **31** 5510–9

[12] Chouirfa H, Evans M D M, Castner D G, Bean P, Mercier D and Galtayries A *et al* 2017 Grafting of architecture controlled poly(styrene sodium sulfonate) onto titanium surfaces using bio-adhesive molecules: surface characterization and biological properties *Biointerphases* **12** 02C418

[13] Liu Z C, Zhang X, He N Y, Lu Z H and Chen Z C 2009 Probing DNA hybridization efficiency and single base mismatch by X-ray photoelectron spectroscopy *Colloids Surf.* B **71** 238–42

[14] Tougaard S 2019 Surface analysis *X-ray Photoelectron Spectroscopy Encyclopedia of Analytical Science* (Amsterdam: Elsevier) pp 400–9

[15] Stevie F A and Donley C L 2020 Introduction to x-ray photoelectron spectroscopy *J. Vac. Sci. Technol.* A **38** 063204

[16] Easton C D, Kinnear C, McArthur S L and Gengenbach T R 2020 Practical guides for x-ray photoelectron spectroscopy: analysis of polymers *J. Vac. Sci. Technol.* A **38** 023207

[17] McArthur S L, Mishra G and Easton C D 2014 Applications of XPS in biology and biointerface analysis *Surface Analysis and Techniques in Biology* (Cham: Springer) 9–36

[18] Prasath V, Kulandaivelu R, Narayanan S and Nellaiappan T S 2018 New core–shell hydroxyapatite/Gum-Acacia nanocomposites for drug delivery and tissue engineering applications *Mater. Sci. Eng.* C **92** 685–93

[19] Hadavi M, Hasannia S, Faghihi S, Mashayekhi F, Zadeh H H and Mostofi S B 2017 Novel calcified gum Arabic porous nano-composite scaffold for bone tissue regeneration *Biochem. Biophys. Res. Commun.* **488** 671–8

[20] Radhakrishnan S, Nagarajan S, Belaid H, Farha C, Iatsunskyi I and Coy E *et al* 2021 Fabrication of 3D printed antimicrobial polycaprolactone scaffolds for tissue engineering applications *Mater. Sci. Eng.* C **118** 111525

[21] Holzapfel B M, Reichert J C, Schantz J T, Gbureck U, Rackwitz L and Nöth U *et al* 2013 How smart do biomaterials need to be? A translational science and clinical point of view *Adv. Drug Deliv. Rev.* **65** 581–603

[22] Park K, Hong H Y, Moon H J, Lee B H, Kim I S and Kwon I C *et al* 2008 A new atherosclerotic lesion probe based on hydrophobically modified chitosan nanoparticles functionalized by the atherosclerotic plaque targeted peptides *J. Control. Release* **128** 217–23

[23] Dash M, Chiellini F, Ottenbrite R M and Chiellini E 2011 Progress in polymer science chitosan—a versatile semi-synthetic polymer in biomedical applications *Prog. Polym. Sci.* **36** 981–1014

[24] Almeida D, Attik N, Amalric J and Abouelleil H 2017 Chitosan coating as an antibacterial surface for biomedical applications *PLoS One* **12** e0189537

[25] Rostam H M, Singh S, Vrana N E, Alexander M R and Ghaemmaghami A M 2015 Impact of surface chemistry and topography on the function of antigen presenting cells *Biomater. Sci.* **3** 424–41

[26] Gonzalez Garcia L E, Macgregor-Ramiasa M, Visalakshan R M and Vasilev K 2017 Protein interactions with nanoengineered polyoxazoline surfaces generated via plasma deposition *Langmuir* **33** 7322–31

[27] Francis P J J 2018 Biomedical applications of polymers—an overview *Curr. Trends Biomed. Eng. Biosci.* **15** 44–5

[28] Smejkalová T, Ţălu Ş, Dallaev R, Částková K and Sobola D 2021 SEM imaging and XPS characterization of doped PVDF fibers *E3S Web Conf.* **270** 01011

[29] Zhu L, Yu J, Xu Y, Xi Z and Zhu B 2009 Surface modification of PVDF porous membranes via poly (DOPA) coating and heparin immobilization *Colloids Surf.* B **69** 152–5

Chapter 20

AI and IOT for biomedical smart applications

Shilpa Bhatkande, Hirak Mazumdar and Hardik Gohel

In today's advanced technology, artificial intelligence (AI) and the internet of things (IOT) are being used to automate almost everything. One of areas most in need of this technology is healthcare which is reaching its peek on adopting new computing concepts. Therefore, integrating AI into the IoT is becoming a common practice. The healthcare system has become a requirement for everyone and business process and finding one's way around is equally important for all. Healthcare is a very sensitive area in all aspects, and certainly the machines and technology used should be rigorously trained to perform tasks successfully where there are limits on human mental and physical performance. The need to go beyond an individual's maximum limits must be assigned to technologies like the IoT and AI. The importance of implementation of innovative solutions in healthcare has become popular, meeting many challenges and the IoT together with AI have proved to be strong drivers of the digital transformation regardless of what field the technologies are applied to. A few business areas are (but not limited to) retail, municipal infrastructure, supply chain, smart homes, manufacturing, education, and healthcare. In short, the entire digital ecosystem, an IoT ecosystem of connected devices, has been created and is growing stronger with each passing day. Empowered with AI and machine learning, among other things, the IoT is used as a means of equipping people with intelligent assistance. Gradually, it is taking over both minor and major processes in several industries. Healthcare is no exception.

20.1 Introduction

The healthcare sector began leveraging information technology in recent years to develop modern applications and enhance the diagnostic and treatment processes. Advanced techniques and scientific theory are the major entities that generate huge volumes of digital data. These are followed by advanced clinical applications which are the brainchildren of information technology which have been developed in recent times. Also, advanced healthcare is assumed to have simple, elegant, and

doi:10.1088/978-0-7503-3379-5ch20

multi-tasking applications. These modifications are incorporated as clinical model extension (from disease-based to patient-based care), informatization development changes (from medical data to regional medical data), extension in clinical management (general management to personal management), and modifications from prevention and treatment (shifting of concentration from disease treatment to preventive medical systems). Hence, the following changes are concentrated to satisfy the basic requirements of individuals to enhance the proficiency of healthcare which in turn improves health service knowledge and implies the future deployment of smart medicine [1].

Advanced medical services are comprised of several stakeholders such as doctors, patients, clinical and research centers. Multiple dimensions should be considered such as disease preventive measures and observation, prognosis and treatment, clinical management, health decision-making, and medical studies. For instance, mobile internet, cloud computing (CC), big data, 5G systems, microelectronics, and artificial intelligence (AI), along with smart biotechnology are assumed to be the milestones of modern healthcare [2]. These methodologies are employed in every stage of advanced healthcare. From the patients' viewpoint, wearable or portable devices can be applied for monitoring their health condition whenever required. They can look for clinical guidance through virtual support and control their homes remotely using remote facilities. From the perception of doctors, smart clinical decision support systems can be applied to guide and enhance the diagnostic procedures.

An extensive diffusion and deployment of effectively incorporated hardware and modern medical sensors for unique healthcare has intended to develop a new concept called the internet of medical things (IoMT). It modifies the healthcare process and number of medical devices that use the internet of things (IoT) to achieve better profit in the future. The data, captured with the help of portable, ingestible, and incorporated sensors, mobile patterns, and device usage patterns, enable the researcher to track a user's habits. With further data collection, it is possible to reveal their medical status by applying state-of-the-art as well as machine learning (ML) or deep learning (DL)-based methods. Classical cloud technology that relies on structures for big data analysis, is applied to provide optimal performance, scalability, and support non-safety as well as delay based IoT domains [3, 4]. However, if there is a medical emergency and the need for efficient and accessible medical care is high, being disconnected from the main network or experiencing significant latency differences could have serious and potentially fatal consequences due to limited resources. The rapid development of structures that examine the collaboration of cloud, fog, and edge computing still remains a challenging process. The main aim of this method is to apply complete edge nodes and low-level fog nodes to manage functional tasks with regards to data processing, examination, correlation, and inference. Hence, the above-mentioned approaches produce challenging outcomes by implementing scalable medical domain services. This occurs because the smart mapping of processing and resource management operations overcome the nodes to satisfy the fundamental needs of IoMT model.

20.2 Why combine IoT and artificial intelligence?

Under the application of AI models, surgical devices, and mixed reality applications, both diagnosis and disease treatment are highly robust. By using AI, specific outcomes are attained from clinical decision support systems (CDSS) such as the diagnosis of hepatitis, lung tumors, and skin cancer. Further, the accuracy of AI diagnosis has exceeded the accuracy accomplished manually. In addition, ML-based models are precise in comparison with well-trained physicians, particularly pathologists and imaging experts. Therefore, a remarkable and representative product in CDSS was rolled out by IBM's Watson. This product has an effective cognitive mechanism and is used for providing the best solution with the help of in-depth analysis of medical and literature details. As a result, a drastic effect has been experienced by healthcare professionals in diagnosing both diabetes and cancer. The application of CDSS is highly efficient and supports the physicians in enhancing the diagnostic processes, limiting the incidence of unexploited diagnosis as well as misdiagnosis, and enabling the users to receive timely and proper medical treatment. According to smart diagnosis, the state of a patient's health and severity of disease can be defined accurately to follow a personalized treatment procedure.

The current research work presents a new AI and IoT convergence-based disease diagnosis model for smart healthcare system. The aim is to develop a disease diagnosis model using AI and IoT convergence technique for the diagnosis of diabetes and heart disease. The presented model encompasses different stages namely, data acquisition, preprocessing, classification, and parameter tuning. IoT devices such as wearables and sensors perform the data acquisition process whereas AI techniques process this data to diagnose the disease. In addition, the isolation Forest technique is employed in this study to remove outliers. To improve the diagnostic outcome, cuckoo search optimization (CSO) algorithm is applied to tune both 'weights' and 'bias' parameters of convolutional long short-term memory (CLSTM) algorithm model. CSO is utilized here since it helps to improve the diagnostic outcome of the CLSTM method. The effectiveness of CSO-LSTM model was validated using healthcare data. The contributions of this research article are summarized here:

- designing and development of a novel AI and IoT convergence-based disease diagnosis model for smart healthcare system
- proposed a CSO-CLSTM model for diagnosing diabetes and heart disease
- incorporated iForest technique-based outlier detection process to improve the classification results
- performed parameter tuning of LSTM model using CSO algorithm
- validated the performance of CSO-LSTM model on two benchmark datasets.

20.2.1 Principles and foundations of IoT and AI

The new trends in the current market are the IoT, big data, and AI, which have shown exponential growth in the number of devices connected to the internet, and the huge volume of data is generated by them, which demonstrates the use of analytical and predictive techniques of AI and DL [5].

20.2.2 What is IoT?

The IoT, sometimes called the fog network refers to a wide range of things such as, smartphones, sensors, actuators, refrigerators, health devices, washing machines or even a coffee machine that is connected to the internet, or any day-to-day useable devices. These are physically connected to the world and can be sensed, stored, processed, and accessed. Basically, the IoT is the infrastructure to the information system that enables advanced services to interconnect physically and virtually based on existing information and communication technologies [6–14] (figure 20.1).

The existence of IoT applications has large scope in the health industry to optimize processes and implement remote monitoring capabilities to increase efficiency and productivity [11–13].

20.2.2.1 IoT reference model

The IoT architecture is defined just like the open systems interconnection (OSI) model. There are two vertical layers management and security, they are spread over all four horizontal layers (figure 20.2).

The device layer is the bottom layer also called the perception layer. This layer contains all physical things that can control the physical world and gather data.

The network layer is the layer that provides the networking support and transfer of data over either wired or wireless network. The layer securely transmits the information from the devices in the device layer to the information processing system.

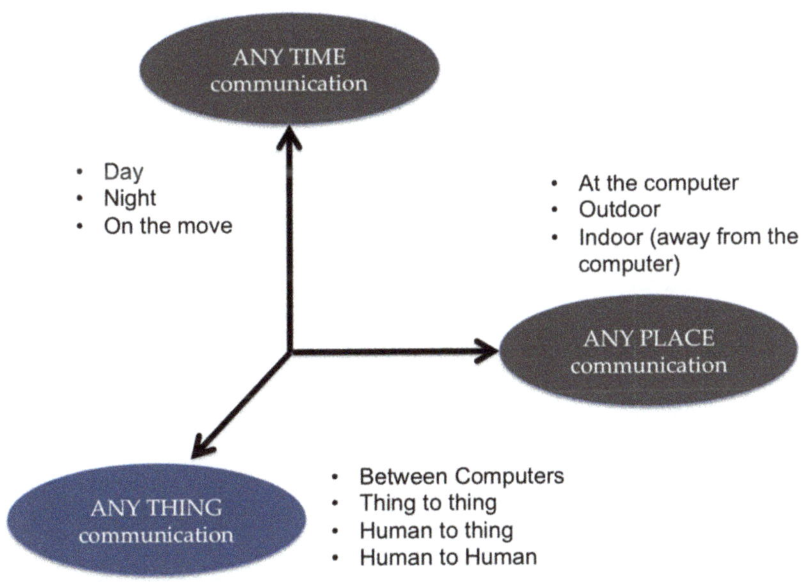

Figure 20.1. IoT dimensions. Adapted with permission from [11]. Copyright Packt Publishing Pvt Ltd.

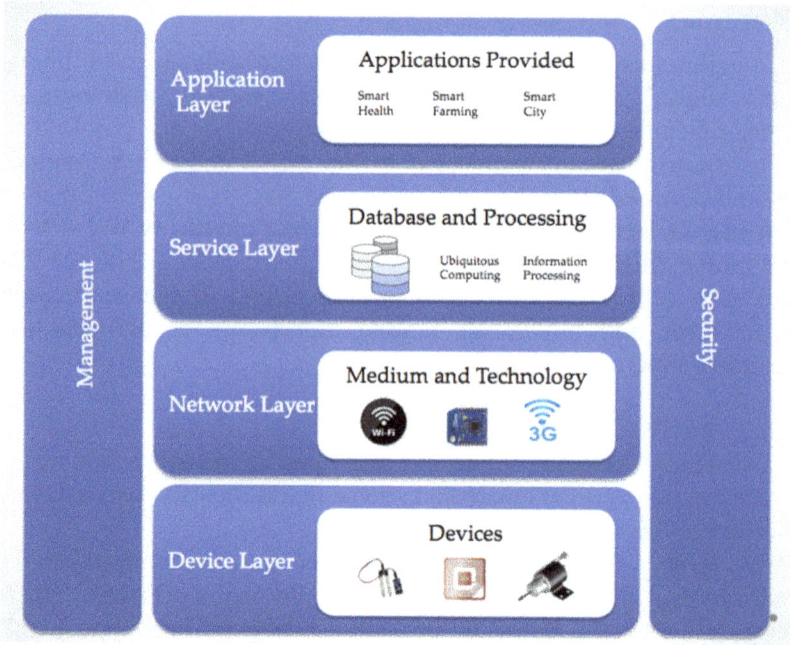

Figure 20.2. IoT layers. Adapted with permission from [11]. Copyright Packt Publishing Pvt Ltd.

The service layer is the layer responsible for service management. It receives information from the network layer, stores it in the database, processes that information, and can make an automatic decision based on the results.

The application layer is the layer that manages the applications dependent upon the information processed in the service layer.

20.2.3 IoT platforms

Information from the network layer is often managed with the help of IoT platforms. Many companies today provide IoT platform services, where they help not only with data but also enable seamless integration with different hardware. Since they function as a mediator between the hardware and application layer, IoT platforms are also referred to as IoT middleware and are part of the service layer in the IoT reference stack. IoT platforms provide the ability to connect and communicate with things from anywhere in the world. The IoT platforms are selected based upon following criteria.

Scalability Addition and deletion of new devices to the existing IoT network should be possible.

Ease of use The system should work perfectly and deliver all its specifications with minimum intervention.

Third party integration Heterogeneous devices and protocols should be able to inter-network with each other.

Deployment options It should be workable on a broad variety of hardware devices and software platforms.

Data security The security of data and devices is ensured.

Before sending the data to the cloud, some form of IoT data transformation is performed. This may involve the following:

- temporal or spatial analysis
- summarizing the data at the edge
- aggregation of data
- correlating data in multiple IoT streams
- cleaning data
- filling in the missing values
- normalizing the data
- transforming it into different formats acceptable to the cloud.

20.2.4 Infusion of AI—data science in IoT

The IoT generates an enormous amount of data; presently, 90% of the data generated is not even captured, and out of the 10% that is captured, most is time-dependent and loses its value within milliseconds. Manually monitoring this data continuously is both cumbersome and expensive. This necessitates a way to intelligently analyze and gain insight from this data; the tools and models of AI provide us with a way to do exactly this with minimum human intervention. The major focus in this chapter will be on understanding the various AI models and techniques that can be applied to IoT data using both ML and DL algorithms. Figure 20.3 explains the relationship between AI, ML, and DL.

By observing the behavior of multiple things, IoT (with the help of BD and AI) aims to gain insight into the data and optimize underlying processes. This involves multiple challenges:

- storing real-time generated events
- running analytical queries over stored events
- performing analytics using AI/ML/DL techniques over the data to gain insights and make predictions.

20.2.4.1 Cross-industry standard process for data mining

For IoT problems, the most used data management (DM) methodology is cross-industry standard process for data mining (CRISP-DM) proposed by Chapman et al [14] It is a process model that states the tasks that need to be carried out for successfully completing DM. It is a vendor-independent methodology divided into six different phases:

- business understanding
- data understanding
- data preparation
- modeling
- evaluation
- deployment.

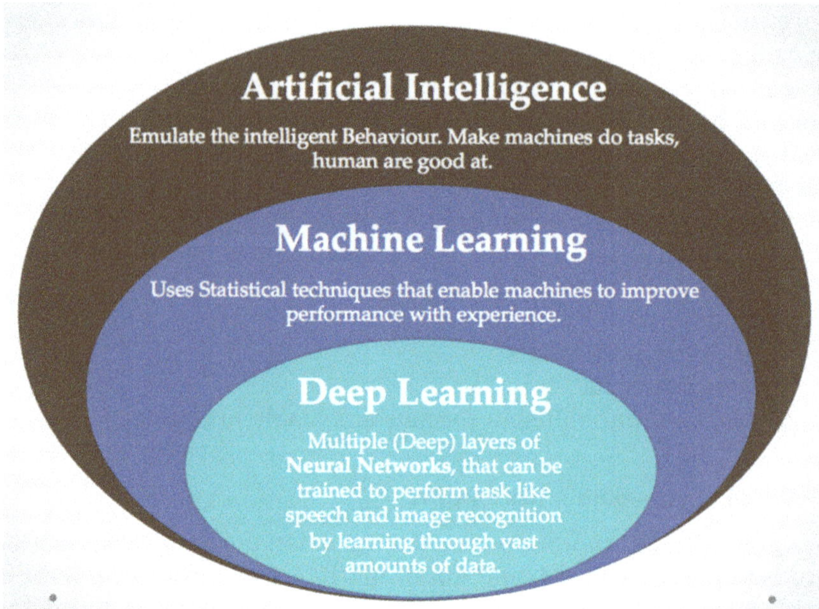

Figure 20.3. AI/ML/DL techniques. Adapted with permission from [11]. Copyright Packt Publishing Pvt Ltd.

20.2.4.2 AI platforms and IoT platforms

Many cloud platforms with both AI and IoT capabilities are available today. These platforms provide the capability to integrate the sensors and devices and perform analytics on the cloud. There exist more than 30 cloud platforms in the global market, each targeting different IoT verticals and services. Figure 20.4 lists the various services that AI/IoT platforms support.

The following is a list of some of the popular cloud platforms:

IBM Watson IoT Platform Hosted by IBM, the platform provides device management; it uses the message queuing telemetry transport (MQTT) protocol to connect with IoT devices and applications. It provides real-time scalable connectivity. The data can be stored for a period and accessed in real time. IBM Watson also provides Bluemix Platform-as-a-Service (PaaS) for analytics and visualizations. We can write code to build and manage applications that interact with the data and connected devices. It supports Python along with C#, Java, and Node.js.

Microsoft IoT-Azure IoT suite It provides a collection of preconfigured solutions built on Azure PaaS. It enables a reliable and secure bidirectional communication between IoT devices and the cloud. The preconfigured solutions include data visualization, remote monitoring, and configuring rules and alarms over live IoT telemetry. It also provides Azure Stream Analytics to process the data in real time. The Azure Stream Analytics allow us to use Visual Studio. It supports Python, Node.js, C, and Arduino, depending upon the IoT devices.

Google Cloud IoT This provides a fully managed service for securely connecting and managing IoT devices. It supports both MQTT and HTTP protocols. It also

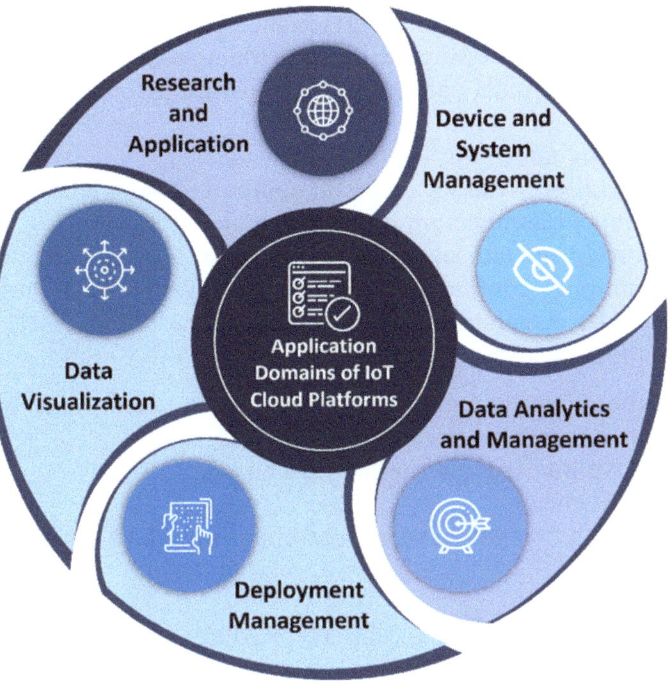

Figure 20.4. Services that different AI/IoT platforms support.

provides bidirectional communication between IoT devices and the cloud. It provides support for Go, PHP, Ruby, JS, .NET, Java, Objective-C, and Python. It also has BigQuery, which allows users to perform data analytics and visualization.

Amazon AWS IoT This allows IoT devices to communicate via MQTT, HTTP, and WebSockets. It provides secure, bidirectional communication between IoT devices and the cloud. It also has a rules engine that can be used to integrate data with other Amazon Web Services (AWS) services and transform the data. Rules can be defined that trigger the execution of user code in Java, Python, or Node.js. AWS Lambda allows us to use our own custom trained models.

The neural networks based on multiple layered models, also known as deep learning models. They have become a buzzword in the last few years and an absolute favorite of investors in the field of AI-based startups.

20.2.5 Distributed AI for IoT

The advances in distributed computing environments and an easy availability of internet worldwide have resulted in the emergence of distributed artificial intelligence (DAI). There are two frameworks, one by Apache the machine learning library (MLlib), and another H2O.ai, both provide distributed and scalable ML) for large, streaming data. IoT systems generate a lot of data; while in many cases it is possible to analyze the data at leisure, for certain tasks such as security, fraud detection, and so on, this latency is not acceptable. What we need in such a situation is a way to handle large data within a specified time—the solution—DAI, many machines in the cluster processing the big data (data parallelism) and/or training the deep learning models (model parallelism) in a distributed manner.

20.2.5.1 Apache MLlib

Apache Spark MLlib provides a powerful computational environment for ML. It provides a distributed architecture on a large-scale basis, allowing one to run ML models more quickly and efficiently. That's not all; it is open source with a growing and active community continuously working to improve and provide the latest features. It provides a scalable implementation of the popular ML algorithms. It includes algorithms for the following:

- classification: logistic regression, linear support vector machine, naive Bayes
- regression: generalized linear regression
- collaborative filtering: alternating least square
- clustering: K-means
- decomposition: singular value decomposition and principal component analysis.

It has proved to be faster than Hadoop MapReduce. We can write applications in Java, Scala, R, or Python.

20.2.5.2 Introducing H2O.ai

H2O is a fast, scalable ML and DL framework developed by H2O.ai, released under the open source Apache license. According to the company-provided details, more than 9000 organizations and 80 000+ data scientists use H2O for their ML/DL needs. It uses in-memory compression, which allows it to handle a large amount of data in memory, even with a small cluster of machines. It has an interface for R, Python, Java, Scala, and JavaScript, and even has a built-in web interface. H2O can run in standalone mode, and on Hadoop or Spark cluster.

H2O includes many ML algorithms like generalized linear modeling, Naive Bayes, random forest, gradient boosting, and deep learning algorithms. The best part of H2O is that one can build thousands of models, compare the results, and even do hyper parameter tuning with a few lines of code. H2O also has better data preprocessing tools. With the ubiquitous status of the IoT, the data being generated is growing at an exponential rate. This data, mostly unstructured and available in vast quantities, is often referred to as big data. Many frameworks and solutions have been proposed to deal with the large set of data. One of the promising solutions is DAI, distributing the model or data among the cluster of machines.

20.2.6 Computing in the cloud

Applying AI algorithms to IoT-generated data requires computing resources. With the availability of many cloud platforms offering service at competitive prices, CC offers a cost-effective solution. Out of the many cloud platforms available today, we will talk about three main cloud platform providers that occupy most of the market share: Amazon Web Service (AWS), Google Cloud Platform (GCP), and Microsoft Azure.

20.3 AI and IoT in healthcare

When it comes to combining AI and IoT in healthcare, the chances are that together they will improve operational efficiency in this field. Tracking (collecting), monitoring (analyzing), control, optimization (training), and automation (modeling, predicting)—these are the key steps that provide for the smart and efficient application of AI algorithms in IoT devices.

Acting in concert, they can reduce the burden of administrative work for clinical staff. Having clinical workflows improved, medical officers will be able to spend more time with their patients and the healthcare service-delivery is consequently bound to take a more patient-centric approach.

Therefore, the main use cases of AI-enabled IoT are the following:

Medical staff, patients, and inventory tracking
Chronic disease management
Drug management
Emergency room wait time reduction
Remote health control

20.3.1 IoT operational principles in the medical field

The best way to explain why one needs to use AI-enabled IoT in healthcare is to provide a more detailed analysis of the IoT operational principles enabling a more nuanced understanding of potential fields of its application in the healthcare system.

20.3.1.1 Devices with physical interfaces to/from the real world

Fundamentally, in healthcare, any service a client requests is related to the physical world. Besides, the use of services involves the physical interaction of caregivers, patients, and the devices. These connected devices as robotics in medicine interact with the physical environment through multiple physical interfaces. Developing intuitive physical interfaces with different communication technologies (i.e., Bluetooth, NFC, Wi-Fi, USB) is thus bound to level up the quality of this interaction, lead to a better information flow among IoT robots and improved service representation and tracking for people. The reason is that, given an IoT-based solution, the physical interfaces can create wireless networks. Apparently, the IoT nodes that stand behind certain sensor devices are being grouped together in such a way to get devices easily connected to the Internet architecture and to get exchange processes well established.

20.3.1.2 Structured data input through sensors

IoT technology produces wireless sensor networks. As previously stated, these networks are successfully bridging the physical and digital worlds. What prevents

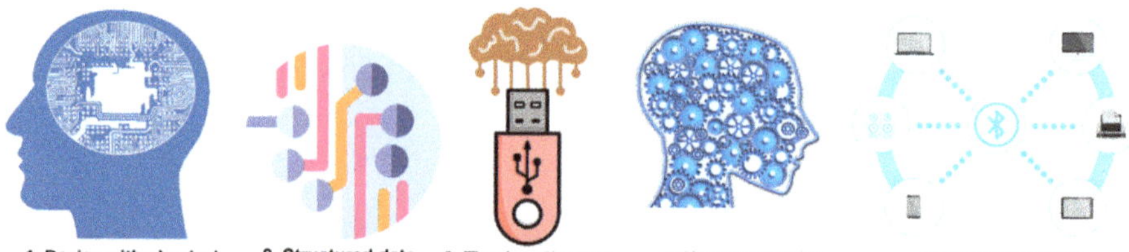

Figure 20.5. IoT operational principles in the medical field.

the performance of the data exchange between these two worlds from becoming a mess is the structured information flow. Input data is collected by the sensor devices and sent to the data control center for further feedback. There might be several data channels involved in parallel, nevertheless, multiple sensor data collection is executed with minimal latency. Also, despite the fact that the number of data sources is typically enormous, the data records remain small and well-structured due to the edge analytics while high dynamism of IoT devices allows deducing missing information from the neighboring gadgets to fill the gaps.

20.3.1.3 Tiny input/output devices

There are certain requirements for the appearance and size of the physical IO devices. Moreover, the requirements should be adjusted to the environmental conditions in which the device is operating. So, in contrast to human interfaces that need relatively big input/output devices, physical interfaces of IoT devices receive input through sensors (which are tiny due to the use of micro-electro-mechanical systems (MEMS) [6] technology) and send data back to mobile/cloud computers through wired or wireless interfaces. Consequently, there is not only a need for but there is also a real possibility of having the size of sensors as well as the IO devices reduced. Consider such instances as implanted heart-rhythm monitors and devices continuously measuring and monitoring biochemical data (figure 20.5).

20.3.1.4 Human–machine–environment system drivers

Evidently, human–machine interaction refers to the process of communication between people and automated systems. However, the IoT is built on the foundation of a more complex relationship among the human, machine, and environment. In healthcare, the environment is a highly important parameter that implies the sum of physical and social factors; and the real-time monitoring of the environmental factor is even more critical for this industry once the IoT technology is in operation. IoT data generated by multi-modal sensors should be, consequently, used as inferable information and made sense of relying on the powers of AI.

20.3.1.5 Real-time action and decision control

One of the main advantages the interoperability of AI and IoT is bringing is that there is an opportunity to keep track of what is going on and to react upon it on the spot. It means the shift towards active patient involvement; customized treatment plans real-time adjustment and a more intelligent approach to data management. Real-time analysis is only possible when a stream of data is continuous. However, it is hardly possible that a system doing complex processing can cope with the nearly continuous data stream from multiple sensors. It is a real-time AI system that can reduce the amount of data and enable intelligent data management. Eventually, embedded AI technology will be of paramount priority for IoT systems, especially in healthcare. Importantly, the desirable action here is making sense of the data at the edge, close to the device, with the edge and fog computing. Again, data analysis performed at the edge instead of a centralized location (i.e., a cloud server or a data center) enables a near real-time analysis right on the IoT devices.

The capacity of AI to meet or exceed the performance of human experts in medical data analysis can, in part, be attributed to the continued improvement of high-performance computing platforms such as graphics processing units (GPUs) and customized ML hardware. These can now process and learn from a large amount of multi-modal heterogeneous general and medical data. This was not readily achievable a decade ago. While there are significant advances in tailoring deep network models and algorithms for various healthcare and biomedical applications, most computationally expensive deep networks are trained on either GPUs or in data centers. The latter typically requires access to CC services which is not only costly and comes with high power demands, but also compromises data privacy. This is distinct to the effective deployment of DL at the edge on an increasing number of medical IoT devices. Edge learning and inference enables the option to move processing away from the cloud. This is critical for highly sensitive medical data and offline operation. Edge-based processing must combine compactness, low-power, and rapid (high-throughput) at a low-cost, to make smart health monitoring viable and affordable for integration into human life.

20.3.2 Principles of artificial and spiking neural networks

Deep neural networks with rate-based neurons have exhibited tremendous progress in the last decade. However, the same level of progress has not been observed in research on spiking neural networks (SNN), despite their capability to handle temporal data, energy-efficiency and low latency. This could be because the benchmarking techniques for SNNs are based on the methods used for evaluating deep neural networks, which do not provide a clear evaluation of the capabilities of SNNs. Particularly, the benchmarking of SNN approaches with regards to energy-efficiency and latency requires realization in suitable hardware, which imposes additional temporal and resource constraints upon ongoing projects. This review aims to provide an overview of the current real-world applications of SNNs and identifies steps to accelerate research involving SNNs in the future. Like artificial neural networks (ANN), SNNs are also inspired by the neural networks observed in biology. However, unlike ANNs, SNNs employ processing units that process information using neuronal units that are much closer to their biological counterparts. Biological neurons process and transmit information using action potentials, also known as spikes, which underlie the incredible energy-efficiency exhibited by the brain. These similarities between spiking neurons and biological neurons also imply that SNNs with similar power requirements as the human brain could potentially be developed. This has motivated several studies to compare ANNs and SNNs from different perspectives. Despite these capabilities, SNNs have not seen the same level of advances as observed in ANNs. The natural capabilities of spiking neurons to represent temporal information renders them suitable for processing spatial–temporal data arising in various domains such as brain and cognitive data analytics, brain–computer interfaces, knowledge transfer between humans and machines, brain-like robotics, incremental and transfer learning of multisensory streaming data. Further evaluation and appreciation of the advantages of SNNs are expected in terms of energy-efficiency, response latency and explanations [7].

20.3.3 Role of AI to investigate a material for biomedical application

Advances in AI, especially ML, provide enormous tools for processing complex data generated from experimental and computational materials research. With the rapid development of AI methods and the complex nature of interdisciplinary research, a challenge is posed as to which methods to choose for different material systems or context and which steps of the material discovery process would stand to benefit. It shows how AI strategies are applied through material discovery stages (including characterization, property prediction, synthesis, and theory paradigm discovery).

This focused edition highlights the latest advances in the application of AI techniques to the field of medical informatics, with a particular emphasis on the improvements achieved in recent years. The basis of evidence-based medicine is to establish clinical correlations and insights via developing associations and patterns from the existing database of information. With highly measurable improvements, the MAI issue demonstrates the great potential and promises of applying AI techniques to pragmatic clinical procedures and analytical medical informatics, especially in the following areas:

(i) AI techniques in medicine
(ii) DM and knowledge discovery in medicine
(iii) medical expert systems
(iv) ML-based medical systems
(v) medical signal and image processing techniques

Apart from continuing to apply ML in different material systems to achieve different goals, these five major key areas can be treated as the future directions for the community to advance into: (1) insightful choice of informatics descriptors; (2) suitable models for dealing with specific materials' data structure; (3) efficient labeling by implementing ML in the loop; (4) high-level design to simplify the complex research problem; and (5) the integration of data and methods from different research groups. By solving the challenges in these directions, our

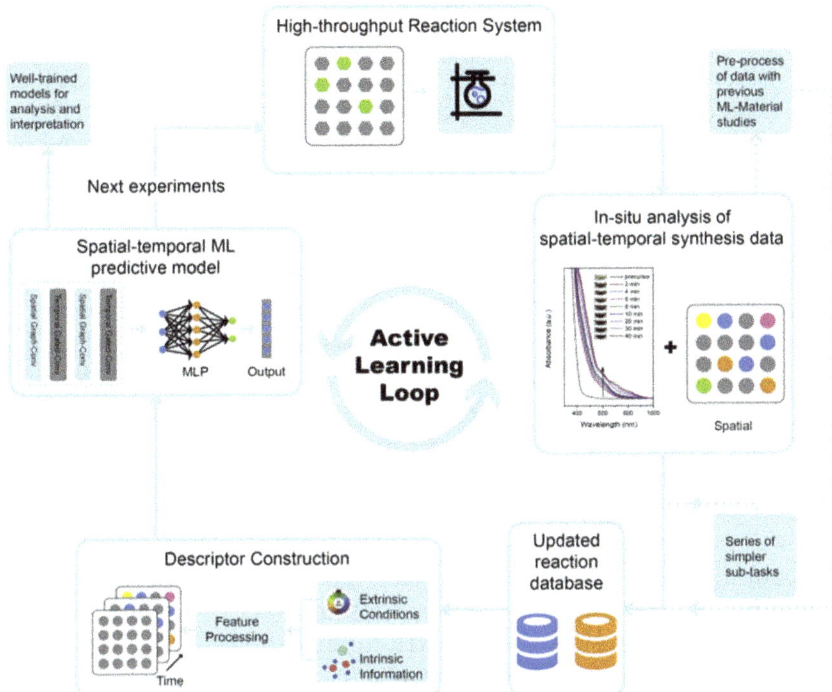

Figure 20.6. An illustration of AI study in a high-throughput material synthesis system with spatial–temporal complexity. Reprinted from Jiali Li et al, Copyright (2002), with permission from Elsevier.

community can discover materials knowledge that was previously not possible to find. For example, solving the challenges can enable us to study complex material synthesis systems that are far from equilibrium with both spatial and temporal complexities (figure 20.6).

Achievements in these five areas will push our community one step closer to realizing next generation material research as shown in the figure. Advancements in each of these five areas hold the potential to drive the material research field towards the next generation. By making progress in these directions, we can improve the material discovery workflow from various perspectives. In particular, the development of material-based ML algorithms capable of analysing spatial-temporal material synthesis data is of significant importance.

20.3.4 ML algorithms' challenges in complex material synthesis systems

For complex material systems with little first-principle understanding, a statistical predictive model might be trained to predict material properties or synthesis results. Most material systems are constrained by the lack of available data, with machine learning models typically trained on only a few hundred data points or less. This is due to the expensive, labor-intensive, or time-consuming nature of laboratory work. However, the recent development of high-throughput experiments would be likely to alleviate this problem to a certain extent. We can take a step forward and imagine ways to further utilize the high volume of data of complex material systems generated by high-throughput experiments in the future. Currently, most complex material systems-based ML models use both the intrinsic materials' information and the extrinsic materials' information. Such information sets are both commonly time-independent information. However, most complex reactions of interest are dynamic, far from equilibrium, and spatially heterogeneous. Thus, with better data collection and characterization approaches, we might be able to incorporate the time dimension into the models. Hence, the intrinsic information and extrinsic information can be time-varying and fed into our ML model at each time step to achieve better performance. Certain neural networks such as recurrent or attention-based neural networks could be used to process such time-series features. Meanwhile, how to better incorporate chemical information into these ML methods in the materials field is still a topic worth exploring. For example, there can be discrete information of molecular structures as well as continuous information such as temperature, pH, and so forth at each time point. Various methods have been implemented to convert discrete information into continuous data and then combine this with other continuous information to realize the prediction and inverse design tasks of materials or material devices. However, analyzing these mixed information forms together with a temporal element can be a challenging problem.

Moreover, characterization methods such as attenuated total reflection Fourier transform infrared spectroscopy with focal plane array detectors can capture information for a two-dimensional space. As a result, not only could the bulk properties during the synthesis process of the material be considered, but more detailed spatial information could also be taken into consideration. For example, the spatial information of a material synthesis process as well as materials with heterogeneous structures can be studied. There exists some good work analyzing spatiotemporal chemical information, although there is still much room for improvement. Finally, when temporal and spatial chemical information are analyzed together, we should expect to understand the complex system much better. Methods such as graph dynamical networks and spatiotemporal graph convolutional networks can be possible solutions to this challenge, while multiple efforts and advances are still needed in methodologies, especially in the fitting materials research domain.

20.3.5 Decomposition of complex tasks in material discovery

To perform good predictions as well as gain understanding of mechanisms of complex systems, decomposition of a complex task is usually needed. Some material properties or synthesis prediction tasks, as well as the data preparation process, are complex in nature. For example, the prediction of perovskite with high Curie temperature and the multiclass classification of genomic silver nanocluster with specific fluorescence color are difficult tasks to achieve with a single prediction model. A clever approach is to decompose this final task into simpler tasks, which normally need fewer efforts in collecting data, whereby the underlying relationships are clearer. As a result, these tasks are easier to train and could reach a higher prediction accuracy than the straightforward approach to analyze the complex task. For example, to synthesize perovskite with high Curie temperature, the formation of the perovskite structure needs to be ensured. The composition suggested by one-step regression Curie temperature prediction failed due to the presence of secondary phases (not pure perovskite structures). To fix this problem, a two-step approach is proposed to decompose the high Curie temperature prediction problem into firstly constructing an SVM classifier to predict whether a perovskite can be synthesized or not to limit composition space, followed by regression for the Curie temperature. This two-step approach realizes the final target to synthesize high-temperature ferroelectric perovskites. In addition, if the final task is not achieved easily, we can try to first complete studies for simpler tasks. For example, the brightness prediction for DNA-templated Ag nanocluster can be studied first and then used as a hint to the design of DNA-templated Ag nanocluster within specific color bands. The motif mining method, high-throughput experimental procedures, and ML implementation experience developed in brightness prediction studies have become the base bricks in realizing the more complicated multiclass classification of fluorescence color of the same material system. Although ML methods can find complex information directly from data, the decomposition of tasks can improve the prediction ability of the whole system as well as adding more transparency to the whole process. Instead of mapping the relations between process variables and device performance of photovoltaics directly, a two-step ML framework is proposed to connect target variables to material descriptors first, then to process conditions. Such transparency can enable a better understanding of the whole prediction workflow, which in turn gives more interpretability. For different material systems, the detailed decompositions of tasks are different; however, there will be several general frameworks that could guide different material systems. This is potentially a valuable research direction [8].

20.3.6 Integration of different applications of AI in material discovery

There are many different applications of ML in materials discovery. However, there is a gap between studies of applications during different stages, since each subcommunity normally specializes in their own topic. This gap should be bridged in the long term. Promising methods used in characterization should be effectively combined with ML framework in the property prediction and synthesis component to accelerate the whole process. Several ML frameworks in property prediction should be compiled together to substitute different computationally expensive simulations and be integrated into a single platform. The learned weights of well-trained property prediction models can be transferred to more complex synthesis study models with limited data to achieve better performance. The standardization of different work is preferred to ensure this level of integration. Finally, an integration of efforts through characterization, property prediction, synthesis, and theory should be compiled in high-throughput experimental systems to realize the next generation of materials laboratories.

Imaging plays an essential role in the fields of biology and biomedicine. It provides information about the structural and functional mechanisms of cells and the human body. Biological and biomedical imaging covers microscopy, molecular imaging, pathological imaging, optical coherence tomography, nuclear medicine, ultrasound imaging, x-ray radiography, computed tomography, magnetic resonance imaging, etc. AI has been applied in biological and biomedical imaging research to address imaging reconstruction, registration, detection, classification, lesion segmentation, diagnosis, prognosis, and so on. The purpose of this special issue is to provide diverse and up-to-date contributions of AI research in this field. Hence, it is important to train the new generation of medical trainees regarding the concepts and applicability of AI and how to function efficiently in a workspace alongside machines for better productivity along with cultivating soft skills like empathy in them [9].

20.4 Biomedical and health informatics

Wearable, implantable, mobile, and remote healthcare have rapidly entered the era of digital health across various IoT applications such as monitoring, recording, and tracking the key signs of people's health to improve their lifestyle and health disorders. Innovations in IoT devices play a vital role in assisting patients in managing their health conditions. Thanks to the advent of modern communication technologies and IoT paradigms that have made the implementation of biomedical devices nearly universal. Now with the evolving industrial revolution, patients and healthcare providers are expecting something more. Practically speaking, healthcare wearables have experienced tremendous growth in the past few years, and it is expected to grow even more shortly, making it an ideal space for the biomedical informatics research community to solve complex healthcare problems and more informed decision-making to improve human health. One of the most renowned applications of mobile healthcare technologies includes implantable devices. Wearables are generally used for preventative and recreational wellness management. Simultaneously, implantable techniques are applied towards the management of chronic conditions (blood pressure, diabetes) (figure 20.7).

Furthermore, in the current scenario of the COVID-19 pandemic, research on wearables and connected healthcare is more important than ever, as it greatly assists patients with chronic conditions and other individuals to monitor their health without having direct contact with physicians. Thus, effectively preventing the spread of a pandemic situation and acting as a lifeline to the end-users. Despite the vast benefits of wearables and mobile healthcare technology and sensor informatics, its real-time growth is hindered due to various barriers. Some of the typical challenges include higher cost, complexity in access to wearable device data, medical errors, privacy, security, and network connectivity concerns (figure 20.8).

The new scope of designing, developing, and assessing innovative sensor informatics tools and algorithms is needed for remote and electronic healthcare

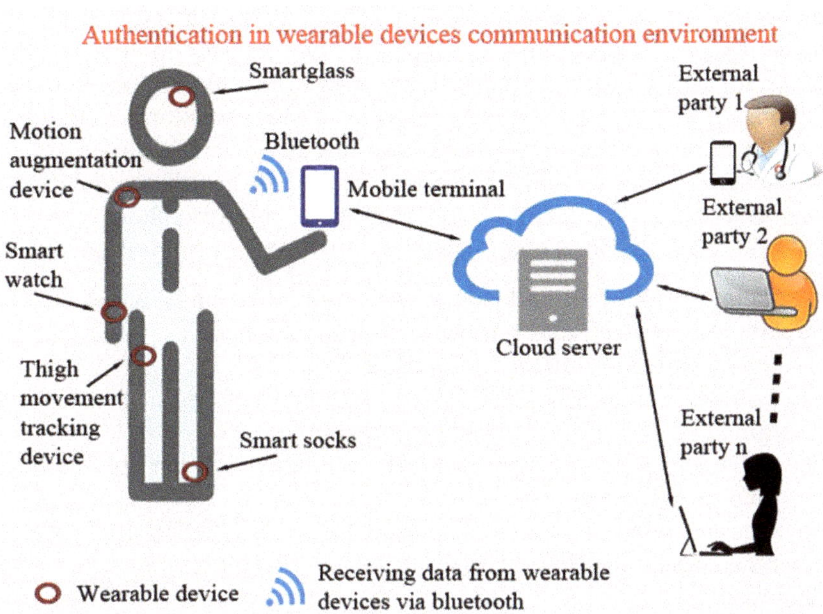

Figure 20.7. Authentication in wearable devices communication environment. Reprinted from Ashok Kumar Das et al, Copyright (2017), with permission from Elsevier

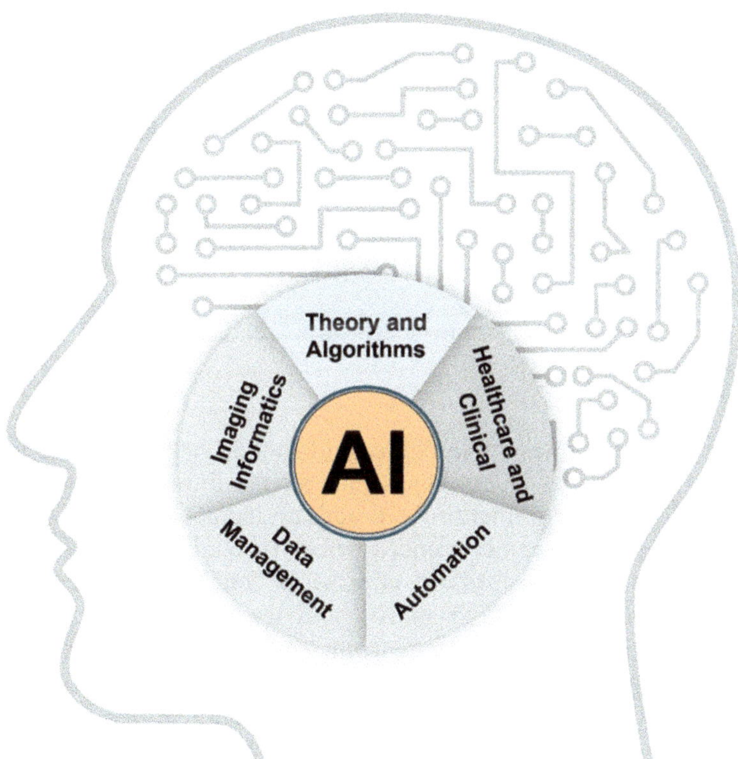

Figure 20.8. AI applications.

and well-being. The major scope is to apply innovations in informatics and data analytics in the practice of remote healthcare and patient monitoring. The key objective is to improve remote healthcare outcomes and services and fulfill the unique application needs of the end-users (ease of use, precision healthcare, safety, privacy, trust, etc). Suitable submissions that discuss system advances, techniques, and approaches relating to health informatics and IoT healthcare device analytics are most welcomed. We particularly encourage interdisciplinary and applied research in this stream [10]. Topics of interest include, but are not limited to:

- enhancing healthcare and social well-being with IoT assistive wearable, implantable, mobile, and remote healthcare informatics
- future of healthcare informatics with BD and AI
- ML secure, and privacy preserving data analytics solutions for emerging wearable and connected healthcare systems
- new advancements in distributed ML techniques for remote healthcare and personal monitoring
- advances in federated learning and CC for mobile health applications
- emerging trends in BD and ML for decision support in healthcare and risk analysis
- challenges in adopting wearable healthcare informatics and its adaptive measures
- prospects of user-centered AI in wearable, implantable, mobile, and remote healthcare informatics
- advances in IoT assisted wearable sensor technologies and its impact on healthcare informatics
- movel applications of IoT and BD analytics to enhance user experience and evaluation methods for healthcare applications
- role of IoT assisted innovative AI and ML technologies in interactive healthcare applications (speech summarization, dialog management, etc)
- innovations in IoT and sensor informatics for monitoring patients with chronic health conditions
- IoT and sensor informatics in healthcare: trends and future directions.

20.5 Conclusion

Looking forward, wearable, implantable, and mobile health monitoring systems, IoT and sensor informatics technologies such as distributed machine learning and 5G networks will play a prominent role. It adds an increased level of convenience to the end-users that they never experienced before by enabling efficient organization and analysis of the health records to improve patient health outcomes. The new wave of technological innovations in IoT and sensor informatics will lead to a multidisciplinary approach that ranges from vital sign and activity monitoring to dealing with emergency situations. More than ever, advanced research on this background paves the way for an efficient healthcare integrated technology that is both simple and trustworthy to be used in real-time. Hence, we can conclude that the future of healthcare applications will create a breakthrough through advancements when they effectively implement innovative IoT and sensor informatics paradigms. The goal should be to strike a delicate mutually beneficial balance between effective use of automation and AI and the human strengths and judgment of trained primary carc physicians. This is essential because AI completely replacing humans in the field of medicine is a concern which might otherwise hamper the benefits which can be derived from it.

References

[1] Kirch D G and Petelle K 2017 Addressing the physician shortage: the peril of ignoring demography *JAMA* **317** 1947–8

[2] Bhavin M, Tanwar S, Sharma N, Tyagi S and Kumar N 2021 Blockchain and quantum blind signature-based hybrid scheme for healthcare 5.0 applications *J. Inf. Secur. Appl.* **56** 102673

[3] Jain S, Nehra M, Kumar R, Dilbaghi N, Hu T, Kumar S, Kaushik A and Li C Z 2021 Internet of medical things (IoMT)-integrated biosensors for point-of-care testing of infectious diseases *Biosens. Bioelectron.* **179** 113074

[4] Manickam P, Mariappan S A, Murugesan S M, Hansda S, Kaushik A, Shinde R and Thipperudraswamy S P 2022 Artificial intelligence (AI) and internet of medical things (IoMT) assisted biomedical systems for intelligent healthcare *Biosensors* **12** 562

[5] Mazumdar H, Kim T H, Lee J M, Kum E, Lee S, Jeong S and Chung B G 2021 Sequential and comprehensive algorithm for fault detection in semiconductor sensors *Appl. Sci.* **11** 10419

[6] Mazumdar H, Kim T H, Lee J M, Ha J H, Ahrberg C D and Chung B G 2018 Prediction analysis and quality assessment of microwell array images *Electrophoresis* **39** 948–56

[7] Wong B K and Selvi Y 1998 Neural network applications in finance: A review and analysis of literature (1990–1996) *Inform. Manage.* **34** 129–39

[8] Thyrhaug E, Bogh S A, Carro-Temboury M R, Madsen C S, Vosch T and Zigmantas D 2017 Ultrafast coherence transfer in DNA-templated silver nanoclusters *Nat. Commun.* **8** 15577

[9] Chung B G, Mazumdar H, Kim T H and Lee J M 2019 Method of establishing image analysis algorithm for microwell array *US Patent App. 16/237* 249

[10] Mujawar M A, Gohel H, Bhardwaj S K, Srinivasan S, Hickman N and Kaushik A 2020 Nano-enabled biosensing systems for intelligent healthcare:20-20 towards COVID-19 management *Mater. Today Chem.* **17** 100306

[11] Kapoor A 2019 *Hands-On Artificial Intelligence for IoT: Expert Machine Learning and Deep Learning Techniques for Developing Smarter IoT Systems* (Birmingham: Packt Publishing Ltd)

[12] Li J, Lim K, Yang H, Ren Z, Raghavan S, Chen P-Y, Buonassisi T and Wang X 2020 AI applications through the whole life cycle of material discovery *Matter* **3** 393–432

[13] Das A S, Sherali Z and Mohammad W 2017 Lightweight authentication protocols for wearable devices *Comput. Elec. Eng.* **63** 196–208

[14] Chapman P, Clinton J, Kerber R, Khabaza T, Reinartz T P, Shearer C and Wirth R 2000 CRISP-DM 1.0: Step-by-step data mining guide

Chapter 21

Summary and aspects of techniques for biotechnology

Ajeet Kaushik, Sesha S Srinivasan and Yogendra K Mishra

The introduction of nano-biotechnology and smart analytical systems in biomedical research is improving everyday lifestyle via specially developing specific systems, personalized health management based on diagnostics, prognosis, and therapeutics. Efforts are being made continuously to reduce form factors of analytical systems for optimization components via advanced characterization for monitoring environment and health at in-field, on-site, and point-of-care (POC). Such generated health informatics and data analytics with the help of artificial intelligence will be useful for developing the strategies needed for better health and related access. This book will be the key educational platform globally for the exploration of fundamental and applied aspects of widely employed analytical techniques to develop advanced prototypes, materials, and technologies in the field biomedical applications. This book explores the potential of nano-enabled multidisciplinary science to design and develop smart platforms and analytical techniques for personalized health care management.

Chapter 1 covered the emergence of analytical techniques, explored the advances in nano-enabled approaches which have improved quality of life significantly and opened an era to explore novel materials, system, therapies, etc. However, the timely testing of a developed system's components is always recommended by experts to make sure that technology is performing well and as it was designed. To achieve this task, novel analytical techniques are always in demand. The overview and state-of-the art of such of technologies was described and discussed in this chapter.

Chapter 2 described electrochemical techniques for biomedical nanotechnology, exploring electrochemical systems that are emerging as being suitable analytical methods to explore electro-activity of a material/nanostructure involving polymer, metal, metal oxide, hybrids, and organic–inorganic nanocomposite systems. Such techniques have also been explored to design and develop effective and sensitive electrochemical gas/biosensors for health wellness. This chapter covered the

doi:10.1088/978-0-7503-3379-5ch21

fundamentals of electrochemical techniques and their potential applications in the field of materials characterization, system fabrication, and technology development. It covers cyclic voltammetry (CV), differential pulse voltammetry (DPV), square wave voltammetry (SWV), and electrochemical impedance spectroscopy (EIS) investigated for various biomedical applications.

Chapters 3 discusses UV–Vis spectroscopy in biomedical nanotechnology, describing UV–Vis (ultraviolet–visible) spectroscopy as a very useful tool to understand electron transition in a nanostructure, mainly polymeric system, and developing absorbance-based sensing assays. This is one of the conventional spectroscopic methods for functional characterization of polymers and band gap estimation of metallic platforms. This approach is also useful to develop optical density-based methods to estimate percentages binding and release of a drug in the process of making a therapeutic cargo. All fundamental and applied aspects of UV–visible spectroscopy were covered in this chapter.

Chapter 4 covers FTIR spectroscopy and microscopy in biomedical nanotechnology, and explains that Fourier transform infrared (FTIR) spectroscopy is one of the most promising functional characterization tools to confirm the available functional groups, drug functional characterization in pharmaceutical science, materials' characterization, tissues analysis including functional and morphological assessment, and confirmation of bindings between two active moieties. This approach is one of the potential methods to develop efficient optical sensors to detect a target analyte selectively. This chapter covers the fundamental understanding of FTIR along with advanced biomedical applications.

Chapter 5 is based on Raman spectroscopy and microscopy in biomedical nanotechnology, justifies that Raman spectroscopy has emerged as one of best vibrational spectroscopic techniques for materials' characterization, functional assessment of materials, tissues integration analysis, and developing analytical diagnostics system. Due to recent advances in electronics and Raman-active materials, this technology is emerging as a potential miniaturized system to understand progression of biological procedures and develop diagnostics tool as well. This chapter covers the fundamental principles of Raman spectroscopy, multi-directional approaches for various applications, improvements in performance using a combinational approach involving spectroscopy and microscopy.

Chapter 6 discusses quartz crystal microbalance for biomedical nanotechnology, and explains that developing a highly sensitive sensing detection system is crucial for monitoring the progression of a disease and developing therapies. The quartz crystal microbalance (QCM) is emerging as one such diagnostic methodology which has been found to be very suitable to detect a target analyte at very low concentration. This is a well adopted method for developing affinity-based bioassays such as biosensors. The basics and applied aspects of QCM are discussed in this chapter.

Chapter 7 covers nuclear magnetic resonance (NMR) in biomedical nanotechnology, describing that various synthetic and natural materials have been proposed for various biomedical application. Prior to introducing these materials in targeted application, the accurate characterization of such materials is a key factor. Among various methodologies, NMR is a well-known spectroscopic technique used to explore the construction of molecules which have NMR active nuclei such as 1H, 2H (or 2D), 13C, 15N, 31P, etc, probing of interactions, probing of molecular dynamics, biomolecule structural understanding, drug target sites, and diagnostics. All aspects of NMR are covered in this chapter.

Chapter 8 is based on mass spectroscopy in biomedical nanotechnology, and proposes that mass spectroscopy (MS) is a very sensitive analytical tool in biomedical research which provides qualitative and as well as quantitative analysis of materials (synthetic and natural), drugs, metabolites, and bio-actives such as proteins, peptides, oligosaccharides, lipids, nucleic acids, etc. Mass spectroscopy, a top-down approach, significantly contributes to the exploration of proteomics and various integrations between the molecules such as protein–protein and drug–molecule. This chapter covers fundamental and applied aspects mass spectroscopy.

Chapter 9 discusses magnetic measurement systems for biomedical nanotechnology and explain that for decades magnetic nanostructures have been the platform of choice to develop magnetically guided system such as sensors, nanomedicine, and drug delivery. The selection of a magnetic nanostructure for a targeted biomedical application is always dependent on its magnitude of magnetism at room temperature and tunability as a function of external stimulation. The complete understanding of magnetism is assessed using vibrating sample magnetometer (VSM), which is the focus of this chapter.

Chapter 10 covers x-ray diffraction for biomedical nanotechnology applications, and justifies that the evaluating material's purity is essential to decide whether the material can be a selected for a targeted biomedical application or not. To achieve this, x-ray diffraction (XRD) is a well-recommended one of potential analytical and non-destructive technique. The XRD has been utilized to explore crystalline/nano-crystalline/amorphous structure and phase purity of materials and biomaterials. In addition to phase or structural evaluations, XRD is also useful to calculate the average crystallite sizes and lattice strain etc of the candidate materials for biomedical applications. All aspects of XRD are discussed in this chapter.

Chapter 11 on scanning electron microscopy for biomedical nanotechnology explains that scanning electron microscopy (SEM) is one of classic and effective imaging techniques used to understand and explore the surface/interface morphology and microstructural analysis. SEM analysis is useful to confirm surface morphology of nanostructures, thin films, and biomolecules. Moreover, various bindings among material–materials, materials–cells, and cell–cell have also been studied using SEM. This chapter explains the fundamental and applied aspects of SEM technology.

Chapter 12 discusses transmission electron microscopy for biomedical nanotechnology, explaining that transmission electron microscopy (TEM) is the only analytical method to explore the purity of a material at atomic level. TEM study is recommended to confirm the preparation of a nanostructure without impurity. This is an authentic technique, along with XRD, to estimate the particle size of a molecule. Exploring the features at atomic levels, this technology has been used to analyse biological samples for morphological understanding, biomolecule (proteins, virus, bacteria, etc) structure evaluation, cell-uptake of nanomaterials, etc. The fundamentals and biological applications of TEM are described in this chapter.

Chapter 13 covers energy dispersive spectroscopy for biomedical nanotechnology, describing that the energy dispersive spectroscopy (EDS) is a well-known analytical technique for elemental analysis of a material and tissue. The EDS-assisted elemental analysis is associated with the generation of characteristic x-rays that reveal the presence of elements contained in the specimens. The EDS is in practice used to detect nanoparticles, which has significance in therapy development, in tissues and biological samples. The fundamental and applied aspects of EDS are covered in this chapter.

Chapter 14 dicsussing atomic force microscopy for biomedical nanotechnology, projects atomic force microscopy (AFM) as a three-dimensional topographic technique with high resolution features to measure surface properties, mainly roughness at the nanoscale. Significant efforts have been made to develop AFM of improved performance to study the various phenomena of material science, biomedical research, and optimizing materials for targeted biomedical research. AFM provides useful and necessary information at the nanoscale for example quantification of a single molecule. AFM has been used to develop nano-enabled drug delivery systems, and examine tissues. The basic and applied aspects of TEM are the topics of this chapter.

Chapter 15 is based on microfluidic systems for biomedical nanotechnology, exploring those microfluidic systems that have been developed as potential analytic platforms to perform automated measurement with high precision and accuracy. Such systems are complex to fabricate but easy to scale-up, and operate. The cell profiling at single level and the separation of cells has been achieved using smart and affordable microfluidic systems. Significant efforts have been made to improve the state-of-the-art microfluidic system to meet the requirements of future research planned for health wellness. This chapter discusses the basics of microfluidics system development and their application in biomedical research.

Chapter 16 discusses the dynamic light scattering particle size analysis for biomedical nanotechnology and justifies that the introduction of nanostructures in biomedical application is increasing rapidly. Significant efforts are being made to design nano-systems of desired solubility and suspension in media or electrolyte recommended for targeted biomedical research field. To understand these features perfectly, dynamic light scattering (DLS), i.e., photon correlation spectroscopy study explores diffusion behavior of macro/nano molecules in a solution. This technique is also useful to calculate diffusion coefficient and hydrodynamic size. DLS is the recommended methodology in pharmaceuticals to study homogeneity of proteins, nucleic acids, and complexes of protein–protein or protein–nucleic acid preparations, as well as to study protein–small molecule interactions. The descriptive explanation of DLS is covered in this chapter.

Chapter 17 is based on zeta potential measurements and analysis for biomedical nanotechnology, it explains that complementary to the homogeneity and hydrodynamic size, another parameter which is also very important to decode materials application in biomedical research is the estimation of surface charge. Surface charge estimation of a nano-system is generally performed using zeta potential measurement via electrophoretic light scattering (ELS). Besides, electrophoretic mobility interpretation of a nano-system can be explained using zeta potential experiments. Presently, this is one of the essential measurements in colloidal science to explore molecule dynamics. Both fundamental and applied aspects of zeta potential technology are described in this chapter.

Chapter 18 on electron paramagnetic (spin) resonance spectroscopy for biomedical nanotechnology, explains that electron paramagnetic resonance (EPR) spectroscopy is used to study the free radicals and paramagnetic species in nano-biomaterials. The biomedical applications such as oximetry, where the EPR is employed to measure the level of oxygen in tissues. The direct detection of transition metal ions such as copper ion or iron ion will allow to detect the neurodegenerative diseases due to the formation of amyloid- or amyloid like fibrillary structures. The EPR imaging demonstrates an unparalleled tool for the 3D mapping of the spatial distribution of paramagnetic species and reactive oxygen species (ROS) and hence widely applicable to clinical and biomedical research applications.

Chapter 19 explores XPS as an analytical technique suitable for surface analysis that can provide intricate information about the chemical environment at atomical and elemental levels on the surface layers of the specimen. XPS has demonstrated various applications in the field of material sciences, life sciences, nanotechnology, electronics, and bioengineering. General information about the instrumentation, data interpretation, and tackling challenges for different aspects of applications in biomedicine is briefly discussed in this chapter. Some of the innovations with this technique like imaging, which are to happen in the near future will be of immense help in biomedical nanotechnology.

Chapter 20 based on artificial intelligence (AI) and the internet of things (IoT) for smart biomedical application, explores the introduction of computer simulation/numerical modelling including AI and the IoT is increasing in materials science and biomedical research to predict patterns and reduce associated risks. This chapter focusses on describing the importance of AI and bioinformatics related to the selection of analytical techniques with respect to a targeted biomedical application.

This book gives a broad understanding of relevant analytical techniques, which provide significant contributions to developing reliable systems of higher efficacy to improve the health wellness. The main objective of this book is to bridge the gap between experts with different subjective knowledge and working in identical fields. Keeping targeted biomedical applications as the key motivation, this book will certainly connect the experts to explore appropriate analytical techniques and procedures for optimization of a nanomaterials for biomedical applications

- assessment of developed system for health wellness.
- discussion of challenges to develop next generation systems
- strategies to calibrate along with validate developed systems; and
- approaches needed for health wellness at personalized manner.

This book will be a key motivation with new ideas to invent the advanced methodologies/analytical techniques and will be a boon in the biomedical research and nano-biotechnological fields.

www.ingramcontent.com/pod-product-compliance
Ingram Content Group UK Ltd.
Pitfield, Milton Keynes, MK11 3LW, UK
UKHW051910100926
8556IPUK00005B/832

9 780750 333771